# Cochlear Implants

Sandra DeSaSouza
Editor

# Cochlear Implants

## New and Future Directions

Springer

*Editor*
Sandra DeSaSouza
Otorhinolaryngologist
Jaslok Hospital
Mumbai, Maharashtra, India

ISBN 978-981-19-0451-6 ISBN 978-981-19-0452-3 (eBook)
https://doi.org/10.1007/978-981-19-0452-3



This Springer imprint is published by the registered company Springer Nature Singapore Pte Ltd.
The registered company address is: 152 Beach Road, #21-01/04 Gateway East, Singapore 189721, Singapore

# Foreword

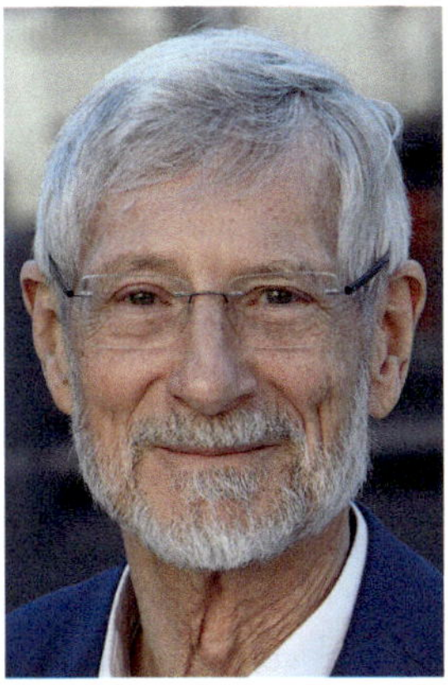

Severe to profound hearing loss affects the quality of life, disrupting the essential needs for communicating and, consequently, the belonging to and participating in society. For neonates, if not rehabilitated, it leads to reduced speech and language development with ensuing severe effects on education. Adults faced with losing their hearing may experience isolation, stigma, inability to perform their job, and even loss of independence. In older people, severe and profound hearing loss leads to an increase in cognitive decline and risk of dementia. It is estimated that 50 million people worldwide are faced with a degree of hearing loss where hearing aids do not provide sufficient speech understanding. One out of 2000–4000 newborns suffers from such a high degree of hearing impairment that they cannot be sufficiently rehabilitated with hearing aids to allow them to follow mainstream education. Up to now, more than three-quarters of a million people have received a cochlear implant (CI), and many millions more will benefit in the future.

My experience with CIs dates back to 1975 when we, my later wife Ingeborg and myself, explored the possibilities of electrically stimulating the auditory nerve to elicit sound sensations in a deaf ear. This work at the Vienna Technical University resulted in the worldwide first implantation of a microelectronic multichannel cochlear implant in December 1977.

In the course of our work, I learned to appreciate CIs as fascinating devices, not only because of the challenging research, engineering, and medical aspects involved, but, first of all, because of their life-changing potential.

Just watching a deaf born child during first switch on is extremely motivating, as well as observing its rapid development after implantation. I am sure, Sandra DeSaSouza experienced similar feelings during her career.

She started implanting CIs as early as 1987, when CIs were still in their infancy. Despite widespread skepticism as well as unavoidable setbacks she remained firm and indomitably pursued her goal, always determined to achieve the optimum outcome for her patients. Our team from MED-EL established a trustful, intensive, and fruitful relation with her and her clinic.

She is one of the leading ENT head and neck surgeons in India. Her expertise covers a wide range of ENT, head, and neck surgery. She was Director of ENT at Jaslok Hospital in Mumbai. She still runs the CI surgery program there, where she has performed more than 2000 CI surgeries.

Her professional life is adorned by a large number of firsts: she, e.g., pioneered CI surgery in India, performed the first implantation of HiRes 90K in Asia, and was the first woman worldwide to implant CIs. Her vast experience enabled her to initiate a number of CI centers throughout India, and she was the first surgeon to operate difficult cases like ossifications and Mondini cases, implanted the youngest deaf child at that time, and performed sinuscopy using image-guided equipment. She has published more than 40 research papers and is the author or coauthor of several books.

I know her for many decades as a very charming person, warm-hearted, and caring. She has also been active in doing social work for the deaf. At present, she is the trustee of "The Stephen High School for the Deaf and Aphasic."

Her exceptional achievements have been honored by a number of highly prestigious national and international awards, the most recent one being the renowned Padma Shri Award in 2020.

She is thus uniquely destined to edit this compendium, which assembles contributions on all aspects of CIs, written by most renowned surgeons and researchers in their field. Furthermore, her unprecedented experience is fundamental to guide the reader through the history of CIs in India.

This book is a compelling testimony about the benefits of cochlear implantation. After just some little browsing the reader will be convinced of the benefits of CIs, their life-changing capabilities providing new career possibilities following implantation.

Despite their spectacular performance, surpassing the boldest dreams of the early proponents, CIs are not spared from the unyielding human quest for perfection. A glimpse into the future is ventured in the last chapter, discussing e.g. the upcoming totally implantable CI, as well as the combination with pharmaceutical agents, and the more remote, but most likely powerful, impact of genetic engineering on the future treatment of hearing loss, or the introduction of stem cells aiming to generate new hair cells.

However, not all severely to profoundly deaf and hard of hearing children worldwide have access to a CI, and only under 5% of adult candidates receive one. It is a moral imperative to ease the access to implantations, and it makes sense for economic reasons as well. Besides the private market, a growing number of governments are beginning to also accept their responsibility, seeing both the immediate benefits for the implantee and the long-term benefits for the community by providing the chance of integration and better education via the CI.

Faculty of Natural Sciences
University of Innsbruck
Innsbruck, Austria

Department of Applied Physics and Microelectronics
University of Innsbruck
Innsbruck, Austria

MED-EL GmbH
Innsbruck, Austria

Erwin Hochmair

# Foreword

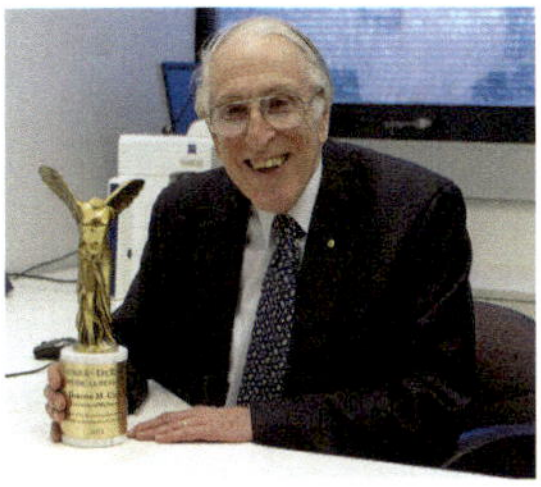

It is a special honor to have been invited to write a foreword to the book *Cochlear Implants: New and Future Directions* edited by Dr Sandra DeSaSouza. I had the pleasure of meeting Dr DeSaSouza at the XVI World Congress of Otorhinolaryngology Head and Neck Surgery in Sydney in March 1997 when there was a major section on cochlear implants. To have a complete section on cochlear implants at a world conference showed there was a seismic shift in the medical profession's acceptance of cochlear implants for the management of severe to profound deafness. Dr DeSaSouza as the lead author presented an excellent poster on cochlear implants in India.

Her paper presented their results from 1987 to 1996. This was at a time when it was only just becoming clear that multichannel cochlear implants gave superior speech results to those of single-channel implants. Hers was a timely study on different coding strategies for six languages. Her work demonstrated vision in the value of the cochlear implant. Her poster also highlighted her ability to integrate streams of basic and clinical thought to achieve lasting benefits for deaf people.

In this book, Dr DeSaSouza has brought together appropriate leading experts in their field to create a well-balanced book on cochlear implants. There is a great range of topics presented by masters in their fields. It is a must-read for all those wanting to see where this exciting area of medical bionics or biomedical engineering is leading. It is the first recreation of a human sense, and the means to give spoken language to children with severe to profound sensorineural deafness. My congratulations to Dr DeSaSouza and her team for a wonderful effort that highlights the benefit of cochlear implants and the possibilities this brings to new biomedical engineering areas such as bionic eyes, spinal cord repair, and the management of drug-resistant epilepsy.

University of Melbourne
Melbourne, Australia

Graeme M. Clark

Electrical & Electronic Engineering
University of Melbourne
Melbourne, Australia

# Preface

This e-book on *Cochlear Implants (CI): New and Future Directions* covers the cochlear implant from its inception to recent advances culminating in the cochlear implants in clinical use today. It also covers future horizons.

All the authors of the different chapters are CI surgeons known worldwide, many of them pioneers of their own technique and also prominent audiologists, clinical engineers, and researchers.

The first few chapters deal with historical events: Benjamin Franklin's electric stimulation of hearing followed by many pioneers ending with the first cochlear implant with FDA approval by House in 1984 and by Clark in 1986.

India was part of history and was touched upon as cochlear implantation started in 1987 with mono- and multi-electrode systems. The evolution of the technology of implants took 35 years, and the changes made by CI companies with clinical support are elaborated. The book then turns to medical and surgical issues. Surgical anatomy of the temporal bone and recent advances in CT scan and MRI are illustrated. Candidacy for selection of potential candidates has changed over the years and varies from country to country; therefore, it is discussed in detail. Next we have prognostic modeling and machine learning in cochlear implantation which is a new direction which could be used to look for better audiological and surgical outcomes. The next few chapters are on different CI surgical techniques each one authored by doyens and pioneers, namely CI surgery using posterior tympanotomy and cochleostomy, CI surgery using the Veria technique, and CI surgery using the round window approach.

Also included are cochlear implants in cases with inner ear abnormalities, bilateral cochlear implants, and subtotal petrosectomy with cochlear implantation. In recent times with new indications we have chapters on CI surgery in case of unilateral hearing loss and hearing preservation in implants with residual hearing, children undergoing cochlear implant surgery, explantation, and reimplantation, and complications of cochlear implant surgery. Robot-assisted cochlear implant surgery is the most recent advance, as it can be used for direct cochlea access, cochleostomy, and precise insertion of electrodes. Image-guided cochlear implant surgery and recent advances in CAS are discussed.

The next chapter deals with recent trends in cochlear implant programming and rehabilitation, and it is followed by a chapter on implant reliability which is highly relevant for counseling patients and for CI manufacturers. Finally, the last chapter is on recent advances and future horizons. A totally implantable cochlear implant and stem cells are still under research.

Almost every author has added a video to their chapter.

Mumbai, India Sandra DeSaSouza

# Contents

1 **A Historical Review of the Development of Cochlear Implants** ...... 1
Sandra DeSaSouza

2 **History of Cochlear Implants in India** ........................... 9
Sandra DeSaSouza

3 **Evolution of Cochlear Implant Technology over the Last 35 Years** ... 19
Anandhan Dhanasingh and Sandra DeSaSouza

4 **Surgical Anatomy and Imaging of the Temporal Bone with Cochlear Implant Imaging** ............................... 35
Shrinivas Desai, Shraddha Sinhasan, and Ritu Kashikar

5 **Cochlear Implants in Clinical Use Worldwide Today** .............. 109
Sandra DeSaSouza

6 **Candidacy and Evaluation of Potential Candidates for Cochlear Implantation** .................................... 165
Nandini Dave Maingi and Sandra DeSaSouza

7 **Prognostic Modelling and Machine Learning in Cochlear Implantation** ..................................... 177
Haroon Shakeel Saeed and Iain A. Bruce

8 **Cochlear Implantation Using Posterior Tympanotomy and Cochleostomy** ........................................ 193
Jacques Magnan and Fathi Baki

9 **Cochlear Implant Surgery Using the Veria Technique** ............. 215
Trifon Kiratzidis

10 **Cochlear Implantation Through the Round Window Approach** ..... 237
Mario Sanna, Anna Lisa Giannuzzi, and Antonio Caruso

11 **Classification and Management of Inner Ear Malformations** ....... 245
Levent Sennaroglu

12 **Bilateral Cochlear Implants** ..................................... 265
Joachim Mueller

**13 Subtotal Petrosectomy and Cochlear Implantation** . . . . . . . . . . . . . . . . 285
Mario Sanna, Gianluca Piras, and Lorenzo Lauda

**14 Cochlear Implants for Single-Sided Deafness** . . . . . . . . . . . . . . . . . . . . 303
Emily Kay-Rivest, J. Thomas Roland Jr, and David R. Friedmann

**15 Hearing Preservation and Electro-acoustic Stimulation in Cochlear Implants** . . . . . . . . . . . . . . . . . . . . . . . . . . . . . . . . . . . . . . . . . 315
Emily Kay-Rivest, J. Thomas Roland Jr, and Daniel Jethanamest

**16 Endoscopic-Assisted Cochlear Implantation** . . . . . . . . . . . . . . . . . . . . . 329
Davide Soloperto, Daniele Marchioni, Nicola Bisi, and Alessia Rubini

**17 Robot-Assisted Cochlear Implantation** . . . . . . . . . . . . . . . . . . . . . . . . . . 345
Daniele De Seta, Yann Nguyen, Renato Torres, Isabelle Mosnier, and Olivier Sterkers

**18 Structure Preservation of the Inner Ear in Cochlear Implantation** . . . 363
William Crohan and Gunesh P. Rajan

**19 Candidacy Considerations and Other Medical and Surgical Issues for Cochlear Implantation in Children** . . . . . . . . . . . . . . . . . . . . 387
William P. R. Gibson and Catherine S. Birman

**20 Explantation and Reimplantation of Cochlear Implants** . . . . . . . . . . . 403
Clarós Pedro and Koniewska Anna

**21 Surgical Complications Following Cochlear Implantation** . . . . . . . . . . 427
Ryan-William Grech and Iain A. Bruce

**22 Recent Trends in Cochlear Implant Programming and (Re)habilitation** . . . . . . . . . . . . . . . . . . . . . . . . . . . . . . . . . . . . . . . . . . . 441
Colleen Psarros and Yetta Abrahams

**23 Cochlear Implant Reliability** . . . . . . . . . . . . . . . . . . . . . . . . . . . . . . . . . . 473
Manfred Pieber and Sandra DeSaSouza

**24 Cochlear Implants: Recent Advances and New Horizons** . . . . . . . . . . . 501
Anandhan Dhanasingh and Claude Jolly

# About the Editor

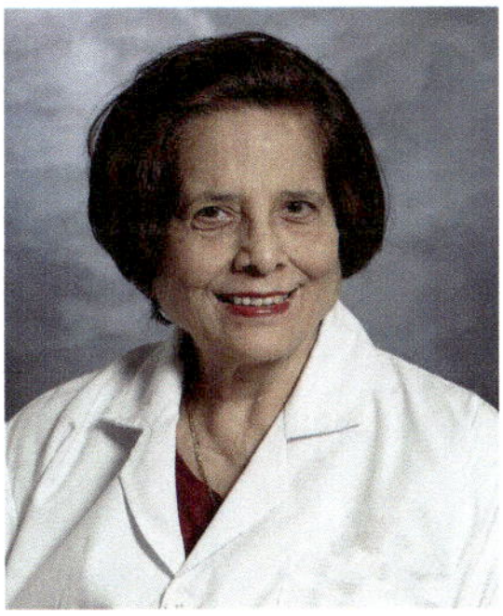

**Sandra DeSaSouza** obtained her Master's Degree in ENT in 1969 and has a diploma in ENT from CPS College in Bombay. She is a fellow of the International College of Surgeons, the American Academy of Otolaryngology—Head and Neck Surgery, and the American Otological Society. She held the position of a Professor Emeritus and Head of the Atmasingh Jethasingh ENT Municipal Hospital. She was also an Emeritus Head of the ENT Department in Jaslok Hospital and Research Centre, where today she is a Consultant Surgeon. She is also a Consultant at Desa's Hospital and Breach Candy Hospital.

In India, she was the president of the Bombay Branch of AOI in 1994, the all-India branch of NES in 1995, and the first women president of AOI in 2002.

In 1987, she was the pioneer of cochlear implant surgery in India, the first women cochlear implant surgeon in the world, the first surgeon to start other centers in India, the first surgeon to use Nucleus, Med-EL, and Clarion Cochlear Implants. She was also the first surgeon to use implants in ossified cochlear and Mondini cases and perform sinuscopy with image-guided equipment. She was the first Asian surgeon to use the Clarion Advanced Bionics HiRes 90K.

She was on the editorial board of the International Tinnitus Journal and has published over 40 research papers and articles and written two booklets, "Modern trends in cochlear implants" and the "Cochlear implant program." She is the co-author and publisher of a textbook titled "*Modern concept of Neurotology*."

She has also been active in doing social work for the deaf and is the present trustee of "The Stephen High School for the Deaf and Aphasic," which has 70 children studying for the standard SSC.

She is listed in "The International Register of Profiles," the "Twentieth Century Admirable Achievers," "Distinguished Who's Who," and "The Limca Book of Records."

The American Biographical Institute has awarded her Lifetime Achievement Award for the Women of the Year 2002. She was Awarded International Scientist of the Year in 2003 for her outstanding contribution to Neurotology and leading scientist of the World in 2005 for her Research in Cochlear Implants. In 2022, the AOI India awarded her the Lifetime Achievement Award.

Dr. Sandra DeSaSouza was conferred the prestigious Padma Shri award on 26 January 2020, on the 71st Republic Day of India. She has deservingly received this honor thanks to an illustrious career as one of India's leading ENT Surgeons and a pioneer of Cochlear Implant Surgery in India.

# List of Videos


Video 2.1 Evolution of cochlear implant surgery in India
Video 2.2 Semicircular canal approach for dysplastic cochlea
Video 3.1 Diametric magnet rotation
Video 3.2 Electrode insertion
Video 4.1 AXIAL CISS MRI images of left cochlea
Video 4.2 Oblique coronal CISS MRI images of left cochlea
Video 4.3 3D MRI of bilateral cochlea
Video 5.1 Working of a cochlear implant
Video 8.1 Cochlear implantation using posterior tympanotomy
Video 9.1 Veria technique
Video 10.1 Cochlear implantation using the round window approach
Video 13.1 Subtotal petrosectomy with cochlear implantation in a case of cochlear ossification
Video 15.1 Implantation with a short hybrid implant
Video 16.1 Endoscopic assisted cochlear implantation
Video 17.1 Robot-based cochlear implant insertion
Video 19.1 Right ear cochlear implantation in an infant
Video 20.1 Facial nerve stimulation
Video 20.2 Explantation reimplantation
Video 20.3 Cochlear implant revision, implant fixed too anteriorly
Video 21.1 Perilymphatic gusher in cochlear implant surgery
Video 22.1 Remote check
Video 22.2 Remote mapping
Video 22.3 Remote rehabilitation
Video 23.1 Test for implant reliability
Video 24.1 OtoPlan recent advances and new horizons

# A Historical Review of the Development of Cochlear Implants

1

Sandra DeSaSouza

Auditory sensation as a result of electrical stimulation dates back as far as 1751, when Benjamin Franklin was the first to suggest that electricity could produce hearing sensations in the deaf. Later Count Alessandro Volta (1800) [1] passed metal rods in both his ears and connected them to a circuit containing his newly developed electrolytic cells. It produced a sensation of sound described as "Boiling of viscous fluid" (Luxford and Brackmann 1985) [2], after which he lost consciousness and did no repeat the experiment.

In the latter half of the nineteenth century, interest in this subject was revived. Politzer treated a series of cases of tinnitus with electrical stimulation. Another well-known otologist of this time to use electrical methods of diagnosis was Gradenigo, who felt that auditory sensation did not result from electrical stimulation of the normal ear, and when it did, it was an evidence of disease. In 1930 Wever and Bray discovered that electrical potential arose in the cochlear as a result of acoustic stimulation. Their important theory that the cochlea acted as a transducer of acoustical to electrical energy, paved the way for the feasibility of artificial hearing through direct eighth nerve stimulation. At about the same time, several radio engineers discovered that tones could be produced by passing an alternating current through electrodes applied near the ear. Stevens termed this the "electrophonic" effect in 1937, and produced tones by passing an alternating electrical current in the audible frequency range from an electrode onto the skin surface. The electrode and skin surface then acted as two plates of a condenser microphone, the resulting vibration being transmitted by air and bone conduction to the cochlea causing auditory

S. DeSaSouza (✉)
ENT Department, Jaslok Hospital & Research Centre, Mumbai, Maharashtra, India

Breach Candy Hospital and Desa Hospital (ENT Section), Mumbai, Maharashtra, India


S. DeSaSouza (ed.), *Cochlear Implants*,
https://doi.org/10.1007/978-981-19-0452-3_1

sensation. However, as electrophonic hearing requires a normal or near-normal cochlea, no practical implication could be found for the hearing impaired.

At the end of the nineteenth century, unscrupulous doctors and characters used this technique, referred to as "Electro-Otiatrics", as a supposed means of preventing or curing deafness. At the same time, there was so much controversy over electro-therapy for other ailments that established doctors dared not become associated with it. At the turn of the century, it died out.

It is difficult to ascertain who first successfully produced true direct stimulation of the auditory nerve. In all probability it was the Russians, as in 1934, Andreef, Gersuni and Volokhov [3] published their results where the patient described various hearing sensations ranging from separate short noises to smooth buzzing sounds on being stimulated with an electrode in the round window.

Later Jones, Stevens and Lurie (1940) [4] reported similar findings on placing a saline-soaked cotton ball electrode on the round window in nine subjects.

The modern era in the electrical stimulation of the auditory nerve was ushered in by two Frenchman, Djurno and Eyries (1957), when they reported the first "Cochlear Implant". They inserted a single copper wire inside the cochlea of a 50-year-old man who was totally deaf and used an electrophonic stimulator producing pulsed stimuli at a rate of 100/s. Later a second implant was performed in a girl with total hearing loss after streptomycin therapy, with the stimulating electrode placed in the round window niche against the membrane. Both patients were able to differentiate several frequencies and also a few words with training. On long-term studies neither subject developed speech discrimination. According to Zollner and Keidel (1963) [5] the implants were still functioning 4–5 years, but the auditory sensations remained unchanged. This was a remarkable report and it spread to the USA stimulating three pioneer researchers, House, Michelson and Simmons, who began independent studies in the 1960s bringing further credibility to the auditory prostheses.

In Los Angeles, House began with studies of electrical stimulation in patients undergoing middle ear surgery, and in 1961 implanted two subjects with a single gold electrode placed in the scala tympani. Later in the same year a multi electrode system was inserted for 2 weeks in one of his patients but removed when a possible allergic reaction occurred (House, 1976) [6].

In 1964, Simmons et al. from the Stanford University Medical School performed bipolar stimulation of the auditory nerve in an 18-year-old male undergoing surgery for a recurrent posterior fossa tumour, using square wave stimulation for 25 min. The patient was able to distinguish between 20 and 900 pulses/s.

Later in May 1964 (Simmons 1966) [7], they implanted a six electrode array directly into the modiolus of a 60-year-old man who reported auditory sensations when 0.1 ms square waves were used at frequencies from 2000 to 4000 Hz. The pitch varied according to the electrode stimulated. The patient was investigated extensively, but research faced an unforeseen difficulty when the patient's vision was lost due to retinitis pigmentosa and he could no longer lip read. In October 1965, the device was removed for fear of infection.

The criticism on this report where leading specialists felt the patient's life could have been at risk, effectively stopped clinical work for several years. Some important animal studies were undertaken and Michelson (1968) [8] confirmed long term functioning and safety of Intracochlear electrodes from animal studies.

Human studies began again in 1969 when House used a six electrode system designed by an engineer Jack Urban, which was hard wired (connected percutaneously) to the external stimulator device). The three patients implanted with this device from 1969 to 1970 were tested extensively for 2 years in the laboratory as a wearable external stimulator was only constructed by House and Urban in 1972. As the results were so encouraging, another ten patients were implanted in 1973 [9]. Meanwhile, in 1971, Michelson reported on four patients implanted with a bipolar electrode system in the scala tympani and a fifth patient with wires embedded in a silastic mould in the basal cochlea. During this period, the National Institute of Health (NIH) in the USA sponsored an independent evaluation of patients then implanted with single-channel implants. The results of this study of 13 subjects using either the House-Urban implant or the Michelson device were published in 1977 (Bilger et al. 1977) [10] and generally confirmed the clinical findings that had been reported by clinics.

Another group in the USA worked with implants at the same time as House in San Francisco (Merzenich 1975) [11]. The next major event in the 1970s was a meeting in 1977 sponsored by what is known now as the House Ear Institute. This first meeting evolved into what became known as the "West Coast Cochlear Prosthesis Workshop" which was held every 12–18 months. Here House proposed that participants agree on a minimum test battery to be performed in common so that results could be more readily compared. The first international Cochlear Implant Conference was held by House in 1977, in which ten teams of surgeon, audiologists and engineers from outside the USA were invited.

Outside the USA, the earliest reported interest in cochlear implantation was by Clark in Australia (Clark et al. 1983) [12]. He first used a multichannel prototype receiver in two cases between 1978 and 1979 at the University of Melbourne. Later this research group developed multichannel Cochlear Implant providing spectral information in addition to temporal and intensity cues, which was considered a second breakthrough in the history of cochlea implants.

Other investigators also developed implants later in Europe. In France, Chouard and Macleod in Paris implanted Europe's first patients in 1973 (Macleod, Chouard and Weber. 1985) [13] Other French, investigators were Portmann in Bordeaus (Daumon, Bebear and Portmann 1990) [14], Fraysee in Toulose, (Fraysee et al. 1987) [15] and Frachet in Bobigny who used the oval window for implantation (Frachet et al. 1987) [16]. In 1978 in Belgium, Marquet developed a multichannel programmable device (Peters et al. 1987) [17]. In UK, research was carried out by Douek, Fourcin and Moore (Moore et al. 1984) [18] and Fraser, who developed a reasonably priced European-made Cochlear Implant (Fraser 1989) [19]. In Austria, the cochlear implant programme was started in Vienna and Innsbruck by Burian, Hochmair-Desoyer and Hochmair in 1975 (Hochmair-Desoyer et al. 1981) [20].

In Switzerland Dillier, Leifer and Fisch first used a modiolar implant (Dillier Spillman, and De Min 1987) [21] and later the round window electrode. In West Germany, Paul Banfai worked with Hortmann and used an extra cochlear

"Hedgehog" in 1981 (Banfai et al. 1984) [22]. In 1987, Hortmann introduced an intracochlear eight electrode array, and a single channel electrode driven by a 12 channel processor became available in 1989.

In Czechoslovakia, Tichy began his developments in 1979, and the first experience with cochlear implants was reported by Valvoda in 1987 [23]. Other single-channel devices were designed in China (Chen Lee and Lin 1985) [24], East Germany (Gerhardt and Wagner 1986) [25] and Thailand (Kanchanarak, Siriratwatanankul and Boonyanukal 1989) [26].

The road from idea to practical clinical application of cochlear has been "Rocky". With new ideas introduced into the practice of medicine perseverance was required in the face of considerable criticism from the professional and scientific community to reach the present state of accepting successful cochlear implants users.

House (1976) wrote "There have been many and varied pressures to abandon the project. If it had not been for the encouragement and stimulation from the deaf patients who are the centre of this project, it would have died long ago".

It is because of this Commercial companies then began to develop cochlear implants and to provide a standard of product reliability. This led to the food and drug administration (FDA) in the USA approving the clinical use of the 3M House device in 1984 (Fig. 1.1). (House and Berliner 1986) and the Nucleus Clark device in 1985 in post lingually deaf adults. Pre-lingual deaf children were first implanted by House in 1980, by Chouard, Banfai and Burian in the early 1980s and by Clark in 1986.

More than 50 cochlear implant devices had been in clinical use throughout the world (Table 1.1), but they all had certain basic components in common. These are a microphone that picks up external sound energy and generates the driving stimulus, so that the processed signal is then transmitted across the skin (transcutaneous) or through the skin (percutaneous) to the implanted electrode array.

However, they all had different processor strategies.

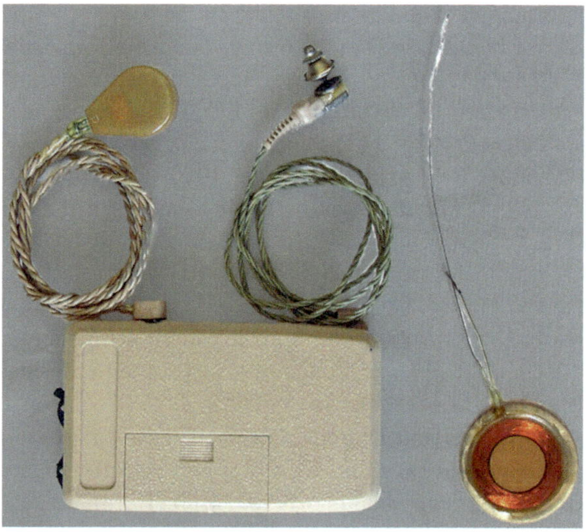

**Fig. 1.1** The 3 M house device

**Table 1.1** List of cochlear implants used worldwide in the past

| Group and device | Commercial manufacturer | Speech processor strategy | Electrode position |
|---|---|---|---|
| 1. Banfai | EMG GmbH | Analogue | Multi (16) |
| (Cologne, Germany) | | | Extra |
| 2. Bonding/Lauridsen | – | – | Multi |
| (Copenhagen, Denmark) | | | |
| 3. Bosch/Colomina | | | Multi (6) |
| (Barcelona, Spain) | | | Intra |
| 4. Chen | | Analogue | Multi (4) |
| (Guanghoi, China) | | | Intra/Extra |
| 5. Chouard | Chorimac | Analogue | Multi (12) |
| (Paris, France) | | | Intra |
| 6. Clark | Nucleus/ | Feature | |
| (Melbourne, Australia) | Cochlear pty | Extraction | Multi (22) |
| | | (F0 F1F2) | Intra |
| 7. Dillier/Fischh | | | Single |
| Spillmann | | | Extra |
| (Zurich, Switzerland) | | | |
| 8. Douek/Fourchin/ | | Feature | Single/Multi (3) |
| (London, EPI, | | Extraction | Extra |
| Group UK) | | (F0) | |
| 9. Eddington | Symbion | Analogue | Multi (4) |
| (Utah) | | | |
| 10. Frachet | | | Intra |
| (Bobigny, France) | | | Single |
| 11. Frasser | Finetech/RNID | Analogue | Single |
| (London, UCH, UK) | | | Extra |
| 12. Frasser | | Analogue | Single |
| (Toulouse, France) | | Receiver in Chest | Extra |
| 13. Gehardt | | Analogue | Multi |
| (Berlin, GDR) | | | (1) Extra (R.W.) |
| | | | (2) Intra (second Turn) |
| 14. Gersdorff/ | | | Single |
| Schneppe (Brussels, Belgium) | | | Intra |
| 15. Goa | | | Single/Multi (3) |
| (Shanghai, China) | | | Intra |
| 16. Hochmair | 3M | Analogue | Single/Multi |
| (Vienna, Innsbruck, Austria) | | | (2,8) |
| 17. Hortmann | | Analogue | Single/Multi (8) |
| (Neckartanzlingen, (Implex) | | | Intra/Extra |
| West Germany) | | | |

(continued)

**Table 1.1** (continued)

| Group and device | Commercial manufacturer | Speech processor strategy | Electrode position |
|---|---|---|---|
| 18. House | 3M | Analogue | Single intra |
| (Los Angeles, USA) | | | |
| 19. Kanchanarak | | | Single intra |
| (Chaing Mai, Thailand) | | | |
| 20. Marqueet/Peeters/ Laura | | | Multi (6,8) |
| (Antwerp, Belgium) | | | Intra |
| 21. Merzencik/ Midhelson | Storz | | Multi (17,4)' |
| (San Francisco, USA) | | | Intra |
| 22. Morrision/Evans | | Analogue or feature | Multi (6,5) |
| | | Receiver in chest | (4) Intra |
| | | | (1) Extra |
| 23. Portmann | Racal | Analogue | Single extra |
| (Bordeaux, France) | | | |
| 24. Pulec | Hortmann | | Multi (8) |
| (Los Angeles, USA) | | | Extra |
| 25. Simmons | Biostim | Analogue | Single intra |
| (Stanford) | | | |
| 26. Trichy | | | Single intra |
| (Prague, Czechoslovakia) | | | |
| 27. Valvoda | Storz | | Single extra |
| (Prague, Czechoslovakia) | | | |

## References


1. Volta A. On the electricity excited by mere contact of conducting substances of different kinds. Philos Trans R Soc. 1800;90:403–31.
2. Luxford WM, Brackmann D. The history of cochlear implants. In: Gray RF, editor. Cochlear-implants. London: Croom Helm; 1985. p. 1–26.
3. Andreef AM, Gersuni GV, Volokhov AA. Electrical stimulation of the hearing organ. J Physiol USSR. 1934;1:546–59.
4. Jones R, Stevens S, Lurie M. Three mechanisms of hearing by electrical stimulation. J Acoust Soc Am. 1940;12:281–90.
5. Zollner F, Kiedel WD. Geroyermittlung durch elektrishce erregung des neruus acousticius. Archives Fur Der Ohren, - nasena dnKehlkopf heilkunde. 1963;181:216–23.
6. House WF, Berliner KI, Crary WG, Graham M, Luckey R, Mortan N, Selters W, Tobin H, Urban J, Wexler M. Cochlear implants. Ann Otol Rhinol Laryngol. 1976;85(Suppl 27)
7. Simmons FB. Electrical stimulation of the auditory nerve in man. Arch Otolaryngol. 1966;84:24–76.
8. Michelson MP. The crossed cochlear efferent. Trans Am Larygol Rhinol Otol Soc. 1968:626–44.
9. House WP, Urban J. Long term results of electrode implantation and electronic stimulation of the cochlear in Man. Ann Otol Rhinol Laryngol. 1973;82:504–14.

10. Bilger RC, Black FO, Hopkinson NT, Mygers EN, Payne JL, Stenson NR, Vega A, Wolf RV. Evaluation of subjects presently fitted with implantable auditory prosthesis. Ann Otol Rhinol Laryngol. 1977;86(Suppl 38)
11. Merzenich MM. In: Tower DB, editor. Studies on electrical stimulation at the auditory nerve in animals and man: cochlear implants in the nervous system, vol. 3. New York: Raven Press; 1975. p. 537–48.
12. Clark GM, Dowell RC, Brown AM, Luscome SM, Pyman BC, Webb RL, et al. The clinical trial of a multichannel cochlear prosthesis. An initial study on four patients with a profound to total hearing loss. Med J Aust. 1983;2:430–3.
13. Macleod P, Chouard CH, Weber JP. French device. In: InL Schindler RA, Merzenich NM, editors. Cochlear implants. New York: Raven Press; 1985. p. 111–20.
14. Daumon R, Bebear JP, Portmann M. Cochlear implant in Bordeauz: past to present strategy. Paper presented at the Politizer society, Courchevel, France, March 11–16, 1990.
15. Fraysee B, Soulien MJ, Urgell H, Levy P, Furia F, Defreness V. Extra cochlear implantation: technique and results. Ann Otol Rhinol Laryngol. 1987;96(Suppl 128):111–3.
16. Frachet B, Vormes E, Despreux G. Electrical stimulation of the oval window. In: Banfai P, editor. Cochlear implant. Current situation. Proceeding from the international cochlear implant symposium, Durren, West German. 1987. p. 657–662.
17. Peters Marquet J, Offeciers FE, Bosiers W, Kinsbergen J, Van Durme M, Somers T, Depaep K, Van Camp K, Moen Eclaey L. The laura cochlear prosthesis: development and description. In: Banfai P, editor. Cochlear implant: current situation. Proceedings from the international cochlear implant symposium, Duren, West Germany. 1987. p. 547–555
18. Moore, B.C.J Douek, E. Fourcin, A.J. Rose, S.M, Walliker, J.R Howard, D.M Abberton, E. and Frampton, S.: Extra cochlear patterns: experience of the EPI group (UK), Adv Audiol, I, 148-162 1984
19. Fraser JG. The University college Hospital/Royal National Institute for the deaf cochlear implant programme. J Laryngol Otol. 1989;Suppl 18:1–3.
20. Hochmair-Desoyer IJ, Hochmair ES, Burian K, Fischer RE. Four years of experience with cochlear prosthesis. Med Progr Technol. 1981;8:107–19.
21. Dillier NM, Spillmann, Demin, N. Ten years experience with cochlear implants; Results with wingle and multi electrode systems. In: Banfai P, editor. Cochlear implant: current situation. Proceedings from the inter-national cochlear implant symposium, Duren, West Germany. 1987. p. 197–215.
22. Banfai P, Kubik S, Hortmann G. Our extra-scalar operating method of cochlear implantation. Acta Otolaryngol. 1984;411:7–12.
23. Volvoda M, Betka J, Hruby J. The first experience with cochlear implantations in Czechoslovakia. In: Banfai P, editor. Cochlear implant: current situation. p. 289–90.
24. Chen CW, Lee PM, Lin MD. Preliminary results of four electrode cochlear implants. Cochlear implant symposium and workshop. Melbourne. Ann Otol Rhinol Laryngol. 1985;96(Suppl 128):139.
25. Gerhardt HJ, Wagner H. The Berlin Cochlear Implant: Conception and first experience with cochlear prosthesis. Part I: Surgical conception. HNO – PRA X (Lp3). 1986;11:187–94.
26. Kanchanarak C, Siriratwatankul N, Boonyanukul A. Expensive cochlear implant device modified from House-3-M. Cochlear implant device. Paper presented at the XIV World Congress of Otol, Madrid, September 10–15, 1989.

# History of Cochlear Implants in India

# 2

Sandra DeSaSouza

## 2.1 History

Indian otolaryngologists had a keen interest in cochlear implants as early as in the mid-1980s, when Dr J N Gurtu delivered lectures on cochlear implants at the AOI conference in 1984, and also at the Maharashtra state conference in 1984. This was followed by the First National workshop on cochlear implants at PGIMER Chandigarh organized by Dr Y.N. Mehra in 1986 at which Carolyn Dobsen from Cochlear Australia had delivered lectures.

Finally in 1987, the first national surgical workshop was organized by Dr Sandra DeSaSouza, (Henceforth referred to as the author) at Jaslok Hospital, Mumbai during which Dr Jack Pulec from the USA was the guest faculty and participants, namely otolaryngologists and audiologists from all over the country participated (Fig. 2.1).

**Supplementary Information** The online version contains supplementary material available at [https://doi.org/10.1007/978-981-19-0452-3_2].

S. DeSaSouza (✉)
ENT Department, Jaslok Hospital, Mumbai, Maharashtra, India

Breach Candy Hospital and Desa Hospital (ENT Section), Mumbai, Maharashtra, India


S. DeSaSouza (ed.), *Cochlear Implants*,
https://doi.org/10.1007/978-981-19-0452-3_2

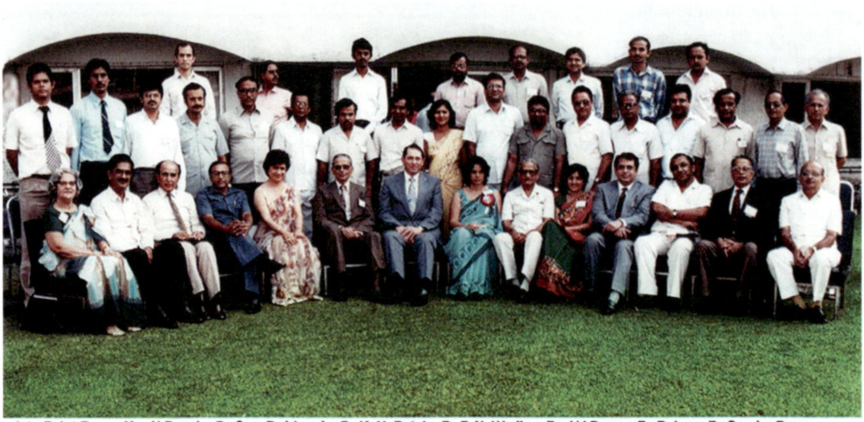

L to R 1st Row • Mrs N Desai • Dr Oza, Dr Idnani • Dr K. N. Patel • Dr P. N. Wadia • Dr J V Desa • Dr Pulec • Dr Sandra Desa • Dr K. U. Shah • Mrs Parulkar • Dr A. B. R. Desai • Dr V. Shah • Dr Gadre • Dr Bhargava
2nd Row • Dr Pradhan • Dr Chandasekhar • Dr Singh • Dr Baburao • Dr Sadera S. S. • Dr Memon • Dr Chaudhari • Dr Kasbekar • Mr P. Mahajan • Dr Borkar D. M. • Dr Bose • Dr M. Kumarsen • Dr D. M. Kalambi • Dr K. S. Parsaram • Dr A. Sorak • Dr Ranade
3rd Row • Dr A. Bhaskar • Dr Ravishankar • Dr Bhole • Dr S. C. Sharma • Dr K. C. Prakasn • Mr Malikarjun • S. S. Sansgiri • Mr Chaudhari • Dr C. E. Desouza

**Fig. 2.1** First National Cochlear implant surgical workshop, Jaslok Hospital 1987

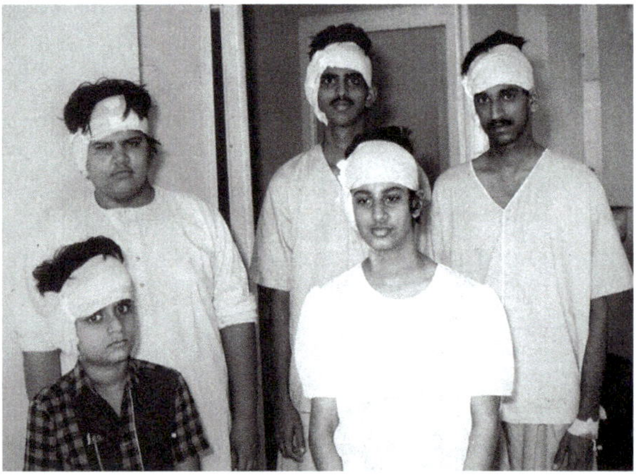

**Fig. 2.2** Group of five children operated at during the first workshop

At the workshop Dr Jack Pulec operated on four children. The fifth child was operated by the author who thus became the pioneer of Cochlear Implants in India (Fig. 2.2). As per the verification of the CI companies, the author was also the first woman Cochlear Implant surgeon in the world.

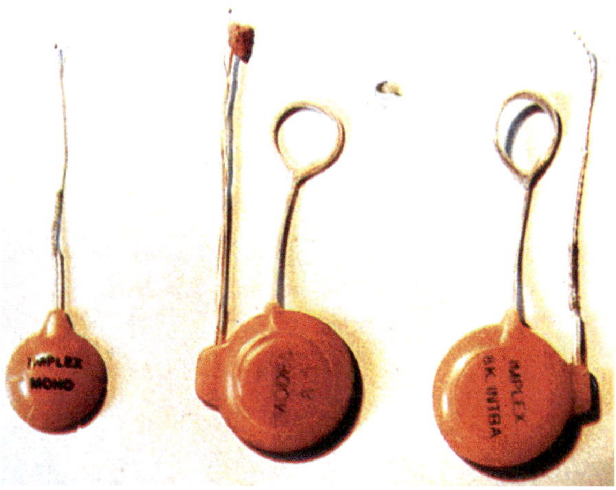

**Fig. 2.3** Hortmann mono, eight extra and eight intra multi electrode Implants

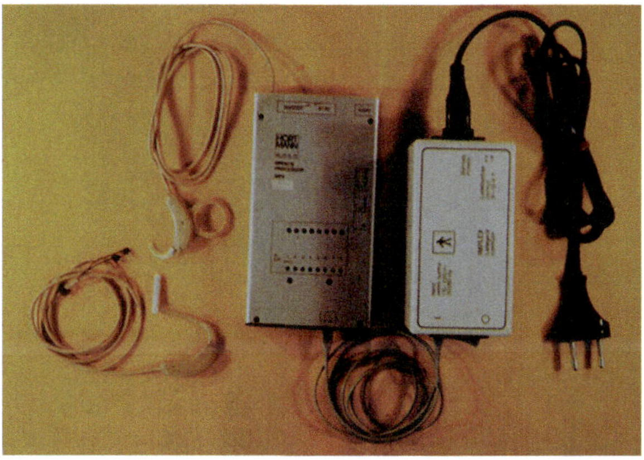

**Fig. 2.4** Hortmann speech processor, battery and charger, stick and ring antenna

This way a clinical trial was started in India, followed up by Hans Leysieffer the Hortmann GmbH and Simplex AG hearing technologist. The implants were from Hortmann GmbH which had 8 channel and later 12 channel Implex implants. The system has mono single electrode, eight extra and eight intra multi electrode implants (Fig. 2.3).

The Hortmann speech processor was large and had a battery pack with a battery charger. There was a stick antenna worn in the ear to transmit signals to the circular coil implanted under the canal skin and connected to the implanted receiver (Fig. 2.4).

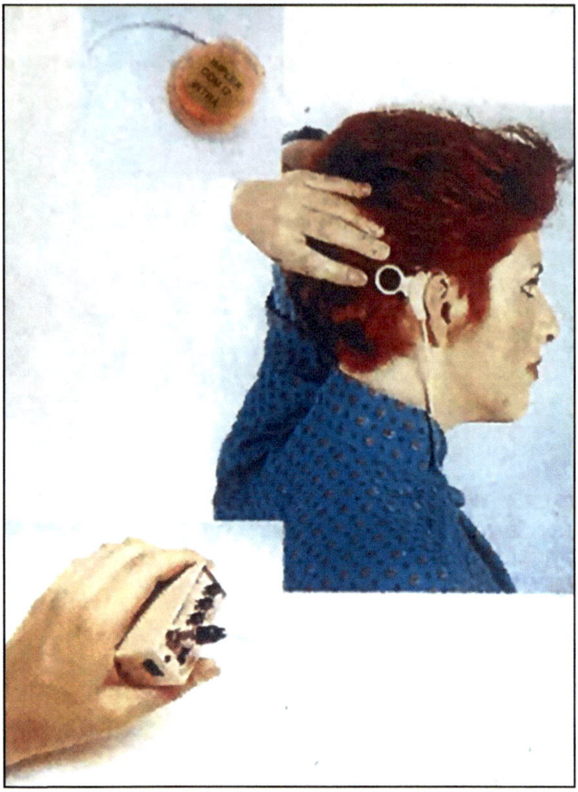

**Fig. 2.5** Speech processor and headset without a magnet

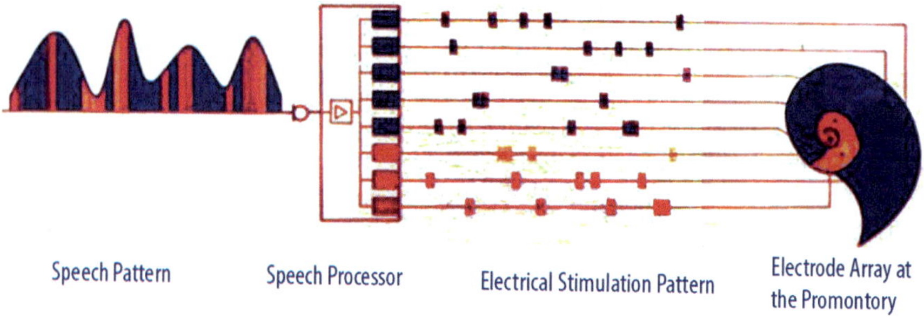


**Fig. 2.6** The single electrode system

In 1989, Hortmann then manufactured a smaller Implex Speech processor and headset without the magnet (Fig. 2.5). The extra and intra electrode systems helped to achieve frequency to place transformation. The single electrode used frequency to time resolution (time delay) by working with multi channels (Fig. 2.6). The multi electrode extra and intra systems worked with place and pitch stimulation strategy (Fig. 2.7).

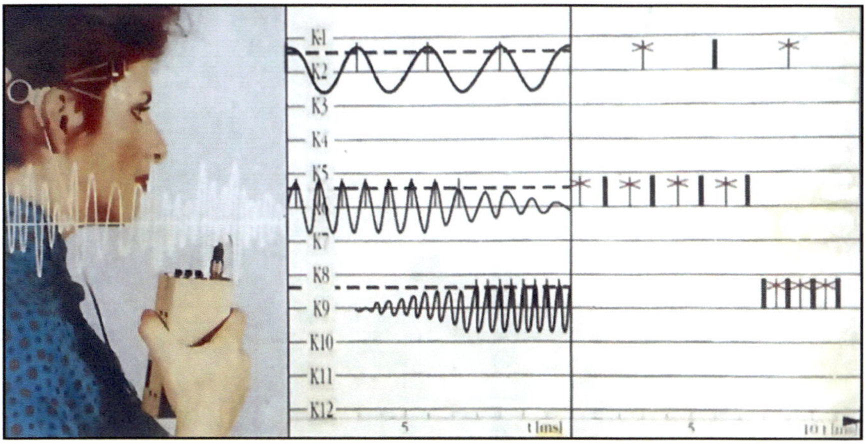


**Fig. 2.7** The multi electrode system

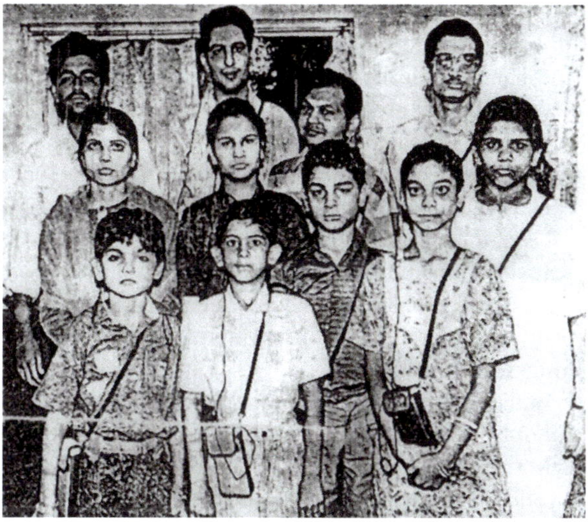

**Fig. 2.8** Group of 11 children

The cochlear implant surgeries done in Mumbai with the first surgical workshop, it created turmoil in the minds of ENT surgeons' audiologists and teachers of the deaf. The author then visited centres in Europe who were using Hortmann implants in Frankfurt, in Denmark with Dr Brad Peterson, in Paris with Dr Andre Sultan, and in Beziers with Dr Jean Bernard Causse. After her return to India the author operated 11 cases (Fig. 2.8), children and adults pre and postlingual along with Hans Leysieffer the clinical technologist from Hortmann who gave technical support [1].

All the implantees were rehabilitated by Dr Vijay Shah who was the first audiologist in India to habilitate and rehabilitate such cases [2]. In the next few years, the author operated 50 deaf patients with Hortmann and Hortmann Implex implants [1].

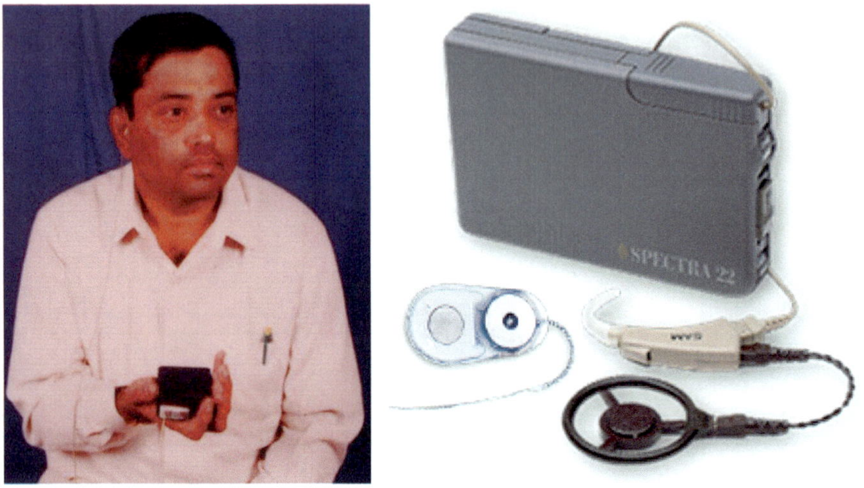


**Fig. 2.9** Dr Sonavane, Nucleus 22 implant and MSP body worn speech processor

All patients were subjected to preoperative promontorium cochlear nerve test with Hortmann cochlear nerve tester [3], later however and also with other companies this test was not used.

In 1993, the author was visited by Albert Sorrel who introduced the Nucleus system from Cochlear and was the first in India to operate in 1993 on Dr Sonavane a post lingual general practitioner with a Nucleus 22 under local anaesthesia as he had a cardiac problem (Fig. 2.9).

In 1994, the author operated in Jaslok hospital with Professor Bill Gibson the first ossified cochlea and the first otosclerosis postlingual with a Nucleus implant.

In 1995, KMC hospital in Manipal did their first implant using Nucleus 22 by Professor Hazarika.

In the same year, the CI programme with the Nucleus implant was started by the author by operating for Dr Janardhan Rao at the Apollo Hospital, Hyderabad.

Mr. Sebastian Foidl from MED-EL visited India in 1994 and met the author and introduced all the implants of MED-EL. The author subsequently performed the first MED-EL 2SC analogue single channel implant in a post lingual who was fitted with a comfort body worn speech processor (Fig. 2.10).

Dr M.V. Kirtane did his first implant in 1996 with a Nucleus device at Hinduja Hospital Mumbai.

Dr H. M. Hans did his first cochlear implant in 1997 and he was also the first person in India to use the Veria technique.

Dr Mohan Kameswaran at MERF Chennai did his first implant using Nucleus in 1997, later became a pioneer in brainstem implant in India.

The first four pioneers, namely the author, Dr M V Kirtane, Dr Mohan Kameswaran, Dr H M Hans are all recipients of Padma Shree Award.

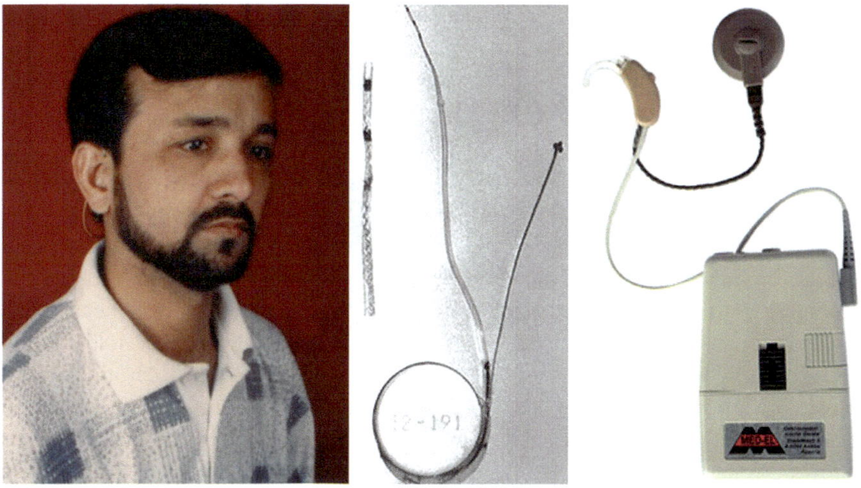


**Fig. 2.10** First patient Asghar Ali with MED-EL implant and comfort speech processor

Dr Vinaya Kumar started CI in early 1996 at Apollo hospital, Hyderabad after which he visited many centres all over India doing cochlear implant surgery.

AIIMS Delhi did their first nucleus implant in 1997 by Dr R.C. Deka.

In AFMC the first implants were done by General V K Singh and General M D Venkatesh in 1997.

Dr Ashish Lahiri did his first CI in Ganga Ram Hospital, Delhi in late 1990.

Habilitation with post lingual and rehabilitation with prelingual were started in Mumbai in 1988 in Jaslok by Dr Vijay Shah who was joined by Shahnaz Shaikh in 1991. Chennai started in 1997 and other centres in Mumbai in 1998. AURED which had started in 1986 for hearing aid users also in late 1990s started training cochlea implantees.

In 1999, the Pune advanced auditory P.A.A.R. did its first cochlear implant with Dr Neelam Vaid and Dr Hemant Dabke and the rehabilitation was done by Dr Kalyani Mandke as the audiologist and speech therapist, a position she still holds today. Dr Neelam Vaid today is a prominent CI surgeon.

In 2000, the first Advanced Bionics implant, the Clarion was used by me (the author) in India (Fig. 2.11).

In 2001, the author visited K. K. Ramalingam Hospital in Chennai where she did their first case using Advanced Bionics implant with Dr Ravi Ramalingam who then became another doyen CI surgeon.

Dr Manoj Manikoth did his first cochlear implant in Kerala in 2001.

In 2003, the Advanced Bionics HiRes 90k was used for the first time in India and Asia by the author (Fig. 2.12).

Dr Sunil Dutt did his first cochlear implant in Bangalore in 2003 and today is the President of Cochlear Implant Group of India (CIGI).

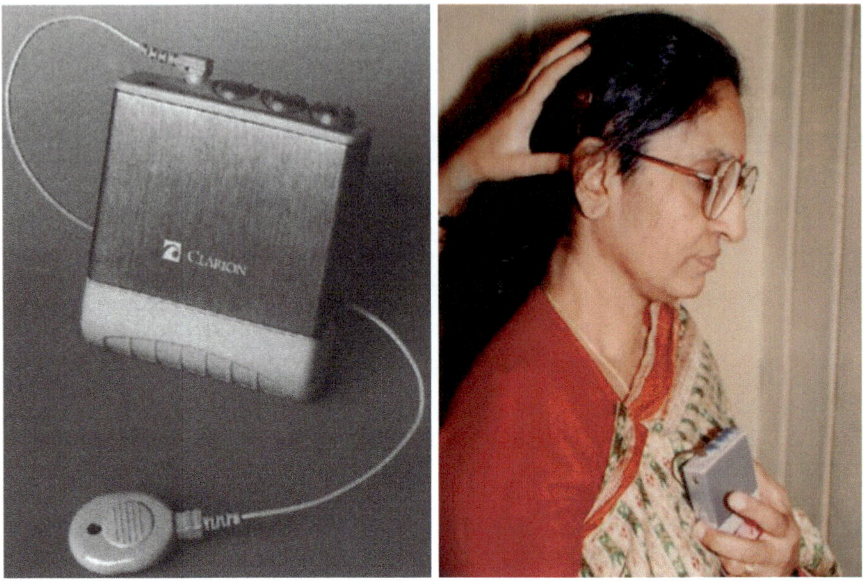


**Fig. 2.11** Clarion processor and the first patient

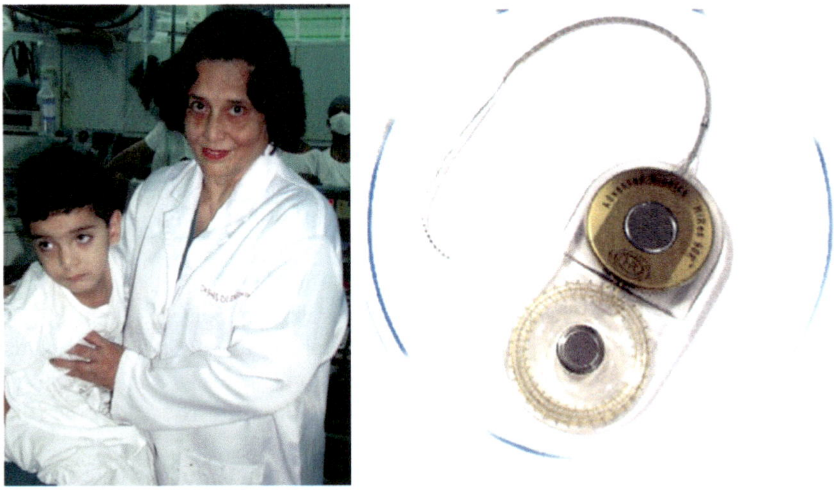

**Fig. 2.12** Advanced Bionics HiRes 90k implant and the prelingual patient

Dr Rajesh Vishwakarma put his first cochlear implant in 2004 at B J Medical College and Civil Hospital and the institution was the first to receive government funding in 2013 for CI surgery in India.

Dr Christopher Dsouza did his first cochlear implant in 2005 at Holy Family hospital Mumbai.

Dr Shabir Indorewalla performed his first cochlear implantation in 2006 at Indorewalla ENT hospital, Nasik.

Dr Amit Kishore did his CI surgery at Apollo Hospital, Delhi, in 2006, he also does BAHA and ABI.

Dr Miklu Senapati put the first South Korean implant in 2008.

Digisonic (Neurelec) implantation was done for the first time in Kannur, Kerala by Dr M V Kirtane in 2008.

Dr M V Kirtane did the first ADIP scheme funded implant at B Y L Nair hospital in December 2014.

Dr Sumit Mirg did his first cochlear implant in 2010 at KGMC Lucknow.

Dr Satyaprakash Dubey put in his first cochlear implant in 2014 and started several state-of-the-art centres.

Dr Dillon Dsouza did his first CI in 1998 at Desa hospital, Mumbai.

Dr Dillon Dsouza with the author did the first CI in Lucknow with Dr Tyagi in the late 1990s. The first CI in Rajasthan hospital was performed by Dr Dsouza, in Ahmedabad in 2003, and he did the first CI in 2005 with Dr Vinod Khandar at Apollo Hospital and at Guwahati with Dr Senapati using Clarion implant in the late 2000. He also did first CI in Central Railway hospital with Dr Dalmia, later Dr Dalmia became a prominent CI surgeon. Dr Dsouza did the first J J Hospital funded implant in 2008.

Dr Shankar Medikiri did his first CI in April 2004, first Mondini in November 2004. He was the first in India to do bilateral simultaneous implant in July 2007.

Cochlear Implant Group of India was founded in 2003. Dr Mohan Kameswaran was the founding member. Today it has 631 members.

The first state funded programme for Cochlear Implant was started by Andhra Pradesh in 2007 by the Late Chief Minister Y S Rajasekhara Reddy.

State funding programmes are now available in Andhra Pradesh, Tamil Nadu, Telangana, Kerala, Rajasthan, Gujarat, Chhattisgarh, and Central government under ADIP scheme.

ADIP scheme (Assistance to disabled persons for purchase/fitting of aids/appliances) funded by Central government for Cochlear implant started in 2014.

Past President of India Dr Abdul Kalam carried out clinical trials for an indigenous implant with Dr Bhujanga Rao to make a cheaper local implant at DRDO (Defence Research and Development Organisation) in 2012–2015.

## 2.2 History of Surgery (Videos 2.1 and 2.2)

Just as there was a history of the various doyens of CI surgery there was a history of different surgical procedures used. In 1987 and 1988, first a small post aural incision later a large C-shaped incision was used followed by an endaural incision with an extended horizontal limb. As the receivers became smaller a postural incision and then a mini postural was used.

While using the Hortmann device in the late 1980s and the early 1990s, the incus was removed and cable introduced through the attic to the cochleostomy. The Hortmann extra cochlear hedgehog for ossified cochlea could only be passed through the attic and after the promontory thinned out pressed onto it and the beak put in the Eustachian tube. For all later devices a posterior tympanotomy and Veria technique was used. The history of development of CI surgery ran parallel with the development of the implant.

## 2.3 Conclusion

Delving into the history of Cochlear implants one finds many hurdles in health and medical schemes which have developed in other countries. India is a subcontinent with millions of people below poverty line. Even after medical insurance were well established by 2000 it could not be made compulsory as the poor could not afford to pay. Moreover, medical insurance companies in India do not pay for or cover cochlear implants. From 2005, innumerable surgeons from all over India as mentioned earlier performed cochlear implantation and also travelled to other cities to start centres so that CI surgery became available throughout the country. There are now more than 35 cochlear implant centres for complete evaluation and rehabilitation all over the country. With awareness increasing government funding around the same time started in almost every state as mentioned earlier. ADIP was the central government of India funding for implantation. Private trusts also started funding for cochlear implantees, but all funding was for prelingual deaf children of 4 years and below. Today thousands of children below the poverty line have been implanted.

This has made the journey truly worthwhile.

For the journey to continue however there should be funding for long-term maintenance and replacement for all non-affording patients.

**Acknowledgements** Cochlear implant professionals.

- Dr. N Vaid for giving me information from her presentation at CIGICON 2015.
- Cochlear implant companies.

**Disclaimer** All information collected from individuals and not written on my own.

## References

1. Desasouza S, Leyseiffer H. The Indian experience with Hortmann Implex implants published in Proceedings of the XIVth World Congress, Madrid, Spain. 1989. p. 1191.
2. Desasouza S, Shah V, Lobo JT. Cochlear implants in prelingual adults and children published in Proceedings of the XIV World Congress, Madrid, Spain. 1989. p. 1179.
3. Desasouza S, Gosavi ND. Promontorium stimulation test published in XVth World Congress of Otorhinolaryngology Head and Neck Surgery, Turkey. 1993. p. 417.

# Evolution of Cochlear Implant Technology over the Last 35 Years

# 3

Anandhan Dhanasingh and Sandra DeSaSouza

## 3.1 Introduction

Cochlear Implant (CI) is the *state-of-the-art* treatment option for severe-to-profound sensorineural hearing loss (SNHL) conditions worldwide. In the early 1990s, only *severe-to-profound* bilaterally deaf hearing loss subjects were considered for CI. But with the advancements in CI technologies in the last 35 years, the indications of CI and the minimum age limit have been expanded liberally. Patients with partial deafness in the high-frequency region who do not benefit from conventional hearing aids (HA) are now considered candidates for CI [1]. Single-sided deafness (SSD)/asymmetric hearing loss (AHL) is another group of patients who are currently treated with CI in many developed countries [2]. With the advancements in the surgical steps, newborn babies as young as <12 months old are now treated with CI [3]. With the advancements in the preoperative image analysis tools, the anatomies of the various inner ear malformation types are now well understood, and these patients are also treated with CI and the results are convincing [4]. The advancements in CI technologies, surgical skills, accessory tools like preoperative image analysis tools are all contributing to the success in safely expanding the CI for various indications

**Supplementary Information** The online version contains supplementary material available at [https://doi.org/10.1007/978-981-19-0452-3_3].

A. Dhanasingh (✉)
MED-EL Medical Electronics, Innsbruck, Austria
e-mail: Anandhan.dhanasingh@medel.com

S. DeSaSouza
ENT Municipal Hospital, Mumbai, Maharashtra, India

ENT Department, Jaslok Hospital, Mumbai, Maharashtra, India

Breach Candy Hospital and Desa Hospital, Mumbai, Maharashtra, India


S. DeSaSouza (ed.), *Cochlear Implants*,
https://doi.org/10.1007/978-981-19-0452-3_3

and age groups. While the surgeons might be aware of the advancements in the surgical steps/skills, it is important to bring out the advancements in the CI technologies. With that aim, this chapter will detail the technological advancements over the last 35 years in the implantable and external components of a CI from a general perspective.

## 3.2 Components of a Cochlear Implant

The *microphone* in the audio processor picks up the acoustic signal from the surrounding environment and the *audio processing unit* breaks it down to digital signals using a *sound-processing algorithm* which will be transmitted to the *receiver stimulator* via an inductive link. Briefly, the inductive link works through an interaction between the external and the receiving antenna when the external transmitter is placed over the *implant magnet*. The implant electronics then convert these signals to electric impulses and transfer them to the inner ear through the intracochlear *electrode array*. All these components of the CI along with the signal processing algorithms have undergone tremendous improvements over the last 35 years and this chapter will bring it to your attention. Figure 3.1 shows the components of a modern CI.

## 3.3 Technological Evolution of the Implant Stimulator Case

One of the key requirements for the overall success of CI is the hermeticity of the implant stimulator. The electronics inside the implant case should be kept dry at all times and any ingress of body fluid could fail the implant electronics. In the late 1970s, the investigational CIs were fabricated using medical-grade epoxy resin to encapsulate implant electronics. In the late 1980s, the epoxy encapsulation of the implant electronics was changed to ceramic housing. The ceramics used in medical applications are commonly based on aluminum oxide ($Al_2O_3$). The advantage of the

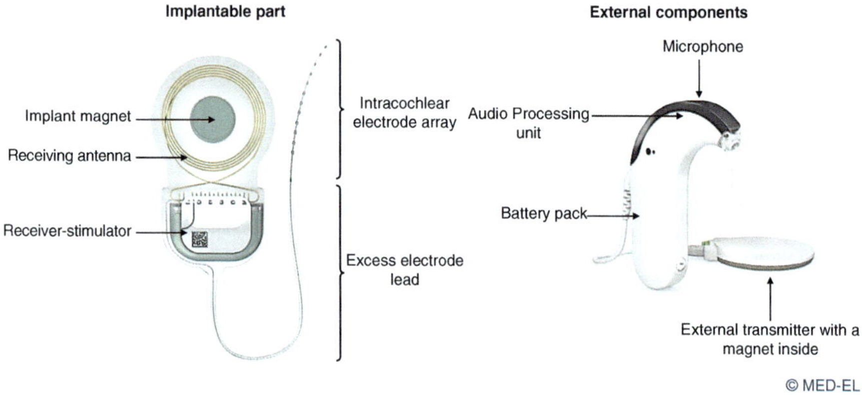


**Fig. 3.1** Components of a modern cochlear implant

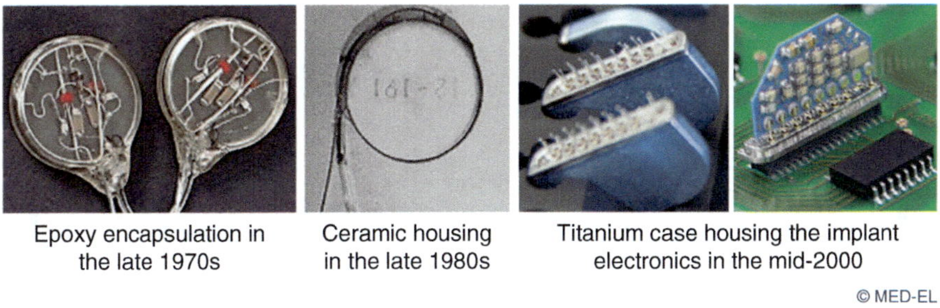


**Fig. 3.2** Different materials used in the fabrication of implant stimulator case over time

ceramic housing is that the receiver coil can be placed within the casing, as ceramics do not greatly affect signal transmission. However, the material is more brittle than titanium and thus more prone to breakage under significant mechanical stress [5]. Figure 3.2 shows the different materials used to encapsulate implant electronics over time.

It is reported that the titanium housing has an impact resistance of up to 2.5 J [6]. Figure 3.2 shows implant electronics casing based on different materials that have evolved over time. Till today (2021), titanium is the *state-of-the-art* material used in the implant case. Recalls from the CI manufacturers due to implant failures are reported from time to time. Cochlear Corporation has recalled its implants in the year 1995 due to internal power supply failure issues and in the year 2011 due to hermeticity failure. Advanced Bionics has recalled in 1995 due to cracked ceramic cases, in 2002, due to suspicion of electrode array positioner being correlated to the risk of meningitis, in 2004, due to moisture trapped inside the implant at the time of manufacturing, in 2006, due to hermeticity failure, in 2010, due to latent short circuit in substrate and in 2020, due to moisture entering the implant causing a decrease in hearing performance [7].

## 3.4 Technological Evolution in the Implant Magnet

The implant magnet plays a key role in keeping the external transmitter in place over the implant, thereby relaying the signals from the external audio processor to the implant. The design of the implant magnet plays a major role in the safety of the CI patient. In the presence of an external powerful magnetic field like a magnetic resonance imaging (MRI) system, the implant magnet could react. If the implant magnet has no freedom to align itself to the external magnetic field, it can pop out of the implant case depending on the implant design, or it can cause the overall implant to shift its location causing pain sensation to the patient depending on the surgical fixation, or the magnet could lose it magnetism [8].

A magnet design with a self-aligning property in response to the external magnetic field could solve several issues. In the absence of a self-aligning magnet design, the magnet can be surgically removed prior to the MRI session, but at the cost of additional surgery and even some damage to the implant.

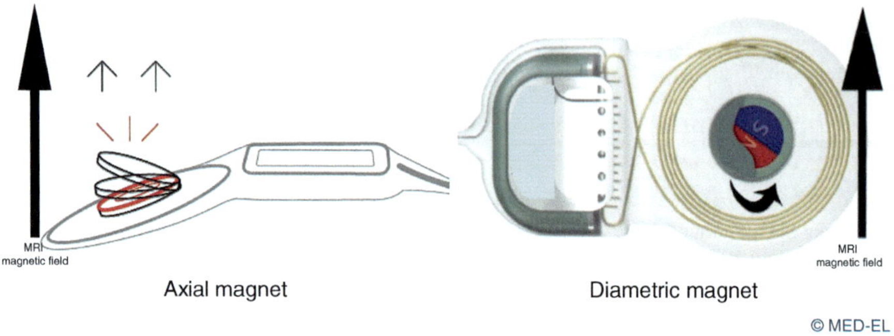


**Fig. 3.3** Implant magnet design. Axial magnet is a regular cylindrical magnet with two magnetic poles on either face of the magnet and could be pulled toward the external magnetic field. The diametric magnet has both the magnetic poles on the same face of the magnet making it to rotate inside the magnet case in response to the external magnetic field (video clip)

In 2014, MED-EL introduced a self-aligning diametric magnet design that revolutionized the CI field when it comes to MRI procedures as shown in Fig. 3.3 (Video 3.1). The diametric magnet design allowed for an unparalleled MRI safety at 3.0 T without the need for magnet removal through an additional surgical procedure [9, 10]. Advanced Bionics and Cochlear Corporation, which are the other two CI manufacturers also came up with a self-aligning magnet concept in the year 2018.

## 3.5 Technological Evolution in the Intracochlear Electrode

Intracochlear structure preservation was not the aim when the first-generation electrode arrays were designed. The first generation of CI electrode arrays were bulky and were designed with ball contacts that protruded out of the electrode array as shown in Fig. 3.4. This was purposefully made with the aim of bringing the stimulating electrode contacts closer to the modiolus wall of the cochlea where the spiral ganglion cell bodies (SGCBs) are housed. It was reported several years after implantation of this first-generation electrode, that the ball contacts were broken and stuck inside the fibrous tissue encapsulation during explantation due to device failure. This warns us that the protruding ball contacts are not the optimal electrode design for CI applications.

Electrode with a positioner pushing the stimulating contacts closer to the modiolus wall was another electrode concept that came into existence in early 2000 [12]. In 2002, the Food and Drug Administration (FDA) reported about 87 cases of meningitis in patients implanted with CI and a total of 17 deaths have resulted mainly in patients implanted with positioner electrodes [13] as shown in Fig. 3.5. After this tragic incident, this electrode type was removed from clinical practice.

Pre-curved modiolar hugging electrode was another concept that was introduced by Advanced Bionics in 1995 and Cochlear corporation in 1999 to the best of author's knowledge. The design of the pre-curved electrode aims at hugging the

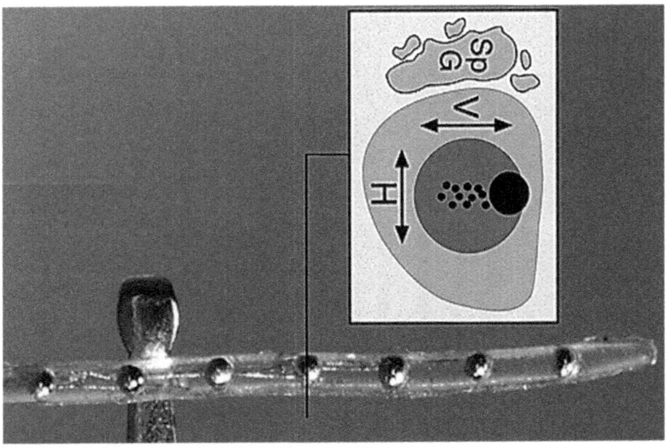


**Fig. 3.4** Electrode with ball contacts protruding out of the electrode surface. Image adapted from Rebscher et al. [11]

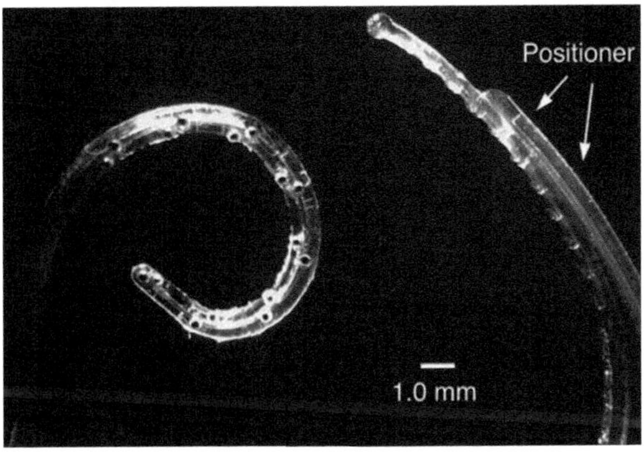


**Fig. 3.5** Electrode with positioner [12]. Image reproduced by permission of Elsevier B.V.

modiolus wall of the cochlea bringing the stimulating electrode contacts close to the SGCBs. These earlier versions of pre-curved electrodes were made bulky with no thoughts on the intracochlear structure preservation but rather on bringing the stimulating electrode channels closer to the SGCBs and on the easiness of insertion fully inside the cochlea. Till today (2021), all the commercially available pre-curved electrodes as shown in Fig. 3.6 are available in a length mainly to cover only the basal turn of the cochlea and not beyond that [14]. This leaves us with the question if pre-curved electrodes have any manufacturing limitations that prevents them to be fabricated longer than what it is now to cover beyond the basal turn of the cochlea with electrical stimulation. The question was answered with yes, in the year 2018 as per the report by Dhanasingh et al. [15].

Since the beginning of MED-EL, its philosophy was to cover the entire population of the neural elements or in other words the entire frequency range with electrical stimulation in profound deaf cochlear conditions and therefore it developed the straight free fitting lateral wall electrode array of length 31.5 mm. Since 2004, MED-EL has introduced electrodes in 31.5 mm, 28 mm, 26 mm, 24 mm, and 20 mm array lengths with the aim of providing electrode solution to any cochlear size and

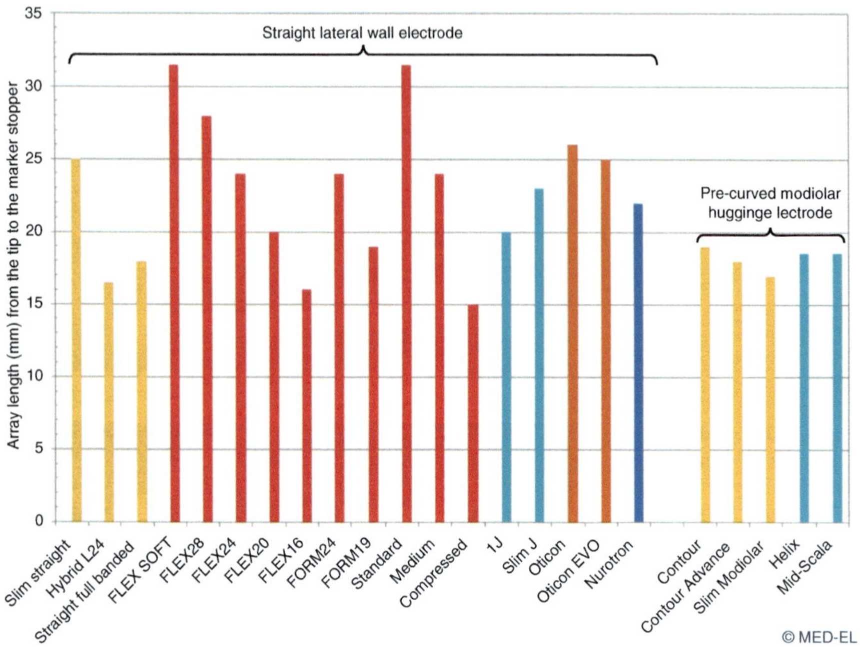


**Fig. 3.6** Chart displays both lateral wall and pre-curved electrode array from all five CI brands. There are 19 lateral wall and 5 pre-curved electrode variants that were developed altogether by all five CI brands. Video clip shows the insertion of a flexible lateral wall electrode goes inside the cochlea

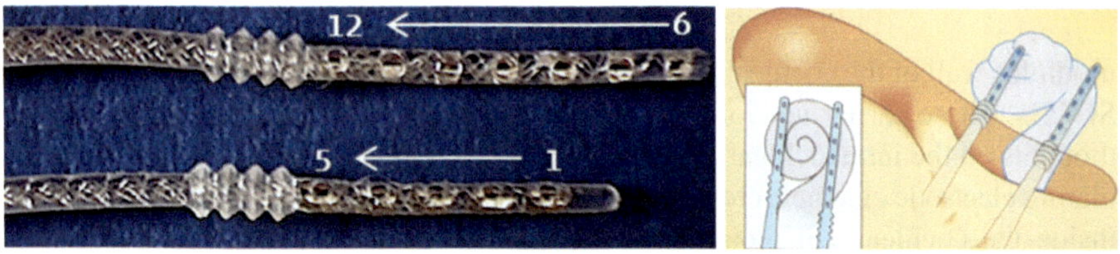


**Fig. 3.7** SPLIT electrode with two branches. The short branch has five channels to be placed in the upper basal turn stimulating the low frequencies and the long branch with seven channels to be placed in the lower basal turn stimulating high frequencies

hearing level [16]. The other CI brands have some varieties on the length of the electrode array within straight lateral wall electrode type to offer different electrode insertion depths. Figure 3.6 captures the electrode types and their variants that are in current (2021) commercial use.

For severely ossified cochlear conditions, any of the regular CI electrode arrays mentioned in Fig. 3.6 may not be suitable. SPLIT electrode is a special electrode design that facilitates the placement of the SPLIT electrode by drilling two channels in the ossified cochlea as shown in Fig. 3.7.

## 3.6 Technological Evolution in the Method of Testing Auditory Nerve

The auditory nerve (AN) must be intact for hearing perception with a CI. In cases of tumor removal from the internal auditory canal (IAC) or in cases with severely malformed cochleae (e.g., hypoplastic cochlear type or hypoplastic IAC, as shown in Fig. 3.8), it may be necessary to assess the viability of the AN to predict the outcome of cochlear implantation [17]. Recording electrically evoked auditory brainstem responses (eABR) via surface electrodes or placing an Intracochlear electrode is a well-established method for determining the integrity of the auditory pathways [18]. This section canvasses through the evolution of such systems over time.

The promontory stimulation test was first conceived by House and Brackmann in 1974, to predict the electrical response of surviving spiral ganglion nerve fiber populations to a cochlear implant. The generation of auditory sensations by preoperative electrical stimulation of the promontory was believed to verify a functioning cochlear nerve and appeared to be predictive of auditory perception following cochlear implantation [19].

The early-days promontory stimulation was performed preoperatively using a trans-tympanic needle electrode placed directly on the promontory at a location close to the round window opening. Electrode impedance confirm the contact with the promontory and the reference electrode was placed on the ipsilateral earlobe.

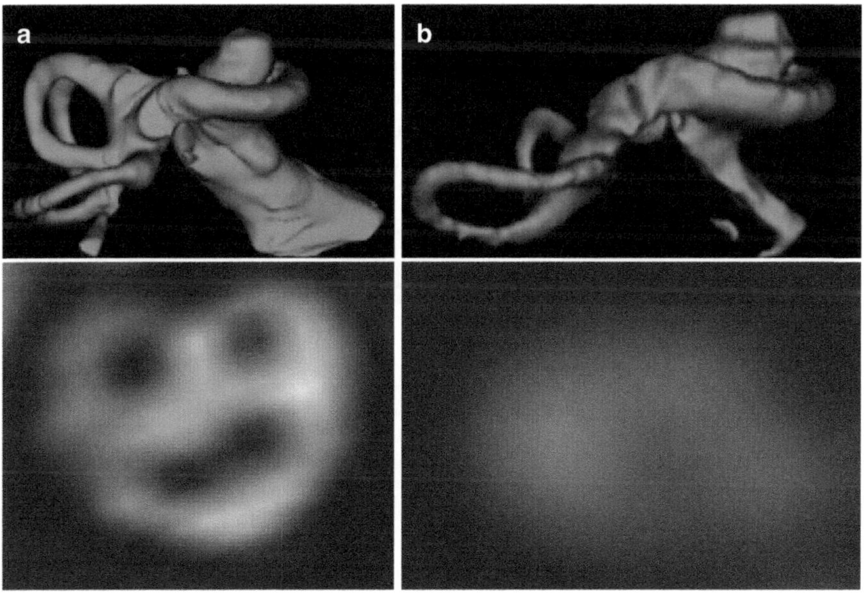


**Fig. 3.8** Three-dimensional (3D) images of normal anatomy and the cross-section of the IAC showing four nerve bundles (**a**) and hypoplastic cochlea and cross-section of the IAC showing just one nerve bundle (**b**)

Promontory thresholds at low frequencies correlate with the percentage of surviving neural elements and therefore it is wise to deliver AC current at frequencies of 50 and 100 Hz. Patients subjectively respond if the electrical stimulation produced a sensation of sound and the data were collected on the smallest current detected [17]. One of the key disadvantages of the subjective promontory test is if the patient is congenitally deaf and how the first hearing sensation can be differentiated from sensation resulting from the side effects of electrical stimulation. The spread of excitation can cause “co-stimulation” affecting the facial nerve or vestibular nerve branches. Some patients will not be able to distinguish a vibrotactile sensation from an electrical auditory sensation, which makes the subjective interpretation of this test difficult.

To overcome the downsides of the subjective promontory test, the objective promontory test was introduced in the late 1980s and in the early 1990s. Objective promontory uses the electrically evoked auditory brainstem response (eABR) to verify the function of the auditory system from the auditory nerve response elicited either from the promontory stimulation or via cochlear implants.

As a further fine-tuning of the objective promontory test, the needle electrode was modified to a golf-club type electrode to be atraumatically placed at the RW as shown in Fig. 3.9. This was originally conceived by Dr. Peter Gibson in the early 1990s. This golf club electrode along with eABR recording makes the objective promontory test safer and more reliable.

In situations where an individual shows no response or is expected to have no response to the sound, and where imaging tests show normal or abnormal anatomy, or where the individual has already been selected for either a CI or an ABI, as an advanced method, an intraoperative test of nerve functionality is currently used. This test includes placement of the cochlear test electrode into the scala tympani (ST) to provide electrical stimulation followed by the eABR recordings.

MED-EL recently developed its own auditory nerve test system (ANTS) as shown in Fig. 3.10. The intracochlear test electrode contains four electrode contacts.

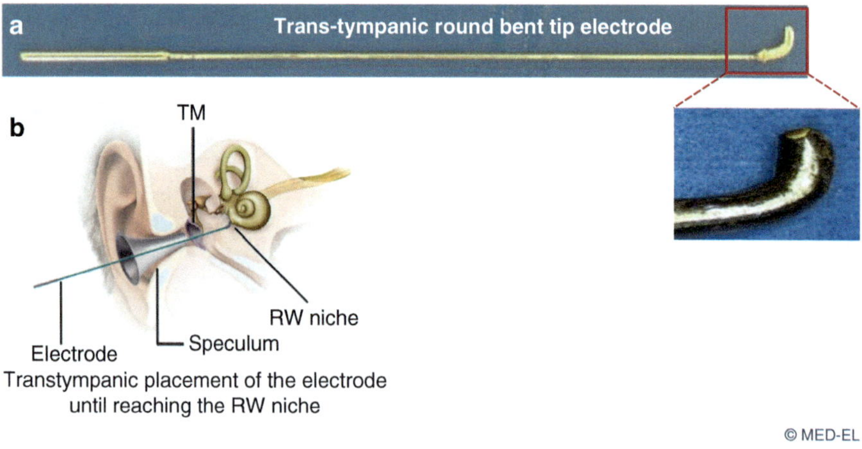


**Fig. 3.9** The “golf club” electrode used in the promontory stimulation (**a**), Illustration of the placement of golf club electrode on the RW niche through the external ear canal (**b**)

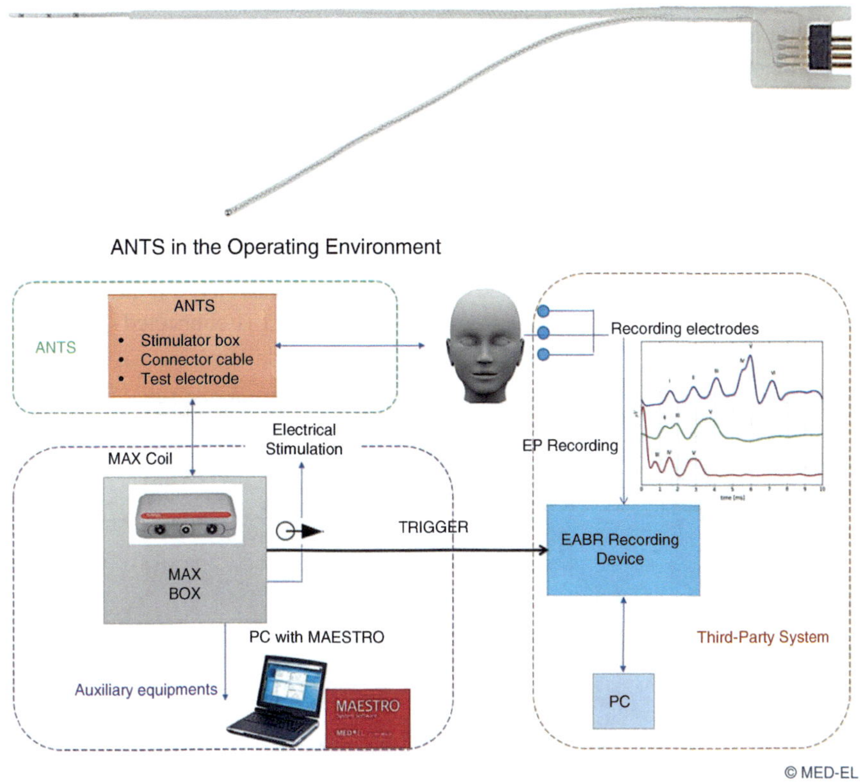


**Fig. 3.10** Intracochlear test electrode and test set-up in recording the eABR responses

It is intended to be inserted into the ST during surgery. The length of the electrode is 18 mm, as indicated by the marker ring. Three of the electrode contacts are placed directly into the ST, and the fourth electrode contact is placed under the temporalis muscle. Biphasic pulses are generated using the MAX interface and delivered to the cochlea. At the time of stimulation, the MAX interface triggers the evoked potential, and eABR response is obtained from the surface electrode as depicted in Fig. 3.10.

This tool is suitable for individuals with questionable functionality of the auditory nerve, individuals with a narrow internal auditory canal and patent or malformed cochlea, in tumor patients to monitor nerve functionality during tumor removal, or in situations where any other tests/methods failed to show CI candidacy, including the use of eABR with the objective promontory stimulation system.

## 3.7 Technological Evolution in the Audio Processor

The routine usage of the audio processor by the CI recipients depends much on the cosmetic look and the design of the audio processor offering wearing comfortableness. Since the beginning of the modern CI, the audio processor is one element of

CI that has advanced a lot over time both in terms of advanced features and the cosmetic look. This section will cover the technological evolution from the early experimental device till 2021.

The very first experimental CI device in the year 1979 had an audio processor in the size of a mini-suitcase as shown in Fig. 3.11. The CI user was made to try a number of speech coding strategies and stimulation field configurations for fundamental research on nerve stimulation.

The audio processor from the mini-size suitcase transformed into a much smaller-sized body-worn type in the year 1979 as shown in Fig. 3.12. The microphone that picks up the audio signal in the body-worn audio processor type is in a different position than the ear pinna. The external transmitter coil is connected to the hear

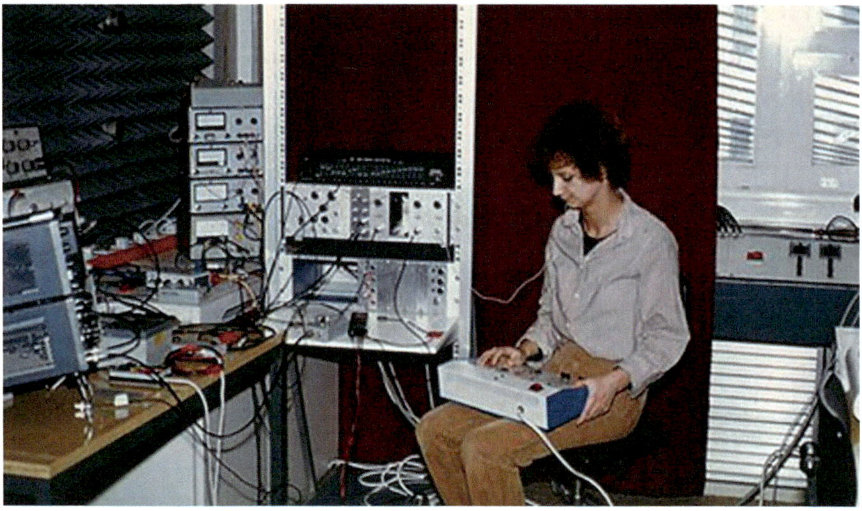

**Fig. 3.11** Mini-suitcase-sized investigational audio processor

**Fig. 3.12** First version of body-worn audio processor

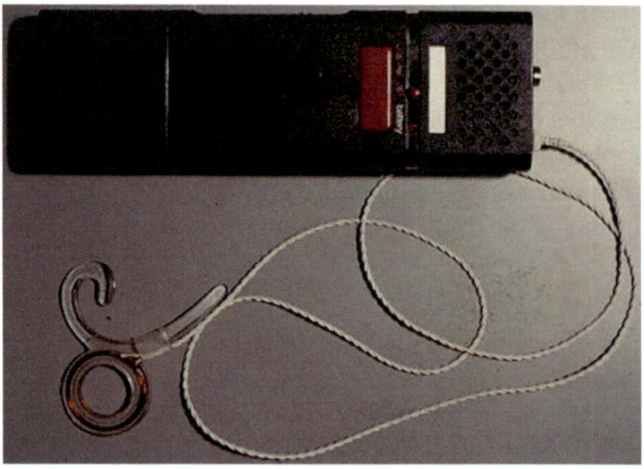

hook to be placed much closer to the implant to communicate with the implant stimulation via an inductive link. Still, it was an investigational device and it lacked a magnet in the external transmitter coil to have a focused inductive link with the implant stimulator.

The first commercial CI audio processor still had the body-worn type having the battery pack and the processing unit. The microphone was however brought to the ear level mimicking ear pinna as shown in Fig. 3.13. The external transmitter coil was designed with the magnet to have a focused inductive link with the implant stimulator. It took 10 years of research and development to bring an audio processor that was more practical to use. This audio processor used an AA battery as the signal processing strategy was high power consumption.

Soon after the development of the first commercial audio processor, the signal processing strategy was fine-tuned to consume less power. As a result, the AA batteries were replaced with zinc-air smaller size batteries allowing miniaturizing the whole audio processor into a much practical and comfortable behind-the-ear (BTE) processor (Fig. 3.14). In 1991, the world's first BTE processor was developed by

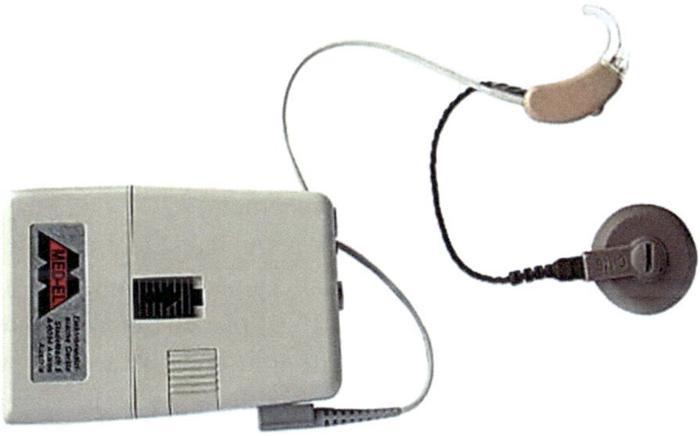

**Fig. 3.13** First commercially available body-worn type audio processor

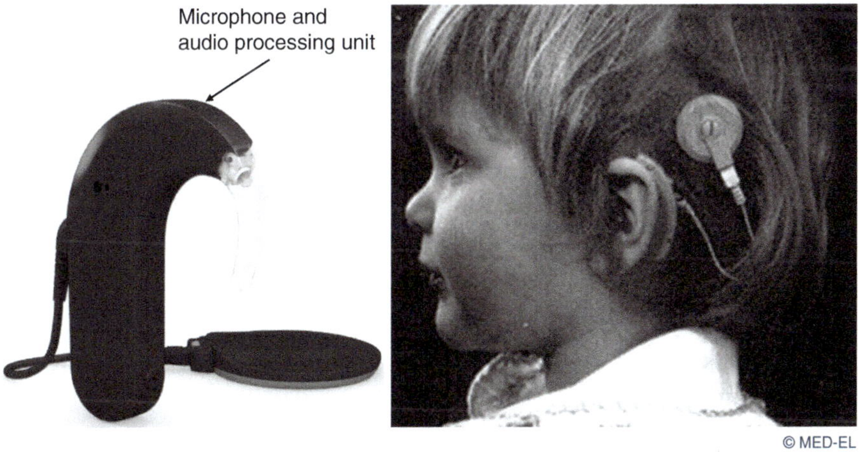


**Fig. 3.14** World's first BTE audio processor

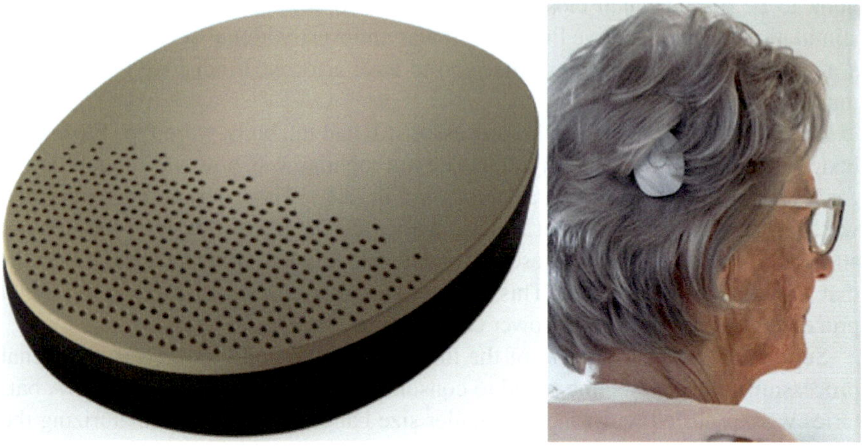

**Fig. 3.15** World's first single-unit audio processor

MED-EL and for the next 20 years, BTE processor was *state-of-the-art*. Dual microphone was one advancement within the BTE processor enhancing the CI recipient to better localize the sound source. Direct audio streaming from external audio devices like mobile phones and media players into the audio processor was a further advancement making the audio processor more practical and up-to-date with the general technological advancement.

Single-unit audio processor is the latest technological advancement in the audio processor that combined the battery pack, signal processing unit, and external transmitter coil as shown in Fig. 3.15. If placed under the hair, it will be highly invisible. In 2013, the world's first single-unit audio processor was introduced by MED-EL, and soon after Cochlear Corporation followed it. Within the single-unit audio processor, wireless charging of batteries, Bluetooth connectivity, water protection case was some of the technological advancements making it more practical to use. The microphone position is shifted from the ear level to more posterior but that did not have any significant effect on the hearing performances as per the published scientific reports [20].

## 3.8 Technological Evolution in Signal Processing Algorithms

Signal processing is a topic that is often seen as difficult to understand. It is the hidden component of the CI and it drives the whole CI system. In simple words, signal processing breaks the acoustic sound signal into frequency-specific smaller components and are converted into electrical signals to be delivered through the individual electrode contacts of the electrode array into the cochlea in a tonotopic pattern.

1991 was an important year in the field of CI, as Prof. Blake Wilson and his colleagues from the Research Triangle Institute in the USA developed the Continuous

Interleaved Sampling (CIS) strategy [21]. Before the introduction of the CIS strategy, it was mainly simultaneous multichannel analog stimulation was in use in which, all the stimulating channels in the electrode array were stimulated at the same time making it highly difficult for the brain to extract information from the stimulation impulse. Therefore, the simultaneous stimulation strategy did not succeed in bringing the complete acoustical input into the cochlea.

In the classic CIS sound coding strategy, the microphone signal is first processed through a pre-emphasis filter that attenuates strong components in the speech above 1.2 kHz and emphasizes signals that are below 1.2 kHz, as the speech information that is needed for normal conversation is around that frequency (stage 1). The output of the pre-emphasis is further passed through multiple channels of processing that include bandpass filters (BPF) (stage 2) for splitting the broadband signal into different frequency bands, rectification, as well as lowpass filtering for envelope extraction (stage 3). The envelope signals are compressed into the narrow dynamic range of electrically evoked hearing (stage 4). Trains of charge-balanced biphasic pulses are sequentially interleaved in time across electrodes to eliminate any overlap across channels, as shown in Fig. 3.16 by the red dotted vertical lines. The pulse amplitudes derive from the envelopes of the bandpass filter outputs and are directed to intracochlear electrodes (EL-1 to EL-12) (stage 5).

All the signal processing strategies that are available in today's CI system from various CI brands are based on the CIS strategy but with some modifications making it compatible with their implant electronics and the number of electrode channels.

The acoustic signal from the ear pinna reaches the middle ear and then to the inner ear where it is converted to electrical potentials by the Organ of Corti and

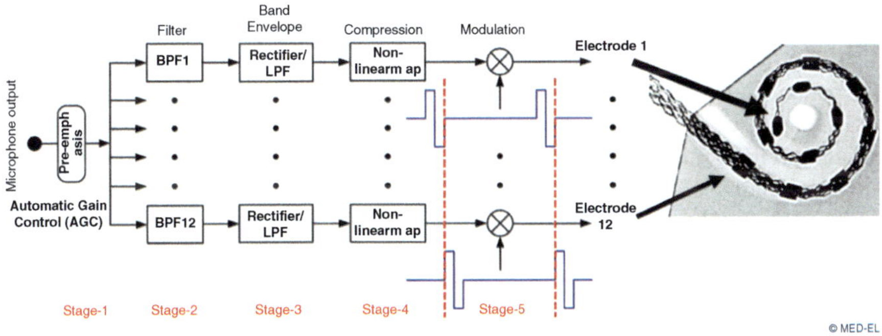


**Fig. 3.16** Block diagram of the CIS strategy. The pre-emphasis filter (pre-emp)/automatic gain control attenuates strong components in the speech above 1.2 kHz. This filter is followed by multiple channels of processing, with each channel including stages of bandpass filtering (BPF), envelope detection, compression, and modulation. The envelope detectors generally use a full-wave or half-wave rectifier (Rect.), followed by a lowpass filter (LPF). Carrier waveforms for two of the modulators are shown immediately below the two corresponding multiplier blocks (circle with an x mark). The outputs of the multipliers are directed to intracochlear electrodes (EL-1 to EL-12). The inset shows an X-ray image of the implanted electrode (in a cochlear model) to which the outputs of the speech processor are directed. Scheme created from Wilson et al. [21]

reaches the auditory cortex where it is perceived as sound. This whole process takes a few milliseconds and it is called traveling wave latency. Whereas with CI, the intracochlear electrode array bypasses the external and the middle ear and reaches the inner ear directly. This makes CI hearing to reach the auditory cortex bit earlier than natural hearing. The latest advancements in the signal processing strategy include a delay compensation feature [22] to adjust for the traveling wave latency making the CI hearing and natural hearing to reach the auditory cortex at the same time, if the patient is using CI in the ipsilateral side and having natural hearing on the contralateral side. This is very crucial in single-sided deafness (SSD) patients.

Conventional hearing aids (HA) take an even longer time to process the acoustic signal and to amplify it. If the patient uses HA on one ear and CI on the other ear, then the mismatch in time delay will be much higher. Bimodal Delay Compensation is a new feature in the signal processing strategy that allows unilateral CI users with HA on the contralateral ear to enjoy much-balanced hearing in both ears.

## 3.9 Future Technologies

Total Implantable Cochlear Implants (TICI) is one concept that carries a lot of potential and was first reported by Cochlear Corporation as a research device in the year 2008 [23]. However, it was never made commercially available till the time of writing this chapter in 2020. In 2020, MED-EL reported their first TICI device implanted in patients within Europe. If TICI is commercially available, the hearing loss will then be completely made invisible and it may not be far from achieving it soon.

The CI electrode array loaded with corticosteroids is another future concept that could come into commercial use soon as there are several research studies on the intracochlear application of corticosteroids by major CI manufacturers [24].

Robot-assisted CI surgery has already come into clinical practice and more than 20 patients are reported to have received a CI using the minimally invasive robot-assisted CI surgical approach [25]. While this robot-assisted surgical approach is limited to mastoid drilling to reach the cochlea, insertion of the electrode was still done manually. HEARO$^{TM}$ is the name of the robotic-assisted surgical system developed by a Swiss company named CAScination in collaboration with MED-EL. ROBOTOL is a robotic arm capable of inserting an electrode array into the cochlea and it was reported recently that few CI surgeries were performed applying ROBOTOL clinically [26]. This was developed by a French company named Collin Medical.

Further miniaturization of the whole CI would be another aim of every CI manufacturer, and something along this line can be expected in the near future. Complete reversing of hearing loss is the aim of some pharmaceutical companies. They are highly active in synthesizing novel molecules that could regenerate the neuronal elements that were either missing by birth or degenerated over time due to several medical conditions. Along this line, research on combining CI with stem cell were reported [27]. Predicting future hearing loss through gene testing is currently in clinical practice in some hospitals and Prof. Shin-Ichi Usami from Matsumoto University in Japan is one of the active pioneers in this topic [28].

Through a mutual collaboration between the clinicians and the CI companies, the future of CI is certainly going to be very exciting as there exists a healthy competition between the CI companies.

## 3.10 Conclusion

Cochlear Implantation field is unique in its way that there are only three manufacturers worldwide who have received food and drug administration (FDA) approval for their CI devices. Every segment of the CI device has advanced tremendously in the last 35 years and thanks to the strong scientific collaboration between the clinicians and the CI manufacturers that made it possible to bring out the innovation reaching the patients. Continuous engagement of the CI manufacturers with the clinicians is essential as the clinicians could provide valuable feedback on how to further improve the CI device as they are the ones who handle it during and after the CI surgery. While the CI technology has reached its maturity in terms of functionalities after 35 years of dedicated research efforts, the near future will focus on evaluating the patient-related factors that affect the uniformity in hearing performance across CI recipients.

## References


1. Yoshimura H, Moteki H, Nishio SY, Usami SI. Electric-acoustic stimulation with longer electrodes for potential deterioration in low-frequency hearing. Acta Otolaryngol. 2020;140(8):632–8.
2. Marx M, Mosnier I, Vincent C, Bonne NX, Bakhos D, Lescanne E, Flament J, Bernardeschi D, Sterkers O, Fraysse B, Lepage B, Godey B, Schmerber S, Uziel A, Mondain M, Venail F, Deguine O. Treatment choice in single-sided deafness and asymmetric hearing loss. A prospective, multi-center cohort study on 155 patients. Clin Otolaryngol. 2020;
3. Yang Y, Chen M, Zheng J, Hao J, Liu B, Liu W, Li B, Shao J, Liu H, Ni X, Zhang J. Clinical evaluation of cochlear implantation in children younger than 12 months of age. Pediatr Investig. 2020;4(2):99–103.
4. Minami SB, Yamamoto N, Hosoya M, Enomoto C, Kato H, Kaga K. Cochlear implantation in cases of inner ear malformation: a novel and simple grading, intracochlear EABR, and outcomes of hearing. Otol Neurotol. 2020;
5. Stöver T, Lenarz T. Biomaterials in cochlear implants. GMS Curr Top Otorhinolaryngol Head Neck Surg. 2009;8:Doc10. https://doi.org/10.3205/cto000062
6. Baumann U, Stöver T, Weißgerber T. Device profile of the MED-EL cochlear implant system for hearing loss: overview of its safety and efficacy. Expert Rev Med Devices. 2020;17(7):599–614.
7. https://cochlearimplanthelp.com/journey/choosing-a-cochlear-implant/cochlear-implant-problems/recalls/.
8. Srinivasan R, So CW, Amin N, Jaikaransingh D, D'Arco F, Nash R. A review of the safety of MRI in cochlear implant patients with retained magnets. Clin Radiol. 2019;74(12):972.e9–972.e16.

9. Young NM, Hoff SR, Ryan M. Impact of cochlear implant with diametric magnet on imaging access, safety, and clinical care. Laryngoscope. 2020;
10. Wagner F, Wimmer W, Leidolt L, Vischer M, Weder S, Wiest R, Mantokoudis G, Caversaccio MD. Significant artefact reduction at 1.5T and 3T MRI by the use of a cochlear implant with removable magnet: an experimental human cadaver study. PLoS One. 2015;10(7):e0132483.
11. Rebscher SJ, Hetherington A, Bonham B, Wardrop P, Whinney D, Leake PA. Considerations for design of future cochlear implant electrode arrays: electrode array stiffness, size, and depth of insertion. J Rehabil Res Dev. 2008;45(5):731–47.
12. Wardrop P, Whinney D, Rebscher SJ, Luxford W, Leake P. A temporal bone study of insertion trauma and intracochlear position of cochlear implant electrodes. II: Comparison of Spiral Clarion and HiFocus II electrodes. Hear Res. 2005;203(1–2):68–79.
13. Arnold W, Bredberg G, Gstöttner W, Helms J, Hildmann H, Kiratzidis T, Müller J, Ramsden RT, Roland P, Walterspiel JN. Meningitis following cochlear implantation: pathomechanisms, clinical symptoms, conservative and surgical treatments. ORL J Otorhinolaryngol Relat Spec. 2002;64(6):382–9.
14. Dhanasingh A, Jolly C. An overview of cochlear implant electrode array designs. Hear Res. 2017;356:93–103.
15. Dhanasingh A. Why pre-curved modiolar hugging electrodes only cover the basal turn of the cochlea and not beyond that? J Int Adv Otol. 2018;14(3):376–81.
16. Dhanasingh A. The rationale for FLEX (cochlear implant) electrode with varying array lengths. 2021. In press. https://doi.org/10.1016/j.wjorl.2019.12.003.
17. Kuo SC, Gibson WP. The role of the promontory stimulation test in cochlear implantation. Cochlear Implants Int. 2002;3(1):19–28.
18. Polak M, Eshraghi AA, Nehme O, et al. Evaluation of hearing and auditory nerve function by combining ABR, DPOAE and eABR tests into a single recording session. J NeurosciMethods. 2004;134:141–9.
19. House WF, Brackmann DE. Electrical promontory testing in differential diagnosis of sensorineural hearing impairment. Laryngoscope. 1974;84(12):2163–71.
20. Dazert S, Thomas JP, Büchner A, Müller J, Hempel JM, Löwenheim H, Mlynski R. Off the ear with no loss in speech understanding: comparing the RONDO and the OPUS 2 cochlear implant audio processors. Eur Arch Otorhinolaryngol. 2017;274(3):1391–5.
21. Wilson BS, Finley CC, Lawson DT, Wolford RD, Eddington DK, Rabinowitz WM. Better speech recognition with cochlear implants. Nature. 1991;352:236–8.
22. Zirn S, Arndt S, Aschendorff A, Wesarg T. Interaural stimulation timing in single sided deaf cochlear implant users. Hear Res. 2015;328:148–56.
23. Briggs RJ, Eder HC, Seligman PM, Cowan RS, Plant KL, Dalton J, Money DK, Patrick JF. Initial clinical experience with a totally implantable cochlear implant research device. Otol Neurotol. 2008;29(2):114–9.
24. Manrique-Huarte R, Zulueta-Santos C, Calavia D, Linera-Alperi MÁ, Gallego MA, Jolly C, Manrique M. Cochlear implantation with a dexamethasone eluting electrode array: functional and anatomical changes in non-human primates. Otol Neurotol. 2020;41(7):e812–22.
25. Caversaccio M, Wimmer W, Anso J, Mantokoudis G, Gerber N, Rathgeb C, Schneider D, Hermann J, Wagner F, Scheidegger O, Huth M, Anschuetz L, Kompis M, Williamson T, Bell B, Gavaghan K, Weber S. Robotic middle ear access for cochlear implantation: first in man. PLoS One. 2019;14(8):e0220543.
26. Daoudi H, Lahlou G, Torres R, Sterkers O, Lefeuvre V, Ferrary E, Mosnier I, Nguyen Y. Robot-assisted cochlear implant electrode array insertion in adults: a comparative study with manual insertion. Otol Neurotol. 2020;
27. Roemer A, Köhl U, Majdani O, Klöß S, Falk C, Haumann S, Lenarz T, Kral A, Warnecke A. Biohybrid cochlear implants in human neurosensory restoration. Stem Cell Res Ther. 2016;7(1):148.
28. Yoshimura H, Moteki H, Nishio SY, Miyajima H, Miyagawa M, Usami SI. Genetic testing has the potential to impact hearing preservation following cochlear implantation. Acta Otolaryngol. 2020;140(6):438–44.

# Surgical Anatomy and Imaging of the Temporal Bone with Cochlear Implant Imaging

4

Shrinivas Desai, Shraddha Sinhasan, and Ritu Kashikar

## 4.1 Introduction

Computed Tomography (CT) and Magnetic Resonance Imaging (MRI) have totally replaced pleuridirectional tomography in the evaluation of bony and soft-tissue abnormalities of the ear. Increasing the resolution of CT and MR provides detailed information about integrity of the auditory pathway. Preoperative imaging is instrumental in determining the feasibility and success of cochlear implantation and preventing complications. The increased spatial and contrast resolution of CT and MRI makes these modalities more accurate in diagnosing ear disorders. Imaging is in addition required for postoperative management of cochlear implant patients. Plain film studies are less expensive but these can be often inaccurate and warrant further detailed study. Conventional Angiography and DSA (digital subtraction angiography) can be useful for the evaluation of vascular tumours. Interventional angiography techniques can be used to treat vascular lesions of the temporal bone. Imaging is of utmost importance even intraoperatively, for image-guided surgeries using c-arm, routinely used for cochlear implantation.

**Supplementary Information** The online version contains supplementary material available at [https://doi.org/10.1007/978-981-19-0452-3_4].

S. Desai (✉)
Imaging and Interventional Radiology, Jaslok Hospital, Mumbai, Maharashtra, India

S. Sinhasan · R. Kashikar
Jaslok Hospital, Mumbai, Maharashtra, India


S. DeSaSouza (ed.), *Cochlear Implants*,
https://doi.org/10.1007/978-981-19-0452-3_4

## 4.2 Plain Radiography

Plain films give information regarding major ear structures and the degree of pneumatization of the mastoids. If the mastoids and petrous bone are markedly pneumatized, the middle ear and internal auditory canal cannot be well seen. Another limiting factor of plain X-rays is the superimposition of other skull shadows over the temporal bone.

There are five views routinely taken for rapid screening of the temporal bone:

1. Lateral (Schuller's) View
2. Transorbital View
3. Oblique Postero-anterior (Stenver's) View
4. Half Axial (Towne's) View
5. Axial or Submento-vertical View

### 4.2.1 Lateral (Schuller's) View (Fig. 4.1)

#### 4.2.1.1 Radiographic Technique

The head of the patient is placed in the true lateral position and the X-ray tube is angled 15 degrees caudally. The incident beam is centered 5 cm above the uppermost external auditory meatus.

Thus, Schuller's view is a lateral projection taken in such a way that it avoids overlap of the opposite mastoid process. Here, the mastoid is superimposed on the petrous and the internal auditory meatus is superimposed on the external auditory

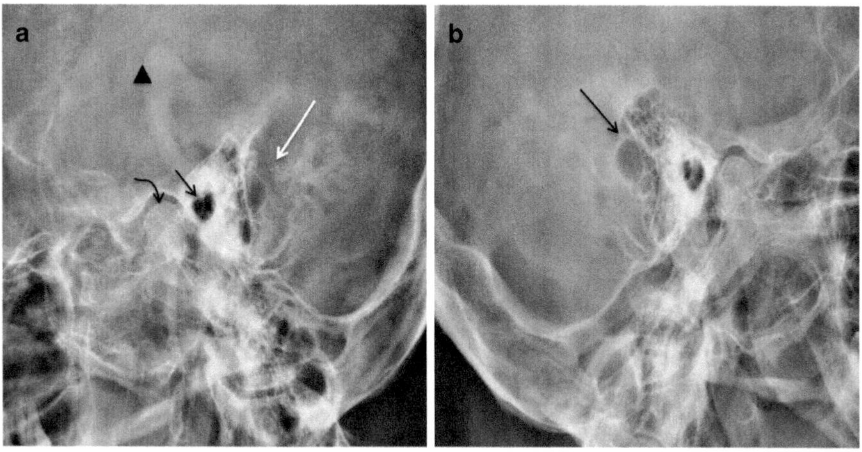


**Fig. 4.1** Schullers view. (**a**) The external auditory meatus appears as a small radiolucent area (short black arrow) with ossicles within. The right mastoid air cells are not well visualized likely to represent hypopneumatization or obliteration due to chronic mastoiditis (white arrow). Shadow of pinna (arrowhead) (**b**) normal mastoid air cells (long black arrow)

meatus. The pneumatization of the mastoid, the position of the lateral sinus, the tegmen tympani, the attic, aditus and mastoid antrum are well visualized.

#### 4.2.1.2 Surgeon's Viewpoint

On this view, extensive erosion of the attico-antral region and of the bony bridge formed by the outer attic wall can be well appreciated. Therefore, the surgeon can assess how much room there is between the external auditory meatus and the middle fossa dura above and the lateral sinus behind, when he makes an approach to the mastoid antrum.

### 4.2.2 Transorbital View (Fig. 4.2)

#### 4.2.2.1 Radiographic Technique

This can be taken with the patient supine or prone. A prone position is preferred to avoid radiation to the eyes. The orbito-meatal line is kept at right angles to the film. The tube is angled 5–10 degrees caudally, centering between the orbits. The internal auditory meati are best seen on this In view of as the petrous pyramids are projected through the orbits.

### 4.2.3 Oblique Postero-anterior View (Stenver's Projection) (Fig. 4.3)

#### 4.2.3.1 Radiographic Technique

The patient lies prone facing the film. The radiographic baseline is horizontal and the sagittal plane of the skull is rotated through 35 degrees and titled 15 degrees away from the side to be examined. The incident ray is inclined at an angle of 12 degrees cranially and is centered on a point 2 cm medial to the mastoid tip.

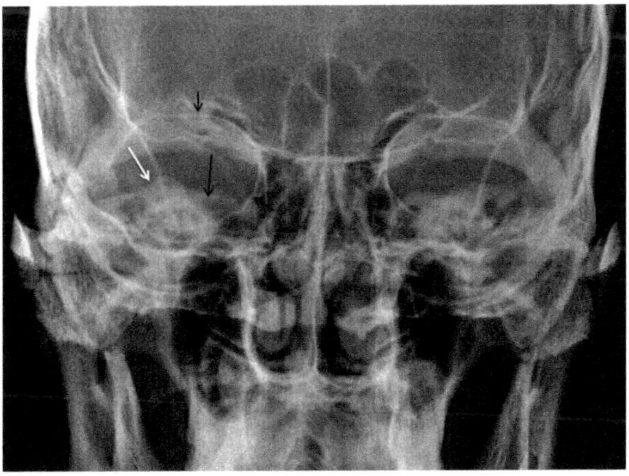

**Fig. 4.2** Transorbital view. The petrous temporal bone (white arrow) is visualized through the orbit (short black arrows), lucent tubular structure is the internal acoustic meatus (black arrow)

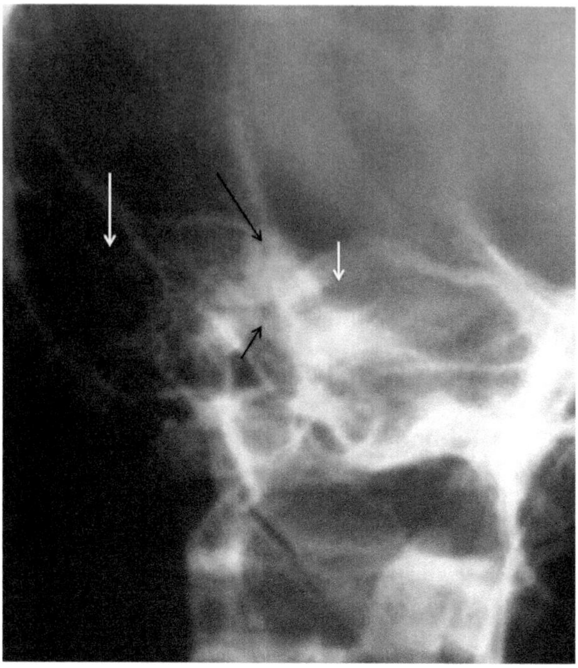

**Fig. 4.3** Stenvers view. The internal acoustic meatus (short white arrow), the vestibule of cochlea (short black arrow), the superior semicircular canal (black arrow) and the mastoid air cells (white arrow) are well visualized on the view

The whole length of the petrous bone is seen on this view as it is placed parallel to the X-ray films.

The petrous tip, internal auditory meatus and canal, the bony labyrinth comprising of the semicircular canals, vestibule and cochlea, and middle ear cleft are well demonstrated in this view.

#### 4.2.3.2 Surgeon's Viewpoint

The presence of erosion of the petrous tip and widening of the internal auditory meatus is looked for in this view. If a cholesteatoma is present, bony erosion is most often seen.

### 4.2.4 Half Axial (Towne's) View (Fig. 4.4)

#### 4.2.4.1 Radiographic Technique

The classical Towne's projection is taken in the supine position. But, this delivers a high radiation dose to the eyes; hence, the reversed Towne's view is done whenever possible.

In the classical Towne's projection, the supine patient is positioned in such a way that the sagittal plane is perpendicular to the table top. The canthomeatal line is also perpendicular to the table top. The incident ray is angled 30 degrees towards the feet centered at the hairline. In the reversed Towne's view with the patient prone, the tube is angled 30 degrees towards the head.

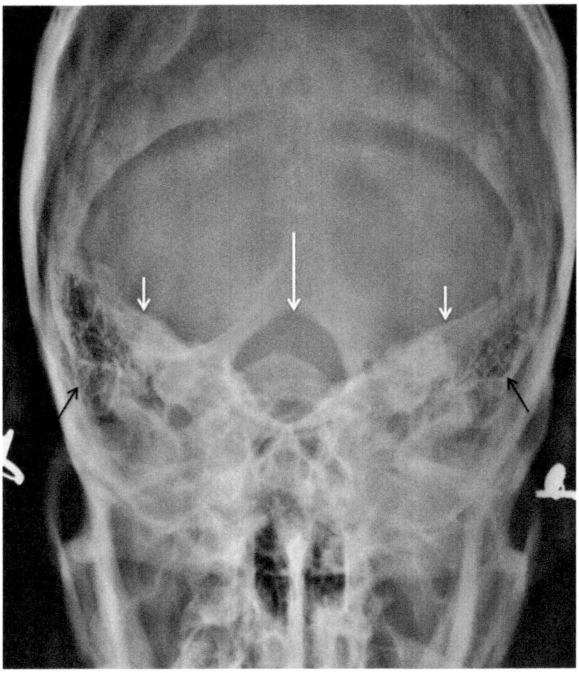

**Fig. 4.4** Towne's view. The foramen magnum (white arrow), the petrous ridge (short white arrows) and the mastoid air cells (short black arrows) are seen in this view

In this view, both petrous ridges, occipital bone, foramen magnum, and dorsum sellae are well demonstrated.

#### 4.2.4.2 Surgeon's Viewpoint

An enlarged attic and antrum can be well identified on this view. Erosion of the lateral spur or scutum by a cholesteatoma is also well seen.

### 4.2.5 Axial or Submento-vertical View (Fig. 4.5)

#### 4.2.5.1 Radiographic Technique

This view is very important and plain studies are incomplete if this is not obtained. Here, the baseline is parallel to the film and the incident beam is centered at a point midway between the angles of the mandible. The middle ear structures, the external and internal auditory meatus, and the eustachian canal are visualized on this view.

#### 4.2.5.2 Surgeon's Viewpoint

The air-containing cavity of the middle ear is well assessed in this view. Air forms a very good contrast which enables clear visualization of the head of the malleus, body of the incus, and the cartilage space of the incudo-malleolar joint. Any abnormality affecting the ossicles is thereby evaluated.

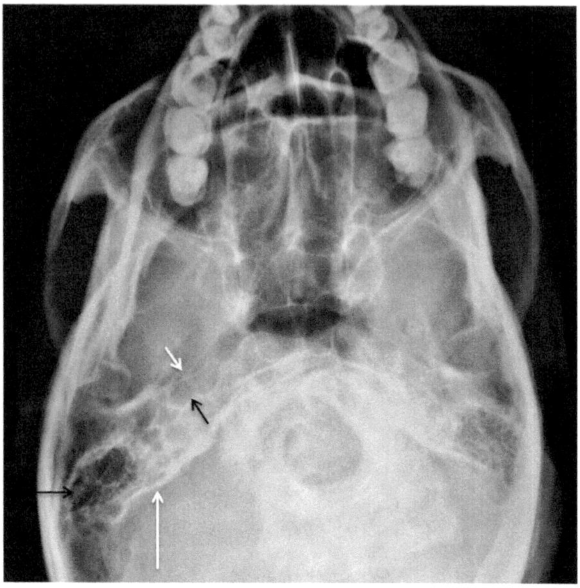

**Fig. 4.5** Axial (base of skull) view. The petrous temporal bone (white arrow) is well visualized. Eustachian tube is seen as linear air filled lucency (short white arrow). The carotid canal (short black arrow) is seen posterior to it. Mastoid air cells (black arrow) are seen laterally

## 4.3 Conventional Tomography (CT)

Before the advent of high-resolution thin-section CT scans, polytomography was used to obtain diagnostic information on the bony portions of the temporal bone. CT added a new dimension by allowing visualization of bony structures, as well as soft tissue structures within and adjacent to the temporal bone. The only advantage conventional tomography has over CT is the ease of obtaining sagittal images and also the cost factor. However, the resolution is far inferior to CT [1].

## 4.4 Computed Tomography (CT) Technique

### 4.4.1 Two (2-D) Dimensional CT (Figs. 4.6 and 4.7)

A high-resolution CT of the temporal bone is obtained. Axial scanning is performed in planes parallel to the infraorbitomeatal line. The axial images are obtained from the superior aspect of petrous bone up to the inferior top of the mastoid bone. The coronal images are obtained from the anterior margin of petrous apex to the posterior margin of mastoid bone. The images are then reconstructed in both the axial and coronal planes, with section thickness as small as 0.3 mm, matrix size of 512 × 512, and a small separate field of view for right and left temporal bones. Thus, the images obtained are of high quality to evaluate abnormalities of small middle ear and inner ear structures [2].

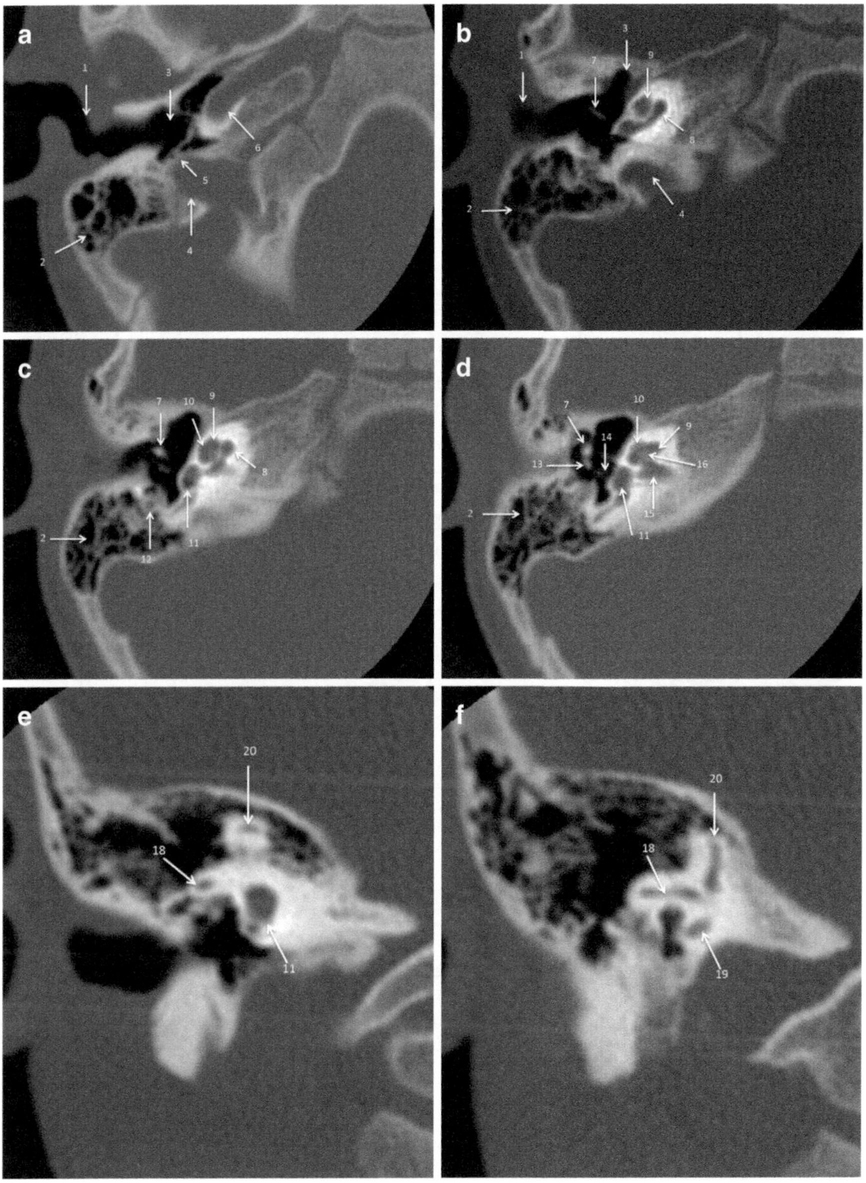


**Fig. 4.6** Axial (inferior to superior) HRCT cuts of right temporal bone. (1) EAC, (2) Mastoid, (3) Middle Ear, (4) Jugular Bulb, (5) Sinus plate, (6) Carotid canal, (7) Malleus, (8) Basal turn of cochlea, (9) Middle turn of cochlea, (10) Apical turn of cochlea, (11) Vestibule, (12) Facial Nerve, (13) Incus, (14) Stapes, (15) IAC, (16) Modiolus, (17) Geniculate Ganglion, (18) Horizontal Semicircular canal, (19) Posterior Semicircular canal, (20) Superior Semicircular canal, (21) Aditus to Antrum, (22) Antrum, (23) Oval Window, (24) Round Window Niche, (25) Aditus to antrum, (26) Antrum

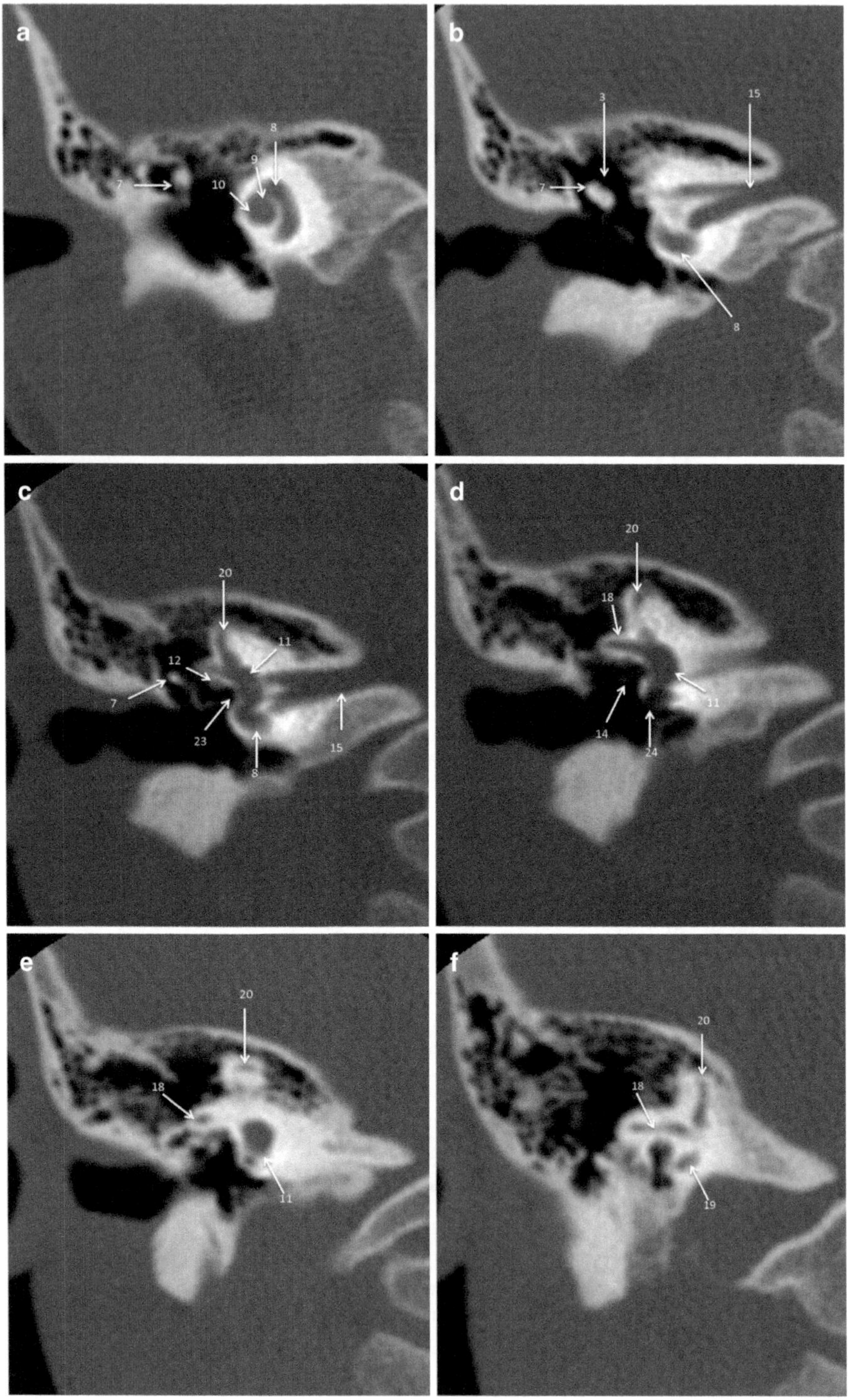


**Fig. 4.7** Coronal (anterior to posterior) HRCT cuts of right temporal bone. See Fig. 4.6 for (1)–(26)

Bone algorithm is used which gives fine details of the complex ear structures. Image quality is also improved by using a low milliampere and a longer scanning time period. Intravenous contrast is given when vascular lesions, soft tissue abnormalities, and intracranial involvement is suspected. However, for primary bone and air space pathology, contrast enhancement is usually not required.

### 4.4.2 Three-Dimensional (3-D) CT (Fig. 4.8)

Three-dimensional reconstruction of CT images of the temporal bone has an important role to play especially for the reconstruction of bony structures. Its most useful application is in imaging congenital abnormalities and trauma as well as some base of the skull and facial tumours.

In congenital bony anomalies, it aids in planning the surgical correction of these anomalies. It essentially helps in the pre-operative and post-operative assessment rather than diagnosis. The sites and sizes of osteotomies and implants can be planned and hands-on manipulation of 3-D images can be done. Surgical simulation can be also performed directly on the computer. This benefits the surgeon to predict the likely outcome of surgery and decreases the intraoperative time.

For injuries to the temporal bone, the 3-D images can be rotated through 360°; hence, the fractures can be viewed from any angle. The degree of displacement of the fracture fragments is well visualized. However, most of the useful information

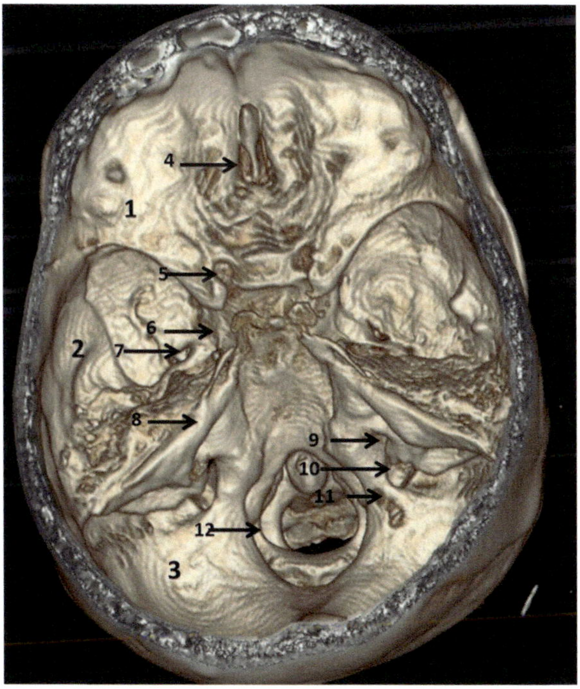


**Fig. 4.8** 3D anatomy base of skull. (1) Anterior cranial fossa, (2) Middle cranial fossa, (3) Posterior cranial fossa, (4) Cribriform plate, (5) Optic canal, (6) Carotid Canal, (7) Foramen Ovale, (8) Petrous bone, (9) Internal Acoustic Meatus, (10) Jugular Foramen, (11) Hypoglossal canal, (12) Foramen Magnum

is best derived from direct axial, coronal, or sagittal sections. Severely comminuted fractures are more easily assessed with 3-D images. Subtle rotational elements of the fracture fragments may only be appreciated on 3-D images. The jugular fossa, hypoglossal canal, and the foramen magnum are also easily appreciated (Fig. 4.8) Therefore, it sometimes does aid in the pre-operative assessment of trauma patients [3–5].

### 4.4.3 Temporal Bone

The four major portions of the temporal bone are petrous, tympanic, mastoid and squamous.

The petrous bone contains the inner ear. The tympanic portion surrounds the tympanic membrane and forms the anteroinferior wall of the external auditory canal. The mastoid portion contributes to the posterior external canal, the posterior middle ear and includes the mastoid antrum and sinus. The squamous portion forms part of the lateral skull.

On CT scan, bony structures are seen as high density, CSF as low density and air spaces appear black. The brain and vascular structures are intermediate in density. Details of the otic capsule contents cannot be well evaluated by CT scans.

### 4.4.4 Inner Ear

#### 4.4.4.1 The Internal Auditory Canal

The internal auditory canal is funnel-shaped and is oriented in the coronal plane as against the 45° off-coronal plane of the petrous pyramid. Its medial opening is the porus acousticus. Laterally, the canal ends at the vestibule. These canals are normally symmetrical. An asymmetry of greater than 2 mm is usually abnormal.

The internal auditory canal is the passageway that transmits the seventh and the eighth nerves from the pontomedullary junction to the inner ear. On coronals, the entire extent of the canal can be seen with the central bony crista falciformis dividing the canal into superior and inferior portions. The superior portion houses the facial and the superior vestibular nerve. The inferior portion houses the cochlear nerve and the inferior vestibular nerve. The individual nerves are well identified on pneumocisternomeatography.

#### 4.4.4.2 The Vestibule

The vestibule is seen as an oval lucency within the dense otic capsule at the level of the internal auditory canal.

#### 4.4.4.3 The Vestibular Aqueduct

It is the bony canal for the endolymphatic duct and is seen as a thin hockey stick-shaped lucency. The duct begins at the common crus of the posterior and superior semicircular canals and ends at the endolymphatic fossa in the epidural space on the posterior margin of the petrous pyramid.

#### 4.4.4.4 The Oval Window

On axial and coronal CT sections, the oval window is seen as a bony defect of the lateral portion of the vestibule along the medial margin of the middle ear.

#### 4.4.4.5 The Cochlea

The cochlea is anteroinferior to the semicircular canals. It has two and a half turns to two three-fourth turns. The cochlear basal turn forms the cochlear promontory which is seen as a smooth bony prominence along the medial wall of the middle ear cavity on both axial and coronal sections. The middle and apical turns appear as a comma-shaped lucency in the dense cortical bone on the coronal sections at the anterior tympanic level.

#### 4.4.4.6 The Cochlear Aqueduct

It lies below and is parallel to the internal auditory canal. Its medial funnel-shaped opening is seen as a triangular lucency at the posteromedial surface of the petrous pyramid facing the cerebellopontine angle. When this opening is large, it may mimic the internal auditory canal.

#### 4.4.4.7 The Round Window (The Fenestra Cochlea)

This is a membrane-covered opening in the cochlear basal turn. The apex of the cochlear aqueduct points towards the round window. On axial sections, the round window is identified as an air-containing niche in the posterior middle ear cavity that extends towards the basal turn of the cochlea. On the coronal CT sections, the round window is seen just posterior to the plane of the oval window.

#### 4.4.4.8 The Semicircular Canals

The lateral semicircular canal is parallel to the axial CT sections and is seen as a semicircular lucency medial to the middle ear cavity above the horizontal portion of the facial canal. On coronal sections, the ampulla of the lateral semicircular canal is seen as a horizontal lucency connecting the vestibule. The convex portion of the canal is seen end-on.

The posterior semicircular canal is parallel to the posterior petrous pyramid. On axial sections at the internal auditory canal level, the ampulla and the adjacent lower convexity of the posterior semicircular canal is visualized as a linear lucency. At the level of the lateral semicircular canal, the posterior semicircular canal is seen end-on.

The superior semicircular canal is perpendicular to the petrous pyramid. On axial sections, the limbs of the canal are seen end-on above the level of the lateral semicircular canal as anterior and posterior corticated rounded lucencies. On a higher axial section, the convexity of the superior semicircular canal is seen as a curvilinear lucency that corresponds to the arcuate eminence.

The complex cavity within the petrous temporal bone housing these structures is called the osseous labyrinth and the membranous sacs, ducts and organs within the osseous portion are called the membranous labyrinth. The osseous labyrinth is seen as a markedly hyperdense structure surrounding the lucent membranous labyrinth [3, 4, 6].

## 4.4.5 Middle Ear (Tympanum)

The middle ear is the air-containing space that lies between the tympanic membrane and the labyrinth.

Vertically, from below upwards, the middle ear cavity is divided into:

- Hypotympanum
- Mesotympanum
- Epitympanum (attic)

The *hypotympanum* is the most inferior portion of the tympanic cavity and connects anteromedially with the bony opening of the eustachian canal. The eustachian canal is inferior and parallel to the semicanal of the tensor tympani muscle.

The *mesotympanum* is the central portion of the tympanic cavity and is bordered laterally by the scutum and the tympanic membrane and medially by the otic capsule. The scutum or spur is a bony crest separating the external auditory canal from the epitympanic space. It is well seen in coronal sections. Prussak's space is located medial to the scutum and lateral to the malleolar neck and is well seen on coronal sections.

The *epitympanum (attic)* forms the superior portion of the middle ear cavity.

The epitympanum and the mesotympanum communicate at the tympanic isthmus, which is at the level of the tensor tympani tendon and stapes. This narrow tympanic passageway is best seen on coronal sections.

The *protympanum* is the anterior triangular portion of the tympanic cavity lateral and adjacent to the carotid canal.

The *postympanum* is the posterior portion of the tympanic cavity that contains the facial recess laterally and sinus tympani medially.

### 4.4.5.1 Walls of the Middle Ear

The bony roof (tegmen) and the floor of the middle ear cavity are well seen on the coronal sections.

The medial wall comprising the cochlear promontory, oval and round windows, cochleariform process, tensor tympani tendon, pyramidal eminence, stapedial tendon and lateral semicircular canal are visualized on axial and coronal sections.

The lateral wall is formed mainly by the thin tympanic membrane (which is sometimes visible on axial CT sections) and partly by the squamous temporal bone.

The anterior or the carotid wall is formed cranio-caudally by the opening of the canal for the tensor tympani, the opening of the eustachian tube and thin plate of bone forming the posterior wall of the carotid canal. The semicanal of the tensor tympani muscle is superior and parallel to the eustachian tube. The opening of the eustachian tube is triangular with the apex extending parallel to the carotid canal. This tube connects the hypotympanum to the nasopharynx and occasionally may contain air.

The posterior or the mastoid wall consists of from above downwards, aditus ad antrum, fossa incudis and the pyramid. The air-filled aditus ad antrum is the narrow communication between the epitympanum and the mastoid sinus antrum [6].

#### 4.4.5.2 Contents of the Middle Ear

- The Ear Ossicles
- Stapedius muscle
- Tensor tympani muscle
- Chorda tympani nerve

**The Ossicles**

The malleus, incus and stapes are normally visualized on axial and coronal sections within the air-filled middle ear cavity as high-density structures. The inherent air-bone contrast on C.T. enables the ossicles to be differentiated from one another.

The inferior axial sections show the handle of the malleus as a linear structure directed backwards along the tympanic membrane. On anterior coronal sections, the handle is seen in its entirely paralleling the tympanic membrane. The neck of the malleus is located between the handle and the head and is seen as an end-on structure on axial sections. A further cranial axial section reveals the head as a rounded structure articulating with the triangular body of the incus giving the appearance of an "ice-cream cone". This ossicular mass is equidistant from the medial and lateral walls of the epitympanum. The long process of the incus is seen medial and parallel to the handle of the malleus on axial and coronal sections. The short process of the incus is directed backwards and is seen to lie below the aditus. In coronal sections, the body of the incus and the incudo-stapedial joint are seen as an L-shaped configuration. The crura of the stapes may occasionally be seen forming an arch over the oval window on high-resolution axial CT scans at the epitympanic internal auditory canal level.

**Tensor Tympani Muscle**

The tensor tympani is seen on coronal sections as a linear soft tissue extending from the malleolar neck to the processus cochleariformis.

**Stapedius Muscle**

The Stapedius tendon is attached to the pyramidal eminence and inserts on the posterior crus of the stapes.

### 4.4.6 External Ear

The medial two-thirds of the external auditory canal is bony. Its anterior and posterior walls have dense sharp cortical margins without soft tissue covering. The anterior margin of the bony external auditory canal forms the posterior lip of the temporomandibular joint. The lateral one-third of the external auditory canal is cartilaginous and is identified as a soft tissue density structure that is surrounded by low-density fat. The tympanic membrane is located at the medial end of the external auditory canal and may occasionally be seen as a thin soft tissue density structure angling medially from top to bottom and laterally from front to back. Its insertion is seen on the drum spur superiorly and the limbus inferiorly.

The tympanic portion of the temporal bone surrounds the tympanic membrane and forms the anteroinferior wall of the external auditory canal. The mastoid portion contributes to the posterior wall of the external auditory canal [6].

#### 4.4.6.1 The Carotid Canal and Jugular Foramen and Fossa

The carotid canal lies just anterior to the jugular fossa, both forming a snowman-like configuration. The carotid canal is usually smaller than the jugular fossa. Both demonstrate sharp cortical margins. Inferiorly a small bony spine separating the two is seen as a high attenuation density. The roof of the jugular fossa is formed by the floor of the tympanic cavity. The jugular foramen is bounded auteriorly by the temporal bone and posteriorly by occipital bone by the temporal bone and posteriorly by the occipital bone. The jugular bulbs may often be asymmetric.

#### 4.4.6.2 The Facial Nerve and Canal Anatomy (Fig. 4.9)

In axial sections, the labyrinthine portion of the facial canal is seen as a linear lucency as the nerve exits from the internal auditory canal. The geniculate ganglion is located anteriorly and is seen as an inverted V surrounded by the dense bone of the otic capsule. The horizontal portion of the facial nerve is sometimes seen as partial anteroposterior linear lucencies in the medial wall of the tympanic cavity directly inferior to the lateral semicircular canal. The posterior genu is formed near the sinus tympani and the pyramidal eminence. The descending portion is seen as a well corticated circular lucency in the temporal bone posterior to the external auditory canal. The nerve then exits from the mastoid portion of the temporal bone via the fat-filled stylomastoid foramen. On coronal sections, this descending segment of the facial nerve is well identified as a sharply marginated supero-inferior linear lucency running below the lateral semicircular canal [3, 6].

#### 4.4.6.3 The Vestibulocochlear Nerves and Their Central Pathways (Fig. 4.10)

CT pneumocisternomeatography is the technique that was used in the earlier days to study the acoustic pathway. With this technique, the introduced air helps in identifying the individual nerves as linear soft tissue structures in the hypodense

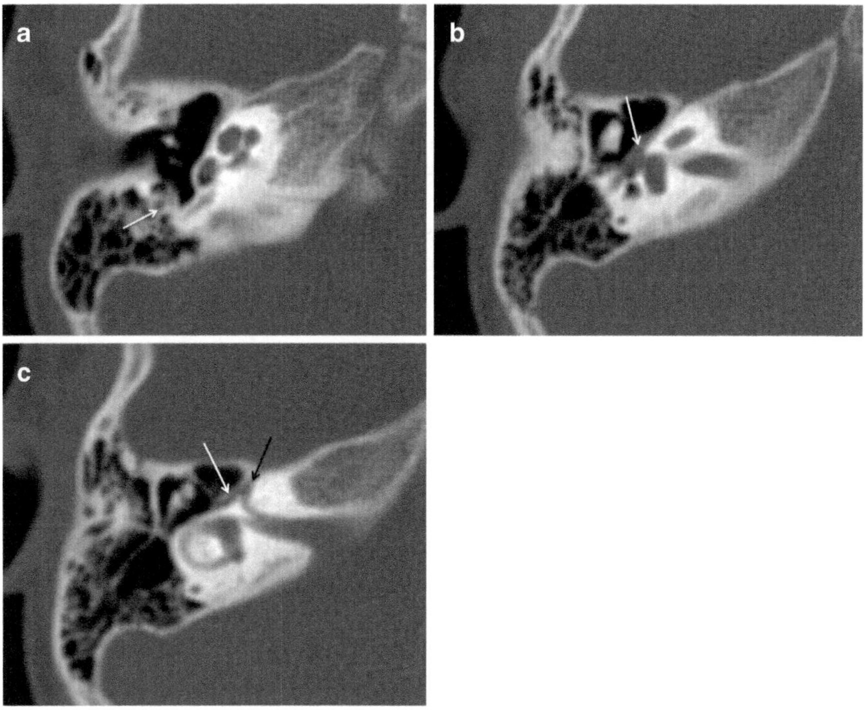


**Fig. 4.9** (**a**–**c**) Facial nerve course. Axial HRCT of right temporal bone (inferior to superior). The facial nerve course in middle ear with geniculate ganglion (black arrow in **c**), horizontal segment along roof of middle ear (white arrow in **c** and **b**) and vertical course in mastoid within the facial canal (white arrow in **a**) are well demonstrated on HRCT temporal bone

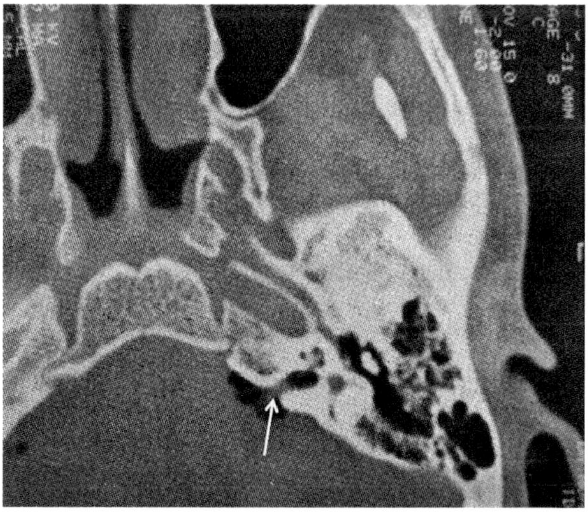

**Fig. 4.10** Air meatography delineating the seventh and eighth nerves in the internal auditory meatii

subarachnoid space and in the internal auditory canal. The cochlear and the vestibular portions of the acoustic nerve join into a common trunk that is seen to enter the internal auditory canal with the facial nerve. If a section is taken at the upper part of the internal auditory canal, a distinct soft tissue density bulge is seen at the lateral end of the internal auditory canal. This bulge is situated on the trunk of the eighth nerve and most likely represents the vestibular ganglion (Scarpa's ganglion).

From the internal auditory canal, these nerves proceed separately towards the brainstem through the subarachnoid space. The acoustic nerve travels behind the facial nerve and in front of the inferior cerebellar peduncle.

The cochlear portion terminates on the restiform body located on the inferior cerebellar peduncle. On CT, the isodense restiform bodies are seen on either side of the fourth ventricle. Most of the fibres of the vestibular nerve end at the pontomedullary junction, though some proceed to the flocculus and the nodule along the inferior cerebellar peduncle. On coronal and axial CT sections, the flocculus is seen as a rounded structure in the cerebellopontine angle that is isodense or slightly hypodense. It is situated posterior to the seventh and eighth nerves and the internal auditory canal and lateral to the choroid plexus of the lateral recess of the fourth ventricle. Part of the anterior inferior cerebellar artery is seen adjacent to the flocculus. On post-contrast CT, the flocculus enhances slightly because of the choroid plexus and anterior inferior cerebellar artery. The nodule is seen posterior to the fourth ventricle in a section taken through the inferior part of the fourth ventricle. The inferior colliculi of the midbrain are primary auditory centers. In a CT section taken at the level of the inferior colliculi, the approximate location of the nucleus where the nerve fibres from the lateral lemniscus terminate is seen. The lateral lemniscus also forms part of the central acoustic pathway [7].

With CT pneumocisternomeatography, not only the seventh and eighth but the fifth, sixth, ninth, and tenth nerves can also be well visualized.

Contrast cisternomeatography with Pantopaque was also a technique performed in the past. The contrast was used to opacify the internal auditory meatii with the seventh and eighth nerve bundles appearing as linear filling defects. Currently, CT cisternography plays an important role in CSF leaks [8]. Accurate localization of the leakage site is essential for treatment planning. Safer non-ionic water-soluble contrast agents are being used for the procedure with a very low incidence of side effects. Similarly, MR cisternography with or without contrast may also be performed by taking 3D CISS sequences.

#### 4.4.6.4 Few Illustrative Diagrams of Anatomy of Ear (Fig. 4.11)

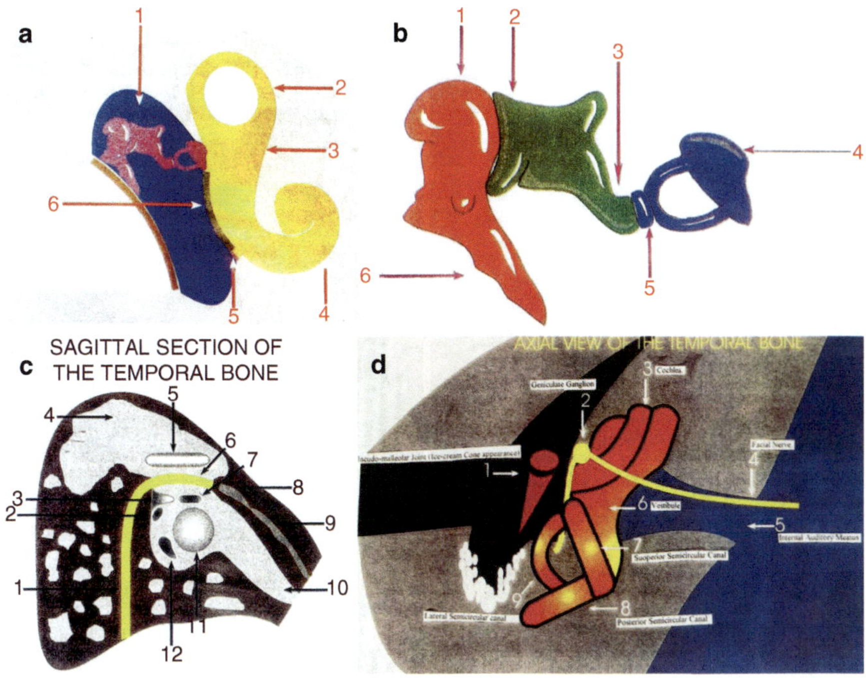


**Fig. 4.11** (**a**): (1) Middle ear cavity, (2) Semi-circular canals, (3) Vestibule, (4) Cochlea, (5) Round window, (6) Promontory. (**b**): (1) Head of Malleus, (2) Body of Incus, (3) Long Process of Stapes, (4) Footplate of Stapes, (5) Head of Stapes, (6) Long Process of Malleus. (**c**): (1) Facial Nerve (vertical portion), (2) Pyramid, (3) Sinus Tympani, (4) Mastoi Antrum, (5) Lateral Semicircular Canal, (6) Facial Nerve (horizontal portion), (7) Oval Window, (8) Processus Cochleariformis, (9) Canal for Tensor Tympani, (10) Eustachian tube, (11) Promontory, (12) Round Window. (**d**) Labelled

## 4.5 Magnetic Resonance Imaging (MRI) (Figs. 4.12 and 4.13; Videos 4.1 and 4.2)

### 4.5.1 MRI Technique

Latest MRI scanners produce beautiful images of the inner ear with very high resolution. A 1.5- or 3-T MR imaging system may be used with section thickness as small as 0.4 mm and small field of view. Sedation is generally required for a paediatric group of patients.

A thin-section gradient-echo sequence that is heavily T2 weighted aids in evaluating fluid-filled spaces of the membranous labyrinth and the eighth cranial nerve. These images (3D-CISS) are obtained to visualize the seventh-eighth nerve complex and internal ear structures. These can be reformatted into sagittal and coronal images as per requirement (Fig. 4.13; Videos 4.1 and 4.2). The cerebellopontine

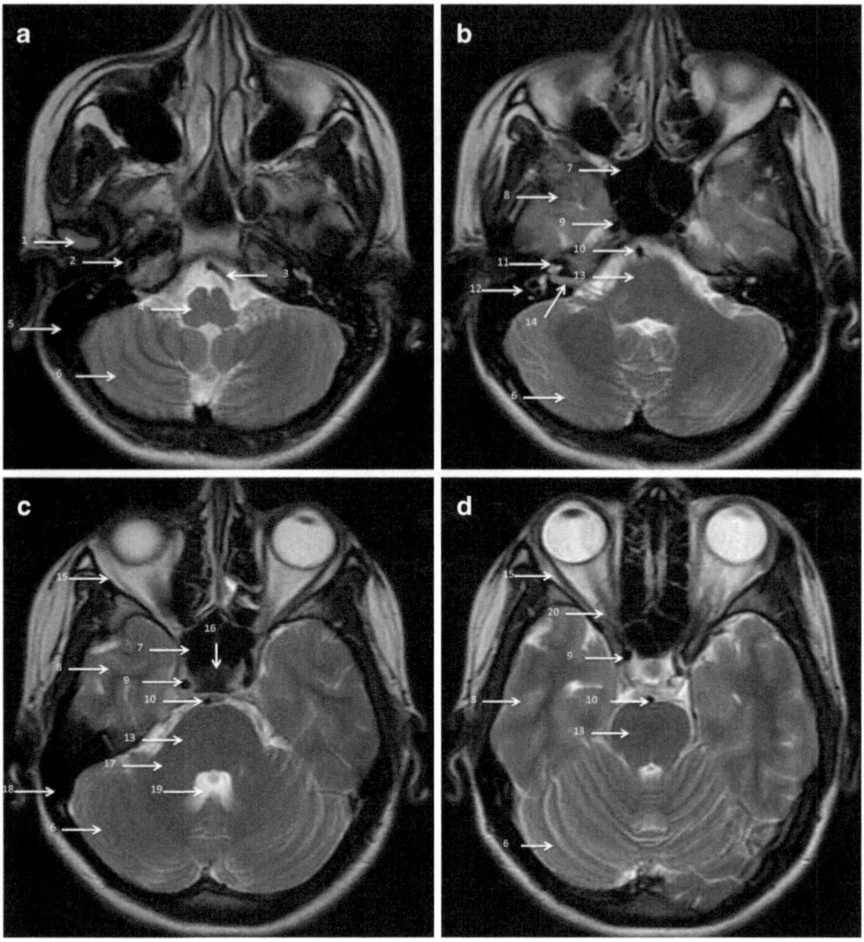


**Fig. 4.12** MRI brain axial anatomy (T2W images). (1) Mandibular condyle, (2) Carotid Canal, (3) V4 segment of left bertebral artery, (4) Medulla, (5) Mastoid, (6) Cerebellum, (7) Sphenoid sinus, (8) Temporal lobe, (9) Carotid artery, cavernous segment, (10) Basilar Artery, (11) Cochlea, (12) Semicircular canals, (13) Pons, (14) IAC containing seventh–eighth nerve complex, (15) Orbit, (16) Pituitary, (17) Middle Cerebellar peduncle, (18) Sigmoid sinus, (19) Fourth ventricle, (20) Optic Nerve, (21) Frontal lobe, (22) MCA, (23) Optic Chiasm, (24) Hippocampus, (25) Midbrain, (26) Occipital lobe, (27) ACA, (28) Frontal horn of right lateral ventricle, (29) Head of caudate nucleus, (30) Internal capsule, (31) Putamen, (32) Globus Pallidus, (33) Parietal lobe, (34) Occipital lobe, (35) Rostrum of corpus callosum, (36) Thalamus, (37) Splenium of Corpus Callosum, (38) Frontal white matter, (39) Centrum Semiovale, (40) Parietal white matter, (41) Intercerebral falx, (42) Superior Sagittal Sinus

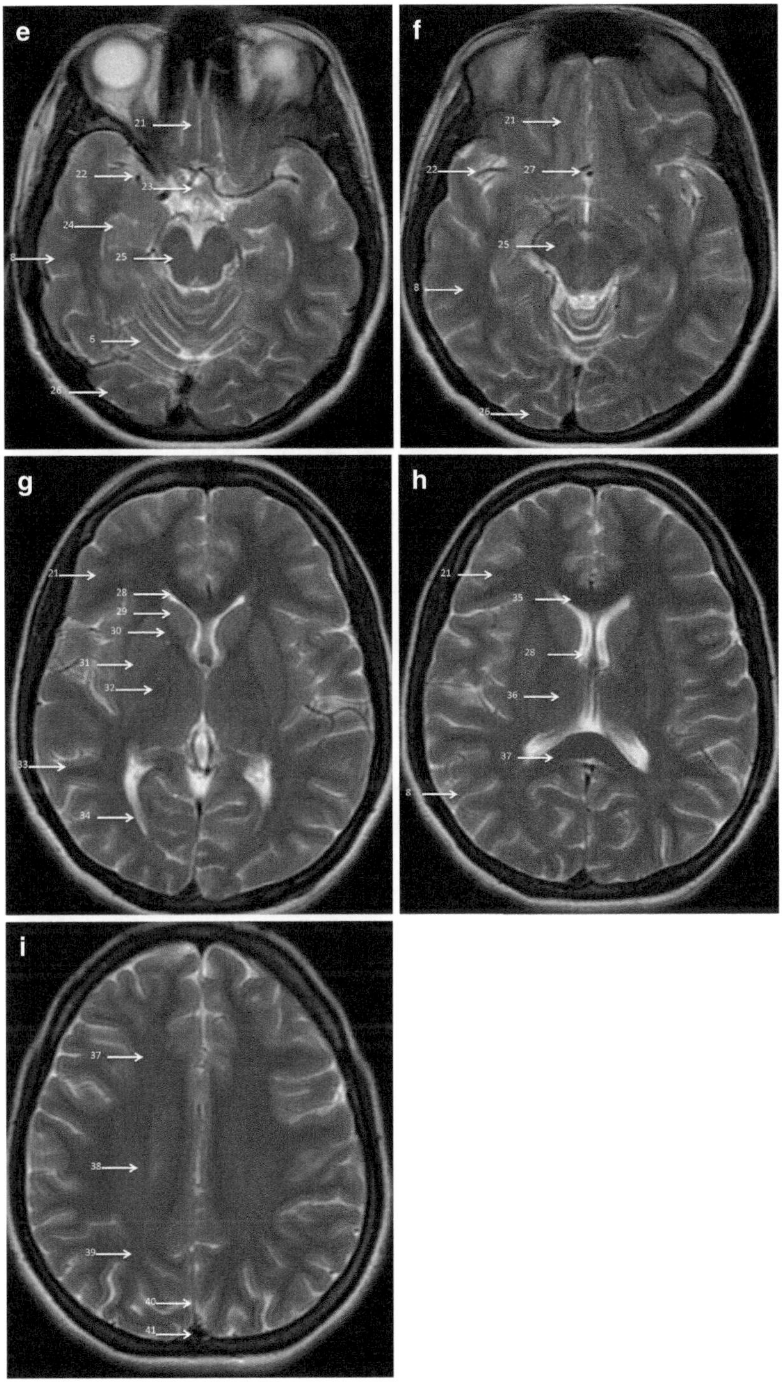


**Fig. 4.12** (continued)

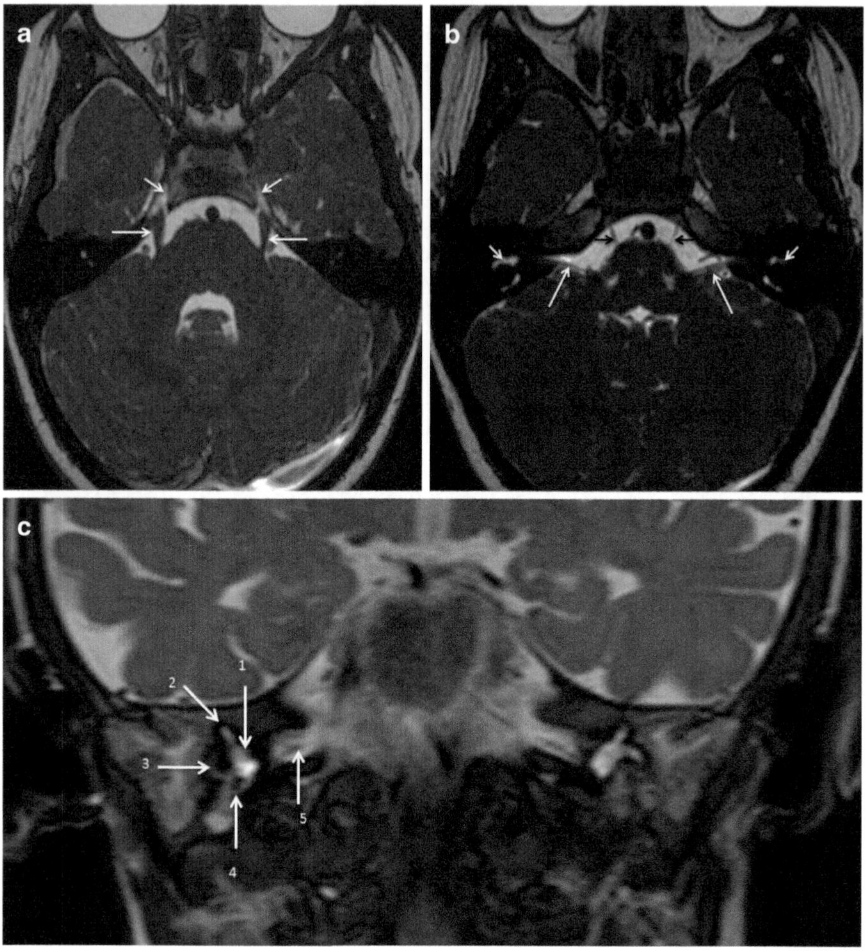


**Fig. 4.13** Heavily T2 weighted sequence axial (CISS/FIESTA). (**a**) The cisternal course of fifth cranial nerves (white arrows) is well visualized. The nerves are then seen entering the Meckels cave (short white arrows). (**b**) The cranial nerves namely, the seventh-eighth nerves (long white arrows) and sixth nerves (short black arrows) are well demonstrated. The semicircular canals (short white arrows) are fluid filled structures and hence appear hyperintense. (**c**)–(**g**): (1) Vestibule, (2) Superior semicircular canal, (3) horizontal semicircular canal, (4) posterior semicircular canal, (5) IAC containing seventh-eighth nerves, (6) Basal turn of cochlea, (7) Middle turn of cochlea, (8) Cochlea, (9) Facial N, (10) Cochlear N, (11) Vestibular N (superior branch), (12) Vestibular N (inferior branch). (**h**) Oblique saggital CISS MRI image of cochlea. Videos 4.1 and 4.2. *IAC* internal acoustic canal, *FN* facial nerve, *CN* cochlear nerve, *SVN* superior vestibular nerve, *IVN* inferior vestibular nerve, *ST* scala tympani, *SV* scala vestibuli, *OSL* osseous spiral lamina, *AT* apical turn, *MT* middle turn, *BT* basal turn, *SSC* superior semicircular canal, *PSC* posterior semicircular canal, *HSC* horizontal semicircular canal. Video 4.3

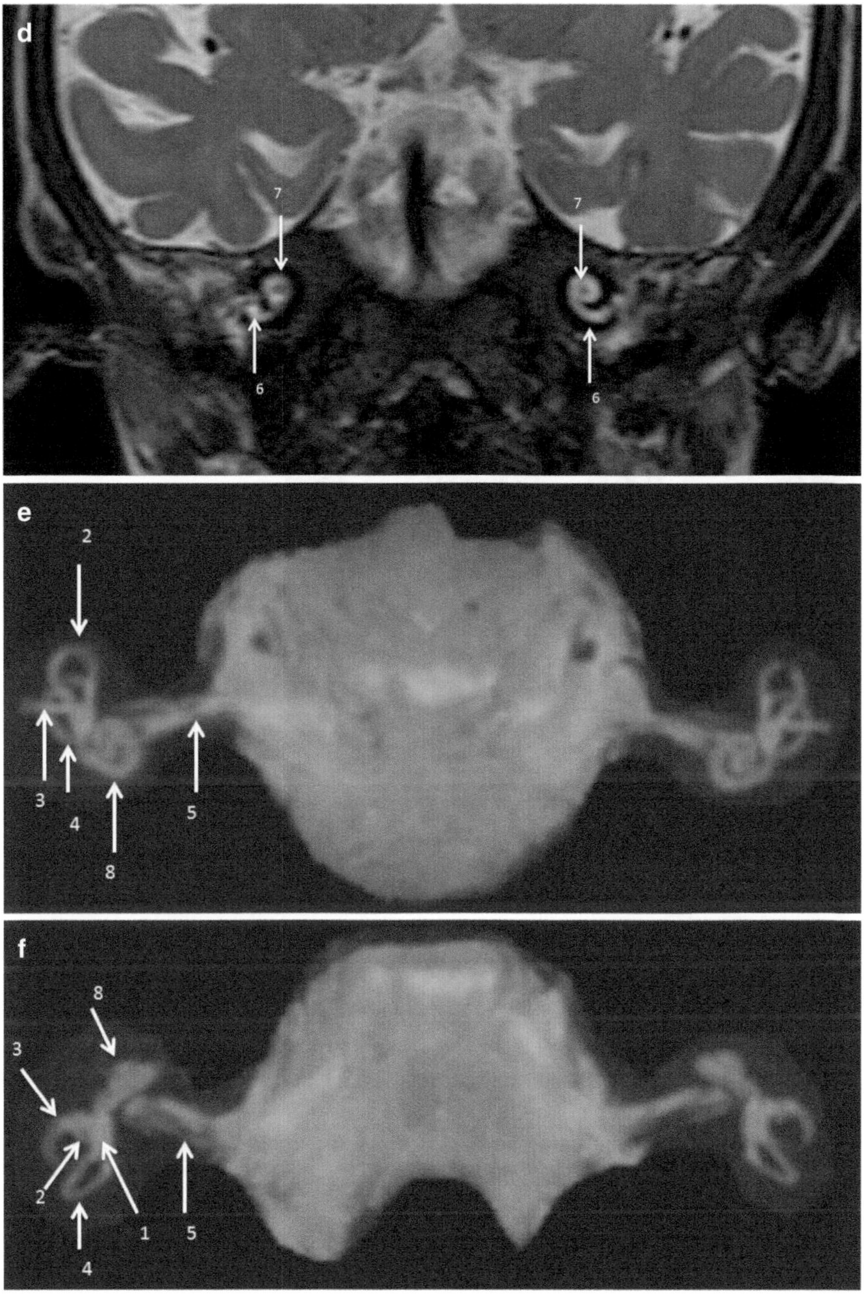


**Fig. 4.13** (continued)

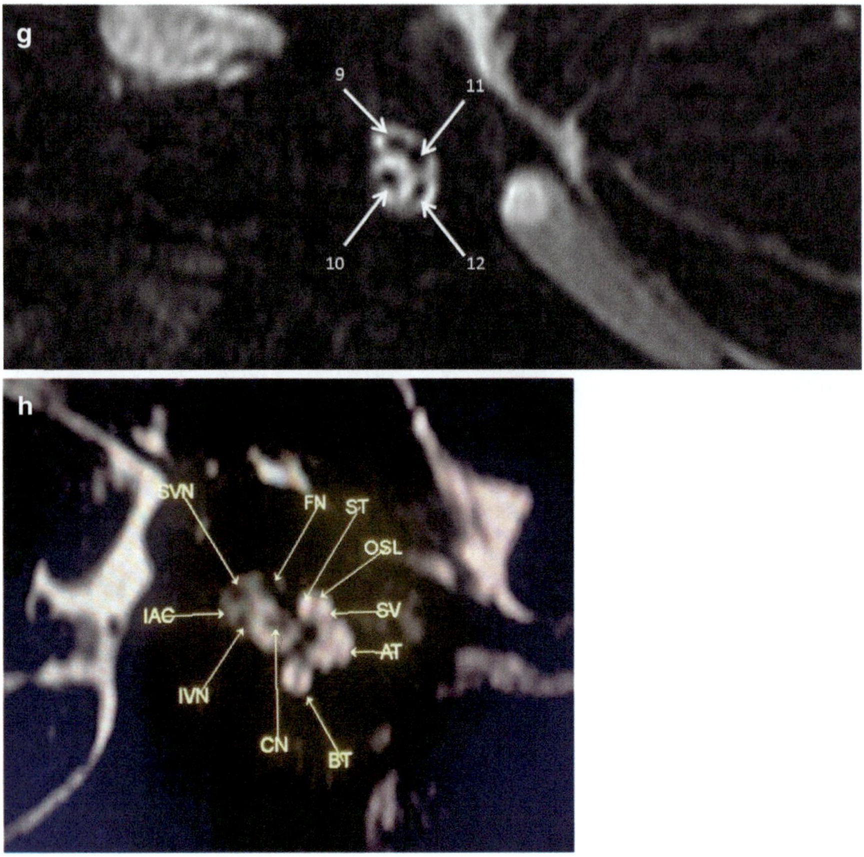


**Fig. 4.13** (continued)

angle is also well evaluated by this sequence. T2-weighted axial imaging of the brain aids in evaluating central nervous system causes of sensorineural hearing loss, if any [2]. A 3D image can also be obtained and rotated in X, Y, and Z planes for better anatomical orientation (Fig. 4.13e; Video 4.3).

T-1 Weighted spin-echo coronal or axial images are routinely performed. Fat shows a high signal intensity and the brain is intermediate in intensity. CSF is low in signal intensity and air and bone spaces appear as signal voids.

T-2 weighted axial spin-echo images accurately display the CSF spaces as high signal intensity regions.

High-resolution thin section 1.5 mm—1 Weighted images can be acquired with I.V. contrast. Gradient-echo images may also be carried out. These have the advantage of high resolution, very thin sections and give information regarding blood flow.

CT and MRI studies are complementary. MRI can characterize the CSF, brain, cranial nerves and blood vessels better than CT scanning. However, MRI studies receive no signal from dense bone or air spaces, so they cannot be used to evaluate these components accurately in the absence of pathology.

MRI is outstanding for the evaluation of blood vessel-related disorders of the temporal bone. Flowing blood is seen as a high signal region with gradient-echo techniques.

Contrast-enhanced MRI is sensitive to detect abnormalities that alter the blood–brain barrier, or to detect vascular lesions. MRI shows contrast enhancement better than CT scans. Also, MRI has a higher resolution and is more sensitive to detect any alternation in the fluid spaces of the inner ear or the cerebellopontine angle [1].

## 4.5.2 Important MRI Anatomy Features

### 4.5.2.1 Axial Sections: Caudad to Cephalad

At the level of the jugular foramen, the gradient-echo images demonstrate the descending portion of the facial nerve lying just lateral to the jugular bulb. The blood vessels are seen as high signal regions because of flow effects.

On T-1 Weighted images, the cartilaginous segment of the external auditory canal is seen as an intermediate density structure surrounded by high signal fat. At this level, the facial nerve is seen as an intermediate to high signal intensity circular structure, surrounded by a large area of signal void of the temporal bone and mastoid air spaces. The carotid canal is seen coursing through the skull base, parallel and medial to the semicanal of the tensor tympani muscle at this level.

On MRI, the medial margin of the middle ear is seen only when there is fluid or a mass within the middle ear. The fluid-filled apical, second and basal cochlear turns are identified by their intermediate signal intensity.

The CSF in the internal auditory canal is well demonstrated on T-1 and T-2 Weighted images with the individual seventh and eighth nerves appearing as filling defects within the CSF. Almost the entire course of the seventh and eighth nerves can be traced from the pontomedullary junction to the inner ear. MRI is more effective than CT in studying the nerves and their nuclei within the brainstem and the cerebellum. The cochlear fluid contents, labyrinthine and horizontal segments of the facial nerve and the geniculate ganglion can all be seen as intermediate signal intensity structures surrounded by the signal void bone.

At the level of the lateral semicircular canal, the endolymphatic duct and sac appear as thin high signal regions [1, 6].

### 4.5.2.2 Coronal Sections: From Anterior to Posterior

Anteriorly, the cochlea and geniculate ganglion can be viewed as fluid and soft tissue intensity structures respectively. Posteriorly, the facial and the vestibulocochlear nerves can be seen together within the CSF in the internal auditory canal, diverging laterally.

### 4.5.2.3 Sagittal Sections: From Lateral to Medial

The important structures looked for are:

The soft tissue components of the descending facial nerve are seen easily as intermediate to high signal intensity. Just medial to this, at the level of the vestibule, the endolymphatic duct and sac are seen as hyperintense structures on T-2 weighed images.

The vestibule is central and the common crus of the superior and the posterior semicircular canals can be seen as CSF intensity structures just posterior and superior to the vestibule. The endolymphatic sac is seen as a triangular area of increased signal at the distal end of the endolymphatic duct. At the internal auditory canal level, the individual seventh and eighth nerves within the canal and their relationship to each other is well demonstrated on sagittal MRI [1, 6].

## 4.6 Angiography and Interventional Radiology Applications

Conventional angiography and DSA (Digital Subtraction Angiography) have a specific role in temporal bone pathology. They are used in the diagnosis and now increasingly aid in the management of vascular masses and pulsatile tinnitus.

DSA has the advantage of higher resolution and definition of vascular pathology by computer-aided subtraction of surrounding bony and soft tissue shadows. This allows the use of smaller catheters and lesser amounts of contrast medium making the procedures much safer than the conventional studies.

Pulsatile tinnitus may be vascular in nature and the causes may be arterial, arterio-venous or venous. The most common causes are paragangliomas, idiopathic and dural AV-fistulas. The common angiographically diagnosed carotid arterial causes are atherosclerosis, fibromuscular dysplasia, styloid compression, aneurysm in the petrous portion, aberrant and lateral displacement of the carotid artery or rarely a persistent stapedial artery. The arterio-venous causes that can be diagnosed include paragangliomas (tympanicum or jugulare), dural AV-fistulas, vertebral AV fistulas, cerebral AV malformations and other vascular tumours. Among the venous causes, a large or exposed jugular bulb may be diagnosed.

Radiologic intervention can help in treating AV fistulas and AV malformations by embolization, which may be pre-operative or may completely cure the disease. The dural AV-fistulas are treated by trans-arterial embolization of the feeding arteries and now, increasingly by the trans-venous approach by retrograde cannulation of the dural sinuses. Permanent liquid embolic agents like IBCA or Histoacryl or particulate agents like PVA sponge or metallic coils especially via the trans-venous route are used. Pre-operative embolization of vascular masses with temporary embolic agents like gel foam has received widespread acceptance as a standard procedure [9–11].

## 4.7 Imaging of Pathologies of the Ear

### 4.7.1 Inflammatory Diseases of the Temporal Bone

CT and MRI are the imaging methods of choice for the diagnosis of petrous temporal inflammatory disease. Axial and coronal CT images accurately detect bony erosions and soft tissue masses involving the temporal bone. MRI with intravenous contrast is the investigation of choice for the identification of intracranial spread of external, middle, and inner ear infections. Contrast-enhanced MRI also differentiates nonenhancing cholesteatoma and fluid from enhancing granulation tissue and tumour [12].

#### 4.7.1.1 Infective Lesions of the External Ear

Simple uncomplicated external otitis is rarely studied by CT/MRI/examination. It is the malignant external otitis that requires complete evaluation either by CT or MRI.

**CT Findings in External Otitis:**

Acute otitis externa (Fig. 4.14) has a 1% annual incidence and a 10% lifetime prevalence. Ninety-eight percent of acute otitis externa is bacterial in origin [13]. Intermediate density soft tissue is seen replacing the black air space within the external auditory canal. Varying degrees of surrounding bone destruction involving the canal wall, skull base, TM joint, petrous pyramid, tympanic cavity or the mastoid process may be seen [6].

**MRI Findings in External Otitis:**

Necrotizing or malignant otitis externa (Fig. 4.14) occurs most commonly in elderly diabetic patients and other patients in immunocompromised states [3]. MRI scores over CT in identifying affection of the bone marrow and occlusion of vessels at the skull base. Bone marrow involvement is seen as the altered signal intensity of the bone and vessel occlusion is seen as loss of normal signal void due to flowing blood on both T-1 Weighted and T-2 Weighted images. MRI displays changes of osteomyelitis earlier than CT. TM joint involvement may also be detected. On contrast-enhanced MRI, a mild central nodular enhancement is sometimes seen in the early cerebritis stage. Meningitis is seen as enhancement along the cerebral convexity underlying the involved temporal bone [14].

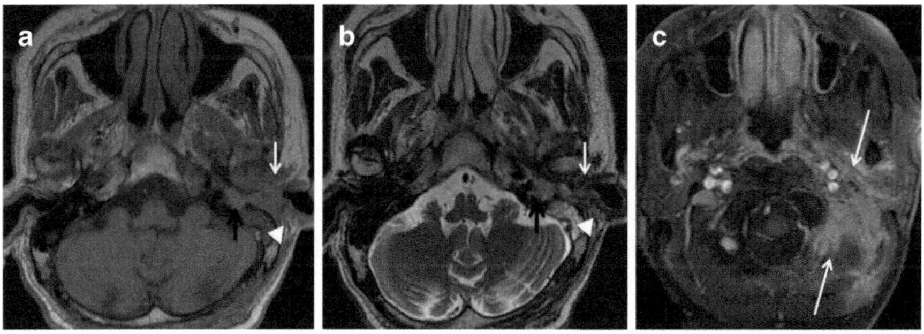


**Fig. 4.14** Malignant otitis externa. Axial T1 (a) and T2(b) MRI scan shows wall thickening involving left external auditory meatus (short white arrow) with extension into the middle ear and osteomyelitis of left petrous bone (shot black arrow). Axial post contrast T1 scan (c) reveals diffuse enhancement on left side extending into suboccipital region, parotid, carotid, parapharyngeal and pterygoid spaces (long white arrows)

*Gradenigo syndrome* consists of the triad of:

1. Petrous apicitis, infection involving petrous apex
2. Abducens nerve palsy, secondary to involvement of the nerve as it passes through the Dorello canal
3. Retro-orbital pain, or pain in the cutaneous distribution of the frontal and maxillary divisions of the trigeminal nerve, due to extension of inflammation into Meckel cave [15].

#### 4.7.1.2 Infective/Inflammatory Lesions of the Middle Ear

These range from acute otitis to chronic otitis and acquired cholesteatomas. These are usually associated with mastoiditis. A spectrum of complications resulting from mastoiditis may occur.

## 4.8 Cholesteatoma

The most common lesion that requires to be imaged by CT is cholesteatoma (Fig. 4.15).

There are two types of cholesteatomas-congenital and acquired. Differentiation between these two types of cholesteatomas is not possible by the imaging methods available today.

(a) Congenital cholesteatomas. These commonly arise in the region of the incudostapedial articulation or the epitympanum.
(b) Acquired cholesteatomas. These are of two types—Pars Flaccida (usually primary acquired) and Pars Tensa (usually secondary acquired). Classically, pars flaccida cholesteatomas displace the ossicular chain medially away from Prussak's space and pars tensa cholesteatomas displace the ossicular chain laterally.

### 4.8.1 Plain Film Findings

Plain films give information regarding the degree of pneumatization of the mastoid air cells. Gross bony destruction by the lesion is seen as rounded radiolucent osseous defects.

The role of CT is to determine the amount of bony destruction and the extent and size of the cholesteatoma [12].

### 4.8.2 CT Findings in Acquired Cholesteatomas

The diagnosis of acquired cholesteatomas is made by the presence of a non-dependent focal or diffuse soft tissue mass in the middle ear with surrounding focal or diffuse bone destruction. The soft tissue is homogenous and is sharply demarcated.

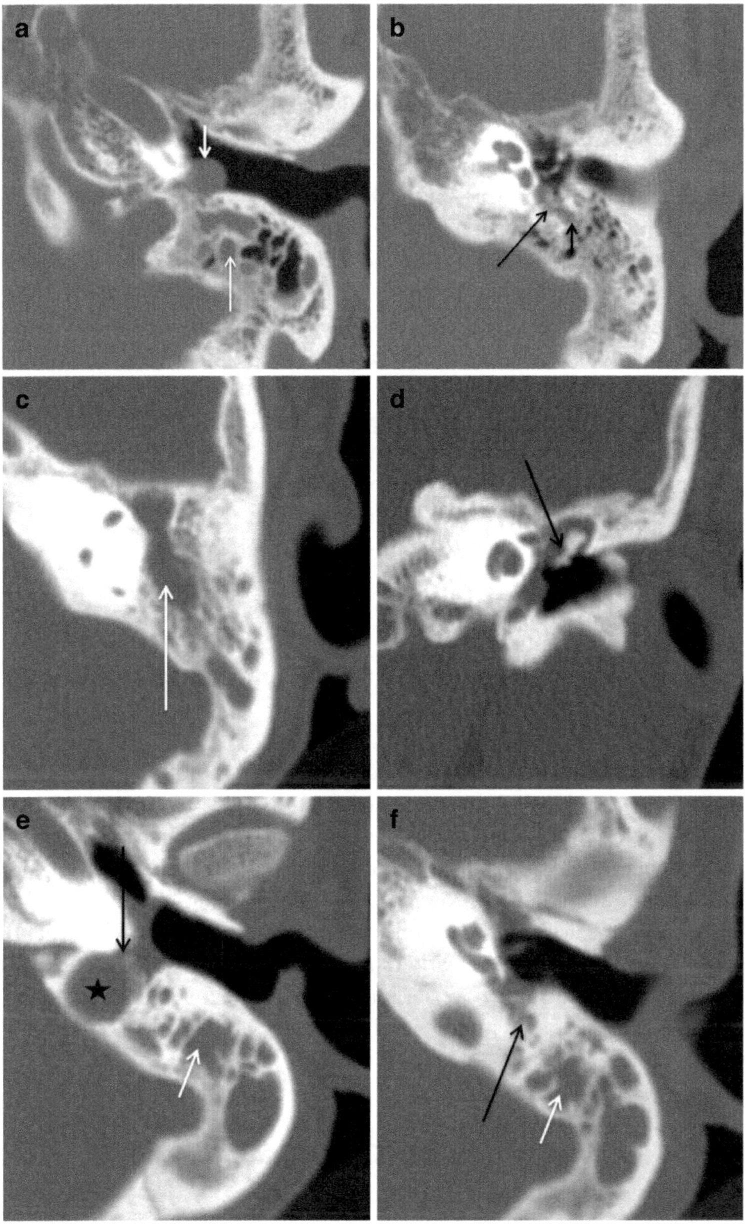


**Fig. 4.15** Cholesteatoma. Axial HRCT of left temporal bone (**a** and **b**) show well defined homogenously hypodense lesion in middle ear (short white arrow). There are underlying erosions seen with extension into mastoid. There is erosion (long black arrow) involving facial canal (short black arrow) also appreciated. There is soft tissue density seen in mastoid suggestive of mastoiditis (**a**—long white arrow). Axial (**c**,**e**,**f**) and Coronal (**d**) HRCT images of left temporal bone of another patient reveals soft tissue density lesion in the attic extending into aditus and antrum of mastoid (long white arrow in **c**) and mastoid air cells (short white arrows in **e** and **f**). Erosions are marked in long black arrows (ossicular erosion in **d**, sinus plate erosion in **e** and facial canal erosion in **f**). Jugular bulb is maked with a black star

Pars flaccida cholesteatoma may show the presence of retraction pocket in the tympanic membrane. Pars tensa cholesteatoma extends directly into the central portion of the middle ear. Extension of the cholesteatoma soft tissue may be seen into the sinus tympani, hypotympanum, attic and then through the aditus into the antrum and the mastoid air cells. Bone involvement is seen as the destruction or dislocation of the ossicles. The short and long processes of the incus are usually eroded. This may be followed by the destruction of the body of incus and the head of malleus resulting in the loss of the normal ice-cream cone appearance. The facial nerve canal, if eroded, appears deficient and the exact relationship of the cholesteatomatous mass and the facial canal is defined. Fistulas of the labyrinth are seen as lucencies in the bone if the lateral or posterior semicircular canals are eroded. Intracranial complications may occur through disruption of the tegmen tympani which is best seen on coronal sections. Bony destruction of the mastoid (automastoidectomy) and petrous pyramid are seen as irregular osseous defects caused by pressure necrosis or enzymatic osteolysis. Occasionally, a large bony defect in the external auditory canal and mastoid is seen secondary to spontaneous extrusion of the cholesteatoma. This appears as an empty air-filled cavity with circumferential soft tissue. Superadded infection may lead to meningitis, intracerebral or epidural abscess and lateral sinus thrombosis [12, 16].

### 4.8.3 Pre-operative Planning of Cholesteatomas: Importance of HRCT to the Surgeon

HRCT of the middle ear and mastoid is valuable to the otologic surgeon before exploration, to stage the cholesteatoma and post-operatively, to assess the response to therapy. It is crucial to determine the presence of ossicular chain destruction, especially stapedial erosion and to exclude perforation of the bony tegmen [16]. This information helps the surgeon to center on removing the diseased tissue and subsequently to preserve and/or reconstruct the conductive hearing function. The greatest value of HRCT is in the early diagnosis of cholesteatoma especially unsuspected lesions within the attic or posterior tympanum beyond otoscopic view. It also aids in diagnosing residual cholesteatoma or regrowth within the mastoidectomy cavity [17].

### 4.8.4 MRI Findings in Acquired Cholesteatoma

MRI is the preferred modality for diagnosing cholesteatoma. Lesions as small as 2 mm can be detected on a 1.5T MRI scanner. The lesion appears hyperintense on T2W images. Non-echo-planar DWI sequence reveals hyperintense signal within the lesion with b value 1000 as compared to b value 0 and shows a corresponding drop in values (hypointense) on the ADC map, confirming diffusion restriction. This sequence is extremely useful to detect recurrence after surgery. CT is performed especially after confirmation of lesion on MRI, for preoperative planning and to exclude perforation of bony tegmen [16].

### 4.8.5 Differential Diagnosis of Cholesteatoma

A non-dependent soft tissue mass when present in an atypical location is unlikely to be cholesteatomas. It is more likely to represent granulation tissue and/or neoplasm. A dependent soft tissue represents fluid.

Paragangliomas of the middle ear (glomus tympanicum) may cause difficulty in the differential diagnosis. These lesions usually arise in the region of the promontory and have a tendency to spare the ossicles. Enhancement of these lesions is usually seen as they are often vascular [9].

## 4.9 Acute and Chronic Otitis Media and Mastoiditis (Figs. 4.16 and 4.17)

### 4.9.1 Plain Film Findings

An overall hazy middle ear and the mastoid is seen due to fluid accumulation and mucosal thickening. The pattern of the air cell distribution and the bony wall of each air cell is not altered.

### 4.9.2 CT Findings

The extent of soft tissue and fluid levels present is well demonstrated by CT. Opacification of the air is seen in the middle ear. There may be thickening and retraction of the tympanic membrane. Bony erosions may be seen (<10%) with occasional tympanic membrane perforation [18]. Fluid levels or opacification is visualized in the mastoid air spaces. As the disease progresses into the subacute stage, focal or diffuse mucosal thickening of the mastoid sinus and middle ear is seen. Demineralization with loss of the trabecular pattern of the mastoid air cells may also occur. The fluid in serous otitis media often cannot be distinguished from pus in purulent otitis media [19].

Three common findings seen in chronic otitis media and mastoiditis (Fig. 4.17) are:

1. Mucosal thickening and occasional fluid levels
2. Non-dependent soft tissue mass in the middle ear, which can represent granuloma and/or cholesteatoma. Both can produce labyrinthine and ossicular destruction.
3. Reduction and destruction of mastoid air cells (hypopneumatization) followed by sclerosis

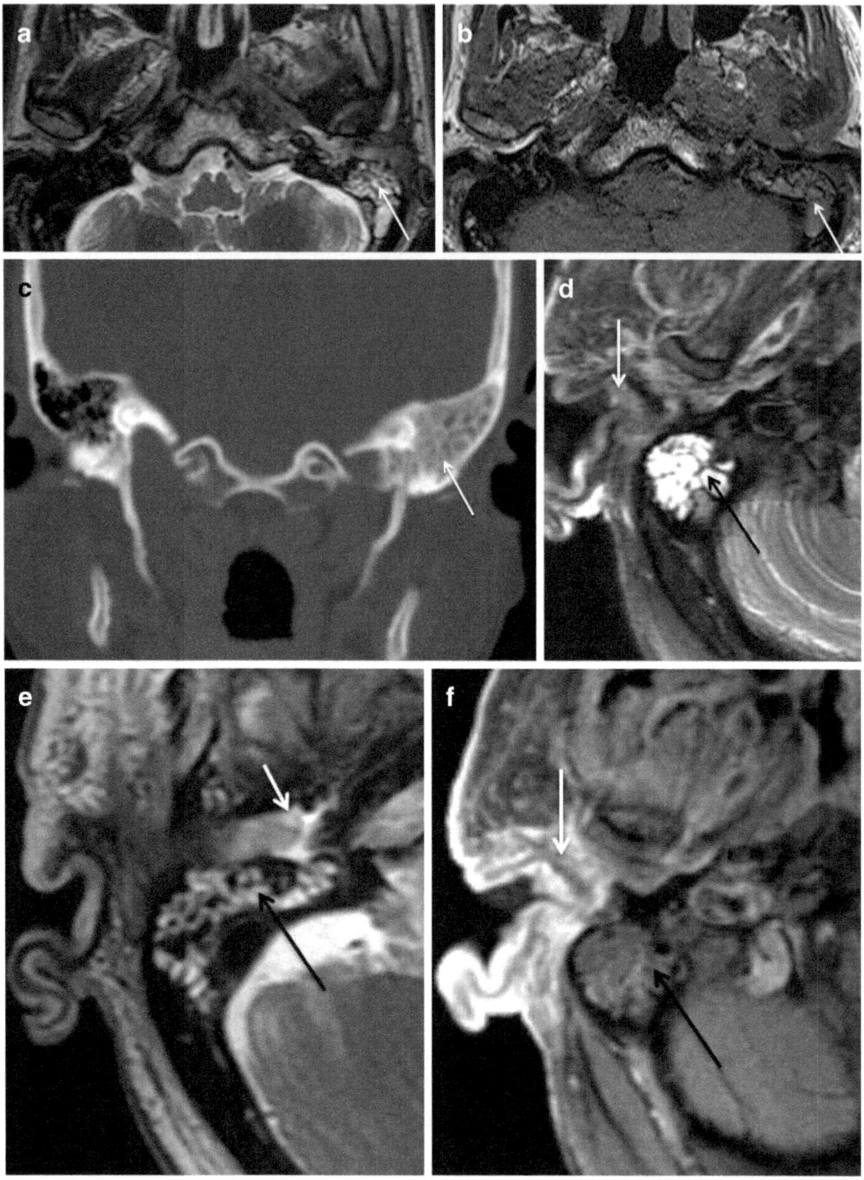


**Fig. 4.16** Acute otitis media with mastoiditis. There is T2 hyperintense (**a**) and T1 iso to hypointense (**b**) signal seen in left mastoid suggestive of mastoiditis. CT coronal image of same patient (**c**) reveals hypodense fluid obliterating the left mastoid air cells suggestive of mastoiditis. T2 fat saturated axial MRI images reveal hyperintense wall thickening involving right external auditory meatus (long white arrow) with diffuse enhancement on T1 post contrast scan (**f**). There is, in addition, T2 hyperintense fluid seen within the middle ear suggestive of acute otitis media (short white arrow) as well as acute mastoiditis (long black arrow)

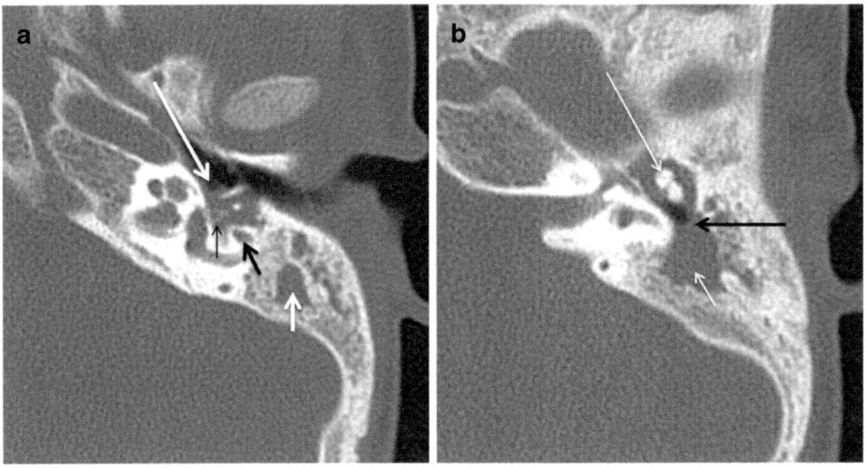


**Fig. 4.17** Chronic otitis media and mastoiditis. Sof tissue density in meso and epitympanum (long thick white arrow), extending into aditus (long thin black arrow) and antrum (short thin white arrow) of mastoid as well as opacifying the mastoid air cells (short thick white arrow). The stapes (short thin black arrow), malleus (long thin white arrow) and facial canal (short thick black arrow) are intact without any obvious erosions

### 4.9.3 MRI Findings

The disease is best identified on T2 images. There is T2 hyperintense inflammatory soft tissue/fluid seen within the middle ear cavity and/or mastoid [18]. Bony erosions are better appreciated on CT as compared to MRI.

## 4.10 Adhesive Otitis Media and Tympanosclerosis

### 4.10.1 CT and MRI Findings

It is a form of chronic otitis media leading to middle ear adhesions as a result of chronic inflammation [20] As the disease progresses, the tympanic membrane can be retracted inwards and become adherent to the promontory. Numerous adhesion bands are seen in the middle ear which appear as irregular linear soft tissue strands. High-density focal deposits may be seen in the middle ear, tympanic membrane and epitympanum as a result of calcific plaques which give rise to tympanosclerosis [14, 19].

## 4.11 Labyrinthine (Perilymphatic) Fistula

It is a pathologic communication between the fluid-filled space of the *inner ear* and the air-filled space of the middle ear, most commonly occurring at either the *round* or *oval window*. It is the result of bony erosion which may follow pathological

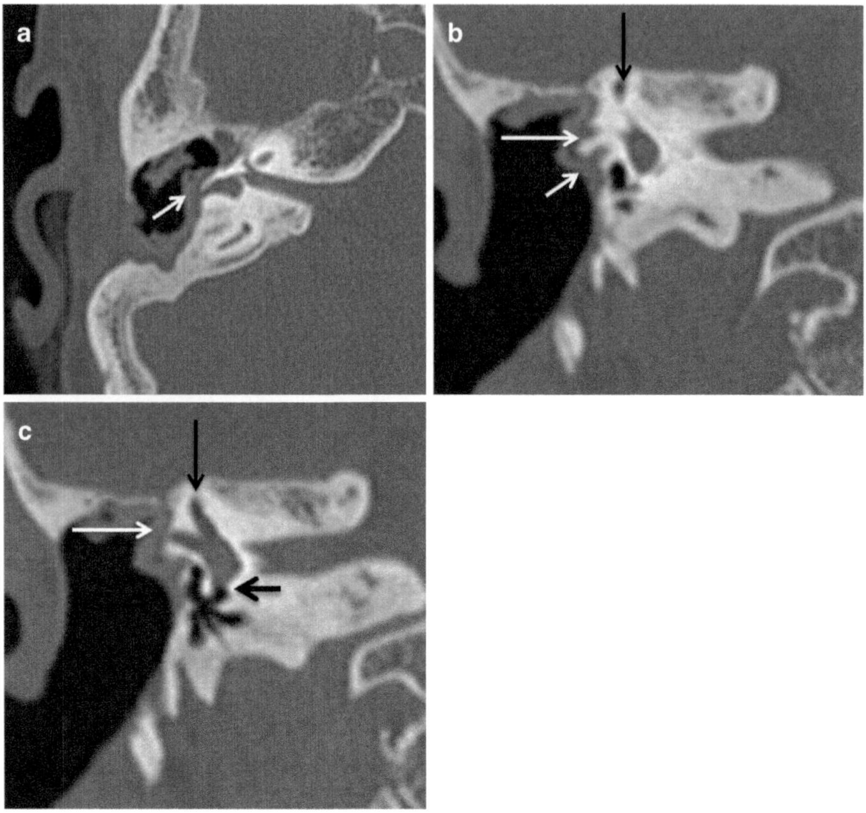


**Fig. 4.18** Labyrinthine fistula. In this patient post mastoidectomy, axial CT images of right temporal bone (**a**)–(**c**) reveal right sided labyrinthine fistula at the level of horizontal semicircular canal (long white arrow). There is adjacent fluid seen within the middle ear (short white arrow) and air within membranous labyrinth (short black arrow). Superior semicircular canal (long black arrow). (*Image Courtesy: Dr. Santosh Gupta, P. D. Hinduja Hospital)*

conditions like chronic otitis media/mastoiditis [20]. Labyrinthine fistula (Fig. 4.18) usually involves the lateral semicircular canals because this structure extends into the middle ear and the mastoid. The osseous covering of the lateral semicircular canal is destroyed.

### 4.11.1 CT and MRI Findings

The bony covering over the lateral semicircular canal is absent as a result of fistula formation. This is best demonstrated on axial CT taken along the orbitomeatal line.

With the improvement in the resolution of computed tomography (CT) and magnetic resonance imaging (MRI), the need for exploratory procedures to identify labyrinthine fistula in traumatic or post-surgical cases has declined. One of the earliest described radiological signs of a PLF is air in the cochlea, vestibule, and/or semicircular canals (pneumolabyrinth) [21]. Small bubbles of air can be hard to visualize on typical CT scans, so high-resolution scans including coronal or sagittal views may be useful in suspected cases [22]. Fluid in the round and oval window is another reliable sign of a labyrinthine fistula. High-resolution CT of the temporal bone has a sensitivity for detection of PLFs of over 80% when compared to intraoperative visualization of leak, and a combination of CT and MRI was reported to diagnose almost 100% of cases [23]. Axial and coronal CISS (constructive interference in steady state) also called FIESTA (fast imaging employing steady-state acquisition) or MPR (magnetic resonance perfusion) sequence are most useful in the diagnosis of this condition.

## 4.12 Sinodural Plate Destruction Intracranial Penetration and Acute Petrositis

Tegmen tympani, tegmen mastoidenum and the sinodural plate act as bony barriers that prevent the spread of infection into the intracranial cavity. Once the osseous barriers are breached, purulent meningitis, sinus thrombosis, cerebritis or abscess formation may result.

When there is pneumatization of the petrous bone, the inflammation may spread to the petrous tip. It may then extend extradurally and give rise to Gradenigo's Syndrome (as described above in malignant otitis externa) due to the involvement of the fifth and the sixth nerves as they cross the petrous tip [19].

### 4.12.1 CT and MRI Findings

The tegmen tympani is normally seen as a thin plate of bone on coronal CT. Erosion is visualized as a discontinuity of this bone which may result in an intracranial extension of the inflammation

Petrous Apicitis reveals opacification of the apical air cells is seen due to the presence of fluid within. Demineralization and bony destruction of the petrous apex are also seen as irregular bony defects.

MRI is more sensitive in detecting dural thickening and enhancement as well as leptomeningitis, cerebritis and cerebral abscess. There may be thickening of fifth and sixth nerves with contrast and the cavernous sinus should be sought, as well as for the findings of cavernous sinus thrombosis. Enhancement appreciated on thin T1 post contrast images. Thickening of the dura of Meckel's cave [24].

## 4.13 Otosclerosis (Otospongiosis) (Fig. 4.19)

Otosclerosis is a disease of the labyrinthine capsule, in which, by an unknown process, the normal lamellar bone is replaced by thick, irregular bone. The initial lytic phase (otospongiosis) is followed by a reparative sclerotic phase (otosclerosis).

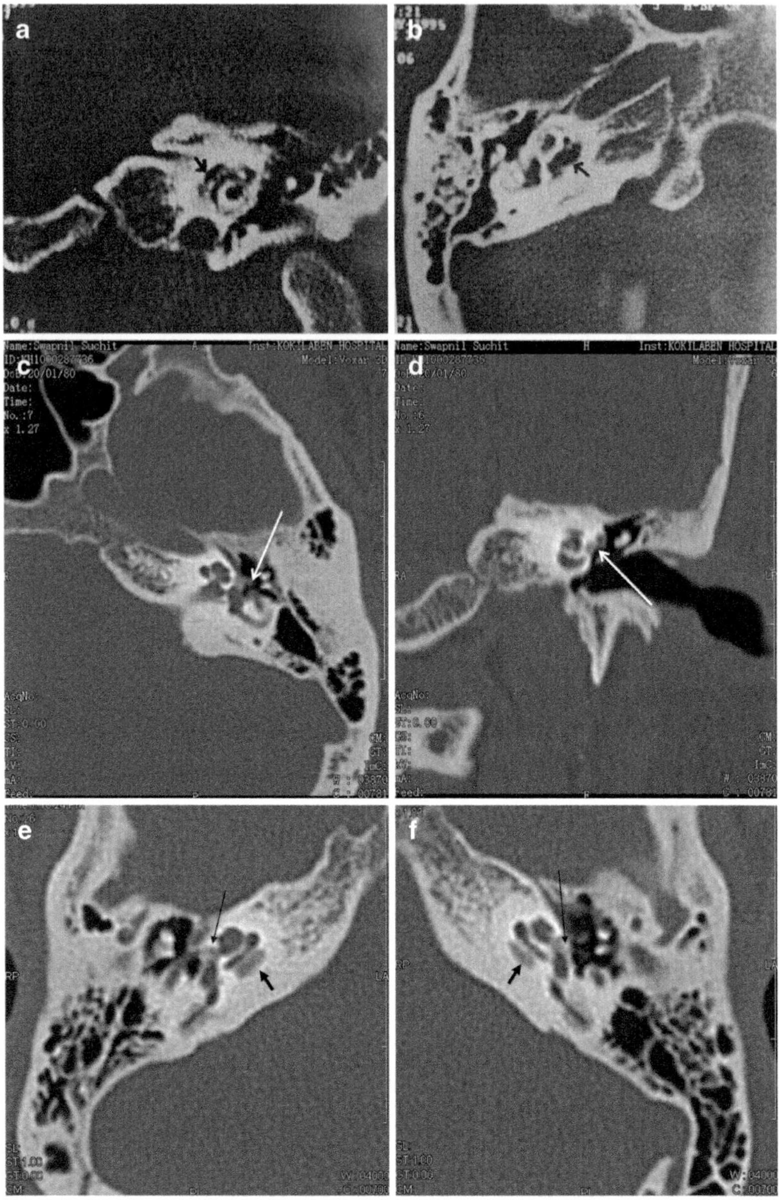


**Fig. 4.19** Otosclerosis (otospongiosis). Cochlear Otospongiosis (**a**). Coronal section of the left temporal bone shows a well demarcated lucent zone following the cochlea coil with normal cortical bone separating the lucency from the cochlea ("The double ring sign" (arrow). Cochlear Otospongiosis (**b**) Axial section of the right temporal bone shows the spongiotic zone merging with the cochlea—"The enlarged cochlea coil" appearance (arrow). Images (**c**) (axial) and (**d**) (coronal) of HRCT temporal bone reveal left sided fenestral otospongiosis. Images (**e**) and (**f**) of another patient very well demonstrates bilateral Fenestral (long black arrows) and Retrofenestral (short black arrows) otospongiosis. Images (**g**) and (**h**) of yet another patient reveal delayed sclerotic phase of Otosclerosis. (*Image courtesy: Dr Abhijit Raut, Kokilaben Dhirubhai Ambani Hospital*)

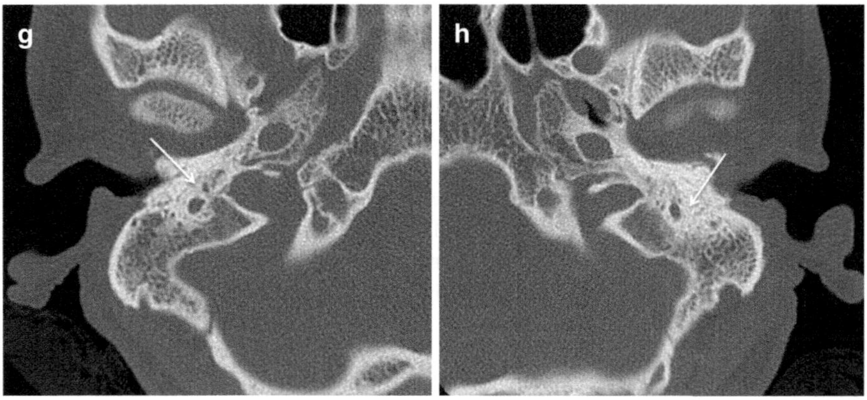


**Fig. 4.19** (continued)

On CT, the lytic phase is seen as lucent areas within the otic capsule or has a more diffuse localization. The sclerotic phase is seen as an obliteration of the normally lucent membranous labyrinth, especially the cochlear first turn (Cochlear Otosclerosis) and/or the oval window-round window niche (Fenestral Otosclerosis). The stapes footplate may also be fixated (Stapedial Otosclerosis). The process of otosclerosis is frequently bilateral. The sites of predilection of otospongiosis in the temporal bone are in the oval window (85%) and around the round window (40%).

The classification for the extent and type of the lesion is as follows:

| | |
|---|---|
| Extent | 1. Limited to the capsule of the first turn of the cochlea<br>2. Diffuse spread throughout the cochlear capsule<br>3. Involvement of the complete labyrinthine capsule |
| Type | 1. Spongiotic changes with possible erosions of the contours of the labyrinthine lumen<br>2. Sclerotic changes<br>3. Mixed appearance of spongiotic and sclerotic bone |

High-Resolution CT axial and coronal contiguous 1.5 mm standard sections are usually enough for detecting the involvement of the oval window by the process of otosclerosis. No contrast is required. The axial sections show the anterior oval window margins well and the coronal sections reveal the superior and inferior margins. Additional scans in six other planes (sagittal, semi-axial, semi-longitudinal, axio-petrosal, longitudinal and inclined sagittal) may be performed. The semi-axial plane is used to study the oval window niche. The semi-longitudinal plane studies the first and the second turns of the cochlea. To look for stapedial otosclerosis, a coronal position is given to the patient and the head is rotated 15° towards the side of interest [25, 26].

### 4.13.1 CT Findings

- *Oval window Otosclerosis*—The changes depend upon the type and extent of the disease.
- *Active Stapedial Otospongiosis*—The oval window margins appear indistinct resulting in a "wide window" appearance.

- *Mature (Inactive) Otosclerosis*—The stapes footplate shows margins or diffuse thickening.
- *Cochlear Otospongiosis*—The bone around the cochlea is resorbed. This is usually seen as a sharply defined, circumlinear lucent zone around the cochlea with normal cortical bone separating the lucency from the cochlea. This lucent halo around the cochlea (in its medial aspect) appears as a characteristic "double ring sign" (Fig. a). Occasionally, the cochlea may merge with lucency. This gives rise to an apparently enlarged cochlear coil (Fig. b). Sometimes this lucent zone does not limit itself to the cochlea, but intersects the lateral semicircular canal or diffusely involves the complete labyrinth or even larger area of the petrous bone. This otospongiotic zone may have a density range from 350 HU to 1550 HU [26].

### 4.13.2 CT Findings in Post-stapedectomy Ear

CT is effective in evaluating the complications of the post-stapedectomy ear with prosthesis insertion. The complications possible include prosthesis ankylosis, prolapse of prosthesis through the oval window, incudo-prosthetic dislocation, reparative granuloma formation, regrowth of obliterative otosclerosis and incus (long process) necrosis. The Teflon and thin wire devices are also identified adequately as thin high density linear structures.

### 4.13.3 Differential Diagnosis of Otosclerosis

Other osteodystrophic conditions like Paget's disease, osteogenesis imperfecta, fibrous dysplasia and osteopetrosis, may affect the petrous temporal bone. Changes in the petrous bone seen in these conditions are similar to otosclerosis but in a setting of diffuse skull changes. Fibrous dysplasias even though seen to involve the petrous bone diffusely may sometimes spare the inner ear (Fig. 4.20).

## 4.14 Neoplasms, Cysts and Other Masses

### 4.14.1 Inner Ear and Cerebello-pontine Angle Neuro-otologic Disorders

Symptoms like dizziness, vertigo and dysequilibrium may be caused by a variety of conditions, such as vascular, metabolic, degenerative and neoplastic lesions within the vestibulocerebellar brainstem complex. Clinically, the lesion is first localized in the cochlear, retrocochlear, vestibular end-organ or central vestibular intracranial region.

CT then evaluates acoustic neurinoma or other posterior fossa lesions in patients suspected of having retrocochlear or vestibulo-cerebellar brainstem complex pathology.

If abnormal vestibular central signs are present, lesions like cerebellar or brainstem infarction or metastases is looked for in the inferior cerebellar peduncular region [11].

Other posterior fossa lesions like meningioma, primary cholesteatoma, hemangioblastoma, brainstem glioma, vascular malformations, etc. can be adequately diagnosed by contrast-enhanced CT and MRI.

### 4.14.2 Acoustic Schwannoma (Fig. 4.21)

It is the most common tumour of the cerebellopontine angle and the most common tumour of the temporal bone. It frequently arises within the internal auditory canal;

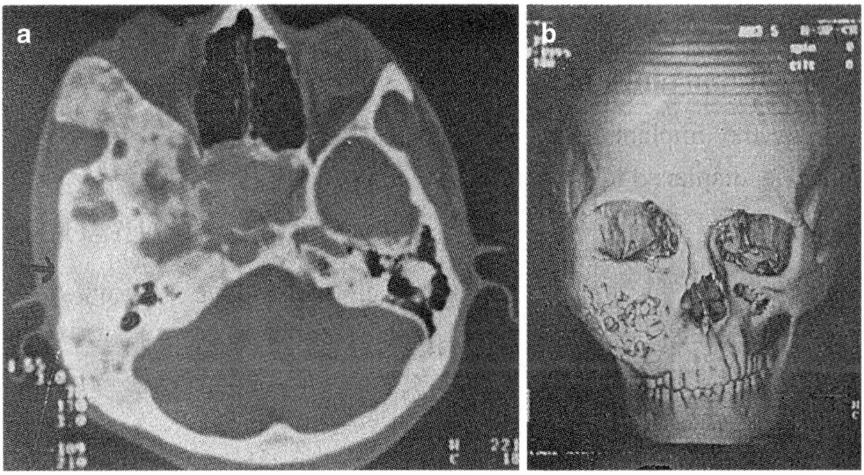


**Fig. 4.20** Fibrous dysplasia. Axial C.T. sections and bony and three-dimensionally reconstructed images show diffuse involvement of the right temporal bone (arrow) and the sphenoid with fibrous dysplasia

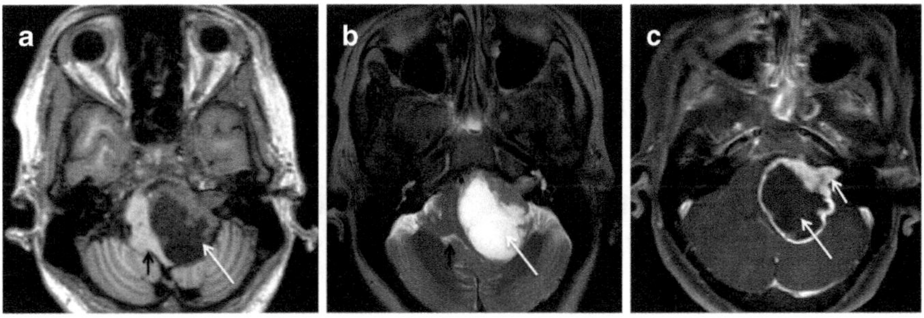


**Fig. 4.21** Acoustic neuroma. MRI brain reveals T1 hypointense (**a**) and T2 hyperintense (**b**) cystic lesion (long white arrow) in the left cerebellopontine angle with peripheral enhancement. The lesion is seen extending into the left IAC, giving 'ice cream cone' appearance. There is mass effect seen on brainstem with rightward displacement and compression of fourth ventricle (short black arrow)

therefore, the internal auditory meatus is first to enlarge. It is usually unilateral. Bilateral cases occur in adults with neurofibromatosis. Purely intracanalicular lesions commonly occur.

MRI is the diagnostic procedure of choice for the investigation of acoustic neurinoma (Fig. 4.21). This is because artefact-free axial, coronal and sagittal images of the brain are obtainable with high resolution and increased confidence of diagnosis. MRI accurately demonstrates both the intracanalicular and extracanalicular portion of the acoustic neurinoma. It is more specific than CT in evaluating intra-canalicular tumours.

T2-weighted and T1-weighted thin (3 mm) axial non-contrast and intravenous contrast MRI scans are taken. Additional coronal T1-weighted thin sections are taken if a lesion is identified. CISS images (also known as FIESTA) is useful in evaluating the CP angles and cisternal segments of cranial nerves.

Axial non-contrast and contrast High-Resolution CT sections can also be used to evaluate the mass. This is an especially preferred imaging modality preoperatively for neuronavigation. Bone window setting detects erosions of the internal auditory canal, if any.

#### 4.14.2.1 MRI and CT Findings

Generally, tumour signals are homogeneous and slightly T1 hypointense compared to the brainstem. These tumours are smoothly marginated with ipsilateral internal auditory canal enlargement. They are more likely to exhibit T2 hyperintensity than a cerebellopontine angle meningioma.

Gadolinium enhancement MRI is better in the evaluation of intra- and extra-canalicular extent of the lesion. Acoustic neurinomas are known to enhance vividly on the administration of intravenous contrast. This feature is important for the detection of intra-canalicular lesions.

CT demonstrates a homogenously enhancing, smoothly marginated, isodense cerebello-pontine angle mass with ipsilateral internal auditory canal enlargement. Sometimes, enhancement may lack in the central portion of the tumour. Cystic changes are common within these tumours and are seen as focal non-enhancing hypodense areas. Bone window setting detects internal auditory canal erosion. If these tumours are large, they widen the cerebellopontine angle cistern and displace the adjacent brainstem and cerebellum. They displace the fourth ventricle contralaterally and compress it from side to side. Non-enhancing hypodense edema may be seen within the cerebellum. If they are very large, they obliterate the cerebellopontine angle cistern.

#### 4.14.2.2 Differential Diagnosis of Acoustic Neuroma

Meningioma: On imaging, it may be difficult to differentiate these tumours from other CP angle tumours, especially meningiomas (Fig. 4.22) which also reveal intense contrast enhancement. Acoustic neurinomas are often centered around the internal auditory meatus and may show "ice cream cone" appearance due to extension into the meatus [27]. They are more rounded and grow upward towards the tentorial notch. Meningiomas, on the other hand, have a more flattened appearance

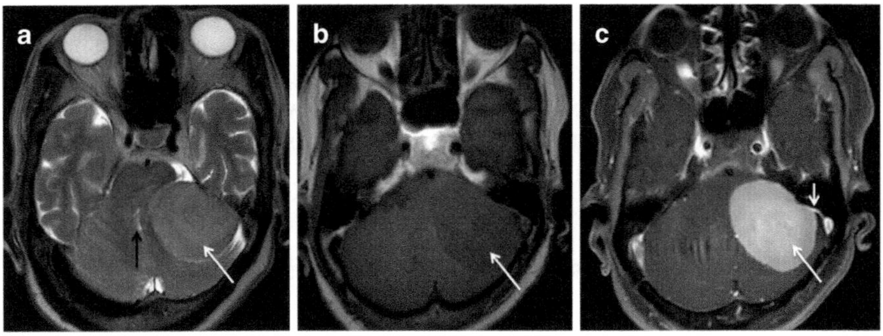


**Fig. 4.22** Meningioma. MRI brain reveals a large T1 hypointense (**a**) and T2 mildly hyperintense (**b**) lesion in left cerebellopontime angle (long white arrow) with homogenous intense contrast enhancement and a dural tai (short white arrow in **c**). There is compression of brainstem and fourth ventricle (short black arrow)

with an “en-plaque” component and are located more anteriorly towards the petrous apex. Also, there is no extension of meningiomas into the internal acoustic meatus.

Fifth Nerve Neuromas: CT demonstrates a well-demarcated isodense or partially cystic contrast-enhancing mass causing bone erosion at Meckel’s cave and, often, of the foramen ovale. The larger ones extend into the cerebellopontine angle and seventh-eighth nerve complex may not be seen separately from the mass.

MRI demonstrates a brainstem-T1 hypointense or isointense and T2 hyperintense mass that enhances well with contrast. Meckel’s cave erosion or identification of the firth nerve branches emanating from the tumour are strong diagnostic clues. These are rare and originate at the Gasserian (trigeminal) ganglion.

### 4.14.3 Petrous Bone Cholesterol Cysts (Cholesterol Granulomas)

They are much less common than acoustic neuroma but are the most common benign lesion of the petrous apex. They are often expansile and quite extensive eroding the petrous apex and adjacent bony structures. They may also involve the labyrinth. *Cholesterol granuloma* (*CG*), also sometimes called a *chocolate cyst* of the ear or *blue-domed cyst,* is a special type of middle ear granulation tissue that is particularly prone to bleeding and is a frequent cause of hemotympanum. Cholesterol granulomas typically affect young to middle-aged patients often with a history of chronic otitis media [28].

#### 4.14.3.1 CT Findings

CT demonstrates a sharply marginated, expansile, petrous apex isodense non-enhancing lesion with a petrous apex epicenter. The mass is principally identified by bone erosion. It usually erodes the internal auditory canal and may extend into the posterior fossa as an extradural cerebellopontine angle mass. It may show thin peripheral enhancement on the contrast scan. These lesions are more erosive when located at the petrous apex as compared to the middle ear where they rarely cause erosions [29].

#### 4.14.3.2 MRI Findings

T1- and T2-weighted images demonstrate a sharply and smoothly marginated tumour mass, MRI is more specific than CT for the diagnosis of petrous cholesterol cysts. These reveal hyperintense signal on T1- and T2-weighted images, which does not get suppressed on fat-saturated sequence. These lesions, unlike cholesteatoma, do not reveal restricted diffusion [28].

### 4.14.4 Primary Petrous Apex Cholesteatomas (Epidermoid Cysts) (Fig. 4.23)

It may just be an extension of a secondary cholesteatoma or an inflammatory cholesteatoma in an unusual location. These may be rarely primarily arising from cellular rests. CT detects petrous apex involvement.

*Congenital cholesteatomas* are identical to epidermoid cysts, differing only in name and location [30]. These occur within the temporal bone (the petrous apex being a common site), at the cerebellopontine angle, or in the middle ear left.

#### 4.14.4.1 CT and MRI Features

The tumours occurring in the cerebellopontine angle are hypodense with respect to the brain and isodense with cerebrospinal fluid. Therefore, the displacement of the

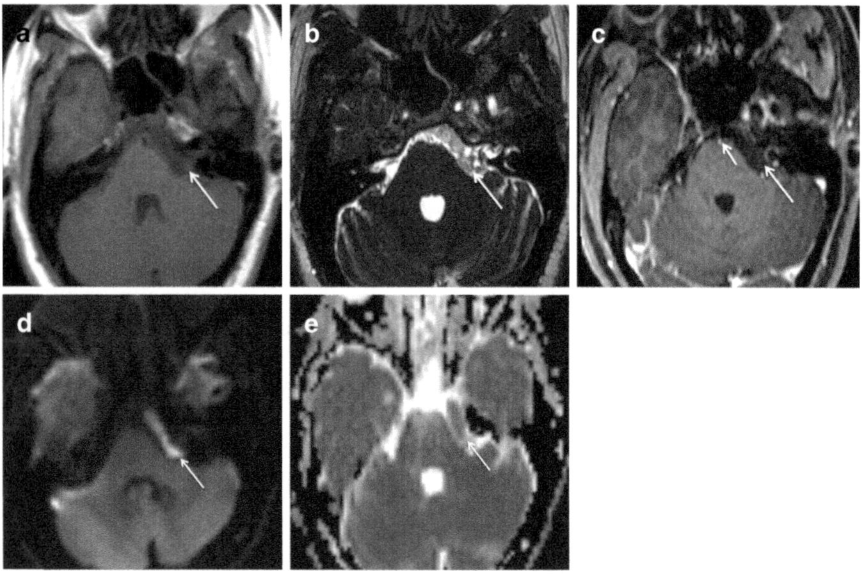


**Fig. 4.23** Epidermoid cyst. Axial MRI brain reveals heterogeneously T1 hypointense (**a**) and T2 hyperintense (**b**) lesion along the posterior petrous cortex. It reveals restricted diffusion with corresponding low ADC levels (**d**). There is no significant contrast enhancement seen within this lesion (**c**). There is partial encasemet of basilar artery with mild attenuation (short white arrow in **c**)

pons and brachium pontis may be the only early signs visible on CT. Intrathecal contrast or gas cisternography were earlier used to make the diagnosis. However, MRI has not replaced these procedures. These lesions, as compared to cholesterol granulomas are iso to hypointense on T2 with restricted diffusion on DWI sequence. They may occasionally reveal peripheral thin enhancement. They mildly attenuate on FLAIR images, unlike Cholesterol granulomas which never attenuate.

The tumours arising within the temporal bone and middle ear are seen on CT and MRI as slowly expansile destructive masses. Middle ear congenital epidermoid cysts cannot be separated from the acquired variety except by the fact that the tympanic membrane is usually spared in the congenital variety [30].

### 4.14.5 Glomus Tumours

Glomus tumours (chemodectomas, paragangliomas) are tumours located in the jugular bulb (glomus jugulare), promontory (glomus tympanicum) and along the course of the vagus nerve below the skull base (glomus vagale) [9].

The glomus jugulare (Fig. 4.24) arises from glomus bodies along Arnold's nerve (auricular branch of cranial nerve X) and the glomus tympanicum arises from glomus bodies along Jacobson's nerve (tympanic division of cranial nerve IX). The glomus jugulare is more common than the glomus tympanicum. These tumours are seen in adults, typically between 40 and 60 years of age, with a moderate female predilection [31].

The glomus tympanicum tumour (Fig. 4.25) is the most common tumour in the middle ear followed by the facial neuroma [9]. It has a female predominance (M:F = 1:3); presentation is most common when patients are more than 40 years old [32].

Axial and coronal thin sections with soft tissue and bone window settings are obtained. I.V. contrast is always required.

#### 4.14.5.1 CT Features

**The glomus tympanicum tumour**

This is seen as a characteristic soft tissue mass (in the hypotympanic recess) with its base along the promontory. It has a high CT attenuation value and enhances markedly, similar to haemangiomas. CT detects hypotympanic recess tumours as small as 3 mm and is more specific than MRI for these small lesions. As the mass grows, it will be detected as a soft tissue lesion completely filling the middle ear air cavity and occluding the eustachian tube. It may extend into the mastoid sinus, grow through the tympanic membrane and protrude into the external auditory canal. Osseous destruction is not typical of glomus tympanicum tumours as it is of glomus jugulare. Despite encasement of the middle ear cavity, the ossicles remain intact.

**The glomus jugulare tumour**

This is the most common bone-destroying tumour arising from the jugular fossa. CT gives the exact extent and size of the tumour mass. The tumour is seen as a soft tissue mass eroding the posteroinferior petrous pyramid and ascending into the

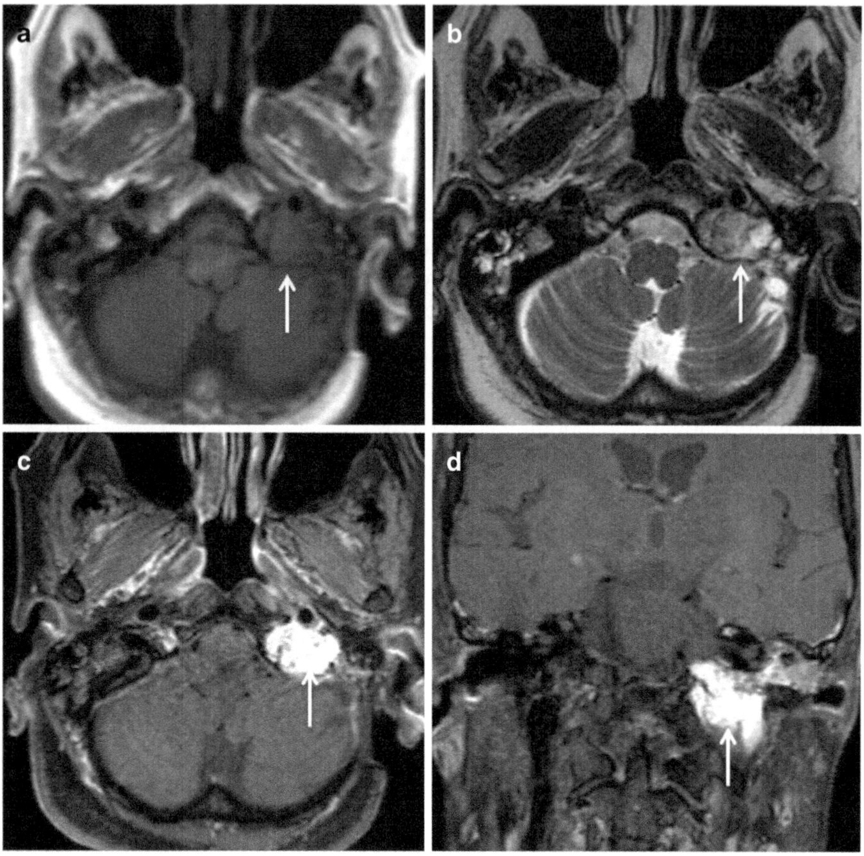


**Fig. 4.24** Glomus jugulare. Axial MRI brain reveals T1 iso to hypointense (**a**) and T2 hyperintense (**b**) lesion in the region of jugular bulb, which is not seen separately. Image (**b**) shows T2 hypointense signal within the lesion giving 'salt and pepper' appearance. Intense heterogenous enhancement is seen within this lesion as demonstrated in axial and coronal contrast MRI scan (**c** and **d**)

middle ear. It is an expansile, permeative tumour destroying the walls of the jugular foramen, the jugular tubercle, and the hypoglossal canal. Frequently, it invades the tympanic cavity typically involving the eustachian tube. The hyperdense ossicles may be destroyed. The tumour often spreads into the parapharyngeal air space. Intracranial extension occasionally occurs through destroyed osteolytic skull base defects. This is usually extradural in location. Caudally, the tumour extension causes destruction of the hypoglossal canal and the occipital condyles. The subtemporal components frequently enhance. Rarely, a patient may have bilateral glomus jugulare tumours. Usually, by the time the tumour is detected, it attains such a large size that it is unresectable [9, 11].

On angiography, the glomus tumours are hypervascular and easily detected with the exception of glomus tympanicum. These are small tumours and superimposition

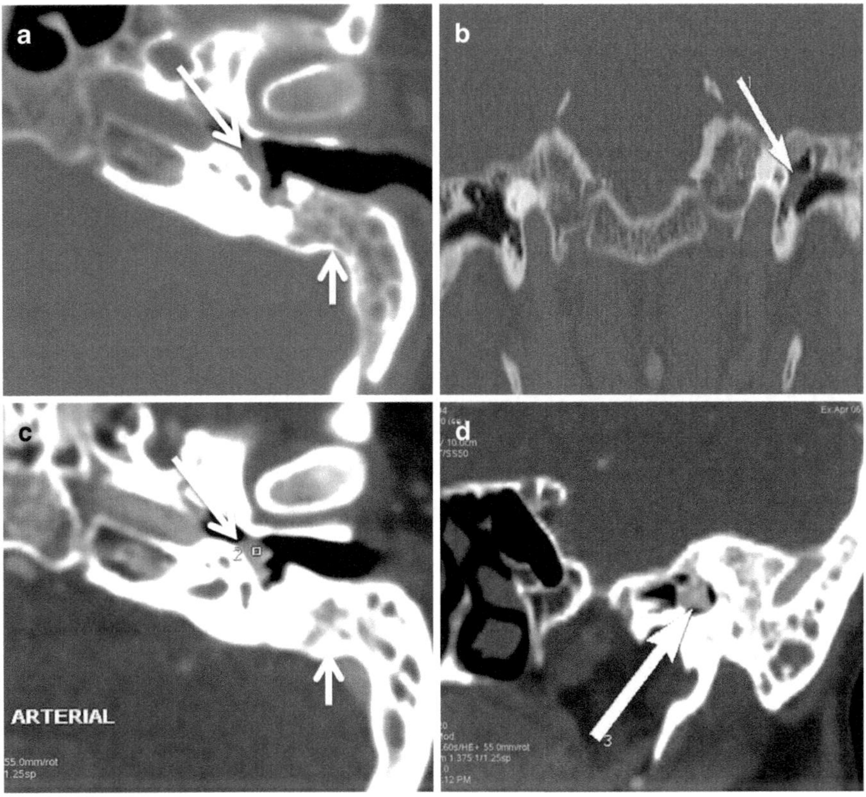


**Fig. 4.25** Glomus tympanicum. Axial and coronal plain CT of left temporal bone shows small isodense lesion (long white arrow) in middle ear cavity (arrows). It shows intense contrast enhancement as seen in axial (**c**) and coronal (**d**) post contrast CT scan. Incidentally seen is left mastoiditis (short white arrow)

of bone makes it difficult to see them adequately on conventional angiography. Hence CT/DSA (digital subtraction angiography) are valuable in the diagnosis of glomus tympanicum.

#### 4.14.5.2 Angiography Findings of Glomus Tumours

The most common vessels to supply the tumour are the inferior tympanic branch of the ascending pharyngeal and the stylomastoid branch of the occipital artery. Typically, a homogeneous stain is seen as these tumours are hypervascular [10].

There are three features that are characteristic of the invasiveness of the glomus jugulare tumour:

1. Permeative destruction of bone, which distinguishes it from neuromas arising in the jugular fossa. Neuromas produce well-defined enlargement of the fossa and arise in the pars nervosa [33]. They are therefore unlikely to erode into the middle ear.

2. Destruction of the caroticojugular spine (Phelp sign) [34]
3. Invasion of the jugular bulb

Clinically, the glomus tumours produce pulsatile tinnitus. Three middle ear vascular anomalies namely high jugular bulb, jugular bulb dehiscence and jugular bulb diverticulum also produce pulsatile tinnitus and therefore, should be looked for carefully in digital subtraction angiography.

Amongst the vascular masses which produce pulsatile tinnitus, glomus tumours especially require angiographic vascular mapping preoperatively. Also, they can be multicentric in about 10% of cases and these can be adequately diagnosed on arch aortography with four-vessel angiography [9–11].

#### 4.14.5.3 MRI Findings of Glomus Tumours

The high flow serpentine tumour vessels of the glomus tumours are seen as signal void areas producing a characteristic "salt and pepper" pattern. This "salt and pepper" appearance is seen as multiple punctate and serpiginous areas of signal void within a matrix of T1 is isointensity and T2 muscle hyperintensity on both T1 and T2 and T2 weighted images. Heterogeneous enhancement can be seen. MRI best shows the tumour relationship to the internal carotid artery and internal jugular vein and intracranial extension. Ipsilateral tongue atrophy is commonly seen. Invasion of the jugular vein can be demonstrated as a soft tissue mass within the normally signal void vein [34].

### 4.14.6 Differential Diagnosis

The differential diagnosis for Glomus Tympanicum includes glomus jugulare extension, aberrant internal carotid artery and cholesteatoma.

- The glomus jugulare extension:

The glomus jugulare tumour extending into the tympanum will be seen arising from the jugular foramen causing regional osteolysis, thus excluding a glomus tympanicum tumour.

- The aberrant internal carotid artery:

The position of the internal carotid artery under and not lateral to the cochlea as detected by CT or MRI coronal technique with an intact medial carotid canal margin excludes the aberrant internal carotid artery.

- Acquired cholesteatoma:

Acquired cholesteatoma (Fig. 4.15) is usually bone destructive and located in Prussak's space. It usually spares the hypotympanic recess, unlike glomus tympanicum.

Major differential diagnoses for Glomus jugulare tumours include a giant jugular fossa, neuromas of cranial nerves IX, X, XI and XII nasopharyngeal malignancies and metastases.

- A giant jugular fossa: A giant jugular canal has smooth margins without any evidence of osteolysis on CT. In contrast study, the enhancement is homogeneous and contiguous with the sigmoid sinus. MRI flow effects seen in spin-echo and gradient-echo images distinguish jugular patency from tumour.
- Cranial nerve neuromas: Neuromas lack the salt and pepper MRI appearance. They produce smooth erosion rather than osteolysis and cause extraluminal rather than intraluminal venous compression. They may be "dumb-bell" shaped seen both above and below the jugular foramen and do not invade the tympanum. Neuromas may have a cystic component.
- Nasopharyngeal malignancies: Nasopharyngeal malignancies usually demonstrate characteristic nasopharyngeal involvement.
- Metastasis: Metastases are very aggressive with respect to osteolysis and rapidly produce cranial nerve palsies. They do not follow typical patterns for glomus jugulare growth. Most often, the primary site is known.

Osteomas, haemangiomas, histiocytoses X, rhabdomyosarcomas, malignant squamous cell carcinoma are amongst the other tumours that involve the temporal bone.

## 4.15 TRAUMA

Temporal bone fracture (Fig. 4.26) is thought to occur in ~20% (range 14–22%) of all calvarial fractures. They have a prevalence of 3% of all trauma patients [35]. Fracture of the petrous temporal bone is usually classified according to the main direction of the fracture plane and/or involvement of the otic capsule [36].

### 4.15.1 Imaging Techniques

The following methods of examination are used for the evaluation of temporal bone trauma:

1. Plain X-ray examination may be the first modality for evaluation of trauma however, not very helpful, except to visualize calvarial fractures, particularly, a linear fracture or squamous temporal bone which may be associated with longitudinal fractures of the petromastoid and is important to detect.
2. Conventional pleuridirectional tomography in the sagittal and coronal planes used to be performed; however, CT has now replaced the need for tomography.
3. High-resolution CT gives precise information regarding the fracture line, the degree of communication and compressive bone fractures. Additional recon-

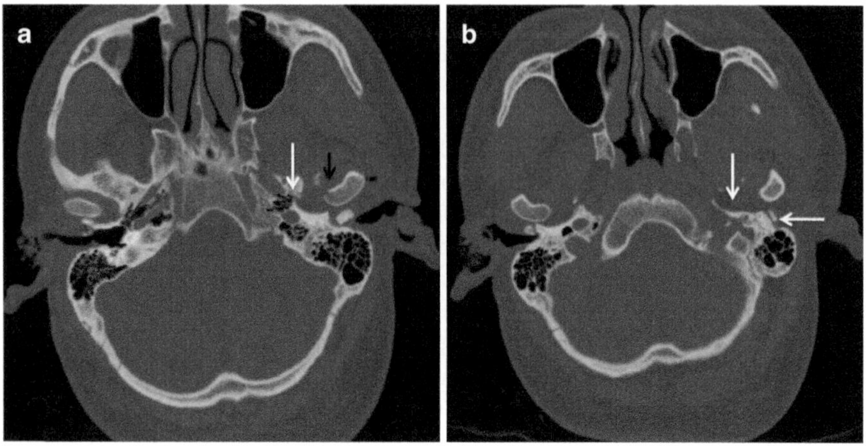


**Fig. 4.26** Temporal bone fracture. Comminuted displaced fracture of left temporal bone (mixed type) is appreciated on bone window of axial CT scan (white arrow). There is fracture of left mandibular condyle also seen (short black arrow in **a**) with displacement at left temporo-mandibular joint

structed sagittal and coronal images are almost always required and give valuable information.

4. Contrast CT cisternography may be needed in patients with suspected or established CSF leak [8].
5. MRI is less useful than CT for the evaluation of fracture. This technique is superior to CT in the evaluation of epidural–subdural hematoma, intracerebral haemorrhage and vascular injuries. MRI cisternography with or without contrast is helpful in diagnosing SCF leak [8].
6. Angiography is indicated to demonstrate internal carotid artery dissection, carotico-cavernous fistula when longitudinal fractures involve the carotid canal.

Temporal bone fractures are classified into three types according to the fracture plane passing through the longitudinal axis of the petrous bone:

1. Longitudinal
2. Transverse and
3. Complex

Three-fourths of the temporal fractures are longitudinal. Facial nerve paralysis occurs in 10–20% of patients. Comminuted bony fragments in the middle ear are seen compressing the intratympanic facial nerve.

Both longitudinal and transverse fractures produce hearing loss but only longitudinal fractures give rise to ossicular damage that are amenable to surgery (transverse fractures tend to pass through the inner ear [37].

Mixed temporal bone fractures are a combination of longitudinal and transverse fracture types, and are probably the most common type. They frequently involve the otic capsule and are associated with both conductive and sensorineural hearing loss [36].

### 4.15.2 Meniere's Disease (Endolymphatic Hydrops)

Ménière disease (or idiopathic endolymphatic hydrops) is an inner ear disorder and as such can affect balance and hearing. Although considered to be idiopathic, there is an association between inner ear effusions and endolymphatic hydrops [38].

It occurs as a result of excessive accumulation of endolymph secondary to either overproduction and/or decreased absorption occurring at the endolymphatic sac.

#### 4.15.2.1 CT and MRI Findings

At high-resolution temporal bone CT, a smaller or obliterated (non-visible) vestibular aqueduct is more often seen in ears affected with Ménière disease compared to controls [39].

During the past decade, the morphologic substrate of Ménière disease, i.e. endolymphatic hydrops, has become visible using high-resolution MRI techniques[9].

Non-contrast MRI technique uses a heavily T2-weighted sequence (such as the vendor-specific sequences CISS or FIESTA-C).

The following findings have been correlated with Ménière disease or at least advanced stages of it [38]:

- Elongation of the saccule (height >1.5–1.6 mm)
- Nonvisibility of the endolymphatic duct and sac
- Reduced fluid length within the cochlear aqueduct

Contrast-enhanced MRI makes use of a 3D fluid-attenuated inversion recovery (FLAIR) sequence or a 3D inversion recovery (IR) sequence, 4 h after intravenous gadolinium administration [40]. The contrast material diffuses into the perilymph but not the endolymph. The sequence can also be obtained 24 h after intratympanic gadolinium administration; however, this method is less preferred.

The following findings on delayed post-contrast 3D FLAIR support endolymphatic hydrops, to detect Ménière disease [40]:

- Vestibular endolymphatic space (saccule and utricle) occupying >33% of the vestibule (significant if >50%)
- Cochlear endolymphatic space (scala media) enlargement displacing Reissner's membrane (significant if endolymphatic compartment exceeds area of the scala vestibuli)
- Saccule larger than utricle

## 4.16 Preoperative, Intraoperative and Postoperative Imaging in Cochlear Implant Surgery

The incidence of Cochlear implant surgery has risen in the last few years. In order to avoid any surgical surprises, it is important to obtain a good temporal bone CT and MRI. Imaging in recent years has shown significant improvement in quality and resolution thereby providing optimum details for surgical planning. CT provides details of temporal bone anatomy and MRI gives information on fluid-filled spaces, vestibulocochlear nerve and also aids in ruling out central neurological causes.

### 4.16.1 Preoperative Imaging

HRCT of temporal bone and MRI of the same region are invaluable modalities for preoperative evaluation of inner, middle and external ear. It is important for the surgeon to be aware of congenital malformation of the ear for patient selection. Information regarding anatomical variations like an aberrant course of facial nerve or carotid artery, dehiscent facial nerve canal or jugular bulb as well as concomitant external or middle ear infections are also essential for surgical planning.

#### 4.16.1.1 Congenital Malformations of the Ear

Developmental insults during embryogenesis can lead to a spectrum of inner ear anomalies and these too can be well evaluated using these imaging modalities.

Congenital sensorineural hearing loss arises as a result of abnormalities in the inner ear, the vestibulocochlear nerve, or the processing centers of the brain. The abnormality may have a genetic cause or be a sequela of infection or injury at birth or idiopathic [41].

CT Imaging and MRI imaging protocols have been discussed at the beginning of this chapter.

**Embryology of Inner Ear**

A good understanding of embryology of the inner ear makes it easier to interpret congenital malformations (Fig. 4.27a–f).

The inner ear arises from the otic placode in a process that begins early in the third week of gestation. By the eighth week, the development of the cochlea is complete. The vestibule is completely developed by the 11th week, and the semicircular canals, between the 19th and 22nd week; the lateral canal or duct is the last to form. Ossification of the labyrinth is complete by the 23rd week, and the development of the inner ear is complete by the 26th week. Various inner ear malformations may result from developmental arrest at any prior stage, with the type of malformation depending on the gestational age at which the arrest occurs [41, 42].

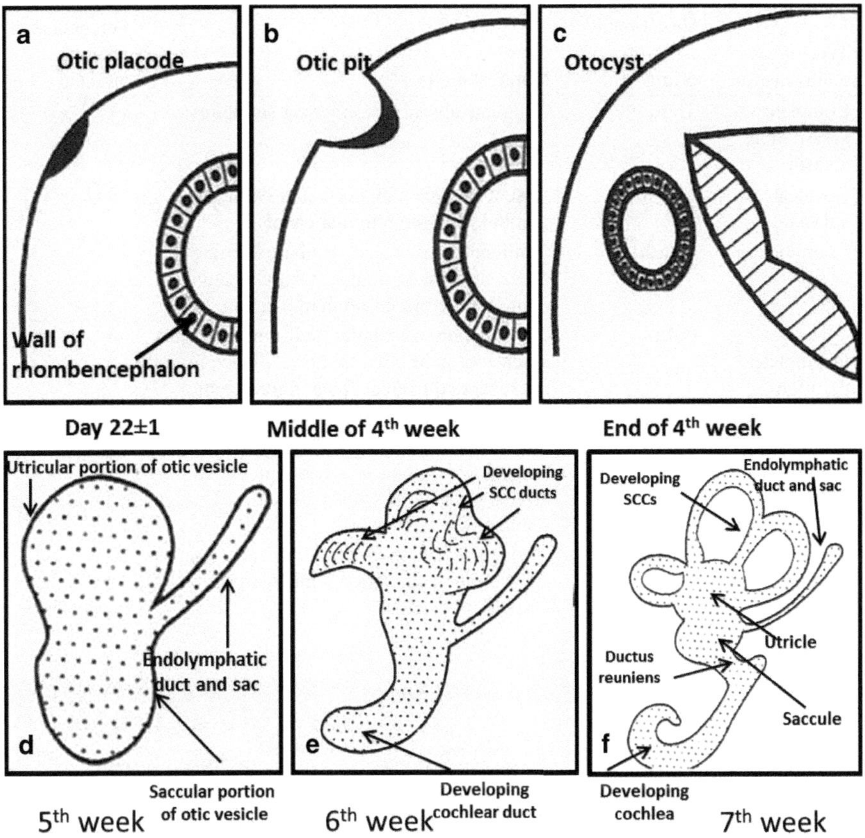


**Fig. 4.27** Embrology of the ear. The images a tof show development of ear in corresponding weeks of gestation. (*Image modified from Inderbir Singh's Human Embryology book*)

(A) *Malformations Involving Membranous Labyrinth*

1. Complete membranous labyrinth dysplasia (Bing–Siebenmann malformation)
2. Cochleosaccular dysplasia (Scheibe malformation)
3. Cochlear basal turn dysplasia (Alexander dysplasia).

(B) *Malformations Involving Osseous and Membranous Labyrinth*

These depend on the time of gestation at which the developmental failure or insult has occurred.

| Type of malformation | Gestational week of origin* | Manifestations | Percentage of patients affected |
|---|---|---|---|
| Complete labyrinthine aplasia | Third | Complete absence of inner ear structures | 1 |
| Cochlear aplasia | Late third | Absent cochlea with normal or deformed vestibule and semicircular canals | 3 |
| Common cavity | Fourth | Confluent cochlea and vestibule forming a cystic cavity with no internal architecture' normal or deformed semicircular canals | 25 |
| Type I incomplete partition | Fifth | Cystic cochleovestibular malformation with absence of modiolus; cystic vestibule present but separated from cochlea; figure-eight or snowman-like appearance on axial CT and MR images | 6 |
| Cochlear hypoplasia | Sixth | Small cochlear bud with less than one turn; normal or deformed vestibule and semicircular canals | 15 |
| Type II incomplete partition | Seventh | Cochlea with normal basal turn and cystic apex; strong association with enlarged vestibular aqueduct | 50 |

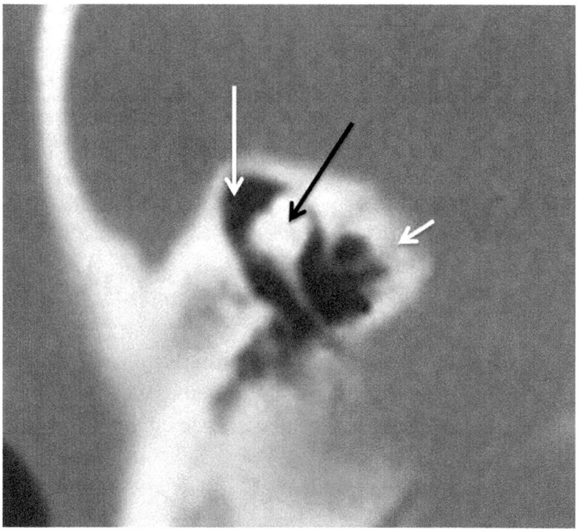

**Fig. 4.28** Complete labyrinthine aplasia. Michel's deformity: CT reveals complete absence of the bony labyrinth (arrow). Note the absence of bulge (promontory) on the medial wall of the middle ear cavity, which is normally seen due to the basal turn of cochlea. *(Image Courtesy: Dr. Akshay Baheti, Tata Memorial Hospital)*

1. *Complete Labyrinthine Aplasia (Michel Aplasia)*
   This is the most severe and rare form of labyrinthine malformation (<1%), first described by Michel in 1863 and hence goes by the name Michel Aplasia [43] (Fig. 4.28). It occurs due to arrest in the development of otic placode at third week of gestation. There is a complete absence of inner ear structures with a narrow atretic IAC on imaging [41, 43, 44]. There is an associated absence of the

eighth cranial nerve. The condition may be unilateral or bilateral with a high incidence of dysplastic opposite side inner ear in unilateral cases.

This condition may also be associated with dysplasia of petrous and mastoid bones and middle ear or skull base and vascular anomalies.

2. *Complete cochlear aplasia*
   Cochlear aplasia (Fig. 4.29) too is a rare anomaly, accounting for 3% of total inner ear malformations. It occurs due to developmental arrest at 3–5 weeks of gestation. The vestibule and semicircular canals may be present or dysplastic [41, 45]. There is dense otic bone identified in place of cochlea and is best appreciated on a CT scan.
3. *Common Cavity*
   It accounts for approximately one-fourth of the total cases of congenital cochlear anomalies. It is characterized by the formation of a common cystic cavity between the vestibule and cochlea without differentiation of internal structures (Fig. 4.30). The average height and width of the cystic cavity are approximately 7 mm and 10 mm, respectively [46]. It is commonly associated with malformations of semicircular canals. CT and MR imaging very well demonstrate the anomaly.
4. *Type I incomplete partition (Cystic cochlea vestibular malformation)*
   This condition occurs due to developmental arrest in the fifth week of gestation [45]. There is a partition seen between the vestibule and cochlea on CT and MR Imaging; however, the cochlea is cystic with absent modiolus, interscalar septum and vestibule are dilated, giving an appearance of figure of "8" [47] (Fig. 4.31). The IAC is dilated with partially dehiscent lamina cribrosa, predisposing the patient to meningitis or perilymphatic gusher during surgery.

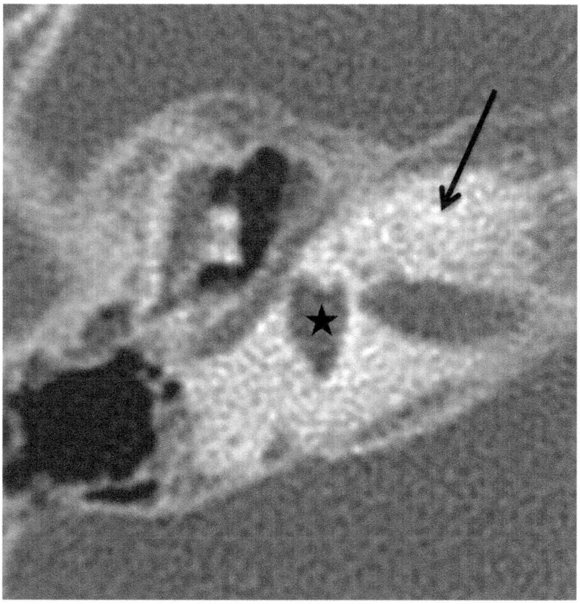

**Fig. 4.29** Cochlear aplasia: CT section reveals complete absence of the cochlea (arrow), with relatively spared vestibule (star), suggestive of cochlear aplasia. *(Image Courtesy: Dr. Akshay Baheti, Tata Memorial Hospital)*

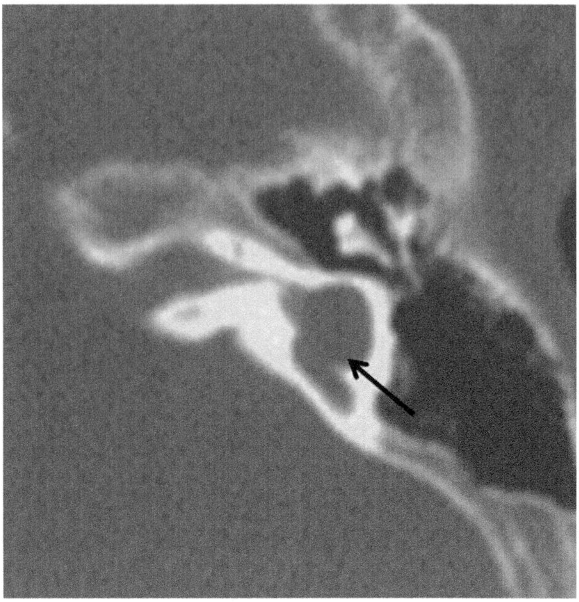

**Fig. 4.30** Common cavity malformation: CT section reveals lack of differentiation between the cochlea and vestibule, with a single common cystic cavity present (arrow). *(Image Courtesy: Dr. Akshay Baheti, Tata Memorial Hospital)*

5. *Cochlear Hypoplasia*
   It is the result of arrest of development at 6 weeks of gestation, involving the cochlear duct [45]. It is characterized by a small cochlear bud with partial or one turn (Fig. 4.32). The IAC is narrow. There may be associated malformations of vestibule and semicircular canals appreciated on CT and MR imaging.
   It accounts for 15% of developmental cochlear anomalies.
   It can be divided into four types:
   (a) Bud-like cochlea (CH-I)
   (b) Cystic hypoplastic cochlea (CH-II)
   (c) Cochlea with less than two turns (CH-III)
   (d) Cochlea with hypoplastic middle and apical turns (CH-IV) [47]

6. *Type II Incomplete partition (Mondini Deformity)*
   It is the most common type of congenital inner ear anomaly and accounts for 50% of total cases (Fig. 4.33). It occurs as a result of developmental arrest at the seventh week of gestation [45]. The cochlea consists of 1 and ½ turns with a normal basal turn and cystic apex [41, 47]. The modiolus is present at the level of basal turn. The condition is described by the following triad:
   (a) Cochlea with normal basal turn and cystic apex
   (b) Enlarged vestibule and vestibular aqueduct
   (c) Normal semicircular canals

MR CISS imaging is valuable in visualizing anatomical details.

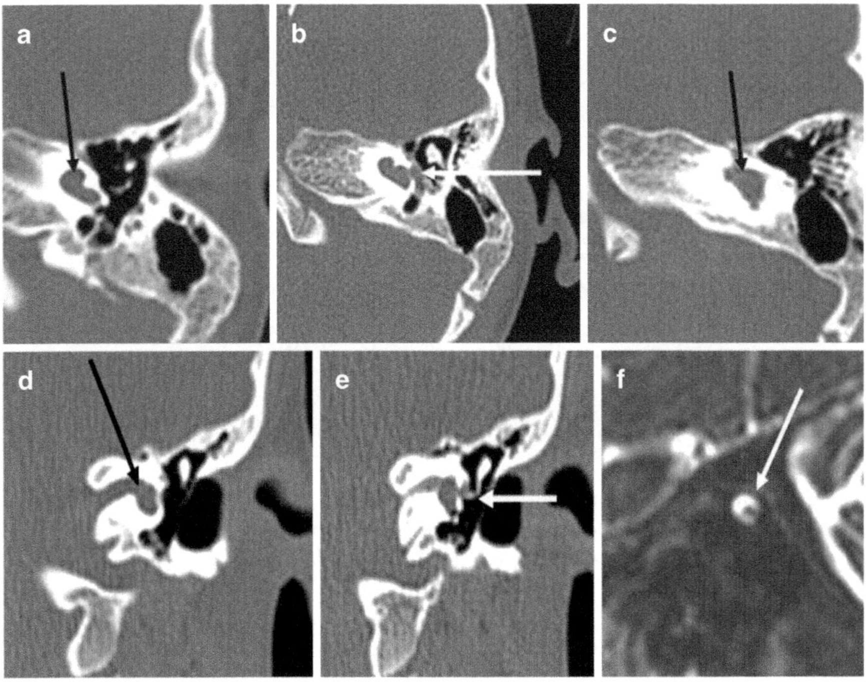


**Fig. 4.31** Incomplete partition type-I defect: Sequential axial CT sections show a cystic cochlea without modiolus (**a**) and dilated vestibule (**c**). The IAC is normal in caliber. There is an associated deficient oval window present (**b**) leading to CSF leak, which is appreciated as minimal fluid adjacent to the defect in the middle ear cavity. The patient had presented with recurrent meningitis and severe left hearing loss. The right ear was normal. IP-I defect: Sequential coronal CT sections of the same patient reveal the lateral aspect of IAC to be deficient (**d**). The deficient oval window and fluid in the middle ear cavity is well visualized (**e**). Oblique sagittal MRI image of the left IAC (**f**) shows the eighth nerve to be absent and the facial N to be more posteriorly located. *(Image Courtesy: Dr. Akshay Baheti, Tata Memorial Hospital)*

7. *Type III Incomplete partition (X linked hearing loss)*
   It is a rare, nonsyndromic type of congenital presenting with mixed conductive and sensorineural hearing loss caused by mutation of gene POU3F4 on the X chromosome. On Imaging, it is characterized by "corkscrew" cochlea with absent modiolus and lamina cribrosa. In addition, there is thinning of the otic capsule, symmetric widening of the fundus of bilateral internal acoustic canals, irregular vestibule with cystic bulges, dysplastic oval and round windows and dilated labyrinthine segment of the facial nerve [47].

(C) *Malformations Involving Vestibule and Semicircular Canals*

The semicircular canals develop between the 6th and 22nd week of gestations [2]. Any insult during this period can lead to various degrees of malformations.

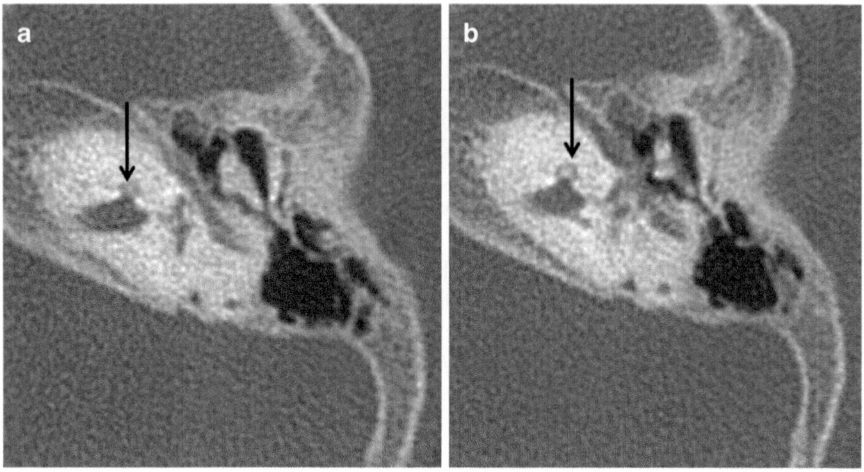


**Fig. 4.32** Cochleovestibular hypoplasia: Contiguous axial CT images show a severely hypoplastic cochlea (arrow) and the cochlear nerve canal with concomitant hypoplasia of the vestibule. *(Image Courtesy: Dr. Akshay Baheti, Tata Memorial Hospital)*

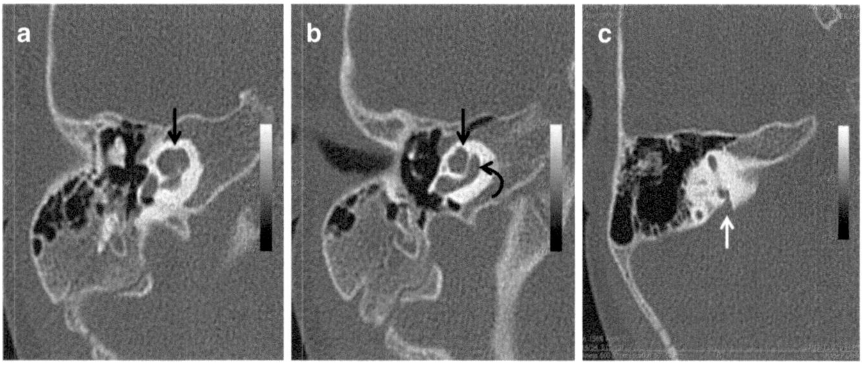


**Fig. 4.33** Incomplete partition type-II defect. Axial CT images show a normal basal turn of cochlea (curved black arrow) and fused middle and apical turns (straight black arrows. Note the dilated VA (white arrow). *(Image Courtesy: Dr. Akshay Baheti, Tata Memorial Hospital)*

## Aplasia of Semicircular canals

There is a complete absence of semicircular canals. It is commonly associated with atresia of oval window, abnormal course of facial nerve, abnormal ossicles and cochlear dysplasia. It is often seen in CHARGE syndrome [48].

## Lateral Semicircular canal dysplasia

The superior semicircular canal is the first to form, followed by the posterior semicircular canal followed by lateral semicircular canal. In this condition, the vestibule is dilated and is continuous with the lateral semicircular canal. It may be associated with cochlear anomalies.

**Vestibular Malformation**
This may include dilatation of the vestibule with partial or complete communication with one of the semicircular canals [2, 41, 45].

**Enlarged Endolyphatic duct and sac**
Enlarged vestibular duct occurs due to developmental insult at 7 weeks of gestation. It is the most common inner ear malformation in patients with early-onset Sensorineural Hearing Loss. It is bilateral in most cases and shows female predominance. CT reveals an enlarged osseous vestibular duct and MRI reveals dilated endolymphatic duct and sac. This can be measured on axial CT and T2-weighted MRI where the diameter should be less than or equal to 1.5 mm. A better way of evaluating this is to compare the diameter of vestibular aqueduct to ascending limb of posterior semicircular canal adjacent to it, which also measures the same [2, 49].

This condition is associated with Pendred syndrome. In addition, there may be other associated inner ear malformations also seen.

**Abnormalities of IAC** (Fig. 4.34) **and Cochlear Nerve:**
The IAC may be atretic, stenostic or may show a bony septum. It is termed stenostic; it measures <2 mm in diameter (normal range: 2–8 mm)

There may be hypoplasia of bony canal of cochlear nerve. Sagittal CISS MR images demonstrate the four parts of the seventh–eighth nerve complex (Fig.)

A normal diameter and appearance of IAC do not exclude eighth nerve anomalies.

There are three types of cochlear nerve anomalies [2]:

- Type 1—Absent eighth nerve with stenotic IAC
- Type 2A—Common Vestibulocochlear nerve with hypoplastic/aplastic cochlear branch and associated other inner ear malformations
- Type 2B—Common vestibulocochlear nerve with hypoplastic/aplastic cochlear branch and normal inner ear structures

**Surgical Point of View**
Inner ear malformations are found in 15–20% of patients with severe sensorineural Hearing loss.

From a surgical point of view, congenital inner ear malformations have been classified into three groups [50]:

1. Gross Malformations (contraindication to surgery)
   Complete labyrinthine aplasia, cochlear aplasia and cochlear nerve deficiency fall under the bracket of gross malformations and are contraindications for cochlear implantation surgery.

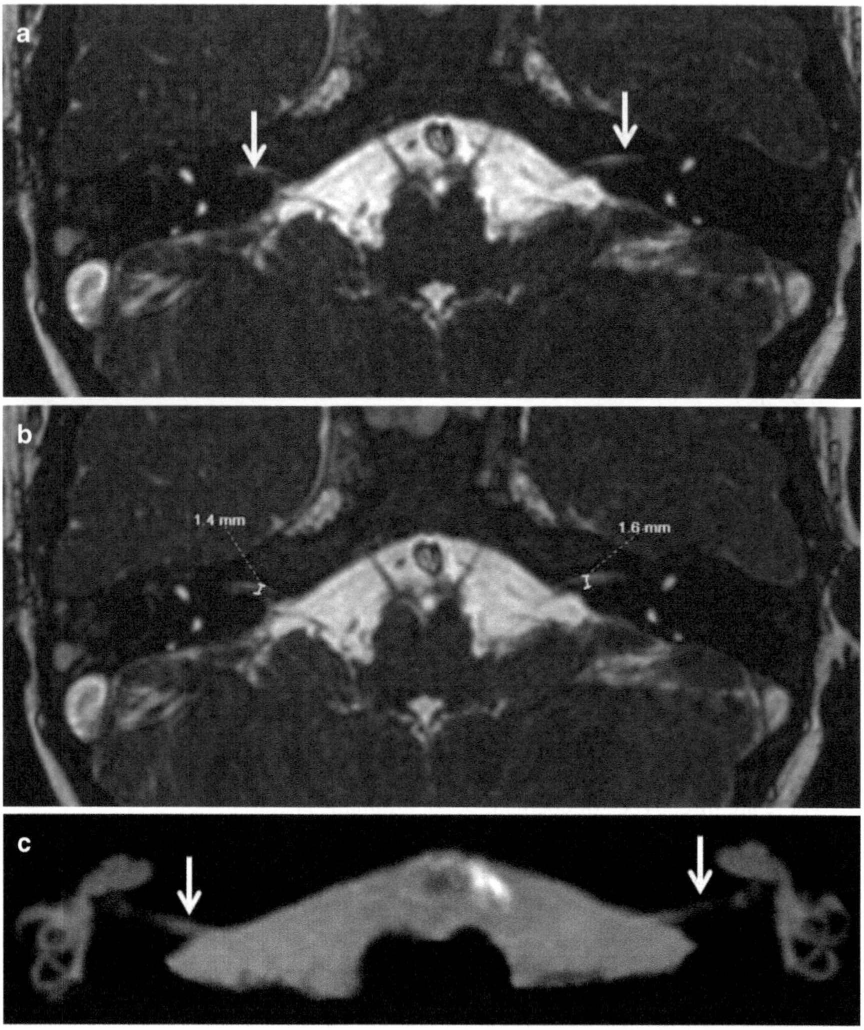


**Fig. 4.34** Bilateral stenotic IAC. Axial highly T2 weighted MRI images (**a** and **b**) reveal bilateral stenotic internal Acoustic Meatii (white arrows) with diameters <2 mm on each side. The 3D reconstructed MRI image (**c**) also well demonstrates the abnormality

In patients with an absent cochlear nerve or thin nonidentifiable cochlear nerve, a detailed presurgical evaluation is validated by an expert in order to be able to predict surgical outcome [51, 52].

2. Major Malformations (increased risk of post-surgical complications)
   Common cavity or severe cochlear hypoplasia are relative contraindications for surgery. These are associated with higher complications of CSF leak, meningitis and electrode displacement. The surgical outcome in these patients is difficult to predict [52].

3. Minor Malformations
   Mild cochlear hypoplasia and malformations of vestibule and vesticular aqueduct are considered.

#### 4.16.1.2 Congenital Malformation of Middle and External Ear

High-Resolution CT is the imaging modality of choice, in malformations of the external and middle ear. Imaging is needed for exact morphological information and presurgical planning.

The external ear, middle ear and ossicular chain develop from the first branchial groove, first and second branchial arches and first pharyngeal pouch.

The development of inner ear structures differs from that of the middle and external ear and hence are more often not associated [53].

**External Auditory Canal Atresia** (Fig. 4.35)

These patients have a deformity of auricle and nonvisualization of external auditory meatus. The deformity of auricle may be associated with a similar degree of ipsilateral jaw deformity. There may be, in addition, systemic abnormalities also present in these patients [53, 54].

One-third of the cases are bilateral with male predominance. Two types have been described:

1. Bony atresia
2. Membranous atresia

HRCT imaging is highly valuable in evaluating this condition as well as any associated middle ear/ossicular chain malformations. It is helpful in visualizing anatomical structures of middle and external ear as well as determining the need for early surgical correction (at 4 years) in patients with bilateral atresia or in patients with concomitant cholesteatoma [55, 56].

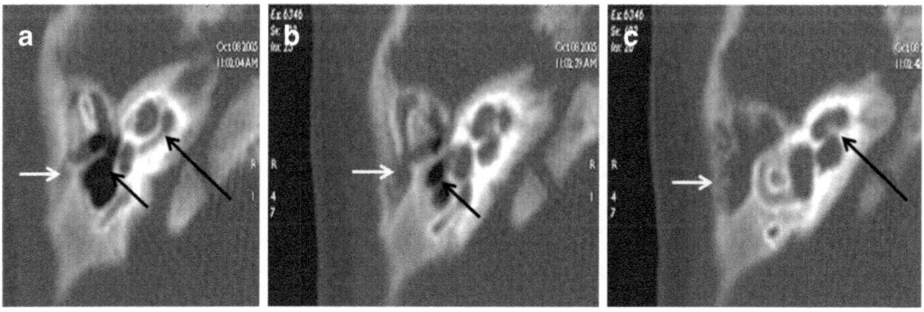


**Fig. 4.35** External auditory canal atresia (complete). Axial CT cuts (**a**–**c**) of patient reveals complete atresia of external auditory meatus (white arrow) with a small middle ear (small black arrow). The inner ear structures are unremarkable on this CT (long black arrow). (*Image Courtesy: Dr. Santosh Gupta, P. D. Hinduja Hospital)*

**TABLE External Auditory Canal Deformity**
*Classification of External Auditory Canal Atresia Slight (small external auditory canal):*

- Hypoplastic tympanic membrane
- Hypoplastic tympanic bone
- Small middle ear cavity
- Varying ossicular deformity
- Well aerated mastoid

*Moderate (absent external auditory canal):*

- Small middle ear cavity
- Atresia plate
- Deformed malleus and incus
- Well aerated mastoid

*Severe (absent external auditory canal):*

- Hypoplastic middle ear cavity
- Severe ossicular deformity
- Poor mastoid aeration
- Modified from [53, 57].

**Isolated Middle ear deformities**
Middle ear deformities are categorized as ossicular, fenestral and cholesteatomatous.

**Isolated congenital Ossicular deformities**
Stapes is most commonly involved. The least involved ossicle is malleus [53, 58].

Ossicular deformities include incudostapedial disconnections, malleoincudal fixations and fusions, stapes fixation, absent stapes and middle ear dysplasia.

Incudostapedial disconnection is seen as a gap between the high-density incus and the stapes. Malleoincudal fixation appears as a linear high attenuation band within the attic attaching malleus and/or incus to the epitympanic wall.

Stapes fixation and absent stapes can be detected with high-resolution CT scan.

Middle ear dysplasia is easily detected by the deformed middle ear cavity and its contents.

A 40–60 dB conductive hearing loss in the absence of a history of trauma or infection indicates congenital ossicular deformity in a child [59].

Imaging is of paramount importance to diagnose and help in the presurgical planning of these surgically correctable conditions.

**Fenestral anomalies**

Fenestral anomalies are rare. Oval window absence/atresia is usually associated with facial nerve canal, ossicular chain and inner ear anomalies. Oval window atresia is seen as an absence of the lucent oval window niche.

**Congenital cholesteatoma**

Middle ear congenital cholesteatoma represents 2% of all middle ear cholesteatomas. These are recognized by the presence of an intact tympanic membrane and the absence of otitis media in contract to acquired cholesteatoma.

CT is the imaging procedure of choice for ossicular, fenestral and cholesteatomatous abnormalities. MR provides only complementary information, especially for cholesteatoma investigation.

#### 4.16.1.3 Brain Abnormalities

Patients with congenital SNHL often reveal T2 hyperintensities in bilateral cerebral white matter (Fig. 4.36). MRI is also helpful in evaluating brain stem, CP angle and diseases in these regions (discussed earlier in the chapter). Congenital CMV infection which leads to SHNL can also be diagnosed on MRI.

#### 4.16.1.4 Few Other Imaging Findings That Can Impact Surgery

**Enlarged Endolymphatic duct and Sac**

The risk of CSF gusher is significantly increased in cases of dilated distal IAC (especially in case of dehiscent bone partition between cochlea and IAC) as well as in cases of dilated endolymphatic duct and sac. CSF gusher predisposes to postoperative meningitis. CT and MRI imaging prior to surgery gives details of anatomy which is essential to treat the condition promptly [60].

**Infections of the ear**

Labyrinthitis: It is important to preoperatively diagnose labyrinthine fibrosis/ossification. It occurs as a sequelae of meningitis. CT imaging of temporal bone helps in evaluating ossification better than MRI. MRI is particularly helpful in viewing labyrinthine fibrosis. In such cases, the surgeries are particularly challenging and may require an implant with a shorter electrode array.

Otitis media and Mastoiditis: It is crucial to rule out infections of the middle ear and mastoid prior to surgery to avoid the potential risk of meningitis. Acute otitis media needs to be treated with medications before surgery. Chronic mastoiditis need not pose a problem for surgery however extensive mastoid sclerosis may interfere with implant well-reservoir and limit exposure to the middle ear.

**Otosclerosis:**

This condition can be diagnosed on CT prior to surgery (Fig. 4.19). Retrofenestral ososclerosis can lead to abnormal facial nerve stimulation after surgery due to the conduction of impulses through otospongiotic bone. This can be corrected by programming out the electrodes causing abnormal stimulation.

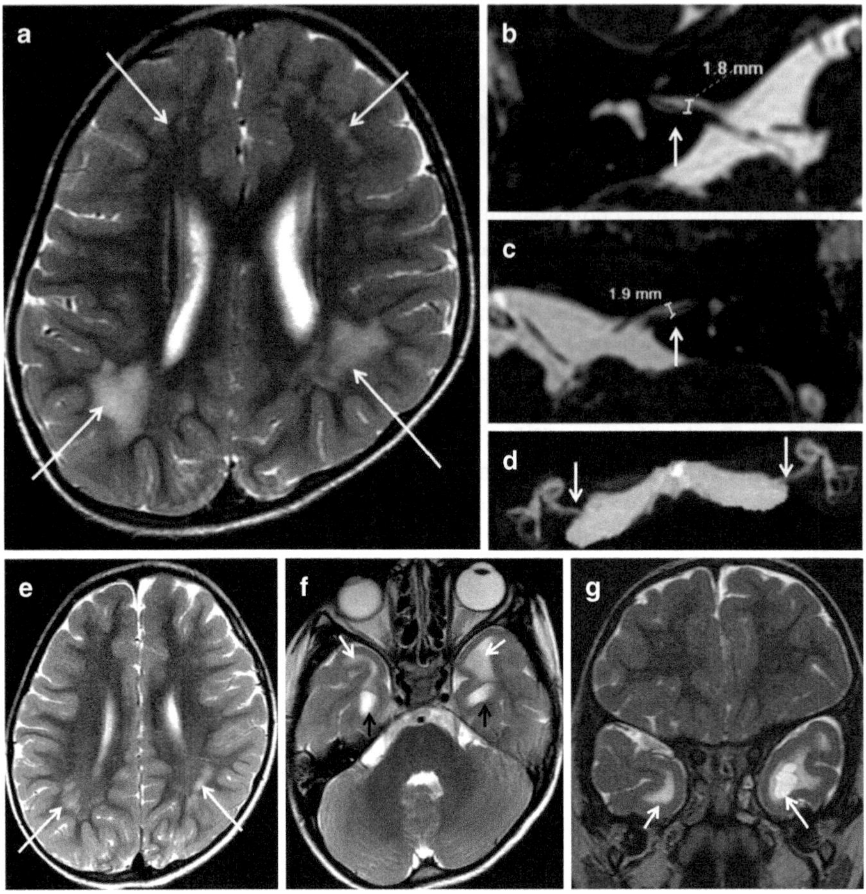


**Fig. 4.36** T2 white matter hyperintensities. Axial MRI image (**a**) of 3 year old patient during preoperative evaluation of cochlear implant reveals patchy T2 hyperintensities in bilateral frontoparital white matter (white arrows). The patient also revealed bilateral stenotic IACs on MRI CISS images (**b**,**c**) and 3D MRI reconstructed image (**d**). Axial (**a**) T2 MRI image of another child of 4 years during precochlear implant surgery showed white matter hyperintensities (long white arrows). The axial (**b**) coronal (**c**) T2 MRI image show cystic encephalomalacic changes in bilateral temporal white matter (short white arrows) with exvacuo dilatation of temporal horns of lateral ventricles (short black arrows)

**Facial Nerve Dehiscence:**
Facial Nerve dehiscence can be identified on preoperative temporal bone CT. It carries a risk of facial nerve injury during surgery and can be prevented with prior imaging.

## 4.16.2 Intraoperative Imaging

### 4.16.2.1 Cochlear Implant

Six decades after the advent of cochlear implants, the world has seen significant improvement in the types and quality of implants, surgical precision, outcomes and imaging. With the recent multichannel devices, there is significantly improved word perception and understanding. This has led to an enhanced rate of language acquisition and thereby literacy in deaf children. Unlike conventional hearing aids, the cochlear implant does not amplify sound but works by directly stimulating any functioning auditory nerves inside the cochlea with an electric field [61].

The first cochlear implantation system was successfully developed by William House in 1960 and approved by US Food and Drug Administration (FDA) in 1990 [62].

Components of cochlear implant (Fig. 4.37):

1. Receiver–Stimulator
2. Headpiece
3. Speech Processor

An external microphone and speech processor are worn behind the ear and convert sound into an electric signal. A magnet-held external transmitter sends the signal via electromagnetic induction through the skin to an internal receiver–stimulator. The receiver–stimulator converts the signal into rapid electrical impulses which are distributed to multiple electrodes on an electrode array implanted within the cochlea. The electrodes electrically stimulate the spiral ganglion cells along the cochlear turns, which then travel along the auditory nerve axons to the brain for sound perception [63].

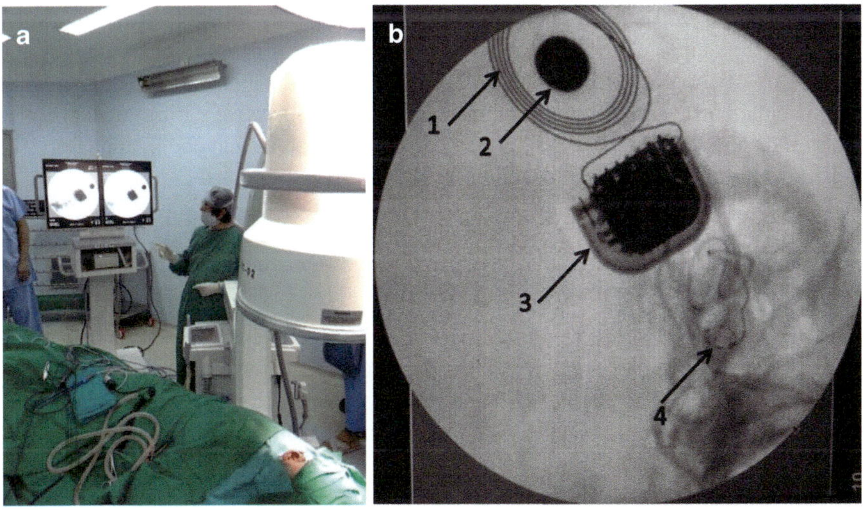


**Fig. 4.37** Intraoperative images during cochlear implant surgery. Image (**a**) is picture of the Operating Room during Cochlear Implant surgery showing utility of C-arm machine to obtain prompt images during the surgery to confirm the position of implant. Image (**b**) shows parts of cochlear implant: 1—Receiver coil; 2—Magnet; 3—Stimulator; 4—Electrode array

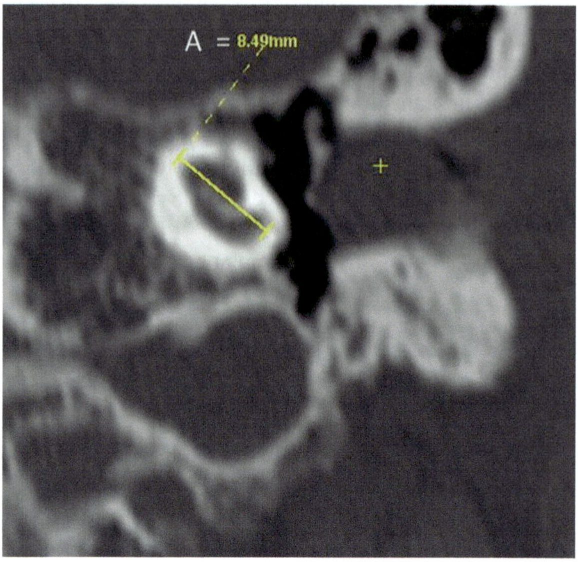


**Fig. 4.38** Cochlear duct length calculation. Evaluation of cochlear duct length (CDL) using the formula CDL = 4.16A−2.7

Preoperatively, the cochlear Duct length can be calculated. Evaluation of cochlear duct length (CDL) using the formula CDL = 4.16A−2.7 (Fig. 4.38). This helps in preoperative planning and selection of implants.

Intraoperative imaging detects unsatisfactory placement of electrodes during CI surgery [64].

Intraoperative monitoring tests during CI surgery play different roles: measurement of impedances and NRI can evaluate the integrity of implant electrodes and the status of the electrode cochlea interface, but they cannot be the only way to confirm the correct positioning of the array. The intraoperative radiological check is helpful during CI surgery (Fig. 4.39), especially with abnormal cochlear anatomy or when the surgeon questions placement [64, 65].

### 4.16.3 Postoperative Imaging

Postoperatively, recognition of scalar dislocation, cochlear dislocation, electrode fold, and malposition of the electrode array (Fig. 4.39c) may have important consequences for the patient such as revision surgery or adapted fitting [63].

Electrode position can be evaluated by any of the following modalities [66]:

1. Conventional Cochlear View X-Ray: routinely used mainly in children due to short investigation time and low radiation dose (Fig. 4.40). It gives projective information if electrode insertion into the cochlea has been, but analysis of the exact electrode position with regard to the topography of the cochlea cannot be evaluated. Modified Stenvers view is commonly used to determine electrode position.

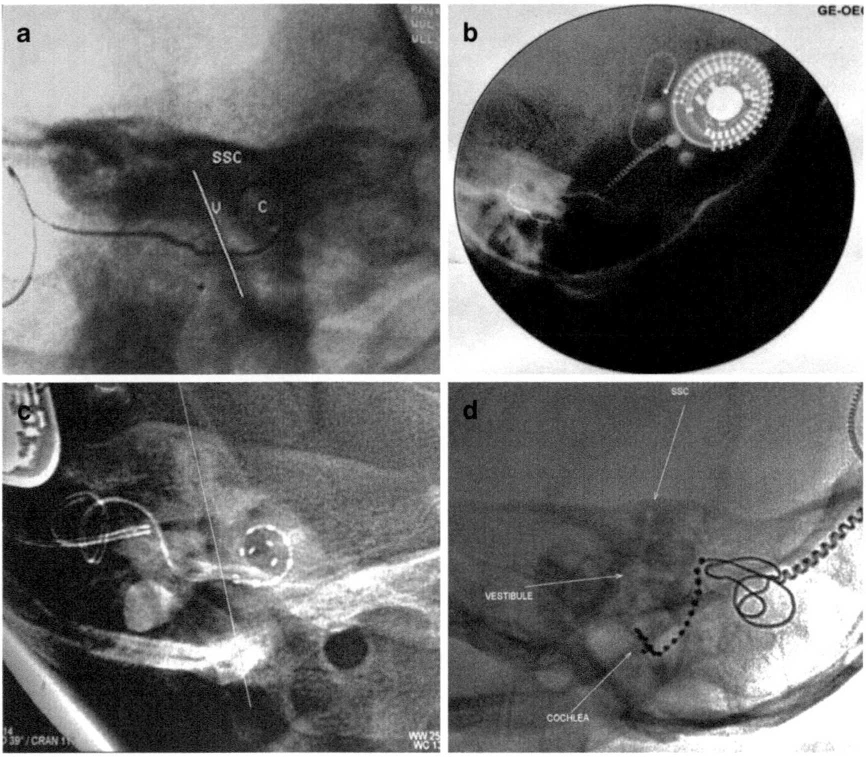


**Fig. 4.39** Post operative images of cochlear implant position. Image (**a**): Optimal placement of electrode array 2¼ turns inside the cochlea of patient with partial Mondini. *v* vestibule, *c* cochlea, *scc* superior semicircular canal. Image (**b**): C-arm picture of cochlear implant in same patient. Image (**c**): Optimal placement of Electrode array in another patient. *v* vestibule, *c* cochlea, *scc* superior semicircular canal. Image (**d**): Malpositioned electrode array

**Fig. 4.40** Postoperative X-ray of cochlear implant. Normal positioning of cochlear implant on Radiograph. 1—Receiver coil; 2—Magnet; 3—Stimulator; 4—Electrodes placed in cochlea. (*Image Courtesy: Dr. Santosh Gupta, P. D. Hinduja Hospital)*

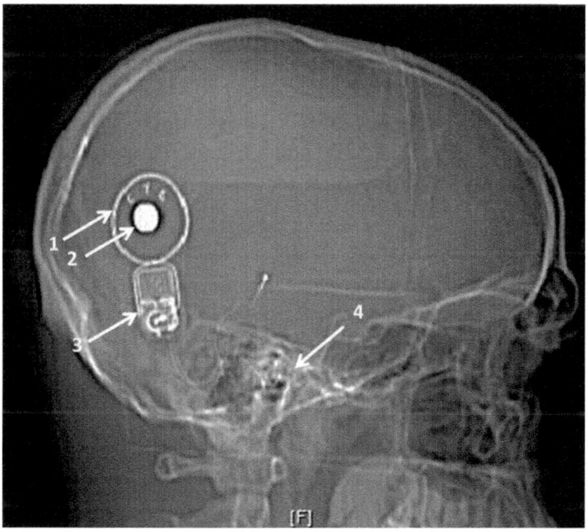

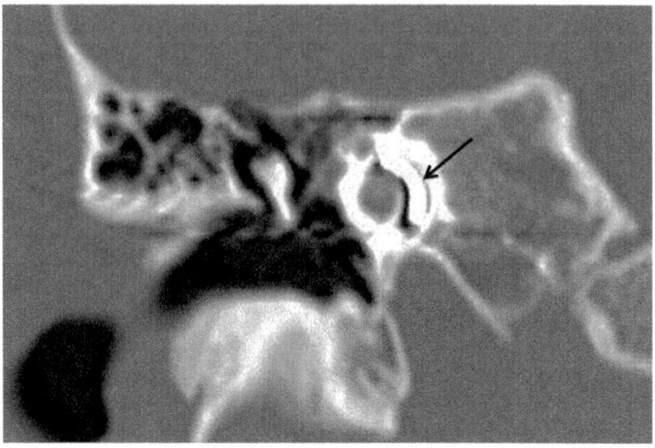

**Fig. 4.41** Post operative CT scan of cochlear implant. Normal positioning of electrode within middle turn of cochlea on CT. (*Image Courtesy: Dr. Santosh Gupta, P. D. Hinduja Hospital*)

2. Multislice CT: It allows for three-dimensional imaging (Fig. 4.41). However, it unfortunately provides metal artefacts; and hence, a more detailed view of the electrodes with regard to the given anatomical structures is desirable.
3. Cone Beam CT (CBCT): It is a low-dose imaging technique for postoperative assessment of cochlear implantation, seems to be promising with fewer artefacts, lesser radiation and higher resolution than multislice CT. But cone beam CT devices are still rare.
4. Rotational computed tomography (RT) is based on three-dimensional digital subtraction angiography. Images are taken with a rotating C-arm in a single rotation. After digital reconstruction, the intracochlear position of an electrode array can be identified. It generates images with lesser artefacts, lower radiation dose compared to MSCT and superior spatial resolution, leading to additional information on the position of the electrode in relation to the modiolus is offered
5. Flat-panel CT—It is a fast and accurate examination in the postoperative imaging of cochlear implants. It is not only superior to conventional X-ray but also superior to MSCT mainly due to fewer artefacts and delivers lower radiation than MSCT.

#### 4.16.3.1 Normal Position of Cochlear Implant

**Radiograph**

Plain radiographs can reliably assess the position and depth of insertion of the electrode within the cochlea, and identify complications.

The modified Stenver's view is used, in which the central beam through the temporal bone is at 45° posteriorly and 12° caudally demonstrates the petrous temporal bone, internal auditory meatus, and bony labyrinth. The oblique beam positions it in the plane of the superior semicircular canal and the electrodes can be visualized within the cochlea [67].

The appropriate placement of a cochlear implant is within the scala tympani, which provides optimum speech discrimination. Radiographic confirmation of intracochlear position and insertion depth is the primary aim of imaging and the gold standard for doing so [68].

All active electrodes are medial to the cochleostomy (Fig. 4.39a, b). Optimal placement is when the most proximal active electrode is as close as possible to the cochleostomy but still within the cochlea [67]. Depth of insertion of the array is important for hearing outcomes.

**CT Scan**

MSCT imaging yields the maximum detail resolution available at present in a clinical setting and provides an (almost) isotropic voxel size when appropriate data acquisition protocols are used. To solve the problem regarding the scan plane, reconstructions can be made to optimize the visualization of the electrode array. Two-dimensional reformations are a useful tool for comprehensive visualization of the electrode array within the complex architecture of the cochlea, because both the electrode contacts and small anatomic structures such as the modiolus and outer cochlear wall can be distinguished [69].

For optimal evaluation of the electrode, a paraxial mid-modiolar plane is selected using multiplanar reconstructions. Maximum intensity projections with variable slice thickness can be used for the entire visualization of the electrode array. The insertion depth of the cochlear implant can be given as the radial position of the tip ranging from 45° to a theoretical maximum of 900° (full two and a half turns) [63, 70] (Fig. 4.42 [69]).

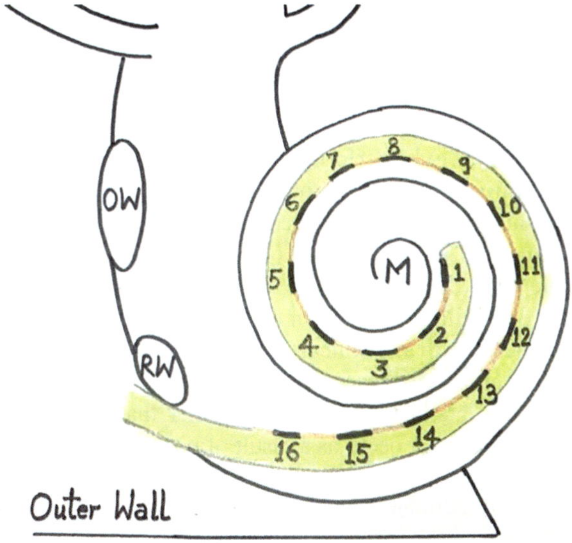


**Fig. 4.42** Schematic representation of electrode array, which is inserted into the scala tympani via a cochleostomy near the round window niche (RW). The electrode array has a reference electrode (R) and 16 equidistantly spaced contacts (black lines), numbered from the tip of the electrode array to the basal end, which are facing the modiolus (M). They are positioned on a silastic carrier (yellow) and are separated by silastic blebs (orange lines). The oval window (OW) and outer wall of the cochlea (outer wall) are indicated. *(Image modified from Reference no 73)*

The electrode array may be placed within the cochlea by three approaches namely, round window, extended round window or cochleostomy (surgical opening) [71]. The normal position of most proximal contact of an electrode is 3–4 mm from round window. The electrode array needs to be placed in scala tympani with close contact with organ of Corti for optimal benefit and hearing preservation [63].

In cases of advanced otosclerosis or labyrinthine fibrosis/ ossification, use of split electrodes may be needed, one in the basal turn and the other in the middle turn. In case of extensive ossification of basal turn, occurring as a sequela of old infective process, a retrograde approach can be used to place the electrode array through the cochlear apex [63].

**Surgical complications:**
Post-cochlear implantation complications are rare and seen in 1% of adults and children. There may be an infection at the site of flap. Some patients may complain of tinnitus and vertigo; however, these tend to resolve spontaneously. Facial nerve stimulation can rarely occur following an aggressive cochleostomy and electrode extrusion through the cochlear wall. Migration of the electrode array is very uncommon but can lead to mechanical malfunction. Imaging is helpful in evaluating these complications (Fig. 4.43a–d). Comparison of serial X-Rays is beneficial [60].

Early complications include unfavourable or malpositioning of electrode array. There may be lifting of basilar membrane seen if the array is placed close to the midline of cochlear lumen, more commonly observed with lateral wall electrodes compared to perimodiolar electrodes [63, 72] The electrode array may be placed in scala vastibuli or may translocate from scala tympani to scala vestibule and lead to a need for increasing the required stimulus charge. Given that the normal position of most proximal contact of an electrode is 3–4 mm from round window, there may be over-insertion or under-insertion of the electrode array. In case of requirement of revision surgery, it needs to be performed within a few days before fibrosis sets in. Other rare complications include electrode pinching (bend) or folding of the base of tip of electrode, which may require the deactivation of electrodes in contact [73].

Rarely there may be malpositioning of electrode array into internal acoustic meatus, tympanic cavity, vestibulum and semicircular canals which require immediate postoperative imaging confirmation for revision surgery. These are more often encountered in patients with anatomical variations and malformations.

Late complications of cochlear implant surgery include electrode migration, more often seen with lateral wall electrodes rather than perimodiolar electrodes [74]. Flap complications may occur as a result of postoperative infections or hematoma or rarely flap necrosis. There may be secondary infections involving the middle and inner ear with/without cholesteatoma [75]. Delayed neural injury due to intracochlear fibrosis may lead to gradual complete hearing loss over time [76].

*Recent imaging studies* are directed towards utilizing the property of human cochlea to transform sound waves into electrical signals in the acoustic nerve fibres with high acuity via vibrating anisotropic membranes (basilar and tectorial membranes) and frequency-specific hair cell receptors.

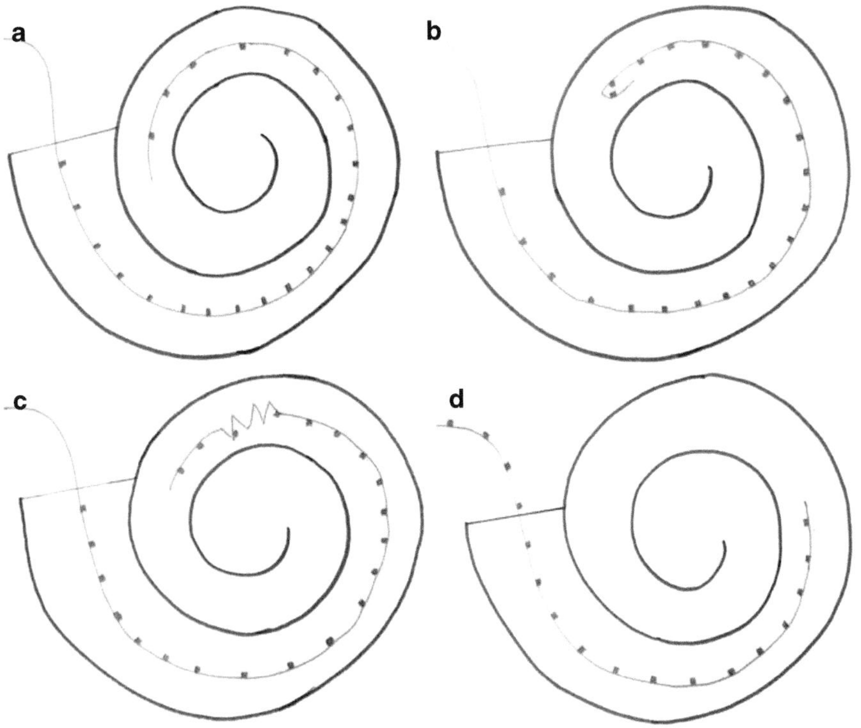


**Fig. 4.43** Schematic representation of intracochlear electrode placement and early complications. Schematic representation of intracochlear electrode placements. The red line represents the electrode array and the red square dots represent active electrodes. The blue line marks the level of the cochleostomy (entrance to the cochlea). (**a**) Full insertion into the cochlea. All active electrodes are medial to the cochleostomy. Optimal placement is when the most proximal active electrode is as close as possible to the cochleostomy but still within the cochlea. (**b**) Electrode tip fold-over. The tip of the electrode has folded back on itself due to resistance to insertion while advancing the electrode. (**c**) Electrode kinking. A portion of the electrode has twisted on itself due to resistance to insertion while advancing the electrode. (**d**) Electrode under-insertion or extrusion. In under-insertion the electrode has not been advanced sufficiently so that all active electrodes are medial to the cochleostomy. Several active electrodes are therefore outside of the cochlea. In the case of extrusion, the electrode has slipped back via the cochleostomy, after insertion, leaving one or more electrodes lateral to the cochleostomy. *(Image modified from Reference no 69)*

The frequency positions in the cochlea can be mapped to create a tonotopic chart. This chart fits an almost-exponential function with the lowest frequencies positioned at the apex and highest frequencies positioned at the cochlear base. Dendritic mapping is used to create a three-dimensional frequency analysis of the cochlea and obtain accurate tonotopic maps of the human basilar membrane/organ of Corti and the spiral ganglion. The three-dimensional tonotopic data based on this new technique called Synchrotron Radiation Phase-Contrast Imaging (SP-PCI) has large implications for validating electrode position and creating customized frequency maps for cochlear implant recipients [77].

In PCI, the phase shifts caused by varying material properties within the sample are transformed into detectable variations in X-ray intensity, which can provide edge contrast to highlight soft tissues. Phase contrast is therefore combined with synchrotron radiation to improve soft-tissue contrast while maintaining accurate visualization of bone [78].

SR-PCI data is used to obtain detailed 3D reconstructions of the human Basilar Membrane, Spiral Ganglion and Cochlear Dendrites. Accurate 3D visualization is particularly important in regions such as the cochlear hook, where dendrites follow a non-radial trajectory and tonotopic compression is observed in the Spiral Ganglion.

To receive accurate frequency-place stimulation with Cochlear Implant, variances in Basilar Membrane band length should be taken into account. Angle-to-frequency correlations can enhance place pitch assessments of cochlear implant contacts according to the neural frequency bands. Previous relationships derived between angular depth and characteristic Basilar Membrane frequencies have relied upon assumptions of the total angular length of cochleae, and in future work, the results presented herein may be used to derive angle-to-frequency relationships that are individualized based on specific Basilar Membrane angular length.

As Cochlear Implant electrode positions are clearly visible in clinical CT, angle measuring would allow clinicians to obtain individualized cochlear implant programming plans using clinically obtainable values [77]. This latest research model paves a path to revolutionize cochlear implant imaging and thereby the surgical outcomes of patients.

## 4.17 MRI Safety in Cochlear Implants

MRI scanners (Fig. 4.44) use strong magnetic fields and radio waves (radiofrequency energy) to make images. This can affect medical implants that contain metal or magnets. When this happens, the implant may move or twist inside of the patient's body, causing discomfort, pain, or injury.

Cochlear implants contain metal as well as a magnet and patients need to be aware of associated risks. It is the responsibility of the patient as well as the health care providers and MR technologists to take proper precautions before an MRI exam.

After cochlear implantation surgery, the patient or caregiver receives may receive an implant card containing important information about the implant and MRI safety. It has the device description, model number, serial number and date of surgery. Each type of cochlear implant has specific recommendations for undergoing MRI exams. Health care providers and MR technologists are expected to follow the cochlear implant manufacturer's recommendations and instructions for use.

The implants can be divided into:

1. *MR Unsafe* means that a patient with that type of implant should not receive an MRI exam while they have the implant.
2. *MR Conditional* means the patient can have an MRI exam under certain specific conditions.

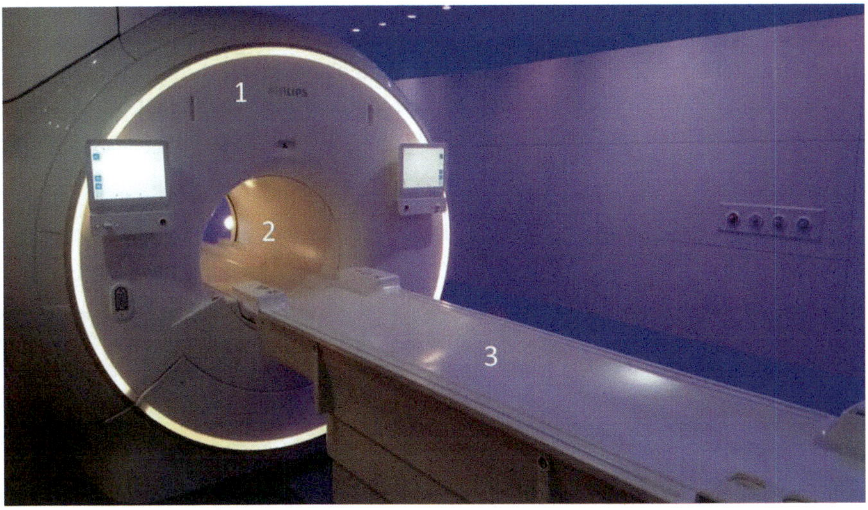


**Fig. 4.44** Image of 3T MRI scanner. 1—MRI Machine; 2—Bore; 3—Patient table

(a) Newer cochlear implants (Fig. 4.45a–d) that are MR Conditional allow the implant magnet to turn and reorient in place. The reorienting of the magnet within the cochlear implant reduces the twisting forces on the implant and surrounding tissue when exposed to the magnetic field of the MRI scanner.
(b) Some MR Conditional cochlear implants may require the magnet to be surgically removed before an MRI can take place. The magnet will need to be surgically replaced following the MRI procedure.
(c) For other MR Conditional cochlear implants, splint/bandaging kits may be available from the manufacturer for use during MRI. If these kits are used, it is important to use the kit designed for the cochlear implant and to follow manufacturer instructions.

With a basic axial implant magnet, the main magnetic field of an MRI scanner is perpendicular to the orientation of the axial magnet. As the patient enters the scanner, the powerful magnetic force of the scanner will attempt to force the implant magnet into alignment.

Many cochlear implant manufacturers use an open "soft silicone pocket" design, which uses a thin lip of silicone to hold a simple axial magnet in place.

With a soft silicone pocket design, there is minimal resistance to this powerful magnetic force, so the implant magnet can easily dislocate. A partially or fully dislocated implant magnet can cause extremely painful concentrated pressure. The adverse effects associated with Cochlear Implants during MRI scan include local pain and swelling, heating of the implant and the requirement of surgical procedure to reposition or replace the magnet or the implant.

If the implant magnet is securely embedded inside of the implant, magnet dislocation is essentially impossible, so the risk for pain or other complications is minimized. These hearing implants are designed to reliably enable 1.5 Tesla MRI scans without the need for surgery or risk of magnet dislocation. The implant has a unique rotatable, self-aligning implant magnet that delivers the highest level of MRI safety available with a cochlear implant. The unique rotatable magnet self-aligns to the magnetic field of the MRI scanner. This neutralizes any adverse effects of magnetic torque—enabling comfortable scans (Fig. 4.45).

Safe, reliable access to MRI is essential for both patients and clinicians. Hence, it is important to be aware of the type of cochlear implant used and its MRI safety.

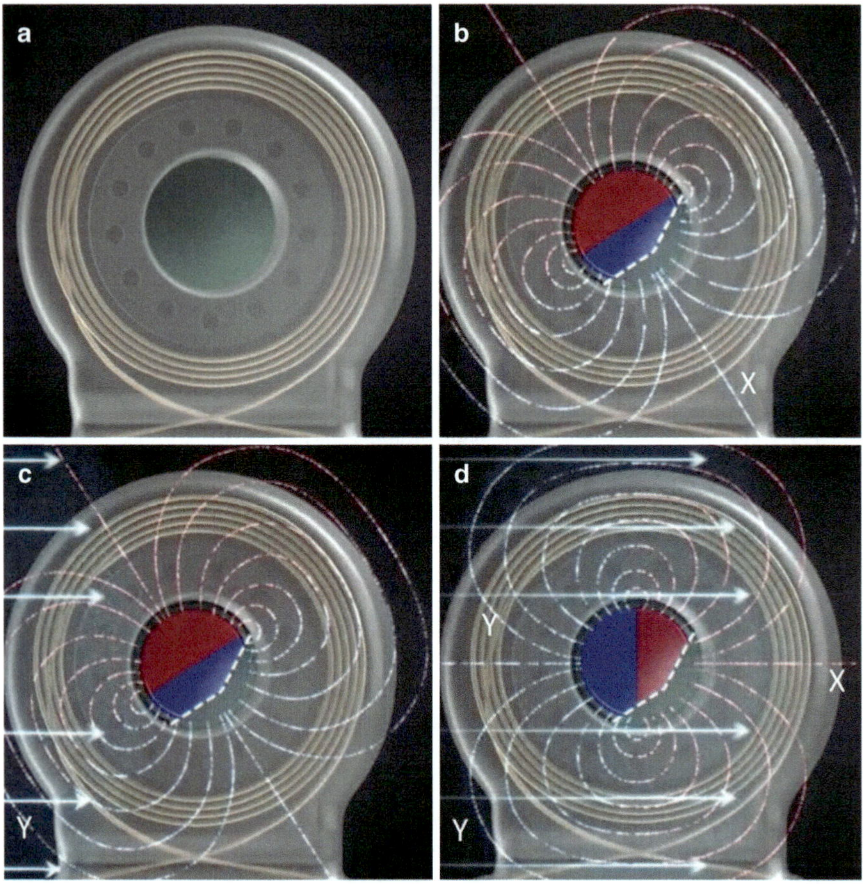


**Fig. 4.45** Mechanism of MR-safe cochlear implant. (**a**) MRI machine with magnet and bore. (**b**) X is the direction of magnetic field of implant magnet. (**c**) Y is the direction of external magnetic field generated by the MRI machine. (**d**) The implant magnet reorients and self aligns itself along the external magnetic field, thereby minimizing twisting forces on implant and surrounding tissue

## References


1. Barrie Grossman C. Magnetic resonance imaging and computed tomography of the head and spine (Ch. 12). 1990. 281–307.
2. Casselman JW, Offeciers EF, De Foer B, Govaerts P, Kuhweide R, Somers T. CT and MR imaging of congential abnormalities of the inner ear and internal auditory canal. Eur J Radiol. 2001;40(2):94–104.
3. Juliano AF, Ginat DT. Gul moonis imaging review of the temporal bone: Part I. Anatomy and inflammatory and neoplastic processes. Radiology. 2013;269(1):17–33.
4. Chakeres DW, Spiegel RK. A systematic technique for comprehensive evaluation of the temporal bone by computed tomography. Radiology. 1983;146:97.
5. Howard JD, Elster AD, May JS. Temporal bone: 3-dimensional computed tomography. Radiology. 1990;177:421.
6. Haaga JR, Charles FL, David JS, Elias AZ. Computed tomography and magnetic resonance imaging of the whole body (Ch. 14). 1994;I(3):428–70.
7. Mahmood FM, Arvind K, Galdino EV, Glen DD, Guy DP, Vlastimil C. C.T. in the evaluation of the vestibulo-cochlear nerves and their central pathways "evaluation of neurotologic disorders". Radiol Clin N Am. 1984;22:45.
8. Foust AM, Nguyen XV, Prevedello L, Bourekas EC, Boulter DJ. Dual-energy CT cisternography in the evaluation of CSF leaks: a novel approach. Radiol Case Rep. 2018;13(1):237–40.
9. Carmody RF, Seeger JF, Horsley WW, Smith JRL, Miller RW. Digital subtraction angiography of glomus tympanicum and jugulare tumors. AJNR. 1983;4(May/June)
10. Murphy A, Glick Y, et al. Digital subtraction angiography. Radiopaedia.org.
11. Taylor S. The petrous temporal bone (including the cerebellopontine angle). Radiol Clin N Am. 1982;20:67.
12. Johnson DW, Voorhees RL, Lutkin RB. Cholesteatomas of the temporal bone: role of computed tomography. Radiology. 1983;148:461.
13. Weerakkody Y, Bullen P, et al. Acute otitis externa. Radiopaedia.org.
14. Juan MT, Joseph TF. Radiology. Diagnosis, imaging, intervention – radiography of the abnormal ear (Ch. 9).
15. Thurston M, Gaillard F, et al. Gradenigo syndrome. Radiopaedia.org.
16. Saber M, Gaillard F, et al. Cholesteatoma. Radiopaedia.org.
17. Swartz JD. Cholesteatomas of the middle ear: diagnosis, etiology and complications. Radiol Clin N Am. 1984;22:15.
18. Rasuli B, Sheikh Z, et al. Otitis media. Radiopaedia.org.
19. Peter DP, Glyn ASL. Diagnostic imaging of the ear. 2nd ed; 1990.
20. Saber M, Wahba M, et al. Perilymphatic fistula. Radiopaedia.org.
21. Mafee MF, Valvassori GE, Kumar A, Yannias DA, Marcus RE. Pneumolabyrinth: a new radiologic sign for fracture of the stapes footplate. Am J Otol. 1984;5:374–5.
22. Sarna B, Abouzari M, Merna C, Jamshidi S, Saber T, Djalilian HR. Perilymphatic fistula: a review of classification, etiology, diagnosis, and treatment. Front Neurol. 2020;11:1046.
23. Venkatasamy A, Al Ohraini Z, Karol A, Karch-Georges A, Riehm S, Rohmer D, Charpiot A, Veillon F. CT and MRI for the diagnosis of perilymphatic fistula: a study of 17 surgically confirmed patients. Eur Arch Otorhinolaryngol. 2020;277(4):1045–51.
24. Deng F, Gaillard F, et al. Petrous apicitis. Radiopaedia.org.
25. Henk D, de Groot JAM, Zonneveld FW, van Waes PFGM, Huizing EH. C.T. of cochlear otosclerosis (otospongiosis). Radiol Clin N Am. 1984;22:37.
26. Mafee MF, Valvassori GE, Deitch RI. Use of computed tomography in the evaluation of cochlear otosclerosis. Radiology. 1985;156:703.
27. Weerakkody Y, Gaillard F, et al. Vestibular schwannoma. Radiopaedia.org.
28. Bell DJ, Gaillard F, et al. Cholesterol granuloma. Radiopaedia.org.
29. Swartz JD, Harnsberger HR. Imaging of the temporal bone. New York: Thieme; 1998.
30. Knipe H, Gaillard F, et al. Congenital cholesteatoma. Radiopaedia.org.

31. Rao AB, Koeller KK, Adair CF. From the archives of the AFIP. Paragangliomas of the head and neck: radiologic-pathologic correlation. Armed Forces Institute of Pathology. Radiographics. 19(6):1605–32.
32. Lee KY, Oh YW, Noh HJ, et al. Extraadrenal paragangliomas of the body: imaging features. AJR Am J Roentgenol. 2006;187(2):492–504.
33. Gupta V, Kumar S, Singh AK, Tatke M. Glossopharyngeal schwannoma: a case report and review of literature. 2002;50(2):190–3.
34. Murphy A, Jones J, et al. Glomus jugulare paraganglioma. Radiopaedia.org.
35. Zayas JO, Feliciano YZ, Hadley CR, Gomez AA, Vidal JA. Temporal bone trauma and the role of multidetector CT in the emergency department. Radiographics. 31(6):1741–55. https://doi.org/10.1148/rg.316115506.
36. Deng F, Di Muzio B, et al. Temporal bone fracture. Radiopaedia.org.
37. Johnson DW, Hasso AN, Stewart CE. Temporal bone trauma: high resolution computed tomographic evaluation. Radiology. 1984;151:411.
38. Deng F, Gerstenmaier JF, et al. Ménière disease. Radiopaedia.org.
39. Miyashita T, Toyama Y, Inamoto R, Mori N. Evaluation of the vestibular aqueduct in Ménière's disease using multiplanar reconstruction images of CT. Auris Nasus Larynx. 2012;39(6):567–71.
40. Bernaerts A. MRI in Menière's disease. J Belg Soc Radiol. 2018;102(S1):13.
41. Joshi VM, Navlekar SK, Ravi Kishore G, Jitender Reddy K, Vinay Kumar EC. CT and MR imaging of the inner ear and brain in children with congenital sensorineural hearing loss. Radiographics. 2012;32(3)
42. Jackler RK, Luxford WM, House WF. Congenital mal formations of the inner ear: a classification based on embryogenesis. Laryngoscope. 1987;97(3 Pt 2, Suppl 40):2–14.
43. Ozgen B, Oguz KK, Atas A, Sennaroglu L. Complete labyrinthine aplasia: clinical and radiologic findings with review of the literature. AJNR Am J Neuroradiol. 2009;30(4):774–80.
44. Marsot-Dupuch K, Dominguez-Brito A, Ghasli K, Chouard CH. CT and MR findings of Michel anomaly: inner ear aplasia. AJNR Am J Neuroradiol. 1999;20(2):281–4.
45. Swartz JD, Mukherji SK. The inner ear and otodystrophies. In: Swartz JD, Loevner LA, editors. Imaging of the temporal bone. New York, NY: Thieme; 2009. p. 298–411.
46. Donaldson JA, Duckert LG, Lambert PM, Rubel EW. Surgical anatomy of the temporal bone. New York, NY: Raven; 1992.
47. Deng F, Gaillard F, et al. Inner ear malformations (classification). Radiopaedia.org.
48. Shin CH, Hong HS, Yi BH, et al. CT and MR imagings of semicircular canal aplasia. J Korean Soc Radiol. 2009;61:9–15.
49. Mafee MF, Charletta D, Kumar A, Belmont H. Large vestibular aqueduct and congenital sensorineural hearing loss. AJNR Am J Neuroradiol. 1992;13(2):805–19.
50. Ramos A, Cervera J, Valdivieso A, Pérez D, Vasallo JR, Cuyas JM. Cochlear implant in congenital malformations [in Spanish]. Acta Otorrinolaringol Esp. 2005;56(8):343–8.
51. Warren FM, Wiggins RH, Pitt C, Harnsberger HR, Shelton C. Apparent cochlear nerve aplasia: to implant or not to implant? Otol Neurotol. 2010;31(7):1088–94.
52. Gupta SS, Maheshwari SR, Kirtane MV, Shrivastav N. Pictorial review of MRI/CT scan in congenital temporal bone anomalies, in patients for cochlear implant. Ind J Radiol Imag. 2009;19(2):99–106.
53. Swartz JD, Faerber EN. Congenital malformations of the external and middle ear: high-resolution CT findings of surgical import. AJR. 1985;144
54. Bellucci RJ. Congenital aural malformations: diagnosis and treatment. Otolaryngol Clin North Am. 1981;14:95–124.
55. Pulec JL, Freedman HM. Management of congenital ear abnormalities. Laryngoscope. 1978;88:420–34.
56. Jahrsdoerfer RA. Congenital malformations of the ear: analysis of 94 operations. Ann Otol Rhinol Laryngol. 1980;89:348–53.
57. Altmann F. Congenital atresia of the ear in man and animals. Ann Otol Rhinol Laryngol. 1955;64:824–57.

58. Hough JVD. Ossicular malformations and their correction. In: Shambaugh GE, Shea JJ, editors. Proceedings of the Shambaugh fifth international workshop on middle ear microsurgery and fluctuant hearing loss. Huntsville, AL: Strode; 1977. p. 186–94.
59. Hough JVD. Congenital malformations of the middle ear. Arch Otolaryngol. 1963;78:335–43.
60. Witte RJ, Lane JI, Driscoll CLW, Lundy LB, Bernstein MA, Kotsenas AL, Kocharian A. Pediatric and adult cochlear implantation. Radiographics. 2003;23(5):1185–200.
61. Bickle I, Jones J, et al. Cochlear implant. Radiopaedia.org.
62. Young JY, Ryan ME, Young NM. Preoperative imaging of sensorineural hearing loss in pediatric candidates for cochlear implantation. Radiographics. 2014;34(5):133–49.
63. Widmann G, Dejaco D, Luger A, et al. Pre- and post-operative imaging of cochlear implants: a pictorial review. Insights Imag. 2020;11:93.
64. Appachi S, Schwartz S, Ishman S, Anne S. Utility of intraoperative imaging in cochlear implantation: a systematic review. Laryngoscope. 2018;128(8):1914–21.
65. Viccaro M, Covelli E, De Seta E, Balsamo G, Filipo R. The importance of intra-operative imaging during cochlear implant surgery. Cochlear Implants Int. 2009 Dec;10(4):198–202.
66. Arweiler-Harbeck D, Mönninghoff C, Greve J, Hoffmann T, Göricke S, Arnolds J, Theysohn N, Gollner U, Lang S, Forsting M, Schlamann M. Imaging of electrode position after cochlear implantation with flat panel CT. ISRN Otolaryngol. 2012;2012:728205.
67. McClenaghan F, Nash R. The modified stenver's view for cochlear implants – what do the surgeons want to know? J Belg Soc Radiol. 2020;104(1):37.
68. Cellik M, Orhan KS, Ozturk E, et al. Impact of routine plain X-ray on post-operative management in cochlear implantation. J Int Adv Otol. 2018;14:365–9.
69. Verbist BM, Frijns JHM, Geleijns J, van Buchem MA. Multisection CT as a valuable tool in the postoperative assessment of cochlear implant patients. Am J Neuroradiol. 2005;26(2):424–9.
70. Fischer N, Pinggera L, Weichbold V, Dejaco D, Schmutzhard J, Widmann G. Radiologic and functional evaluation of electrode dislocation from the scala tympani to the scala vestibuli in patients with cochlear implants. AJNR Am J Neuroradiol. 2015;36:372–7.
71. Richard C, Fayad JN, Doherty J, Linthicum FH. Round window versus cochleostomy technique in cochlear implantation: histologic findings. Otol Neurotol. 2012;33:1181–7.
72. Kamakura T, Nadol JB. Correlation between word recognition score and intracochlear new bone and fibrous tissue after cochlear implantation in the human. Hear Res. 2016;339:132–41.
73. Zuniga MG, Rivas A, Hedley-Williams A, et al. Tip fold-over in cochlear implantation: case series. Otol Neurotol. 2017;38:199–206.
74. Mittmann P, Rademacher G, Mutze S, Ernst A, Todt I. Electrode migration in patients with perimodiolar cochlear implant electrodes. Audiol Neurotol. 2015;20:349–53.
75. Dagkiran M, Tarkan O, Surmelioglu O, et al. Management of complications in 1452 pediatric and adult cochlear implantations. Turk Arch Otorhinolaryngol. 2020;58:16–23.
76. Fayad JN, Makarem AO, Linthicum FH. Histopathologic assessment of fibrosis and new bone formation in implanted human temporal bones using 3D reconstruction. Otolaryngol Head Neck Surg. 2009;141:247–52.
77. Li H, Helpard L, Ekeroot J, et al. Three-dimensional tonotopic mapping of the human cochlea based on synchrotron radiation phase-contrast imaging. Sci Rep. 2021;11:4437.
78. Elfarnawany M, et al. Micro-CT versus synchrotron radiation phase contrast imaging of human cochlea. J Microsc. 2017;265:349–57.
79. Chakeres DW. C.T. of ear structures: a tailored approach. Radiol Clin N Am. 1984;22:3.

# Cochlear Implants in Clinical Use Worldwide Today

# 5

Sandra DeSaSouza

## 5.1 The Working Principles of the Cochlear Implant

The Cochlear Implant consists of externally worn audio processor and the implant that is surgically placed under the skin on the surface of mastoid bone. The audio processor is worn comfortably behind the ear. The flexible electrode array is inserted into the cochlea. The cochlea is the part of the inner ear that converts sound waves into nerve signals which the brain processes as hearing. The apical region of the cochlea is responsible for detecting low-pitched sounds and the basal region is responsible for detecting high-pitched sounds. The cochlea is lined with thousands of sensory cells known as hair cells which detects the sound waves and send the sound information as nerve signals to the auditory nerve to the brain. For individuals with severe to profound sensorineural hearing loss, most of the hair cells do not function normally and are not able to send these nerve signals properly. A CI system bypasses the non-functioning hair cells by using electrical pulses that sends sound signal to spiral ganglia and then to the auditory nerve. To achieve this, the audio processor detects environmental sounds and digitally converts them into coded electrical signals. Audio processor transmits these signals through the skin to the implant by a communication coil. The implant translates these coded signals into electrical pulses which are transmitted along the electrode array to stimulate specific locations of the cochlea responsible for specific pitches. This targeted stimulation across the whole cochlea provides more accurate pitch perception for better sound quality.

**Supplementary Information** The online version contains supplementary material available at [https://doi.org/10.1007/978-981-19-0452-3_5].

S. DeSaSouza (✉)
ENT Department, Jaslok Hospital & Research Centre, Mumbai, Maharashtra, India
Breach Candy Hospital and Desa Hospital (ENT Section), Mumbai, Maharashtra, India



S. DeSaSouza (ed.), *Cochlear Implants*,
https://doi.org/10.1007/978-981-19-0452-3_5

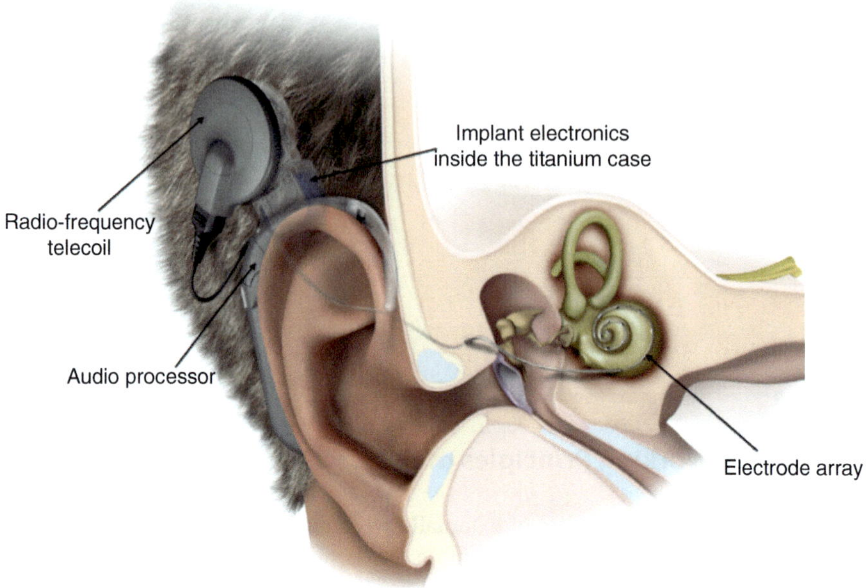


**Fig. 5.1** Working principles of cochlear implant (Video 5.1)

By mimicking the natural function of hair cells, these pulses can deliver sound signals to spiral ganglia and to the auditory nerve. These signals are then transmitted by the auditory nerve to the brain, where they are interpreted as sound (Fig. 5.1).

## 5.2 MED-EL

### 5.2.1 Evolution of Implants and Processors

| | | |
|---|---|---|
| 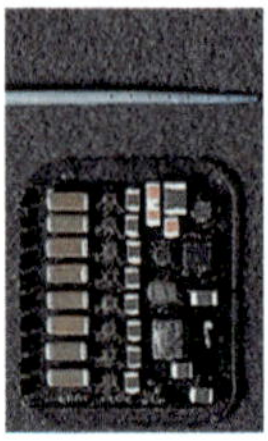 World's first microelectronic multi-channel CI—1977 | 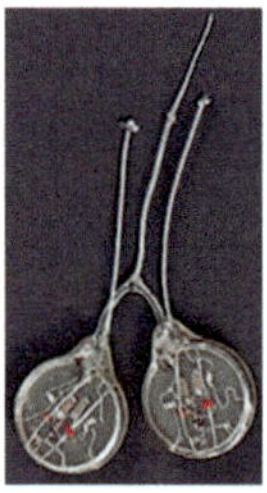 Six- and four-channel implant variants—1978 | 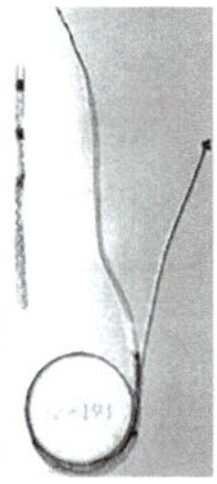 COMBI 40 system with eight channels—1994 |

| | | |
|---|---|---|
| 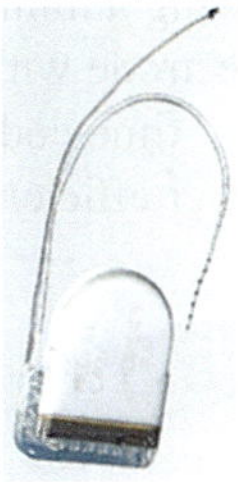 COMBI 40+ with 12 channels—1996 | 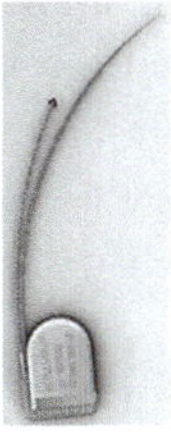 PULSAR CI—2004 | 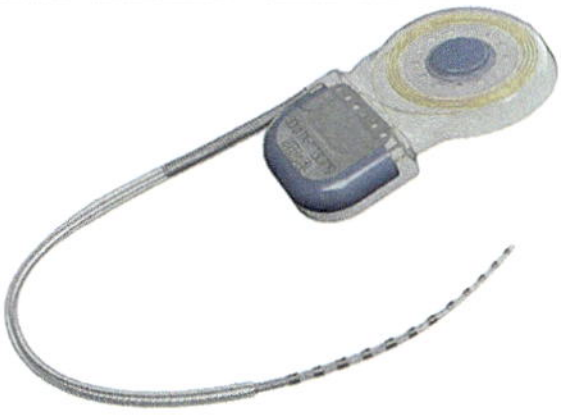 Titanium SONATA CI—2006 |
| 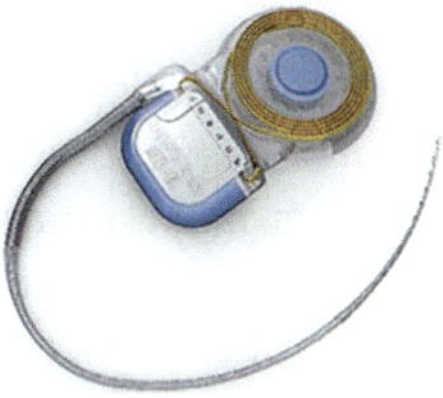 Titanium CONCERTO CI. Titanium case thinner than SONATA—2008 | 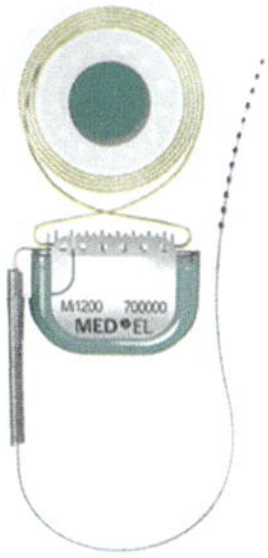 SYNCHRONY CI with MRI compatible implant magnet—2014 | 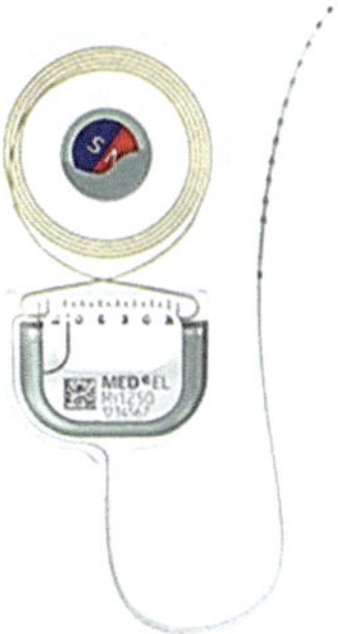 SYNCHRONY-2 CI with central exit electrode lead and MRI compatible implant magnet—2019 |

| | | |
|---|---|---|
| 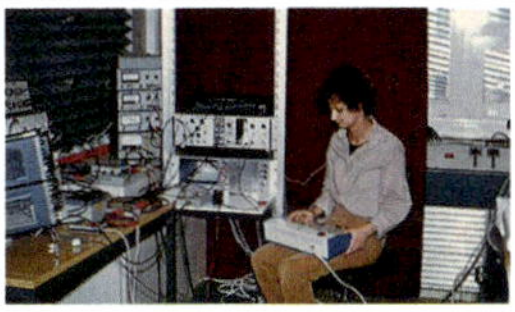 Small portable audio processor—1979 | 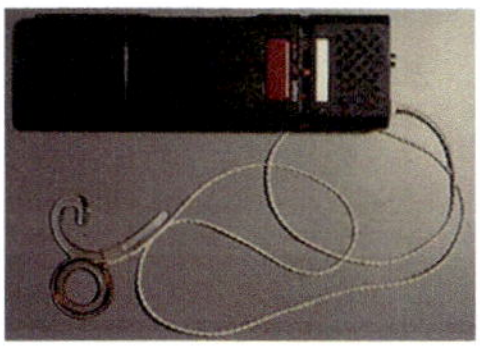 Small body-worn processor—1979 | 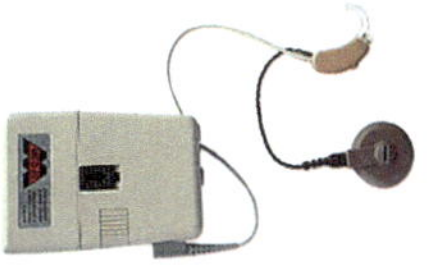 Speech processor featuring an ear-level microphone—1989 |
| 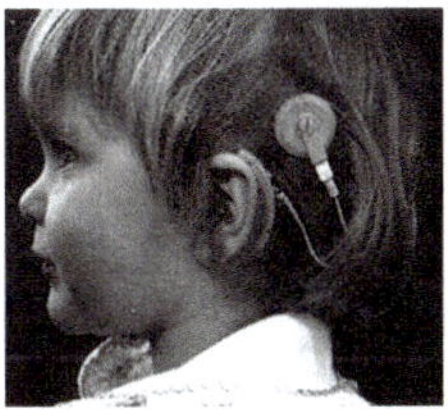 World's first behind-the-ear (BTE) audio processor—1991 | 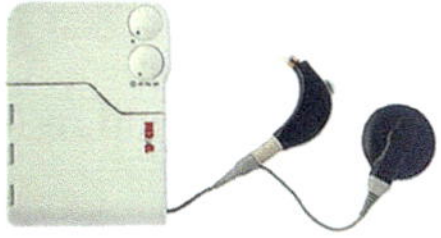 CIS PRO+ processor—1995 | 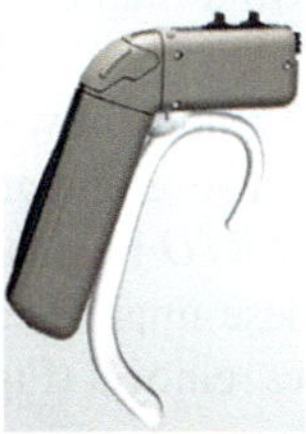 TEMPO+ BTE audio processor—1999 |

| | | |
|---|---|---|
| 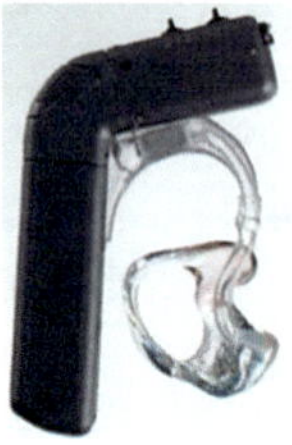 World's first DUET speech processor having hearing aid component to amplify low-frequency sound signals—2005 | 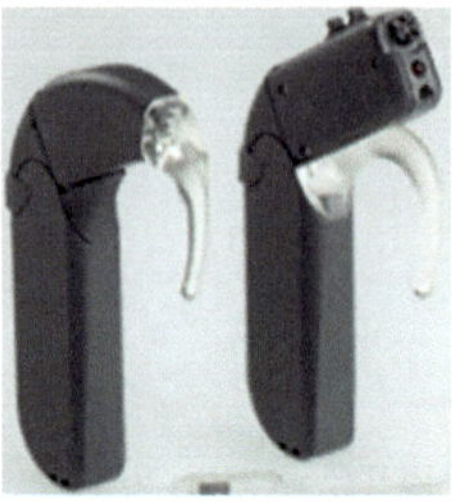 OPUS audio processor having a sleek, switch-free design—2006 | 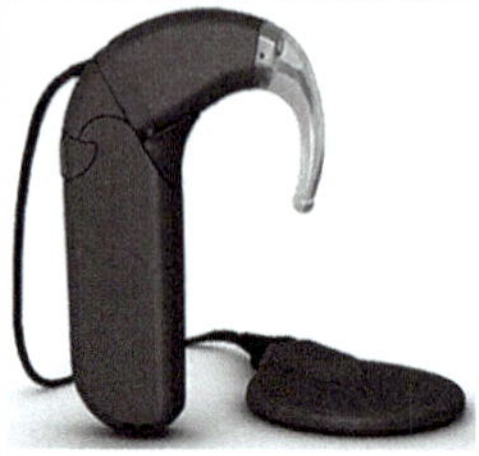 OPUS 2 audio processor—2010 |
| 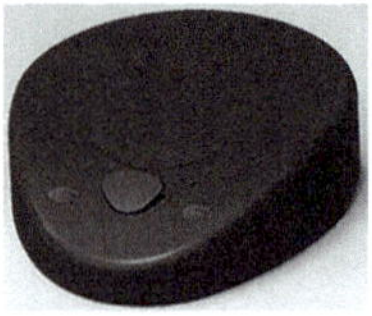 RONDO single-unit processor—2013 | 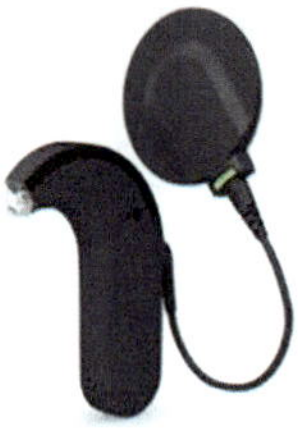 SONNET audio processor—2014 | 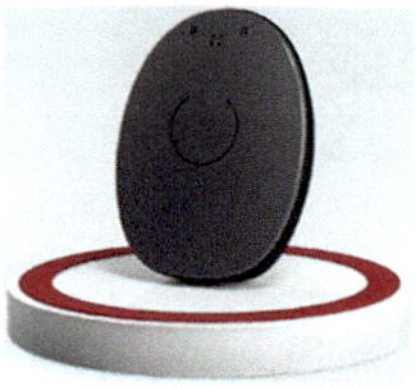 RONDO 2 audio processor—2017 |
| 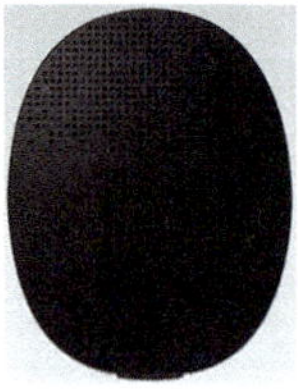 RONDO 3 audio processor—2020 | | |

### 5.2.2 Implants

Like any other CI brands, MED-EL also offers implants with implant electronics protected in a titanium case. The electronics inside the titanium case is of utmost importance.

*SONATA* implant was the first of its kind in MED-EL CI system and it is still in existence in several markets (Fig. 5.2).

*CONCERTO* implant was designed 25% thinner than the SONATA implant and both of these implants are compatible with up to 1.5 Tesla MRI, without the need for magnet removal (Fig. 5.3).

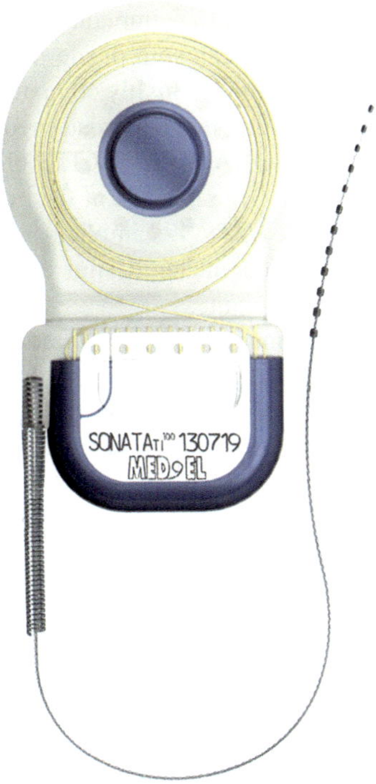


**Fig. 5.2** SONATA

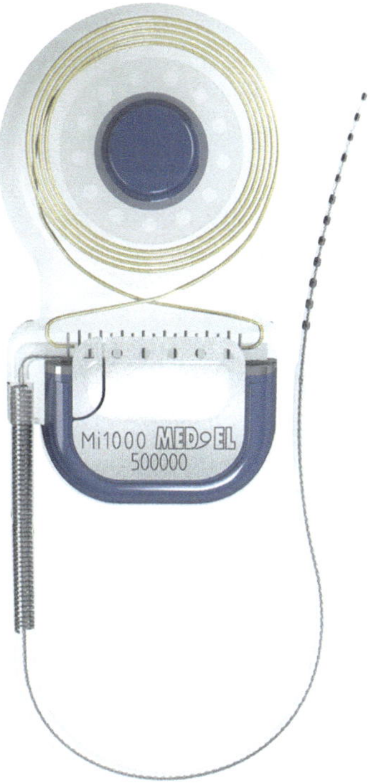


**Fig. 5.3** CONCERTO

*SYNCHRONY* implant was designed with a revolutionized implant magnet design that can spin inside the magnetic case in response to any external magnet field making it a highly compatible magnet design up to 3 Tesla MRI. The rotatable, self-aligning magnet greatly reduces torque to increase patient comfort during MRI scans. SONATA, CONCERTO, and SYNCHRONY implants have the electrode lead exit from the side of the implant (Fig. 5.4).

*SYNCHRONY 2* implant is the latest implant design that has the 3 Tesla MRI compatible magnet design and has the electrode lead exit from the central location of the implant.

The magnet from all these four implants can only be removed from the bottom side of the implant, making dislocation of the magnet due to trauma almost impossible. CONCERTO PIN and SYNCHRONY PIN implants feature titanium fixation pins to secure the placement of the implant for outstanding stability (Fig. 5.5).

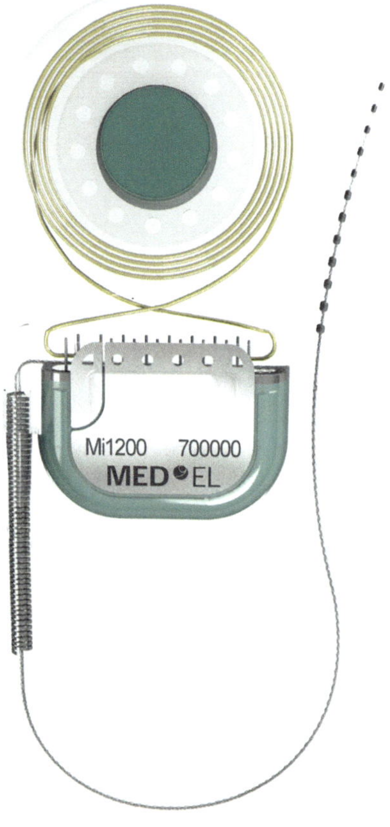


**Fig. 5.4** SYNCHRONY

**Fig. 5.5** SYNCHRONY 2

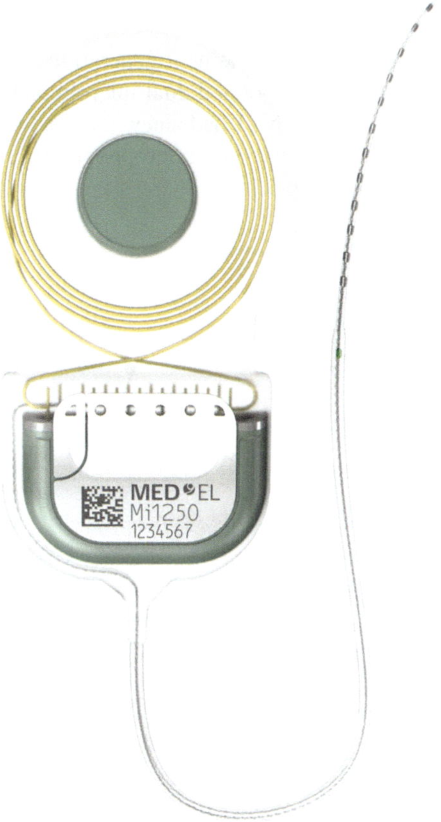


*Safety Capacitors*: All these four implant variants from MED-EL have one thing in common in its electronics design, which is the safety capacitors for every individual stimulating channels. Safety capacitors act like filters in filtering out any unsafe direct current components, if there will be any such component coming out of the implant electronics, safeguarding the intra-cochlear neuronal elements and preventing the platinum contact pads from dissolving.

### 5.2.3 Audio Processors and Accessories

MED-EL offers audio processors in two different variants, namely, *behind-the-ear* (BTE) and single-unit processor as shown. From the body-worn type processor, MED-EL upgraded it to BTE type in the early 1990s.

*OPUS 2* is one of the earliest designs that are in commercial existence since 2010 that carries dual-loop automatic gain control (AGC) function. AGC is essential in attenuating sound signal above 1.2 kHz and enhances sound signals below 1.2 kHz offering better speech understanding to the listeners. OPUS 2 design came up with

XS battery pack making it the thinnest and lightest audio processor in the market at that time (Fig. 5.6).

*SONNET* was the next generation BTE audio processor that was introduced in 2014 that incorporated dual microphone offering better directionality to the users. Also, the SONNET had a new feature, wind noise reduction (WNR) which in combination with the dual microphone, offering a much clearer hearing experience to the users (Fig. 5.7).

**Fig. 5.6** OPUS 2

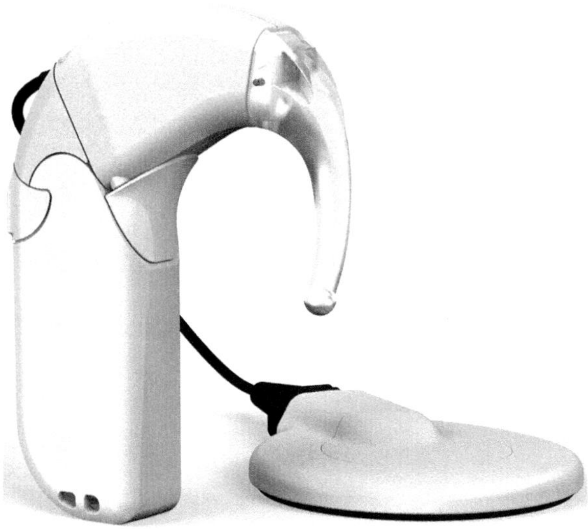

**Fig. 5.7** SONNET

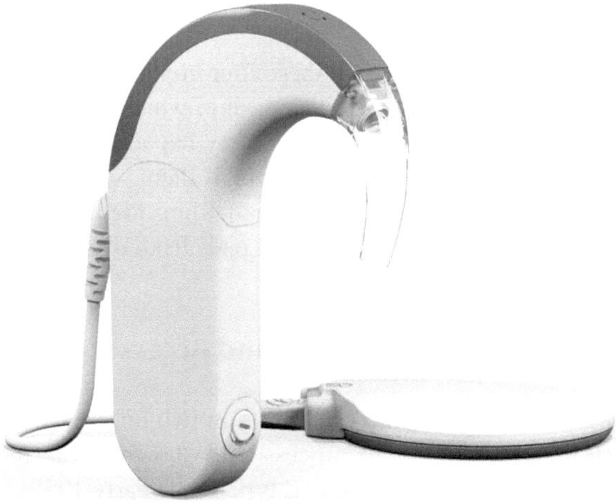

In 2019, *SONNET 2* BTE processor was introduced that incorporated three additional features, namely, transient noise reduction (TNR), ambient noise reduction (ANR), and adaptive intelligence (AI) making it the most advanced BTE audio processor in the market (Fig. 5.8).

*RONDO* was the first all-in-one audio processor, the battery pack, control unit, and the radio frequency telecoil all-in-one unit. MED-EL was the CI company to design the single-unit audio processor and brought it to the market in the year 2013 (Fig. 5.9).

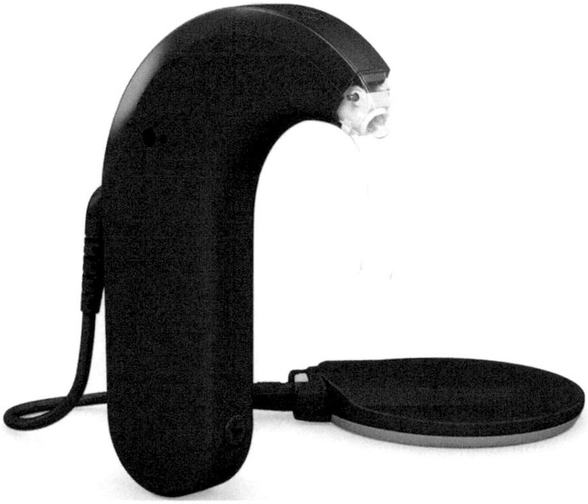

**Fig. 5.8** SONNET 2

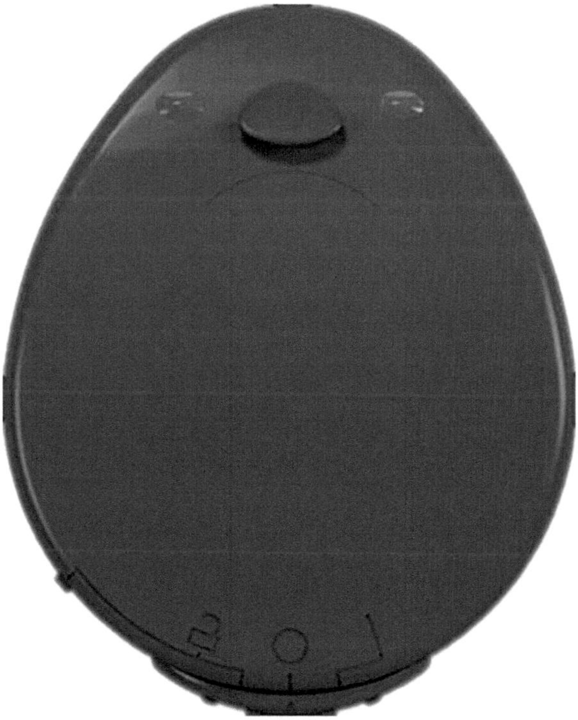

**Fig. 5.9** RONDO

*RONDO 2* was the second-generation single-unit processor that was designed slightly thinner and lighter than RONDO. RONDO 2 was designed for wireless charging of the battery without the need for battery removal and it was again the industry first at that time. Both RONDO and RONDO 2 are implemented with AGC function (Fig. 5.10).

In 2020, *RONDO 3* was introduced in the market that has all the features including AGC, WNR, TNR, ANR, and AI, along with wireless charging of the batteries (Fig. 5.11).

**Fig. 5.10** RONDO 2

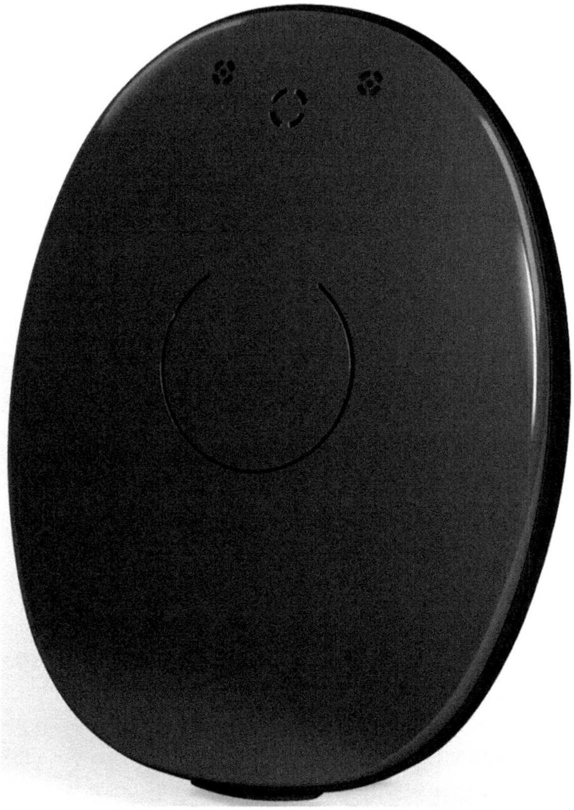

**Fig. 5.11** RONDO 3

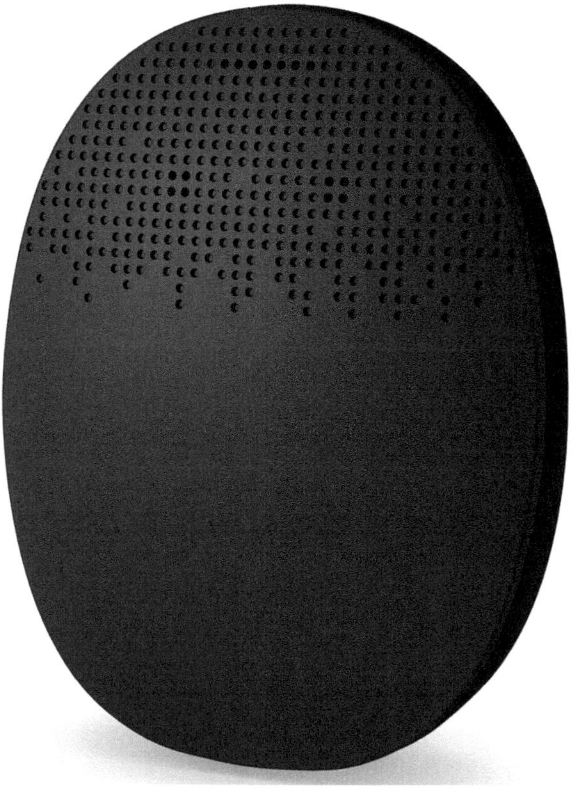

### 5.2.4 Electric-Acoustic Stimulation (EAS)

In some patients, the high frequency (HF) responsible hair cells are permanently damaged. This may occur due to variety of reasons, including aging, noise-related hearing loss (HL), genetics, medication side effects, and different diseases, causing severe to profound HL in the HF region. However, the low-frequency (LF) residual hearing with mild to moderate HL could still be utilized in such patients through a sound amplification device, like hearing aid (HA). The exact frequency range and the degree to which the HL occurs can be detected from the pure tone audiogram of the patient, tested in the quiet condition. Figure is a typical audiogram of an extended indication (indication 2) of a partially deaf patient with severe to profound HL in the HF region which extends from 1500 to 8000 Hz, and mild to moderate HL from LF to mid-frequencies in the range between 125 and 1500 Hz. A normal hearing is referred to when the hearing threshold is within 25 decibels (dB) of HL across all frequencies (Fig. 5.12).

The length of the electrode array must be shorter just to cover the HF region with electrical stimulation leaving the LF region for acoustical amplification using hearing aids (Fig. 5.13).

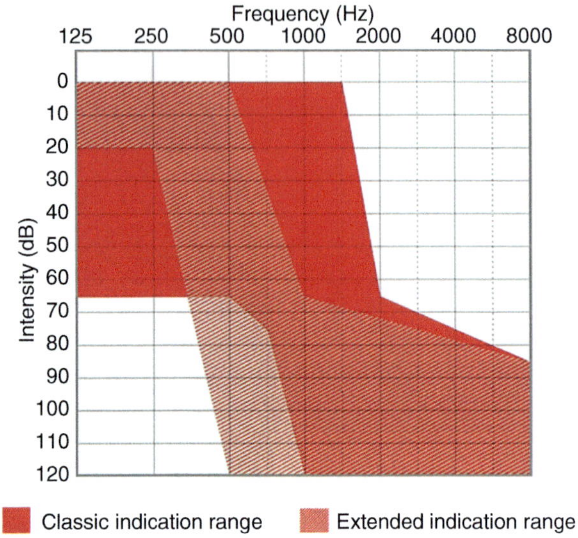


**Fig. 5.12** Typical audiogram of a partially deaf patient with severe to profound HL in the HF region: indication from the earlier times when the functional LF residual hearing cut-off was kept at 500 Hz which was extended to 1500 Hz under expanded indication criteria

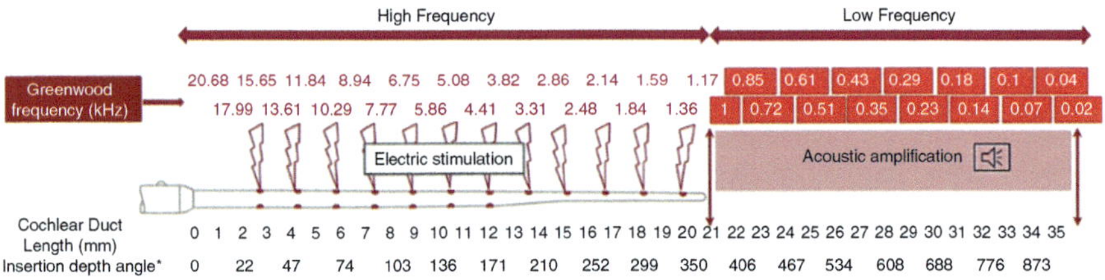


**Fig. 5.13** Schematic representation of electric stimulation in the HF region and acoustic amplification in the LF region in an average-sized cochlea

*MED-EL's EAS* hearing system consists of implant stimulator with a shorter length electrode array in the range of 24 or 20 mm and *behind-the-ear* (BTE) SONNET EAS audio processor that is combined with the hearing aid (HA) as a unified audio processor. The SONNET EAS audio processor sends the amplified acoustic signal through the earmold into the ear canal (Fig. 5.14).

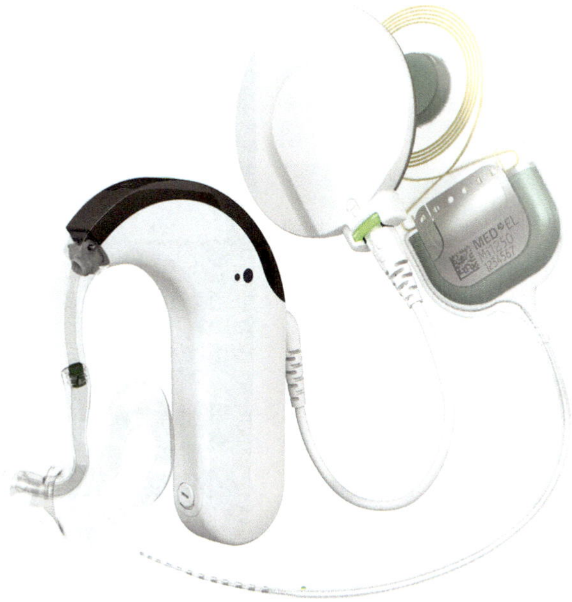

**Fig. 5.14** SONNET EAS

*SONNET EAS* processor offers

- Directional microphones
- Six-channel acoustic amplification
- Gain of up to 48 dB
- Maximum power output of 118 dB SPL.

The timing of both the electric and acoustic signals is matched, which enables a full, rich perception of sound.

### 5.2.5 MED-EL Accessories

MED-El offers accessories to control the audio processors and to link it with other audio streaming devices. In 2010, MED-EL introduced a remote control (*FineTuner*) to control the OPUS 2 audio processor mainly for adjusting the volume and program selection. SONNET, SONNET 2, and RONDO 3 audio processors can be connected to any audio streaming devices using *AudioLink*, a Bluetooth connectivity device (Fig. 5.15).

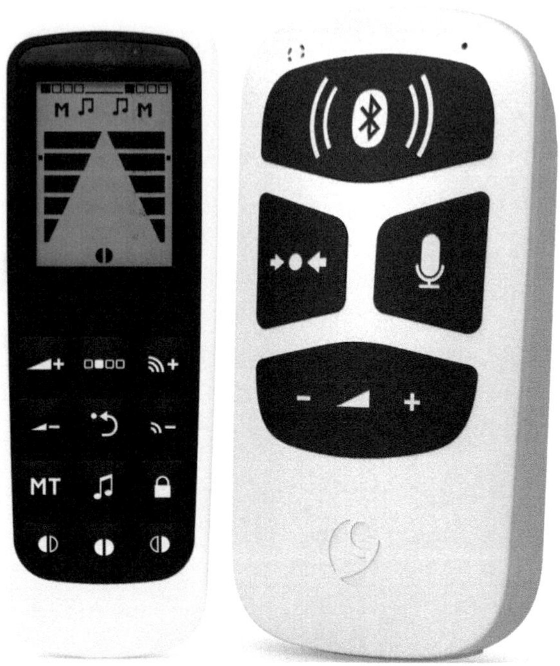


**Fig. 5.15** FineTuner and AudioLink

### 5.2.6 Electrodes

*FLEX series* carries five different electrode array lengths.

- FLEX SOFT is used in patients with profound hearing loss across all frequencies.
- FLEX28 is used in patients with profound hearing loss or with some low-frequency residual hearing.
- FLEX26 is used in patients with profound hearing loss or with some low-frequency residual hearing.
- FLEX24 and FLEX20 are mainly for the patients with good functional low-frequency residual hearing. These two short length electrodes are used to electrically stimulate the basal turn of the cochlea and the low-frequency region is amplified using hearing aid.

The FLEX electrode arrays have the apical five contacts arranged in a single line configuration making the electrode tip highly flexible to minimize the intra-cochlear electrode insertion trauma (Fig. 5.16).

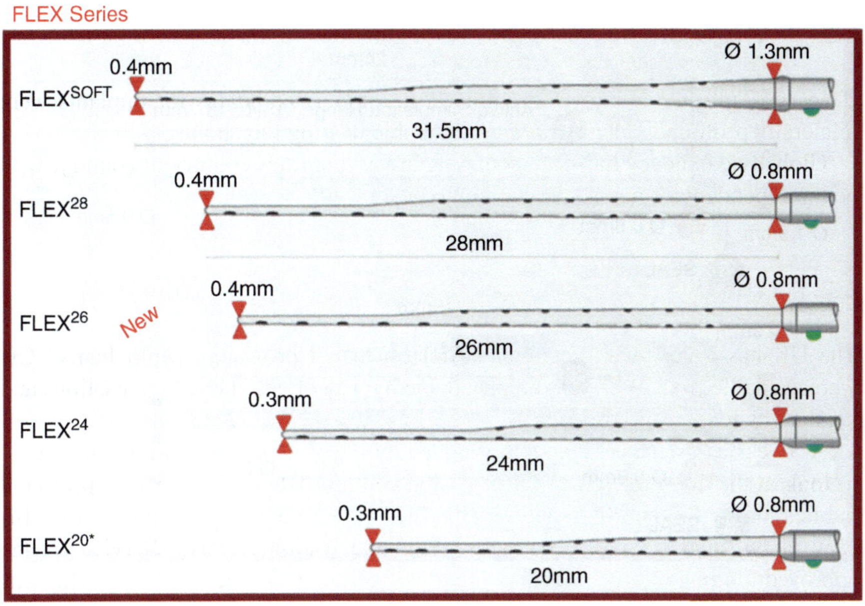


**Fig. 5.16** Flex electrodes

*FORM series* carries two different electrode array lengths.

- FORM24 is mainly for Mondini's deformation type (IP type II) cochlea.
- FORM19 is for severely deformed incomplete partition (IP type I).

Both IP type I and IP type II are mostly characterized with enlarged vestibular aqueduct or enlarged internal auditory canal, posing the risk of cerebrospinal fluid (CSF) gusher. The CORK insertion stopper could assist the operating surgeon to seal the cochlea (Fig. 5.17).

FORM Series

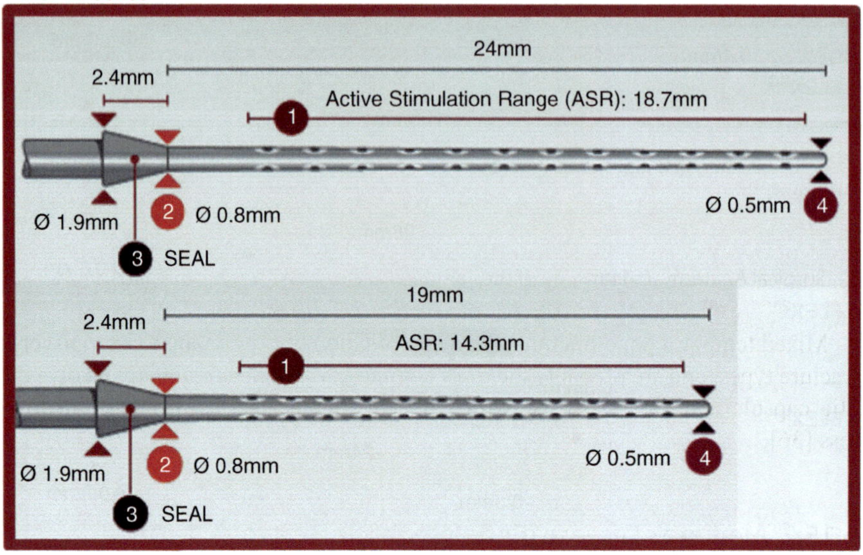


**Fig. 5.17** FORM electrodes

SPECIAL Electrodes

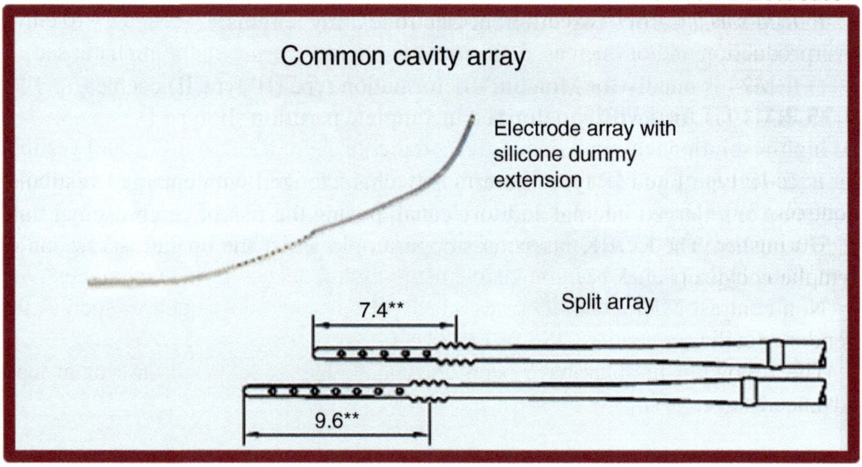


**Fig. 5.18** Special electrodes

*Special electrodes* including the SPLIT array and common cavity array are only available upon a special request (Custom Made Device).

The SPLIT electrode is designed for fully ossified cochlea. Ossified cochlea does not offer a chance for the operating surgeon to place a regular electrode array in the cochlear lumen. For the SPLIT electrode array placement, the surgeon has to drill two channels in the ossified cochlea to place the two branch arrays.

Common cavity array is specifically for the common cavity deformation, where this array would offer a nice loopy placement inside the cavity (Fig. 5.18).

### 5.2.7 Signal Processing Strategies in MED-EL's Audio Processor

MED-EL's audio processors (OPUS 2, SONNET, SONNET 2, RONDO, RONDO-2, and RONDO-3) have front-end processing strategies that model/mimic the functionality of external and middle ear covering the directionality and filtering processes. The sound coding strategies are the ones that model/mimic the inner-ear functionality.

Front-end processing is brought under the term Automatic Sound Management (ASM). OPUS 2, RONDO, and RONDO 2 processors have ASM 1.0, that includes the automatic gain control (AGC), which is essential to attenuate high-level signal and enhances low-level signal, enabling the CI user to hear even a very soft sound signal. ASM 2.0 was the next general front-end processing, which includes new features microphone directionality (MD) and wind noise reduction (WNR) in addition to AGC. ASM 2.0 is available in SONNET audio processor. ASM 3.0 is the current generation front-end processing, which includes ambient noise reduction (ANR), transient noise reduction (TNR), and adaptive intelligence (AI) in addition to AGC, MD, and WNR from ASM 1.0 and 2.0. SONNET 2 and RONDO 3 are equipped with ASM 3.0.

MED-EL's sound coding strategy is based on continuous interleaved sampling (CIS) that was proposed by Prof. Blake Wilson in 1999, from the Duke University. The Fine Structure Processing (FSP) strategy is an advanced version of CIS strategy that includes phase-locking of low-frequency signals to the neurons in the apex of the cochlea where they are naturally tuned to process low-frequency signals. The FSP can be applied to the apical two channels only. FS4 was a next generation sound coding strategy that extended the FSP to the apical four channels. In both FSP and FS4 strategies, only one of the apical channels would fire electrical pulse at a time. FS4-p is the latest sound coding strategy that would enable more than one apical channel to fire electrical pulse at a time. All the audio processors of MED-EL that are in clinical use can be made to use any of the sound coding strategies that are mentioned above.

## 5.3 Cochlear

### 5.3.1 Evolution

- 1979 A medical device group Nucleus, Cochlear, and the Australian government partnered together to develop a commercially available cochlear implant.
- 1982 The first commercial Nucleus implant was released, and the recipient was Graham C
- 1985 The Nucleus Mini22 implant with wearable sound processor was the first multi-channel device to receive FDA approval.
- 1998 ESPrit the first multi-channel behind-the-ear processor was introduced.
- 2000 Nucleus 24 Contour perimodiolar electrode array was introduced.
- 2005 Nucleus Freedom system released.

- 2008 Nucleus freedom available for N22 implants. Cochlear Hybrid Sound processor introduced for electric and acoustic stimulation.
- 2016 Cochlear launched Slim Modiolar Electrode the worlds thinnest lightest full-length perimodiolar electrode.
- 2016 Kanso introduced smallest lightest off-the-ear sound processor.

### 5.3.2 Implant Generations (Figs. 5.19 and 5.20)

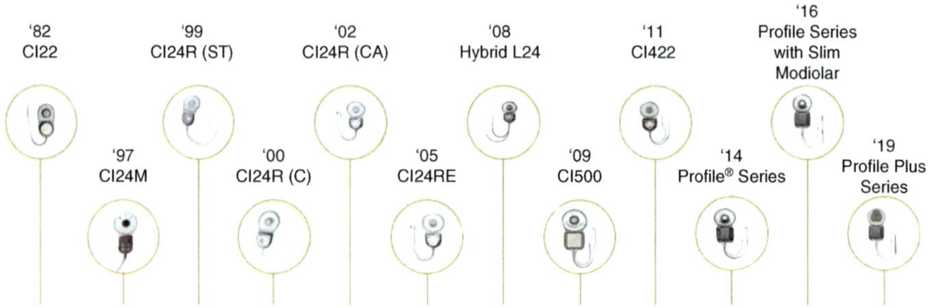


**Fig. 5.19** Implants

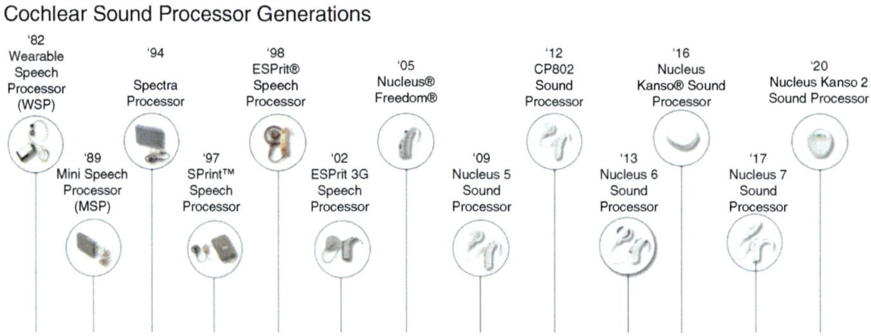


**Fig. 5.20** Processor

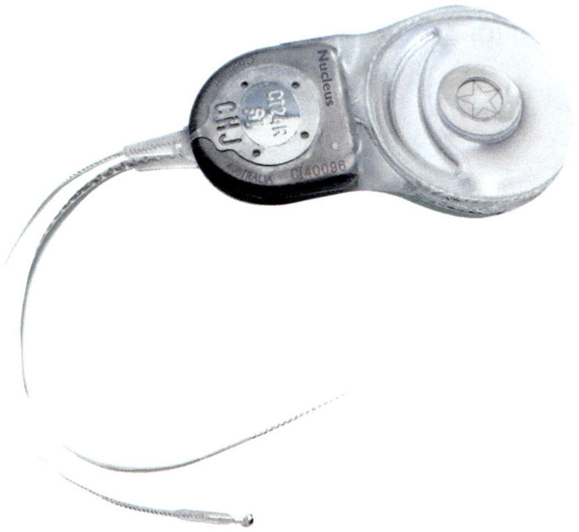


**Fig. 5.21** Nucleus® CI24R(ST)

## 5.3.3 Implants

### 5.3.3.1 Nucleus® CI24R(ST) (Fig. 5.21)

- Simplified for Surgery
- Smaller design
- Re-modeled receiver/stimulator
- Vertically aligned exit leads
- Proven Nucleus® Performance
- Established electrode technology
- Demonstrated recipient performance

### 5.3.3.2 Nucleus® CI24R(C) (Fig. 5.22)

- Contoured for Performance
- 22 half-banded electrodes designed to be safely placed adjacent to the modiolar wall
- Contoured for Safety
- Array designed without invasive bands or positioners
- Simplified for surgery
- Smaller implant with circular pedestal for easier drilling

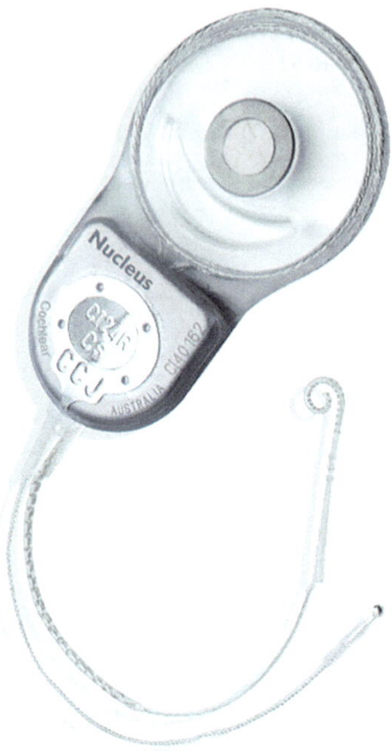


**Fig. 5.22** Nucleus® CI24R(C)

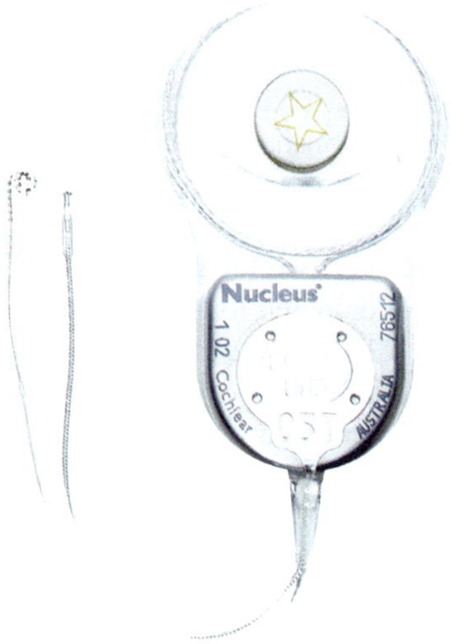


**Fig. 5.23** Nucleus CI24R(CA)

#### 5.3.3.3 Nucleus® CI24R(CA) (Fig. 5.23)

Proven reliability of the CI24R receiver/stimulator [1]

The Nucleus® 24 Contour Advance™ features the unique Contour™ Electrode with Softip™, designed to preserve the delicate structures of the cochlea, and aid in consistent perimodiolar positioning [2, 3]. Intelligently engineered geometry, softness, and flexibility enable the Softip™ to glide smoothly through the lumen of the cochlea while minimizing lateral wall forces [3]. Smooth insertion improves consistency of perimodiolar positioning, as the tip enables the electrode array to easily settle in its resting position.

It is recommended that surgeons use the Advance Off-Stylet™ (AOS) insertion technique (see over) to realize the full benefits of the Softip™ design.

### 5.3.3.4 Nucleus® CI24RE (ST) Cochlear Implant (Fig. 5.24)

- Receiver stimulator in titanium casing
- Removable magnet for MRI safety
- MRI safe at 3.0 Tesla with magnet removed
- Implant coil, enabling telemetry
- Two extracochlear electrodes for different stimulation modes, and high performance.

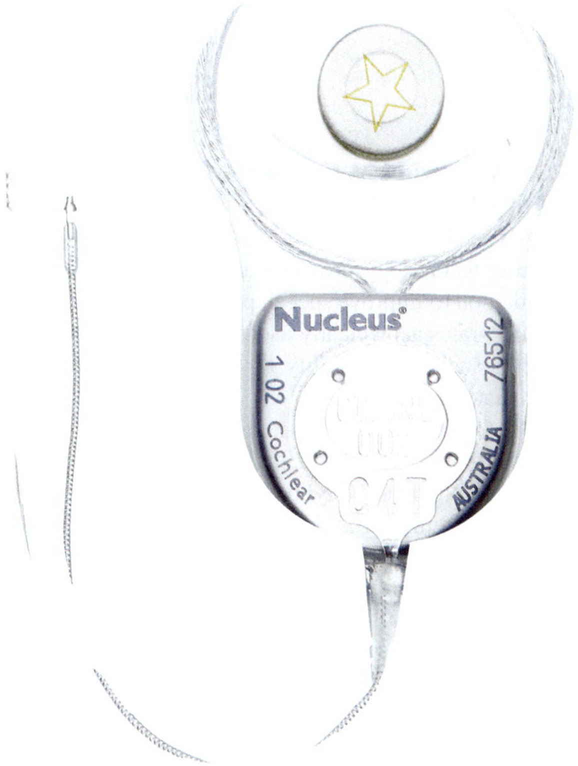


**Fig. 5.24** Nucleus® CI24RE (ST)

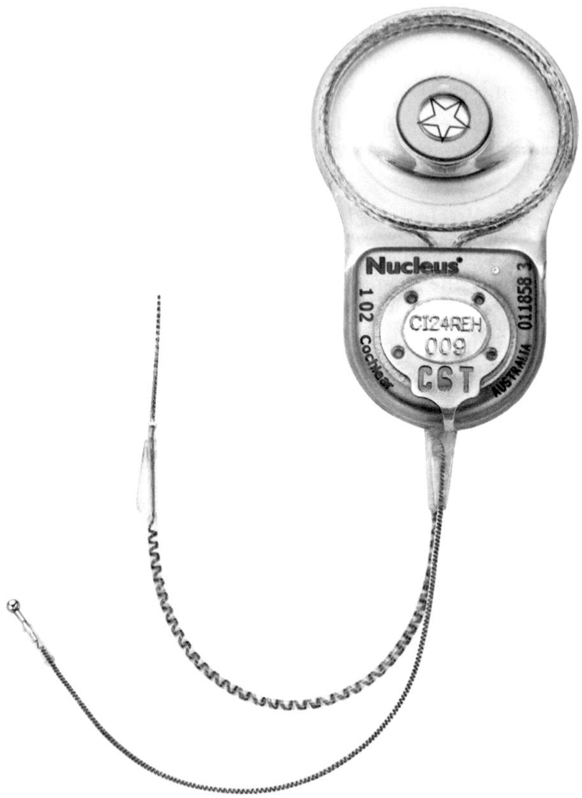


**Fig. 5.25** Hybrid L24

#### **5.3.3.5 Hybrid L24 Cochlear Implant** (Fig. 5.25)

Cochlear™ Hybrid™ System is a new treatment option available to address the unique needs of patients with severe to profound high frequency hearing loss. This exciting technology provides access to high frequency information via electrical stimulation to improve speech perception abilities. At the same time, Hybrid retains and integrates acoustically useful low-frequency hearing that may lead to additional benefits such as the ability to listen in the presence of background noise and to appreciate music.

The Cochlear Hybrid System is the first truly integrated electro-acoustic stimulation solution available for those with severe to profound high frequency hearing loss. The Nucleus® Hybrid L24 is the surgically implanted component of the Hybrid System and is designed to restore hearing in higher frequencies through electrical stimulation. The Hybrid L24 implant uses the same technology as the benchmark setting Nucleus Freedom™ cochlear implant. Since the release of the first multi-channel system in 1982, Cochlear has produced several generations of cochlear implants, with each successive generation of implant being more reliable than the last. Over that time the improvements made in implant technology have resulted in improved hearing outcomes. The Hybrid L24 implant continues in this tradition and provides significant benefit for your patients.

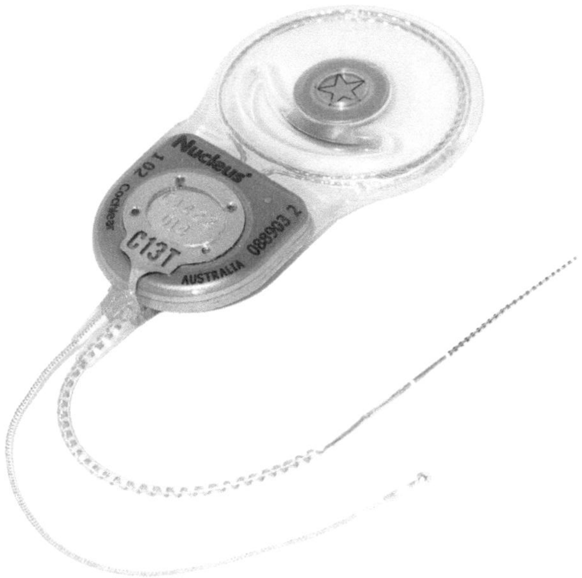


**Fig. 5.26** Nucleus CI422

### 5.3.3.6 **Nucleus CI422 Cochlear Implant** (Fig. 5.26)

- Receiver/stimulator in titanium casing for high impact resistance
- Removable magnet for MRI safety
- MRI safe at 3 Tesla with magnet removed. Non-magnetic plug to assist MRI procedures
- Two extracochlear electrodes for different stimulation modes, and high performance telemetry

### 5.3.3.7 **Nucleus® CI632** (Fig. 5.27)

**Nucleus Profile Plus with Slim Modiolar electrode**

The thinnest implant body with no pedestal designed to minimize bone excavation and skin protrusion

Implant coil enabling telemetry

Titanium casing for impact resistance

Symmetrical side-by-side exit leads from main casing. Same procedure for left and right ear.

Removable magnet for MRI safety to minimize image distortion. MRI at 1.5 and 3.0 Tesla with magnet in place.

**Fig. 5.27** Nucleus CI632

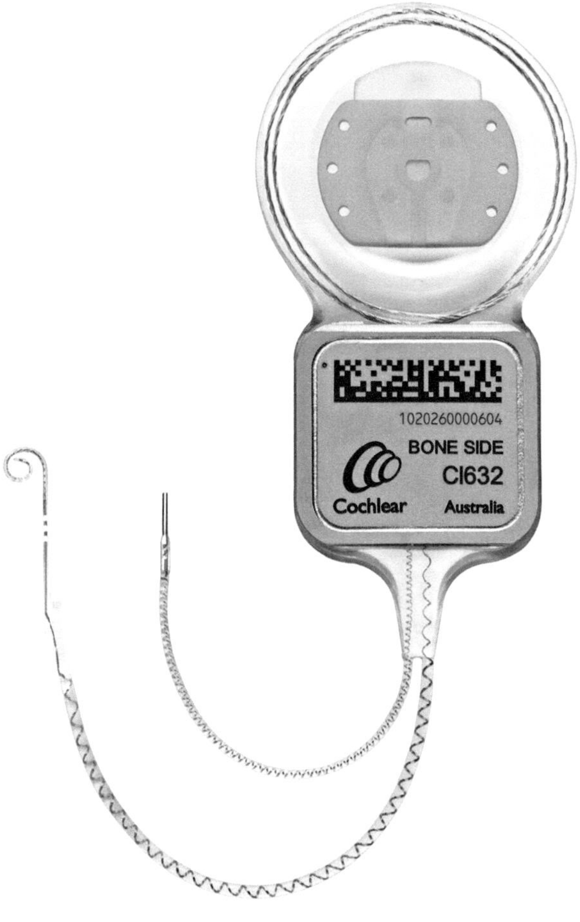


### 5.3.4 Audio Processors

#### 5.3.4.1 Nucleus Freedom Sound Processor

New automatic phone detection through Auto Telecoil for optimized phone use—this unique and patented feature is only available on Cochlear's CP810 Sound Processor.

Dual omnidirectional microphones—these sophisticated microphones capture more sound and enhance directionality, while improving hearing performance outcomes.

#### 5.3.4.2 Nucleus CP802 Sound Processor (Fig. 5.28)

The CP802 Sound Processor has been designed for humid and dusty climates and to withstand the rough and tumble of everyday life. It is tough and reliable.

The CP802 has been designed to be simple, so individuals feel confident wearing and using it in any situation.

Fig. 5.28 Nucleus CP802

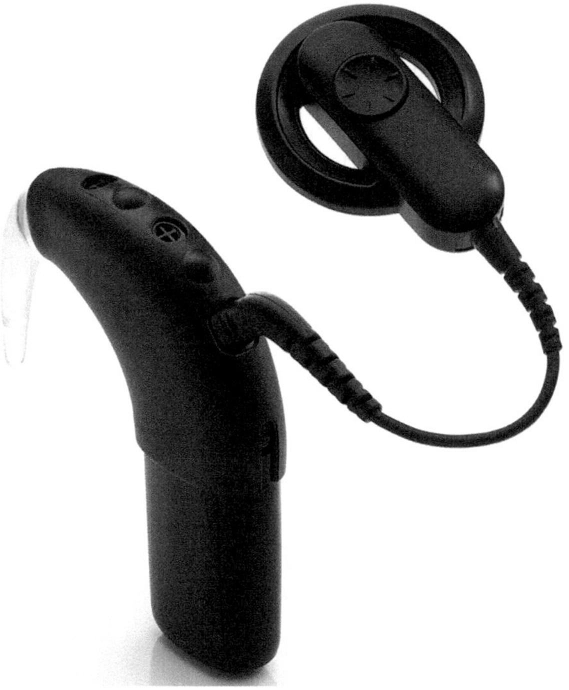

#### 5.3.4.3 Affordable to Use

Cochlear's CP802 Sound Processor has been designed to be affordable. Everyone wants to live their life their way—to talk, laugh, sing, and live without compromise.

So you, or your child can become more involved in everyday life such as sports activities, sharing a joke with friends or telling your family about their day.

#### 5.3.4.4 Connectivity

- Telecoil: This can be used to improve their hearing in a wide range of situations, such as: on the telephone, in cinemas, churches, and meeting rooms (where there is a hearing loop installed).
- FM: The CP802 includes compatible components that allow it to pick up signals from FM systems so your child can hear the teachers voice more clearly.
- Programming: Custom Sound™ Suite 4.3 or higher.

#### 5.3.4.5 Nucleus® CP810 Sound Processor (Fig. 5.29)

*SmartSound*™—offers customized settings for four different listening environments:

- *EVERYDAY*—designed for everyday listening situations such as at home or in the office or classroom.
- *NOISE*—designed for noisy environments such as crossing a busy road, or at a party.

- *FOCUS*—designed for focused listening when the speaker is in front and background noise is present, such as at a café.
- *MUSIC*—designed for listening to live or recorded music.

New automatic phone detection through Auto Telecoil for optimized phone use—this unique and patented feature is only available on Cochlear's CP810 Sound Processor.

Dual omnidirectional microphones—these sophisticated microphones capture more sound and enhance directionality, while improving hearing performance outcomes.

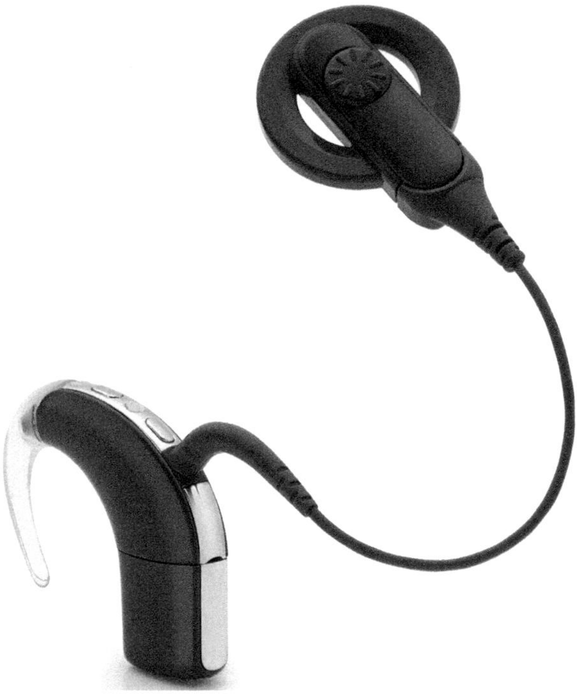

**Fig. 5.29** Nucleus CP810

#### 5.3.4.6 Water Resistance

When using a rechargeable battery module, the CP810 Sound Processor has a dust and ingress protection rating of IP57.

When using a standard battery module (with disposable batteries) the CP810 Sound Processor has a rating of IP44. IP57 and IP44 are rated according to International Standard IEC 60529.

### 5.3.5 Nucleus 6 Sound Processor (Fig. 5.30)

Built on a completely new microchip platform with five times the processing power of its predecessor (the Cochlear Nucleus CP810 Sound Processor), the CP910 is able to support significant advances in sound processing that deliver new levels of hearing performance.

SmartSound iQ, our most sophisticated sound management system yet, has a range of individual technologies that are designed to work together seamlessly to meet the user's needs in every listening environment. Even better, it can do this automatically, so they do not have to worry about it.

**Fig. 5.30** Nucleus CP910

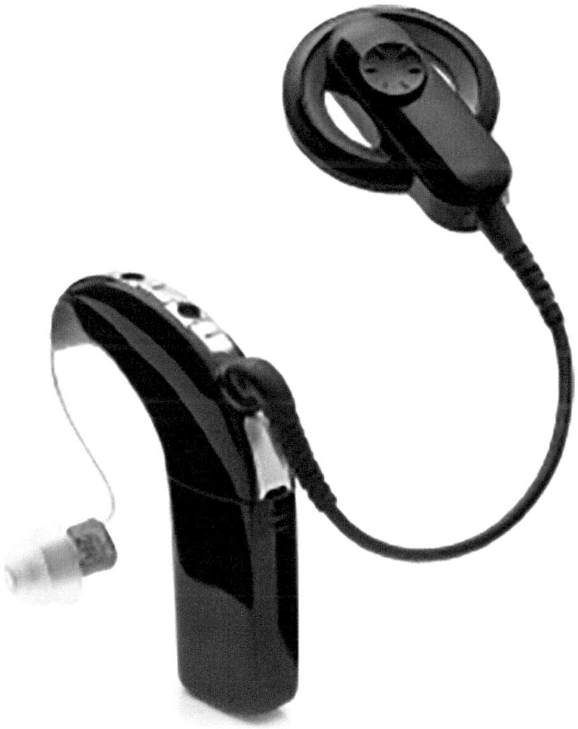

#### 5.3.5.1 Hearing Performance

- *Quiet*: For appreciating soft sounds such as soft incidental speech and environmental sounds in quiet environments.
- *Noise*: For noisy environments such as large crowds, the roar of traffic, or the hum of machinery, when it is still important to hear incidental speech.
- *Speech:* For conversations in relatively quiet environments, like family discussions around the dinner table. Speech in Noise such as a café or restaurant where there is a lot of other competing conversation happening.
- *Wind:* For enjoying the windy outdoors without the distracting noise.
- *Music:* For when the user wants to balance the need to understand lyrics with the broader music experience.

#### 5.3.5.2 Hybrid Mode

For those who have residual hearing, the CP910 is capable of operating both as a hearing aid and cochlear implant system simultaneously and seamlessly.

In a few simple steps, a hearing professional can swap the earhook on the sound processor with one that accommodates the acoustic hearing aid component. Natural hearing is boosted by the hearing aid and complemented by the cochlear implant.

#### 5.3.5.3 Water Resistance

The sound processor has an IP57 rating for protection against failure from dust and temporary immersion in water when it is worn with a rechargeable battery module, a coil and coil cable, a closed accessory socket, and no acoustic component.

When worn in Hybrid mode with an acoustic component and a standard tamper resistant battery module, the sound processor is IP44 rated for protection against failure from splashing water or access of foreign objects 1.0 mm in diameter or larger.

The CP910 also has an advanced water-repellent coating.

#### 5.3.5.4 Nucleus CP920 (Fig. 5.31)

The Cochlear Nucleus CP920 Sound Processor uses sophisticated technology to deliver hearing performance across a range of listening environments automatically.

For those preferring to be more involved in monitoring or managing their hearing, the CP920 Sound Processor can communicate wirelessly with two optional remote management accessories: the Cochlear Nucleus CR210 Remote Control and the Cochlear Nucleus CR230 Remote Assistant.

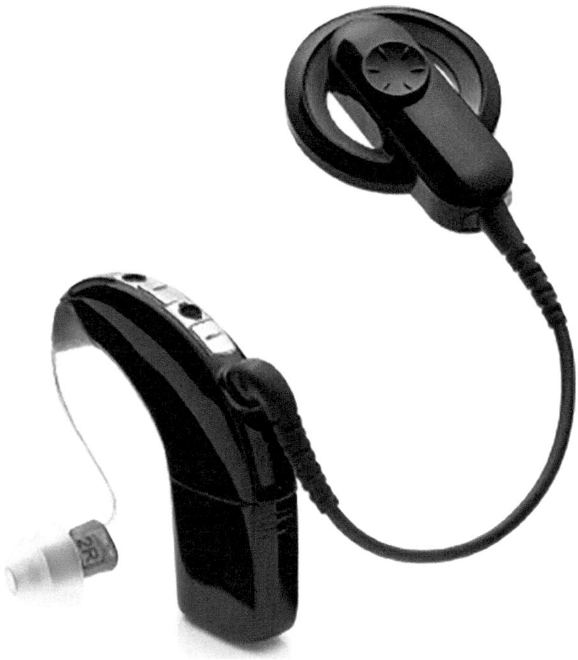

**Fig. 5.31** Nucleus CP920

#### 5.3.5.5 Hybrid Mode

For those who have residual hearing, the CP920 is capable of operating both as a hearing aid and cochlear implant system simultaneously and seamlessly.

In a few simple steps, a hearing professional can swap the earhook on the sound processor with one that accommodates the acoustic hearing aid component. Natural hearing is boosted by the hearing aid and complemented by the cochlear implant.

The sound processor has an IP57 rating for protection against failure from dust and temporary immersion in water when it is worn with a rechargeable battery module, a coil and coil cable, and no acoustic component.

When worn in Hybrid mode with an acoustic component and a standard tamper resistant battery module, the sound processor is IP44 rated for protection against failure from splashing water or access of foreign objects 1.0 mm in diameter or larger.

The CP920 also has an advanced water-repellent coating.

#### 5.3.5.6 Nucleus Kanso Sound Processor (Fig. 5.32)

- Simple, discreet, off-the-ear sound processor with the proven technology of Nucleus 6.
- Kanso helps recipients hear with clarity using SmartSound iQ with SCAN and dual microphones and is compatible with Cochlear True Wireless™ devices.
- Kanso is dust and splash resistant.
- SmartSound iQ with SCAN
- Dual microphones
- IP54 rating for water and dust resistance
- Seven magnet strengths available
- LED status monitoring

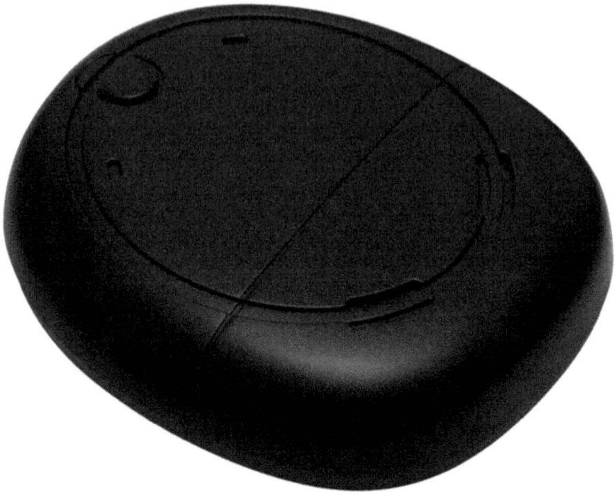

**Fig. 5.32** Nucleus Kanso sound processor

- Compatible with Cochlear Nucleus CR210
- Remote Control and CR230 Remote Assistant
- Compatible with Cochlear True Wireless devices
- FM compatibility available with the Cochlear Wireless Mini Microphone 2+*
- Telecoil optimized for room loops

#### 5.3.5.7 Nucleus 7 Sound Processor (Fig. 5.33)

Delivering clinically proven hearing outcomes, the Nucleus 7 Sound Processor is the smallest, lightest, and only cochlear implant sound processor offering connectivity and control directly from a user's smartphone.

With the Nucleus Smart App, recipients can take control of their hearing like never before. Made for iPhone connectivity allows recipients to stream calls, music, and entertainment directly to their sound processor from their iPhone, or wirelessly from their Android™ device via the Cochlear Wireless Phone Clip.

Meanwhile, Cochlear's most advanced sound management system—SmartSound iQ with SCAN—helps recipients hear their best even in noisy environments.

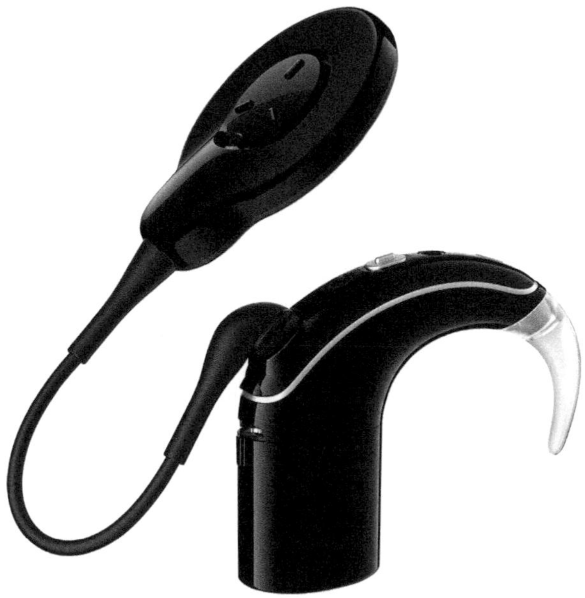

**Fig. 5.33** Nucleus 7 sound processor

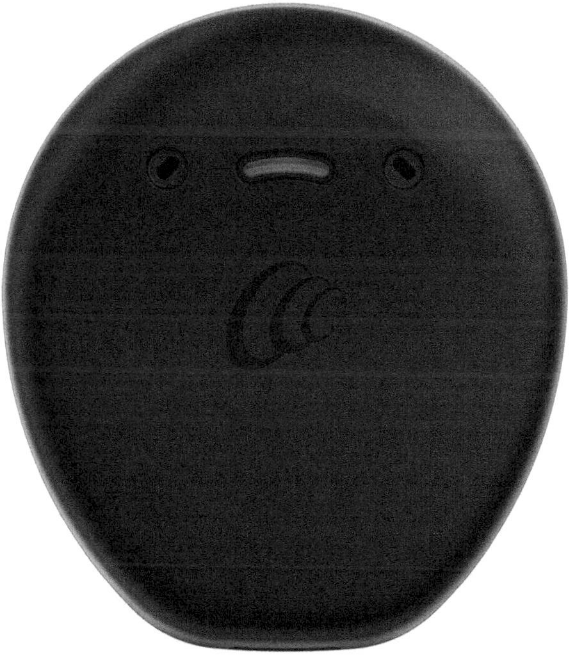

**Fig. 5.34** Kanso 2 sound processor

#### **5.3.5.8 Nucleus Kanso 2 Sound Processor** (Fig. 5.34)

- Smallest off-the-ear cochlear implant sound processor
- SmartSound iQ with SCAN

- ForwardFocus (if enabled by a clinician)
- Dual omnidirectional microphones
- Wireless inductive charging
- Integrated rechargeable lithium-ion battery
- IP rating for water and dust resistance: IP68~
- Waterproof with Aqua+
- Six magnet strengths available with Profile Plus series implant, seven available for compatible prior implant generations
- LED status monitoring
- Compatible with the Nucleus Smart App
- Compatible with Cochlear Nucleus CR310 Remote Control
- Direct streaming from compatible Apple and Android devices#
- Streaming from other Bluetooth®-enabled devices via the Cochlear Wireless Phone Clip
- Compatible with Cochlear True Wireless™ devices

### 5.3.6 Nucleus® Freedom® Sound Processor

The availability of multiple coding strategies and flexible parameter choices, allows clinicians to customize an individual's speech processor program (MAP) which results in significant improvements in hearing performance. The Freedom sound processor delivers a broad range of speech coding strategies including ACE, SPEAK, and CIS for optimal hearing outcomes.

ACE™: Advanced Combination Encoders is a unique family of strategies introduced with the Nucleus 24 implant series, which provides a wealth of both pitch and timing information and has been found to provide the best outcomes for the majority of Nucleus recipients. ACE is a high rate roving strategy using many channels. ACE combines the strengths of SPEAK and CIS to improve both temporal and spectral representation of the speech signal.

CIS: Continuous Interleaved Sampling presents high fixed rate stimulation to a relatively limited set of channels. The use of high rate stimulation provides important information on the timing of speech. CIS is especially useful for recipients with a limited number of available electrodes.

SPEAK: An interleaved pulsatile strategy. It delivers stimulation at a moderate rate and dynamically selects the number and location of electrodes to be activated, depending on the intensity and frequency characteristics of speech. It is rich in spectral information that has been proven to provide excellent outcomes for recipients. SPEAK provides excellent energy efficiency.

In addition to three speech coding strategies, Freedom also offers SmartSound™ pre-processing technologies that have been shown to significantly increase speech intelligibility and perception. SmartSound models natural hearing by adjusting audibility overall, as well as by frequency. Louder frequencies can be reduced for comfort while softer sounds can be increased. This helps ensure that recipients will hear complex sounds like speech and music easily, completely and comfortably.

### 5.3.7 Nucleus CP802 Sound Processor

The CP802 speech processor offers ACE, CIS, and SPEAK digital speech coding strategies.

ACE™: Advanced Combination Encoders is a unique family of strategies introduced with the Nucleus 24 implant series, which provides a wealth of both pitch and timing information and has been found to provide the best outcomes for the majority of Nucleus recipients. ACE is a high rate roving strategy using many channels. ACE combines the strengths of SPEAK and CIS to improve both temporal and spectral representation of the speech signal.

CIS: Continuous Interleaved Sampling presents high fixed rate stimulation to a relatively limited set of channels. The use of high rate stimulation provides important information on the timing of speech. CIS is especially useful for recipients with a limited number of available electrodes.

SPEAK: an interleaved pulsatile strategy delivers stimulation at a moderate rate and dynamically selects the number and location of electrodes to be activated, depending on the intensity and frequency characteristics of speech. It is rich in spectral information that has been proven to provide excellent outcomes for recipients. SPEAK provides excellent energy efficiency.

In addition to three speech coding strategies, CP 802™ also offers SmartSound™ pre-processing technology that results in significant increase in speech intelligibility and perception with the help of inbuilt dual microphones. SmartSound™ models natural hearing by adjusting audibility overall, as well as by frequency. Louder frequencies can be reduced for comfort while softer sounds can be increased. This helps ensure that recipients will hear complex sounds like speech and music easily, completely and comfortably.

### 5.3.8 Early and Recent Speech Processor and Speech Coding

The Nucleus Freedom speech processor consists of the transmitting coil and the BTE processing unit and controller. The modular design of the speech processor allows recipients to use a BTE or Body-worn controller. The main BTE processing unit contains all the relevant speech processing and MAP functions and is therefore unaffected by changing the controller. The controller contains the batteries, user-adjustable controls, and an LCD screen. The BTE controller uses three Zinc Air disposable batteries or a Lithium-ion rechargeable pack. A two-battery BTE controller is also available. The Body-worn controller uses two AAA Alkaline or rechargeable batteries. The BTE processing unit contains a custom digital integrated circuit containing four parallel digital signal processing (DSP) units, a microcontroller, and memory.

The ultralow power custom DSP architecture is capable of performing more than 180 million operations per second, allowing for future input processing and speech coding upgrades. The parallel processing architecture uses much less power than would be required if a single processing unit was used. Up to four MAPs can be stored in the processor. Each MAP is independent of the others, thus can differ in

T-SPL and C-SPL levels, SmartSound options, and other MAP functions. The unit also contains two microphones, an omnidirectional and a directional. In normal operation the directional microphone is used. The new SmartSound beamformer option, Beam, uses both microphones.

The Freedom processor can be programmed with any of the speech coding strategies: SPEAK, ACE, and CIS. The stimulation rate for SPEAK is 250 Hz per channel. Stimulation rates for ACE and CIS are between 250 Hz and 3.5 kHz per channel.

| Year | Sound processor | Speech coding strategy | Reference |
|---|---|---|---|
| 1982 | Wearable Speech Processor (WSP) | F0F2 speech coding strategy F0F1F2 (introduced in 1986) | • Dowell, R. C., Blamey, P. J., Seligman, P. M., Brown, A. M., & Clark, G. M. (1986). Speech recognition performance with a two-formant coding strategy for a multi-channel cochlear prosthesis. Australian Journal of Audiology, (suppl.2), 11. |
| 1989 | Mini Speech Processor (MSP) | MPEAK | • Skinner MW, Holden LK, Holden TA, et al. Performance of postlinguistically deaf adults with the Wearable Speech Processor (WSP III) and Mini Speech<br>• Processor (MSP) of the Nucleus Multi-Electrode Cochlear Implant. Ear Hear 12:3–22, 1991.<br>• Holden LK, Skinner MW, Holden TA. Speech recognition with the MPEAK and SPEAK speech coding strategies of the Nucleus Cochlear Implant. Otolaryngol Head Neck Surg. 1997 Feb;116(2):163–7. https://doi.org/10.1016/s0194-5998(97)70319-x. PMID: 9051058.<br>• Skinner MW, Fourakis MS, Holden TA, Holden LK, Demorest ME. Identification of speech by cochlear implant recipients with the Multipeak (MPEAK) and Spectral Peak (SPEAK) speech coding strategies. I. Vowels. Ear Hear. 1996 Jun;17(3):182–97. https://doi.org/10.1097/00003446-199606000-00002. PMID: 8807261. |
| 1994 | Spectra Processor | SPEAK | • Skinner MW, Clark GM, Whitford LA, Seligman PM, Staller SJ, Shipp DB, Shallop JK, Everingham C, Menapace CM, Arndt PL, et al. Evaluation of a new spectral peak coding strategy for the Nucleus 22 Channel Cochlear Implant System. Am J Otol. 1994 Nov;15 Suppl 2:15–27. PMID: 8572106. |

| Year | Sound processor | Speech coding strategy | Reference |
|---|---|---|---|
| 1997 | Sprint™ Speech Processor | ACE, SPEAK, and CIS | • Pasanisi E, Bacciu A, Vincenti V, Guida M, Berghenti MT, Barbot A, Panu F, Bacciu S. Comparison of speech perception benefits with SPEAK and ACE coding strategies in pediatric Nucleus CI24M cochlear implant recipients. Int J Pediatr Otorhinolaryngol. 2002 Jun 17;64(2):159–63. https://doi.org/10.1016/s0165-5876(02)00075-7.<br>• Skinner, Margaret & Holden, Laura & Whitford, Lesley & Plant, Kerrie & Psarros, Colleen & Holden, Timothy. (2002). Speech Recognition with the Nucleus 24 SPEAK, ACE, and CIS Speech Coding Strategies in Newly Implanted Adults. Ear and hearing. 23: 207–23. https://doi.org/10.1097/00003446-200206000-00005.<br>• Wilson BS, Finley CC, Lawson DT, et al. Better speech recognition with cochlear implants. Nature 352:236–238, 1991a.<br>• Skinner, MW, Arndt, PL, Staller, SJ. Nucleus 24 advanced encoder conversion study: performance versus preference. Ear Hear. 2002;23(suppl): 2S–17S. |
| 1998 | ESPrit® Speech Processor[a] | SPEAK<br>ACE (up to 9 kHz—introduced in 2000) | • Note: N22 ESPrit did not have ACE<br>• Patrick JF, Busby PA, Gibson PJ. The Development of the Nucleus® FreedomTM Cochlear Implant System. Trends in Amplification. 2006;10(4):175–200. https://doi.org/10.1177/1084713806296386 |
| 2002 | ESPrit 3G Speech Processor[a] | ACE, SPEAK, and CIS | • Note: N22 ESPrit 3G did not have ACE and CIS<br>• Patrick JF, Busby PA, Gibson PJ. The Development of the Nucleus® FreedomTM Cochlear Implant System. Trends in Amplification. 2006;10(4):175–200. https://doi.org/10.1177/1084713806296386 |
| 2005 | Nucleus® Freedom® Sound Processor[a] | ACE, ACE(RE)[b], CIS, CIS(RE)[b], SPEAK, MP3000 (introduced in 2010). | • Patrick JF, Busby PA, Gibson PJ. The Development of the Nucleus® FreedomTM Cochlear Implant System. Trends in Amplification. 2006;10(4):175–200. https://doi.org/10.1177/1084713806296386<br>• Balkany T, Hodges A, Menapace C, Hazard L, Driscoll C, Gantz B, Kelsall D, Luxford W, McMenomy S, Neely JG, Peters B, Pillsbury H, Roberson J, Schramm D, Telian S, Waltzman S, Westerberg B, Payne S. Nucleus Freedom North American clinical trial. Otolaryngol Head Neck Surg. 2007 May;136(5):757–62. https://doi.org/10.1016/j.otohns.2007.01.006. PMID: 17478211.<br>• Büchner, Andreas & Beynon, Andy & Szyfter, Witold & Niemczyk, Kazimierz & Hoppe, Ulrich & Hey, Matthias & Brokx, Jan & Eyles, Julie & Van de Heyning, Paul & Paludetti, Gaetano & Zarowski, Andrzej & Quaranta, Nicola & Wesarg, Thomas & Festen, Joost & Olze, Heidi & Dhooge, Ingeborg & Müller-Deile, Joachim & Ramos, Angel & Smoorenburg, Guido. (2011). Clinical evaluation of cochlear implant sound coding taking into account conjectural masking functions, MP3000™. Cochlear implants international. 12:194–204. https://doi.org/10.1179/175476281 1Y0000000009. |

| Year | Sound processor | Speech coding strategy | Reference |
|---|---|---|---|
| 2009 | Nucleus 5 Sound Processor | ACE, ACE(RE)[b], CIS, CIS(RE)[b], SPEAK, MP3000 (introduced in 2010). | • Jace Wolfe, Erin C. Schafer (2010), Basic terminology of Cochlear Implant Programming in Programming Cochlear implants, 1st edition. Plural Publishing. |
| 2012 | Nucleus CP802 Sound Processor | ACE, ACE(RE)[b], SPEAK | • No new speech coding—not specific to speech coding strategies but for performance with CP802, this article is available:<br>• Singh, S., Vashist, S., & Ariyaratne, T. V. (2015). One-year experience with the Cochlear™ Paediatric Implanted Recipient Observational Study (Cochlear P-IROS) in New Delhi, India. Journal of otology, 10(2), 57–65. https://doi.org/10.1016/j.joto.2015.09.002 |
| 2013 | Nucleus 6 Sound Processor[a] | ACE, ACE(RE)[b], CIS, CIS(RE)[b], SPEAK, MP3000. | • Jace Wolfe, Erin C. Schafer (2015), Basic terminology of Cochlear Implant Programming in Programming Cochlear implants, 2nd edition. Plural Publishing. |
| 2016 | Nucleus Kanso® Sound Processor | ACE, ACE(RE)[b], CIS, CIS(RE)[b], SPEAK, MP3000. | • No new speech coding—not specific to speech coding strategies but for performance with Kanso, this Cochlear whitepaper article is available:<br>• D1110229 Philips, B., Plasmans A., Dhoogeb, I (2016) Comfort and listening benefits of the Kanso off-the-ear sound processor in children. (Sponsored by Cochlear). |
| 2017 | Nucleus 7 Sound Processor[a] | ACE, ACE(RE)[b], CIS, CIS(RE)[b], SPEAK, MP3000. | • No new speech coding |
| 2020 | Nucleus Kanso 2 Sound Processor | ACE, ACE(RE)[b], CIS, CIS(RE)[b], SPEAK, MP3000. | • No new speech coding |

[a] Only SPEAK available when used with N22 implants. ACE, CIS, and MP3000 cannot be programmed with N22 implants
[b] Note: CIS(RE) and ACE(RE) only available for CI24RE/Freedom implant models and later

## 5.4 Advanced Bionics

### 5.4.1 History of Implant Evolution (Figs. 5.35 and 5.36)

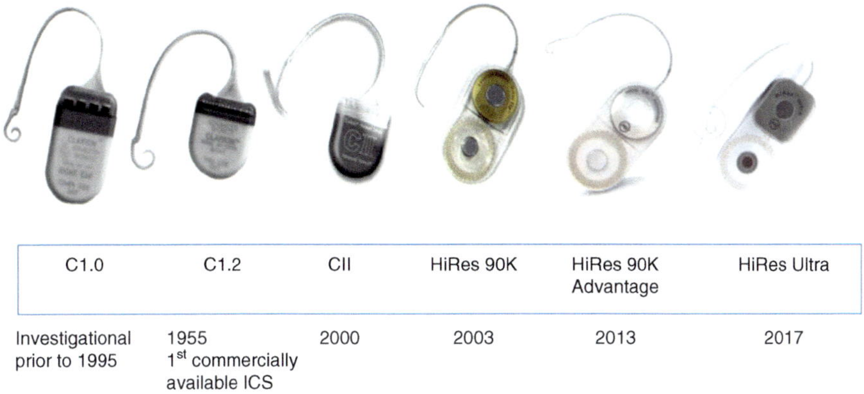


**Fig. 5.35** Implant evolution

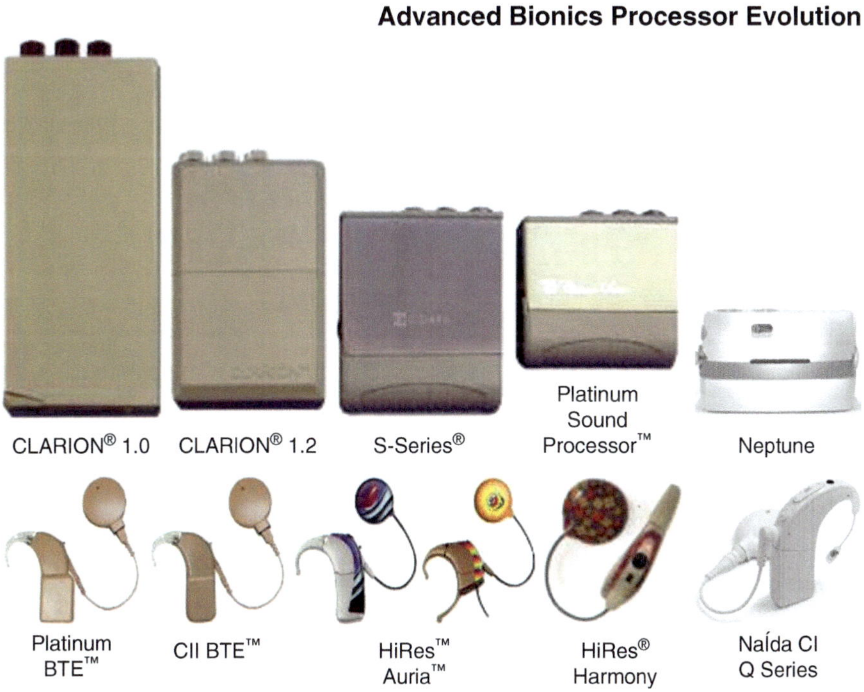


**Fig. 5.36** Processor evolution

#### **5.4.1.1 HiRes™ Ultra** (Fig. 5.37)

- Minimal Drilling: A shallow 1 mm ramped recess or surface mount makes it suitable for all—adults and children
- 3 T MRI Compatible with magnet removal and 1.5 T with magnet in place
- Titanium Implants
- Exceeding the industry standard for impact resistance
- 16 Active electrodes resulting into 120 stimulation sites
- 2 Integrated ground electrodes

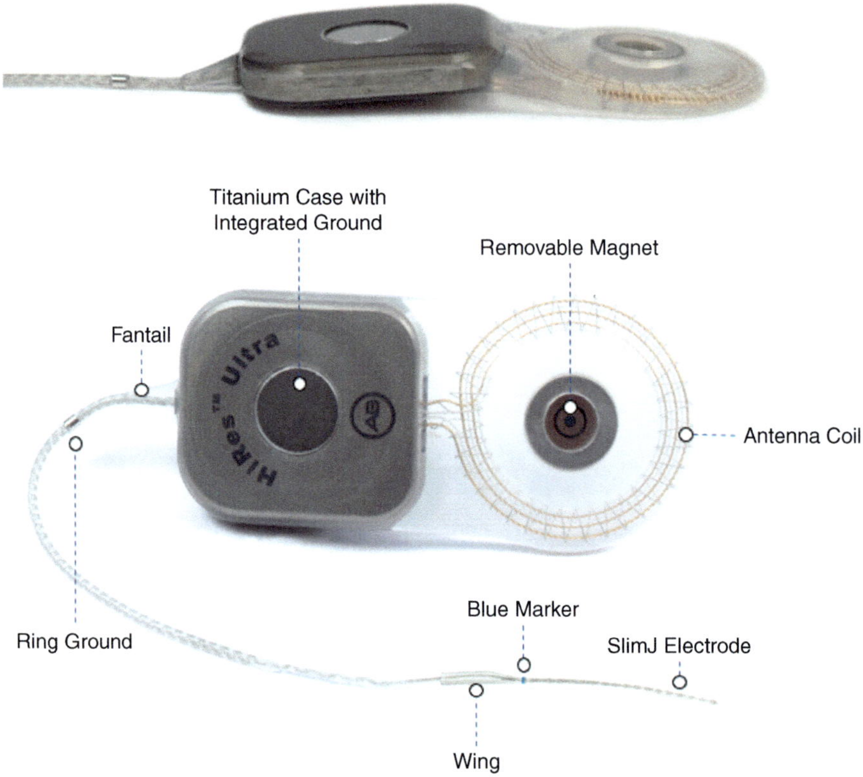


**Fig. 5.37** HiRes Ultra side and front veiw

### 5.4.2 Advanced Bionics Implant's Technology

- The 16 independent current sources allowing stimulation of up to 120 stimulation sites
- A digital processor capable of up to 10 million operation per second
- An update rate of the audio signal of 90K times per second
- Stimulates up to 83,000 pps. Highest in the Industry.
- Widest IDR of 80 dB
- IntelliLink for safety
- Impact resistance up to 6 J Strongest in the Industry
- Upgradeable electronics platform without additional surgery (Figs. 5.38, 5.39 and 5.40)

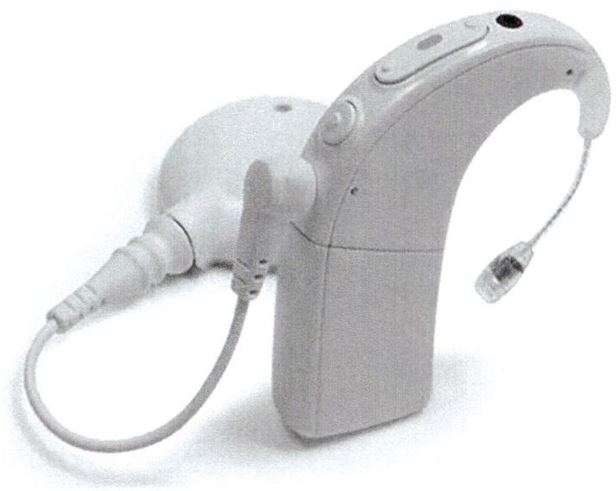

**Fig. 5.38** Naida CI Q Series Sound Processor

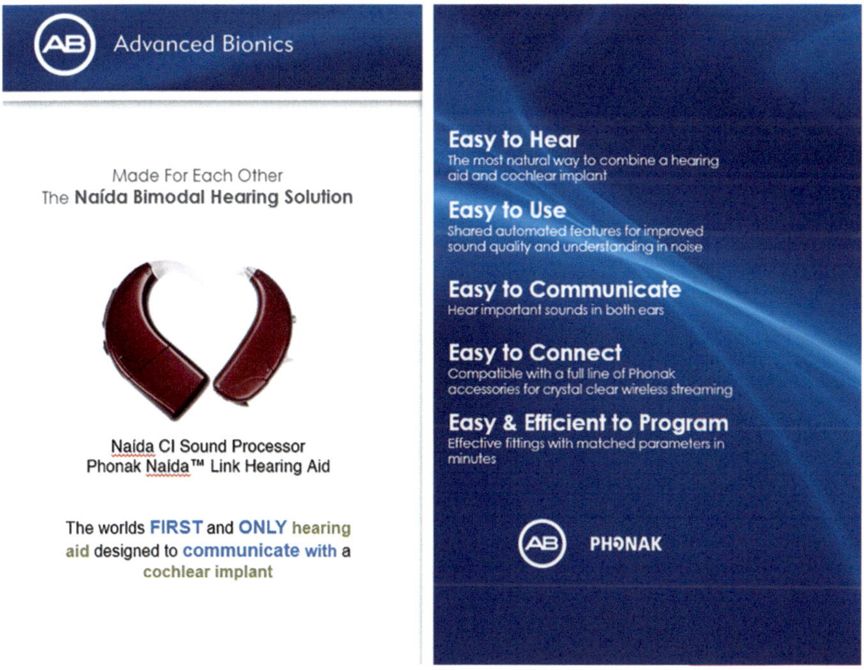


**Fig. 5.39** Phonak

# Phonak Naída™ Link CROS

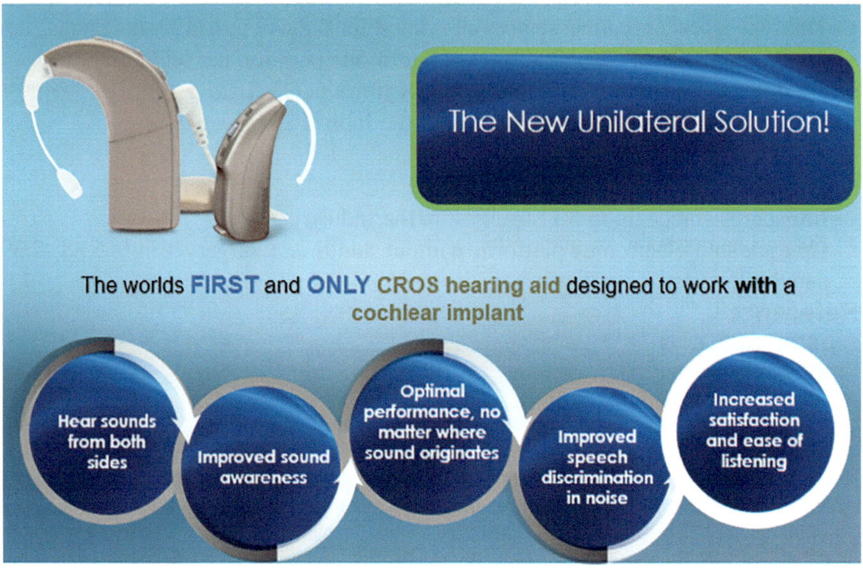


**Fig. 5.40** Phonak

| Naida CI Q90 | Naida CI Q70 | Naida CI Q30 |
|---|---|---|
| Auto UltraZoom | | |
| StereoZoom | | |
| EAS ready | | |
| SoundRelax | SoundRelax | |
| EchoBlock | EchoBlock | |
| WindBlock | WindBlock | |
| QuickSync | QuickSync | |
| DuoPhone | DuoPhone | |
| ZoomControl | ZoomControl | |
| UltraZoom Feature | UltraZoom Feature | UltraZoom Feature |
| ClearVoice | ClearVoice | ClearVoice |
| AutoSound | AutoSound | AutoSound |
| HiRes Fidelity 120 Sound Processing | HiRes Fidelity 120 Sound Processing | HiRes Fidelity 120 Sound Processing |
| HiRes Optima Sound Processing | HiRes Optima Sound Processing | HiRes Optima Sound Processing |
| Most focused binaural Automated beamformer and EAS capabilities | Bilateral and Bimodal technology for hearing with two ears | Outstanding performance in Noise and Wireless connectivity |

### 5.4.3 Electrodes

HiFocus SlimJ : A thin atraumatic lateral wall electrode

HiFocus Mid-Scala : Atraumatic Mid-Scala cochlear placement

Each electrode has:

16 planar electrodes Non-stimulating marker(s)

The ability to reload ALL the electrodes for re-insertion.

HiFocus Electrodes design:

- minimize forces on cochlear tissue
- optimal mid-scala cochlear placement*
- designed for cochlear structure preservation (Figs. 5.41, 5.42, 5.43 and 5.44)

**Fig. 5.41** Electrodes

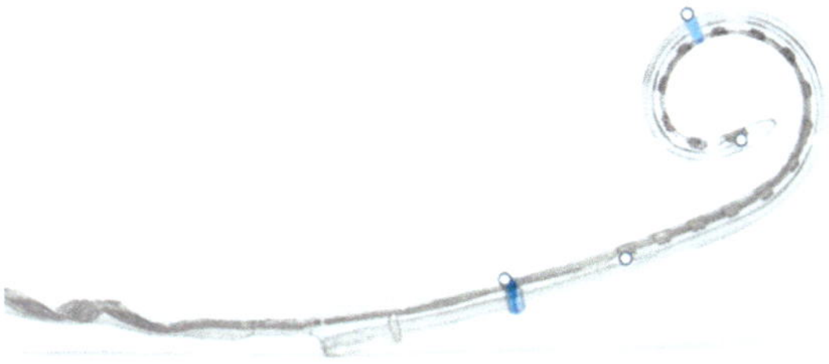

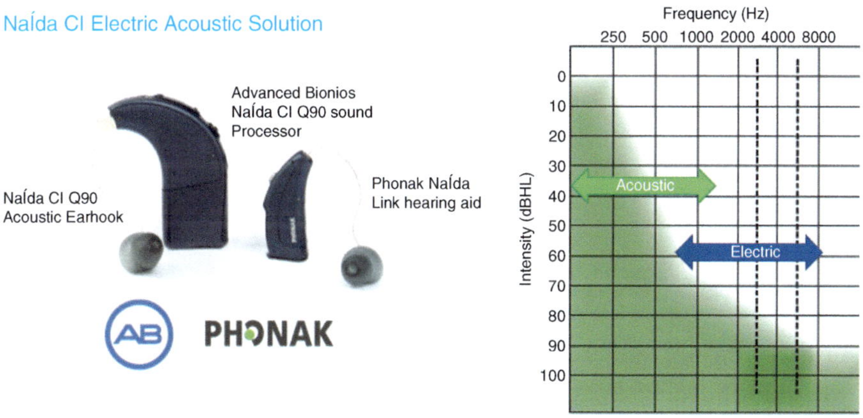


**Fig. 5.42** EAS

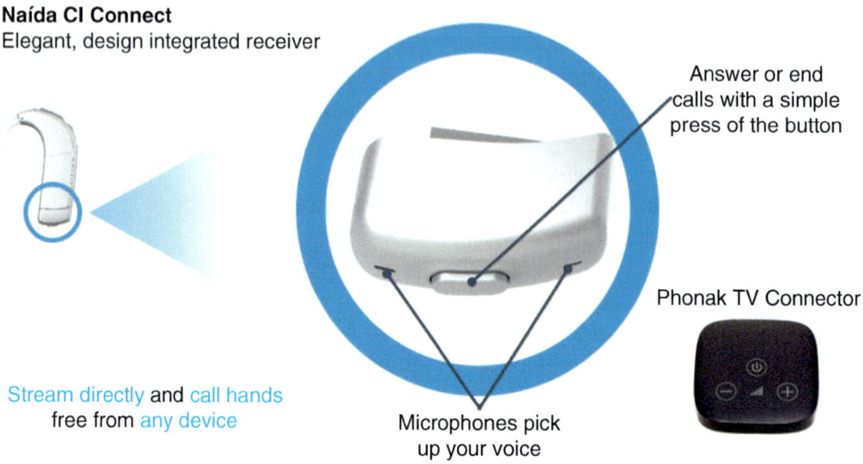


**Fig. 5.43** Naida CI connect

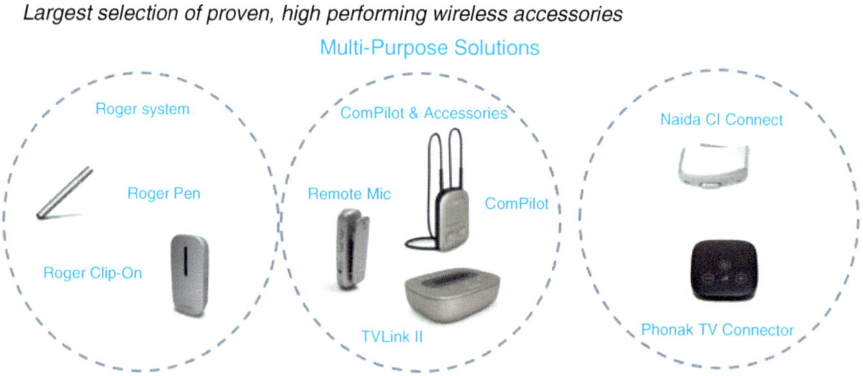


**Fig. 5.44** Accessories

### 5.4.4 Speech Processing

Advanced Bionics (AB) has a gamut of patented cochlear implant technologies. They have the highest number of sound coding strategies as well and kept innovating since 1993 till date. A list of Speech coding strategies by AB are:

- ClearVoice
- SoftVoice
- HiRes Optima-S
- HiRes Optima-P
- HiRes-S with Fidelity 120
- HiRes-P with Fidelity 120
- HiRes-S

- HiRes-P
- CIS
- MPS
- SAS

AB was the first in the world to have included a fast hi-resolution processing strategy which took care of the temporal processing in the sound dimensions. HiRes-P was able to stimulate at 82,500 Pulses Per Second, making it the world's fastest speech coding strategy. AB has a unique option of either stimulating via sequential or paired method. Paired is stimulating two electrodes at a time with a gap of eight electrodes. HiRes-S or P are 16 channel coding strategies.

In 2005, AB became the first again in the CI industry to have virtual channels. They were able to steer the current with independent current sources and have 120 stimulation sites in the cochlea via their strategy of HiRes-S or P with fidelity 120. In 2013, they moved ahead with HiRes Optima which does the same along with battery saving capabilities of 50–109%.

AB is also the first and only in the CI industry to have a noise-reduction algorithm coding strategy called ClearVoice since 2009. It improves the SNR by 6–18 dB and looks to control the steady-state noise in the environment which are continuous in nature. This acts at medium to high noise levels. In 2019, they yet again launched the first and only coding algorithm for soft-noise called the SOftVoice, which acts of soft level noises. Example like the small humming sounds in the environment and it enhances the soft speech or whispered speech in a conversation. These are powerful speech coding strategies to give the widest IDR of 80 dB, highest frequency spectrum of 120 virtual channels, and fastest stimulation of upto 82,500 PPS along with noise-reduction strategies to make the SNR much better.

The legacy and new implants can also run old strategies of SAS, CIS, and MPS. However, they are not used in today's generation implants by matter of choice as 120 virtual channels prove much more beneficial.

## 5.5 Oticon

### 5.5.1 History and Evolution

Oticon Medical has developed a wide range of implants and currently markets Neuro Zti, the latest generation of implants released at the end of 2015. Historically, the implant casings used to be made of ceramics but Titanium and Zirconia, a very resistant alloy, are now widely used.

First multi-channel cochlear implantation in France by Prof. Chouard

The first implant marketed by Oticon Medical (Neurelec at that time) was the Digisonic DX10, the first multi-channel cochlear implant.

*Digisonic DX10*—the first digital multi-channel cochlear implant—1992 (Fig. 5.45).

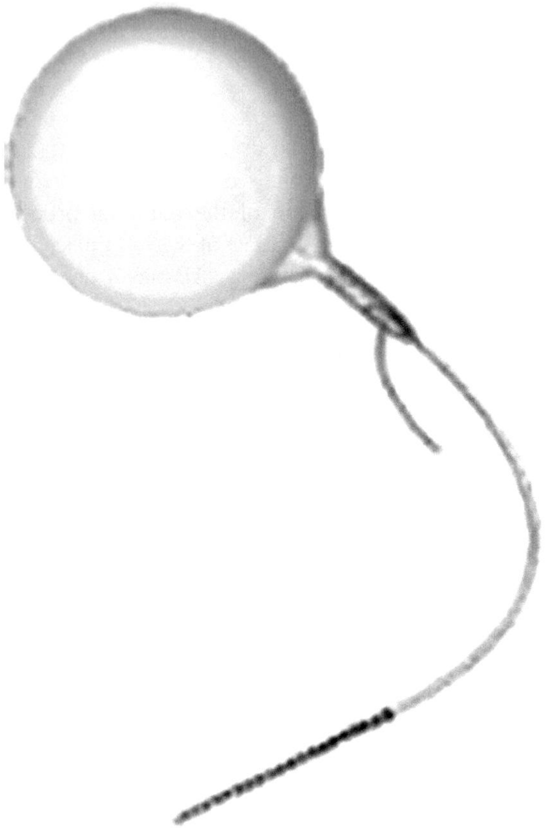

**Fig. 5.45** DX 10

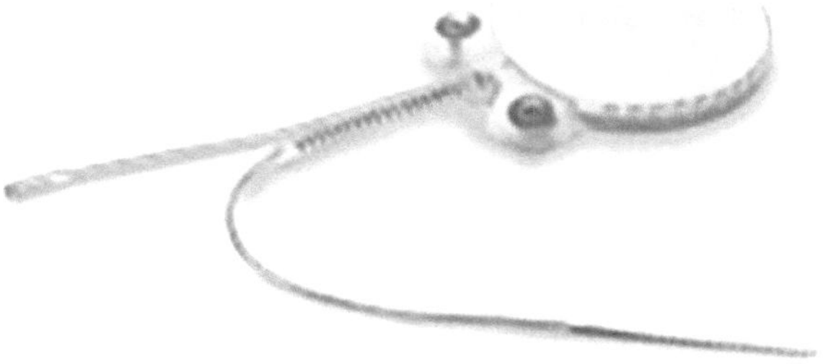

**Fig. 5.46** Digisonic SP—20 channel implant—2004

*Digisonic SP*, with an exclusive first-generation screw fixation system and 20 channels, has been the first worldwide marketed Oticon Medical implant. Production has just stopped in 2020 (Fig. 5.46).

Digisonic Binaural implant has been developed to cover additional user needs.

At last, the most recent implant is Neuro Zti, with a unique second-generation screw fixation system shown to be particularly safe and efficient in a clinical environment (with drilling required to securely fixate the implant). Neuro Zti casing is made of titanium and Zirconia, a very resistant and radiofrequency transparent material, allowing an embedded removable magnet in a rigid monobloc structure making Neuro Zti the implant with the smallest surgical footprint allowing a minimally invasive approach. It provides an extra cochlear ground electrode with a unique stimulation strategy, based on loudness coding in duration (not time coding) and a unique pulse shape to have a safe, precise, effective, and power efficient stimulation.

### 5.5.2 Implants

Oticon Medical has developed a wide range of implants and currently markets Neuro Zti, the latest generation of implants, and released at the end of 2015. Historically, the implant casings used to be made of ceramics but Titanium and Zirconia, a very resistant alloy, are now widely used (Fig. 5.47).

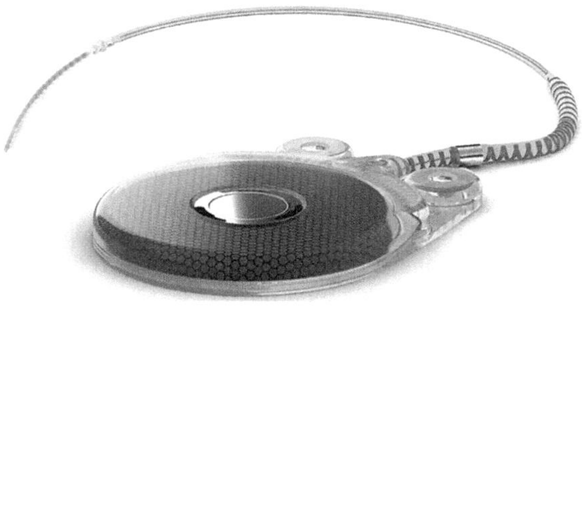

**Fig. 5.47** Neuro Zti

The first implant marketed by Oticon Medical (Neurelec at that time) was the *Digisonic DX10*, the first multi-channel cochlear implant.

*Digisonic SP*, with an exclusive first-generation screw fixation system and 20 channels, has been the first worldwide marketed Oticon Medical implant. Production has just stopped in 2020.

*Digisonic Binaural* implant have been developed to cover additional user needs.

At last, the most recent implant is Neuro Zti, with a unique second-generation screw fixation system shown to be particularly safe and efficient in a clinical environment (with drilling required to securely fixate the implant). Neuro Zti casing is made of titanium and Zirconia, a very resistant and radiofrequency transparent material, allowing an embedded removable magnet in a rigid monobloc structure making Neuro Zti the implant with the smallest surgical footprint allowing a minimally invasive approach [4, 5]. It provides an extra cochlear ground electrode with a unique stimulation strategy, based on loudness coding in duration (not time coding) and a unique pulse shape to have a safe, precise, effective, and power efficient stimulation [6–9].

### 5.5.3 Audio Processors and Accessories

Oticon Medical currently markets two types of CI BTE (Behind-the-ear) sound processors.

*Saphyr Neo* launched in 2013 with additional new coding strategy (Crystalis XDP) with, for the first time, implementation of a post processing compression to avoid sound input distortion due to common AGC systems. This brought a more clear and comfortable hearing. The Voicetrack™ feature, aiming at preserving speech signals by reducing background noise, while still allowing the listener to detect important background information was also implemented in Saphyr Neo.

*Neuro 2*, launched in 2018. It has been carefully designed to be the smallest and the most beautiful CI sound processor. And it is a success, with not less than eight international design awards and significantly smaller than any other CI sound processor ever marketed [10]: Miniaturization to its maximum. The extra long rechargeable battery life, the unique BTE showing highest water and dust protection (IP 68) [11] without any extra protection, the extra strong and discreet antenna cable (reinforced with Aramid fiber, a next generation Kevlar™)...make it very appealing for professionals and patients. The Streamer XM wireless Bluetooth-based connectivity gateway completes the offer.

Based on Oticon Inium sense chipset and Brainhearing (providing high end audiological outcomes while reducing the listening effort), Neuro 2 processing offer uses CAP (Coordinated Adaptive Processing) technology (see next section for further information) and allows to provide an advanced balanced hearing bimodal option and unique directionality possibilities with the Free focus Speech omni mode, an exclusive light directional mode inspired from the natural "pinna effect" with frequency cut-off allowing better performance in conversations.

### 5.5.4 Saphyr Neo Collection

Better speech understanding in noise with Voice Track and Crystalis XDP.

Saphyr Neo launched in 2013 with additional new coding strategy (Crystalis XDP) with, for the first time, implementation of a post processing compression to avoid sound input distortion due to common AGC systems. This brought a more clear and comfortable hearing. The VoicetrackTM feature, aiming at preserving speech signals by reducing background noise, while still allowing the listener to detect important background information was also implemented in Saphyr Neo (Fig. 5.48).

**Fig. 5.48** Saphyr Neo

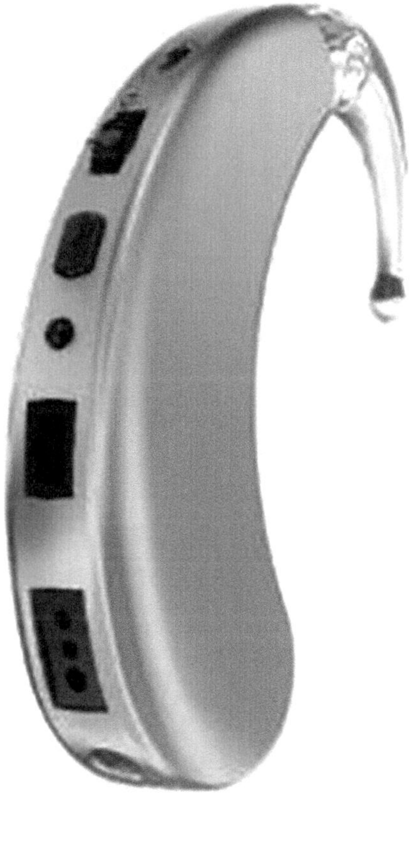

### 5.5.5 Neuro 2 Sound Processor

Neuro 2, launched in 2018. It has been carefully designed to be the smallest and the most beautiful CI sound processor. And it is a success, with not less than eight international design awards and significantly smaller than any other CI sound processor ever marketed: Miniaturization to its maximum. The extra long rechargeable battery life, the unique BTE showing highest water and dust protection (IP 68) without any extra protection, the extra strong and discreet antenna cable (reinforced with Aramid fiber, a next generation KevlarTM)...make it very appealing for professionals and patients. The Streamer XM wireless Bluetooth-based connectivity gateway completes the offer (Fig. 5.49).

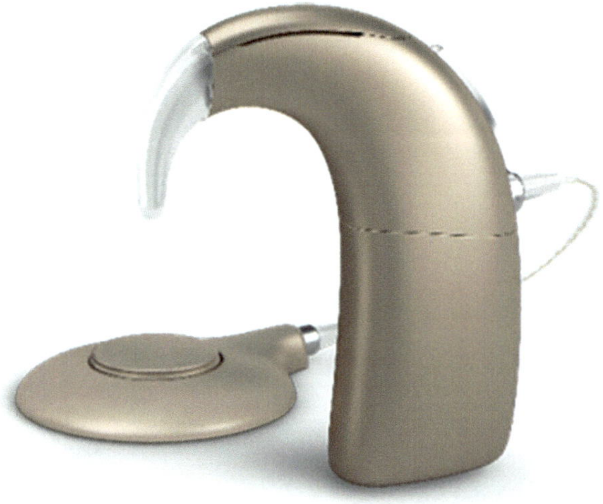

**Fig. 5.49** Neuro 2

### 5.5.6 Neuro 2 Processor and Dynamo Bimodal

Based on Oticon Inium sense chipset and Brainhearing (providing high end audiological outcomes while reducing the listening effort), Neuro 2 processing offer uses CAP (Coordinated Adaptive Processing) technology and allows to provide an advanced balanced hearing bimodal option and unique directionality possibilities with the Free focus Speech omni mode, an exclusive light directional mode inspired from the natural "pinna effect" with frequency cut-off allowing better performance in conversations (Fig. 5.50).

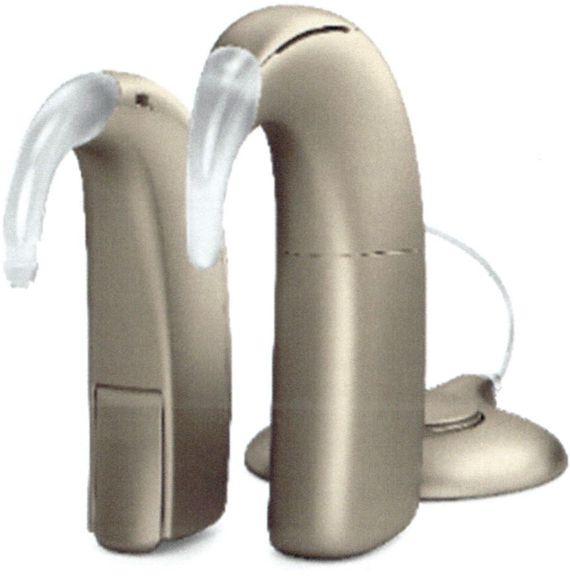

**Fig. 5.50** Neuro 2 DYNAMO BIMODAL

### 5.5.7 Electrodes

#### 5.5.7.1 Neuro Zti$^{EVO}$

Medium sized straight lateral wall electrode array (24 mm active length), EVO designed to preserve the fragile structures of the cochlea with a smooth surface, small diameter, thin end, and a highly flexible apical tip. Evo is typically used in implantations in normal cochleas with residual hearing. Its shape-conforming design goes from 1, 5 mm at the base to 1, 2 mm at the apex and provides push-rings to make it easy to grasp, to push during the insertion, and to mechanically seal the cochlea. The insertion forces are reduced by 32% compared to the CLA version (Fig. 5.51).

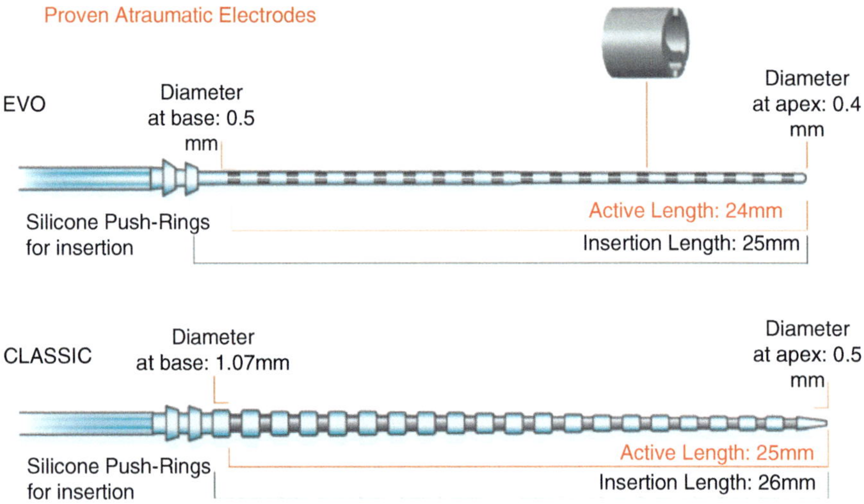


**Fig. 5.51** Zti electrode

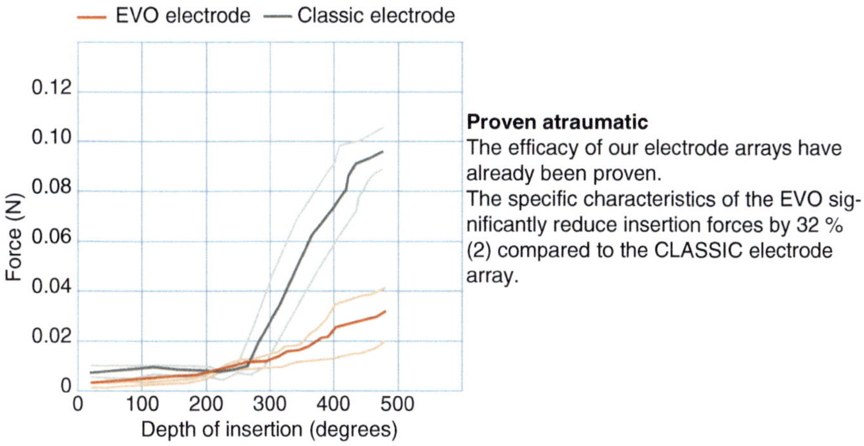


**Fig. 5.52** Comparison EVO and Classic electrodes

#### 5.5.7.2 Neuro Zti^CLA

Medium sized straight lateral wall electrode array (25 mm active length), CLA has an optimized stiffness profile with silicone rings along the electrode array that make it compatible with typical and difficult insertions and/or for ossified cochleas. The push-rings at the base provide a "safe" point to manipulate and hold the array (Fig. 5.52).

### 5.5.8 Signal Processing

Latest Oticon Medical sound processors use the CAP (Coordinated Adaptive technology).

#### 5.5.8.1 Front-End and Back-End Processing

The signal processing chain implemented in Coordinated Adaptive Processing can be seen in (Fig. 5.53) and shown to provide better speech understanding even in challenging situations [12, 13].

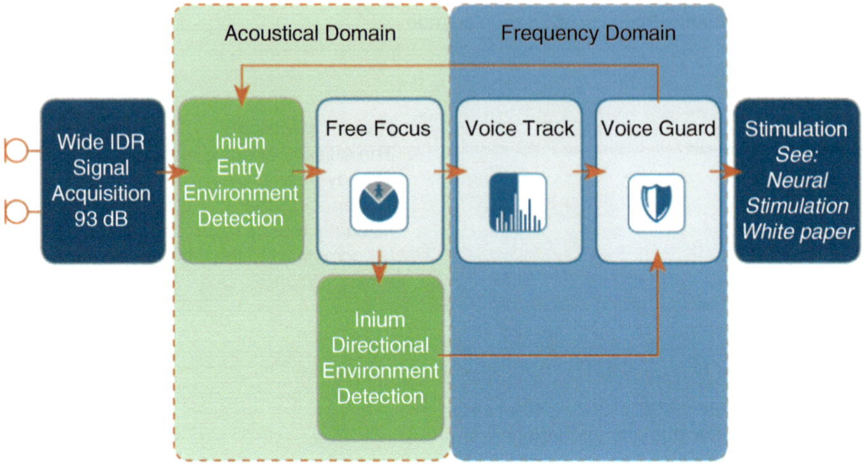


**Fig. 5.53** Signal processing

In CAP, sound processing starts with a wide input Dynamic Range (IDR) dual microphone signal acquisition, in order to benefit from the richest sound possible entering the processing chain. The Inium Sense™ environment detection system then offers real-time analysis of the acoustic environment, selecting the idea directionality mode of the Free Focus adaptive directionality technology, together with a dedicated wind noise-reduction algorithm. The signal is then transformed to the frequency domain and VoiceTrack™ reduces noise in selected spectral channels. Finally, VoiceGuard™ applies dedicated multiband instantaneous output compression, based on the analysis of the environment detection system. The VoiceGuard™ sound compression system preserves 95% of the speech information [12, 14] before processing so the sound signal is enriched in every listening situation.

The entire system is constantly adapting its behavior to the listener's actual acoustic environment. The information is then transferred by forward telemetry to the Neuro Zti implant.

CAP aims to automatically deliver the perfect coordination and balance between its different sound processing tools in order to allow access to maximum speech audibility and sound clarity in every listening situation. Two main ideas led the path to the development of Coordinated Adaptive Processing:

1. Deliver the richest sound experience possible to cochlear implant users by capturing sounds from the environment over the widest possible dynamic range and apply sound processing algorithms without introducing or propagating distortion.
2. Maximize speech and sound quality in every listening situation, by integrating a unique combination of hearing instrument algorithms and cochlear implant dedicated sound treatments, driven by continuous monitoring of the acoustic environment.

### 5.5.9 Sound Coding

Loudness coding, a unique technology, is done in duration. Physiological coding of loudness is naturally using a temporal code, as a higher density of action potentials (with similar amplitude) on the auditory nerve is observed for louder sounds. Auditory nerves do not use amplitude coding, as action potential has similar amplitudes. Loudness coding in durations has shown to be at least as efficient as more commonly used time coding [15].

The coding strategies implemented in a sound processor define how sound is transformed into electrical stimulation and distributed to the various electrodes.

**MPIS CAP** The MPIS CAP strategy (Main Peak Interleaved Sampling) is a multiband spectral extraction strategy coupled with Coordinated Adaptive Processing: An automatic backend multiband compression function (Voice Guard). A preselected number of electrodes are stimulated per acquisition frame. An anti-crosstalk function has also been implemented to minimize interaction between electrodes (so two adjacent electrodes cannot be stimulated at the same time). An environment detection system drives CAP features: directionality, wind noise reduction, and Voice Guard. This strategy is mainly recommended for patients in whom neural survival is thought to be limited.

**Crystalis CAP** The Crystalis coding strategy is a multiband spectral extraction strategy coupled with Coordinated Adaptive Processing: An automatic backend multiband compression function (Voice Guard) and stimulation of a selected number of electrodes per acquisition frame. Stimulation of adjacent electrodes together with an enhanced high pitch frequency filtering mechanism is applied to provide as much information as possible to the patient. An environment detection system drives CAP features: Directionality, wind noise reduction, and Voice Guard.

Recent preliminary results from the MHH Medical School in Hannover [14] indicate that the Coordinate Adaptive Processing (CAP) sound coding strategy allows Oticon Medical CI users to achieve excellent speech understanding in the most critical cases, that is to say in the presence of background noise and after a long period of hearing deprivation.

**MPIS XDP** The MPIS CAP strategy (Main Peak Interleaved Strategy) is a multiband spectral extraction strategy, which has a multiband compression function (XDP). A pre-selected number of electrodes are stimulated per acquisition frame. An anti-crosstalk function has been implemented to minimize interaction between electrodes (so two adjacent electrodes cannot be stimulated at the same time).

**Crystalis XDP** The Crystalis coding strategy is a multiband spectral extraction strategy, which has a multiband compression function (XDP). A pre-selected number of electrodes are stimulated per acquisition frame. Stimulation of adjacent electrodes together with an enhanced high pitch frequency filtering mechanism is applied to provide as much information as possible to the patient.

As shown, XDP strategies resulted in improved intelligibility both in quiet and in noise compared to previous generations of coding strategies [16].

Recently Oticon Medical's parent company Demant announced its intention to divest Oticon Medical and therefore has negotiated an agreement to sell Oticon Medical to Cochlear.

## References


1. Arndt P, Staller S, Arcaroli J, Hines A, Ebinger K, Cochlear Ltd. Within – subject comparison of advanced coding strategies in the Nucleus 24 cochlear implant. 1999.
2. Wolfe J, Neumann S, Marsh M, Schafer E, Lianos L, Gilden J, O'Neill L, Arkis P, Menapace C, Nel E, Jones M. Benefits of adaptive signal processing in a commercially available cochlear implant sound processor. Otol Neurotol. 2015;00:00.
3. Patrick JF, Busby PA, Gibson PJ. The development of the Nucleus® Freedom™ cochlear implant system. Trends Amplification. 2006;10(4):175–200.
4. Data on file at Oticon Medical-Mechanical Overall Feature Doc-00060923.
5. Vanlommel M, Lipski S, Dolhen P. Minimally invasive pocket technique for the implantation of Neurelec Digisonic SP cochlear implant. Eur Arch Otorhinolaryngol. 2014;271:913–8.
6. Cogan SF. Neural stimulation and recording electrodes. Annu Rev Biomed Eng. 2008;10:275–309.
7. Miller CA, Abbas PJ, Rubinstein JT, Robinson BK, Matsuoka AJ, Woodworth G. Electrically evoked compound action potentials of guinea pig and cat: responses to monopolar, monophasic stimulation. Hear Res. 1998;119:142–54.
8. Macherey O, Carlyon RP, van Wieringen A, Deeks JM, Wouters J. Higher sensitivity of human auditory nerve fibers to positive electrical currents. J Assoc Res Otolaryngol. 2008;9(2):241–51.
9. Brummer SB, Turner MJ. Electrochemical considerations for safe electrical stimulation of the nervous system with platinum electrodes. IEEE Trans Biomed Eng. 1977;24(1):59–63.
10. Data on file Oticon Medical, DOC-TX15_MT_0111.
11. Data on file at Oticon Medical (Test report TX15_RES_0046).
12. Segovia-Martinez M, Gnansia D, Hoen M. Coordinated adaptive processing in the neuro cochlear implant system. Oticon Medical White Paper. 2016;M80293
13. Langner F, Gnansia D, Hoen M, Büchner A, Nogueira W. Effect of dynamic range in different stages of signal processing in Cochlear Implant listeners on speech. ENT World Congress, IFOS 2017, June 24–28, Paris, France. 2017.
14. Monocentric data collection performed at the MHH Hannover Medical School in Germany in 2016 by A. Buchner et al. (183351).
15. Adenis V, Gourévitch B, Mamelle E, Recugnat M, Stahl P, Gnansia D, Nguyen Y, Edeline JM. ECAP growth function to increasing pulse amplitude or pulse duration demonstrates large inter-animal variability that is reflected in auditory cortex of the guinea pig. PLoS One. 2018;13(8):e0201771. https://doi.org/10.1371/journal.pone.0201771. eCollection 2018.
16. Segovia-Martinez M, Gnansia D. Design and effects of post-spectral output compression in cochlear implant coding strategy. Oticon Medical White paper. 2013.

## Further Reading

Chambers S, Newbold C, Stathopoulos D, Needham K. Protecting against electrode insertion trauma using dexamethasone. Cochlear Implants Int. 2018;1–11 https://doi.org/10.1080/14670100.2018.1509531.

Ching TY, Incerti P, Plant K. Electric-acoustic stimulation: for whom, in which ear, and how. Cochlear Implants Int. 2015;16(Suppl 1):S12–5.

Dalbert A, Huber A, Baumann N, Veraguth D, Roosli C, Pfiffner F. Hearing preservation after cochlear implantation may improve long-term word perception in the electric-only condition. Otol Neurotol. 2016;37(9):1314–9.

Dazert S, Thomas JP, Büchner A, Müller J, Hempel JM, Löwenheim H, Mlynski R. Off the ear with no loss in speech understanding: comparing the RONDO and the OPUS 2 cochlear implant audio processors. Eur Arch Otorhinolaryngol. 2017;274(3):1391–5. https://doi.org/10.1007/s00405-016-4400-z. Epub 2016 Dec 1

Dhanasingh A, Jolly C. An overview of cochlear implant electrode array designs. Hear Res. 2017;356:93–103. https://doi.org/10.1016/j.heares.2017.10.005. Epub 2017 Oct 18.

Dhondt CMC, Swinnen FKR, Dhooge IJM. Bilateral cochlear implantation or bimodal listening in the paediatric population: retrospective analysis of decisive criteria. Int J Pediatr Otorhinolaryngol. 2018;104:170–7. https://doi.org/10.1016/j.ijporl.2017.10.043.

Dunn CC, Etler C, Hansen M, Gantz BJ. Successful hearing preservation after reimplantation of a failed hybrid cochlear implant. Otol Neurotol. 2015;36(10):1628–32.

Gfeller KE, Olszewski C, Turner C, Gantz B, Oleson J. Music perception with cochlear implants and residual hearing. Audiol Neuro-otol. 2006;11(Suppl 1):12–5.

Gifford RH, Revit LJ. Speech perception for cochlear implant recipients in a realistic background noise: effectiveness of preprocessing strategies and external options for improving sentence recognition in noise. J Am Acad Audiol. 2010;21:441–51.

Gifford RH, Dorman MF, Skarzynski H, Lorens A, Polak M, Driscoll CL, Roland P, Buchman CA. Cochlear implantation with hearing preservation yields significant benefit for speech recognition in complex listening environments. Ear Hear. 2013;34(4):413–25.

Hochmair I, Nopp P, Jolly C, et al. MED-EL Cochlear implants: state of the art and a glimpse into the future. Trends Amplif. 2006;10(4):201–19. https://doi.org/10.1177/1084713806296720.

https://s3.medel.com/pdf/21617.pdf

https://blog.medel.pro/sonnet-2-audio-processor/

https://blog.medel.pro/mri-cochlear-implants-reliability/

https://www.medel.com/hearing-solutions/cochlear-implants/mri-and-cochlear-implants

Jeong SW, Kang MY, Kim LS. Criteria for selecting an optimal device for the contralateral ear of children with a unilateral cochlear implant. Audiol Neurootol. 2015;20(5):314–21.

Kisser U, Wünsch J, Hempel JM, Adderson-Kisser C, Stelter K, Krause E, Müller J, Schrötzlmair F. Residual hearing outcomes after cochlear implant surgery using ultra-flexible 28-mm electrodes. Otol Neurotol. 2016;37(7):878–81.

Mady LJ, Sukato DC, Fruit J, et al. Hearing preservation: does electrode choice matter? Otolaryngol Head Neck Surg. 2017;194599817707167

Nguyen S, Cloutier F, Philippon D, Côté M, Bussières R, Backous DD. Outcomes review of modern hearing preservation technique in cochlear implant. Auris Nasus Larynx. 2016;43(5):485–8.

Parkinson AJ, Rubinstein JT, Drennan WR, Dodson C, Nie K. Hybrid music perception outcomes: implications for melody and timbre recognition in cochlear implant recipients. Otol Neurotol. 2019;40(3):e283–9. https://doi.org/10.1097/MAO.0000000000002126.

Ramos Macias A, Perez Zaballos MT, Ramos de Miguel A, et al. Importance of perimodiolar electrode position for psychoacoustic discrimination in cochlear implantation. Otol Neurotol. 2017;38(10):e429–37. https://doi.org/10.1097/MAO.0000000000001594.

Scheper V, Hessler R, Hütten M, et al. Local inner ear application of dexamethasone in cochlear implant models is safe for auditory neurons and increases the neuroprotective effect of chronic electrical stimulation. PLoS One. 2017;12(8):e0183820. https://doi.org/10.1371/journal.pone.0183820.

Snels C, IntHout J, Mylanus E, Huinck W, Dhooge I. Hearing preservation in cochlear implant surgery: a meta-analysis. Otol Neurotol. 2019;40(2):145–53. https://doi.org/10.1097/MAO.0000000000002083.

Távora-Vieira D, Miller S. The benefits of using RONDO and an in-the-ear hearing aid in patients using a combined electric-acoustic system. Adv Otolaryngol. 2015;2015, Article ID 941230, 4 pp. https://doi.org/10.1155/2015/941230

Wolfe J, Neumann S, Marsh M, et al. Benefits of adaptive signal processing in a commercially available cochlear implant sound processor. Otol Neurotol. 2015;00:00–00.

Wolfe J, Morais M, Neumann S, et al. Evaluation of speech recognition with personal FM and classroom audio distribution systems. J Educ Audiol. 2013;19:65–79.

Young NM, Hoff SR, Ryan M. Impact of cochlear implant with diametric magnet on imaging access, safety, and clinical care. Laryngoscope. 2020. https://doi.org/10.1002/lary.28854. Epub ahead of print.

# 6 Candidacy and Evaluation of Potential Candidates for Cochlear Implantation

Nandini Dave Maingi and Sandra DeSaSouza

What is Candidacy? Traditionally people talk about candidacy as an extended debate of indications that direct a clinician to having cochlear implantation as a step toward treatment and rehabilitation for hearing impairment. In this chapter, we will talk about indications however take the topic of candidacy to a wider level and discuss how it has evolved as time and technology changed.

## 6.1 Who Can Have a Cochlear Implant?

In general, cochlear implantation is the standard of care for severe to profound sensorineural hearing loss. At a closer look there are many factors that exist that determine whether a person is a candidate for a cochlear implant (CI).

The fundamental determination for CI candidacy is audiological, medical (including radiological), and psychological variables. Guidance is needed to set the framework on which professionals base their judgment of a patient. These in general are given as guidelines or recommendations depending on the country, for example, NICE in UK.

N. D. Maingi (✉)
MED-EL India Pvt, New Delhi, India

MED-EL Elektromedizinische Gerate Gesellschaft GmbH, Innsbruck, Austria
e-mail: Nandini.maingi@medel.com

S. DeSaSouza
ENT Municipal Hospital, Mumbai, Maharashtra, India

ENT Department, Jaslok Hospital & Research Centre, Mumbai, Maharashtra, India

Breach Candy Hospital and Desa Hospital, Mumbai, Maharashtra, India



S. DeSaSouza (ed.), *Cochlear Implants*,
https://doi.org/10.1007/978-981-19-0452-3_6

The topic of candidacy is a *fluid* one and is routinely being debated. There are growing international trends of implantation in recipients with residual hearing, asymmetric hearing loss, auditory neuropathy spectrum disorder (ANSD), partial deafness where hybrid implantation can be given (Electric-Acoustic Stimulation, EAS), and single-sided deafness (SSD) [1] (Vickers et al. 2016).

These more complex applications of CIs make the question of candidacy a widely discussed and hotly debated topic.

In this chapter, we look at the history of CI candidacy globally by giving examples of the way policies have been shaped in various countries and the status of things at present.

## 6.2 The Story so Far

If we look into the history of candidacy, the initial candidates for implants were bilaterally profoundly deaf with no measurable hearing thresholds.

Globally candidacy has been changing at varying rates country to country, with heavy dependence being socio-economic factors.

### 6.2.1 The UK

The UK has a very well-documented history of CI provision. Multichannel CIs were available from 1988, funding available by way of charitable organisations and personal funds.

A 3-year assessment was commissioned by the government with the main goal to look at the coordination of CI provision centres. The outcome was a profound publication by Summerfield and Marshall [2] (1992 HMSO) that showed the efficacy of cochlear implantation. As a result, the National Health Service (NHS) approved funding for cochlear implantation [3] (Raine and Vickers 2017). This was an important achievement, but there was a need for guidelines to steer the professionals to identify candidates and to ensure equity of access for people across the country. In the UK, the standards for healthcare are monitored and governed by the National Institute for Care and Excellence (NICE); they set out standards of care for the NHS, Public Health and Social Services. They produce evidence-based guidance and policies [4] (NICE 2021). Initial NICE guidance was that CIs should be administered for all children and adults with profound deafness who do not receive sufficient benefit from hearing aids. This allowed for equal access of funds across the country as long as patients met the strict criteria. The NICE guidelines were then that the hearing had to be 90 dBHL (later 80 dBHL) at 2 kHz and 4 kHz in the better ear and a score of <50% at 70 dBSPL in BKB sentence test presented in quiet. As experience with CI grew, their benefit became more and more evident. Technology also improved rapidly. The British Cochlear Implant Group (BCIG) campaigned for a wider candidacy for CI. The BCIG have met annually since 1990 and have monitored CI use in varied recipients, as a result have campaigned for funding for CI in cases that previously would not have been considered. They persistently said that these guidelines were too restrictive. In 2017, they released a consensus [5] (BCIG 2017), summarising their thoughts, listing who should *not* be side-lined in consideration for CI.

As times and technology have changed, there are many more patients that have been proven to benefit from CIs. Most prominently patients with residual hearing (better than severe-profound as measured on an audiogram), asymmetric hearing loss where the hearing significantly different on both sides, and where only one ear is sufficient for implantation [5] (BCIG 2017). NICE guidelines changed in 2019 to accommodate a wider range of candidates [6] (NICE 2019). New guidelines state paediatric patients with hearing levels greater than 80 dBHL at two or more consecutive frequencies (500 Hz, 1 kHz, 2 kHz, 3 kHZ, and 4 kHz) and show no adequate benefit from hearing aids can be given bilateral CI. Adults meeting the same criteria qualify for unilateral CI unless they have additional disabilities such as blindness. The guidance defines adequate benefit from acoustic hearing aids as: for adults, a phoneme score of 50% or greater on the Arthur Boothroyd word list (AB Word List) presented at 70 dBA and for children, speech, language, and listening skills appropriate to age, developmental stage, and cognitive ability [6] (NICE 2019). The decision is made by a multidisciplinary team consisting of CI surgeon, audiologist, speech therapist, Teacher of the Deaf, and psychologist. Even though the criteria have been widened, the UK is still comparatively stringent with the guidance as compared to other countries such as Germany and candidates must meet the criteria set to qualify.

### 6.2.2 The USA

America is an example of a country that over the years has had strict guidelines in place regarding CI, but a recent study found that *78%* of surgeons have reported to have done 'off label' non-traditional cases of CI [7] (Carlson et al. 2018).

If we look briefly at the journey CI has made here, we can see that though research on CIs started as early as the 1950s, the first CI was approved for use in children over the age of 2 years only in 1990 [8] (Food and Drug Administration FDA, 2021). Thereafter a welcome change of lowering the approved age to 12 months came in 2000 [9] (NIDCD 2021), thanks to many evidence-based arguments. Continued research in the 2000s showed much evidence for further lowering of this age [10] (Waltzman & Roland 2005), [11] (Cosseti & Roland 2010). As a result, the FDA approved the CI for children as young as 9 months who have profound SNHL in 2020.

Currently the FDA allow CI for SNHL in 2–17 year olds with open-set speech score of less than 30% and profound hearing loss in babies as young as 9 months. In cases of SSD and asymmetry approval is for over 5 year olds who have profound loss in the poorer ear [12] (MED-EL 2019), [6] (FDA 2019).

The expanded criteria were welcomed as they showed confidence in findings that early identification and intervention is important for improved speech and language outcomes. Many professionals, however, do believe that while this is a positive step, the lack of FDA approval for the wider range of indications means that there is no uniformity in the paediatric cases getting referred. Children will, therefore, have access at differing times or may not get referred at all [13] (Holcomb and Smeal 2020).

The message that CI advocates are very keen to bring forward is that CI evaluation should *not* be delayed [13] (Holcomb and Smeal 2020). Leigh et al. [14] (2016) recommended that children under the age of 3 years with unaided pure tone thresholds of >60 dBHL would benefit from CI rather than traditional acoustic amplification. In a study akin to this by Zwolan et al. [15] (2020) showed that adults with thresholds >60 dBHL and unaided word recognition score of <60% would benefit from a CI. They called this the 60/60 guideline and suggested it be applicable for older children too [15] (Zwolan et al. 2020). The authors Holcomb and Smeal [13] (2020) state that children with AHL or bilateral hearing loss better than severe to profound *may* be overlooked for CI candidacy if they show an age-appropriate speech and language development, however they may be struggling even with the correct acoustic amplification. The authors say that it is vital that these children are assessed in complex listening environments to appropriately gauge if they are candidates for CI.

The interesting thing about the trends in the USA is that though the FDA has been conservative in its approvals, professionals are going 'off label' and making decisions on candidacy based on scientifically proven outcomes in various patient groups. This results in more and more outcome experience on these varied candidates which further supports the need for a wide candidacy scope.

### 6.2.3 Other Parts of the World

Above are two examples of countries and their historical journey to the current candidacy scenario. The UK is considered quite stringent in its approach to candidacy and the USA seems to be having the trend for a significant number of 'off label' implantations for candidates assessed and considered suitable by their professional teams. Other countries that have been known for their relatively easier access to CI include Australia and Germany [1] (Vickers et al. 2016). This study states the professional team has the final say in the candidate suitability and cases are looked at on an individual case basis. The UK and Belgium have a more conservative approach when it comes to candidacy and the audiometric measures still play a significant role in the final case approval in these countries.

Despite the varied approaches to candidacy, it is very evident that there is a definite step toward widening the gateway to allow for an increasing number of candidates to be considered for cochlear implantation based on their individual needs. This fast-paced and growing trend is changing the CI world rapidly and professionals from every area attached to this field very much support this.

In the next section of this chapter, we will look at the finer points for consideration with regard to CI candidacy approval. As touched on above, audiometric considerations are reducing in importance as the preeminent factor. By now, other areas are being seen as more informative regarding the listening ability of a potential CI recipient.

## 6.3 How Is a Candidate Determined?

In general, new-borns with hearing loss, aided children with poor performance in speech and language, and adults struggling with their acoustic amplification or who have developed a severe to profound loss later in life should all be considered for cochlear implantation. However, from that wide and very general description there are several audiological, medical, radiological, and even psychological assessments to cross before a person is considered a suitable candidate. The earlier text described the global general guidelines as they currently stand; the reader must keep in mind that candidacy is a vast subject that is constantly changing and being updated through new research findings.

Here we shall look at the specifics that a multidisciplinary CI team need to consider before giving the green light.

### 6.3.1 Clinical History

Derived from clinical experience, the first step is an in-depth conversation with the audiological physician, ENT specialist, or audiologist. This is clinical history taking and it aims to collect comprehensive information regarding various aspects of the patient.

The professional can gauge information about the child from the parents or the adult themselves regarding their day-to-day life and hearing. This discussion with the professional will provide:

- overall hearing history of the subject, including hearing aid experience if any
- the medical history in depth including any medications
- the social and educational aspects of their lives
- patient/parental expectations of cochlear implantation.

When a parent or an adult patient comes to be assessed for a CI, they can have a huge variation in knowledge regarding the process. Expectations also vary greatly. So, the initial consultation provides an essential information exchange platform from the professional to the candidate in terms of comprehensive and clear CI knowledge and a good forum for the patient or candidate to express any concerns or questions they may have.

## 6.3.2 Audiology

The audiologist has key goals:

- to determine the pure tone thresholds—(audiometry)
- to determine functional benefit of acoustic hearing aids—(speech perception)
- to test using electrophysiological methods to determine neural efficiency (e.g. Auditory Brainstem Response ABR)

### 6.3.2.1 Audiometry

The actual tonal audiogram is becoming less critical now and CI candidacy is less about this and more about the question of if acoustic amplification provides enough for the patient. Pure tone audiometry (PTA) cut offs vary country to country, *but the average is 75–80 dBHL at frequencies over 1000 Hz*. This used to be a bilateral requirement but now generally with the move to fit more asymmetric losses this cut off is acceptable as a need for one ear [1] (Vickers et al. 2016).

Pure tone threshold levels have a general area on the audiogram for which they must fall for CI to be considered. Illustration 6.1 shows the generalised requirement for severe to profound hearing loss and CI. The pattern for the air conduction and bone conduction thresholds can fall anywhere within the red shaded area.

SSD now more popularly being fitted with CI in some countries like Germany and Switzerland. The audiogram configuration for SSDs given below in Illustration 6.2.

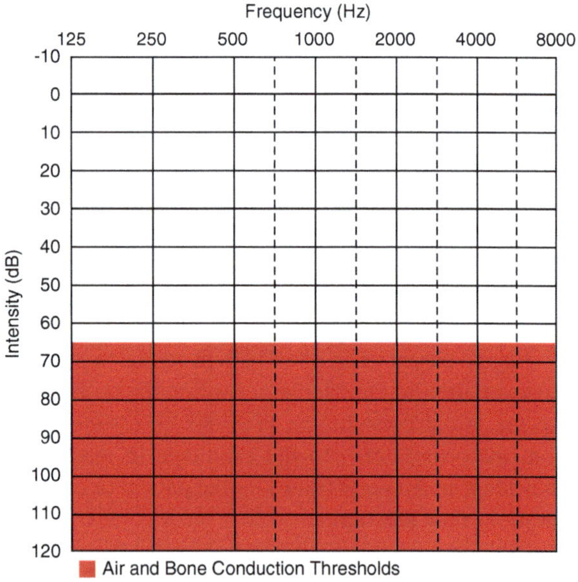


**Illustration 6.1** Audiogram showing the threshold levels considered for CI. Red shaded area highlights the area where the thresholds must fall. The configuration can be any as long as they are in this area

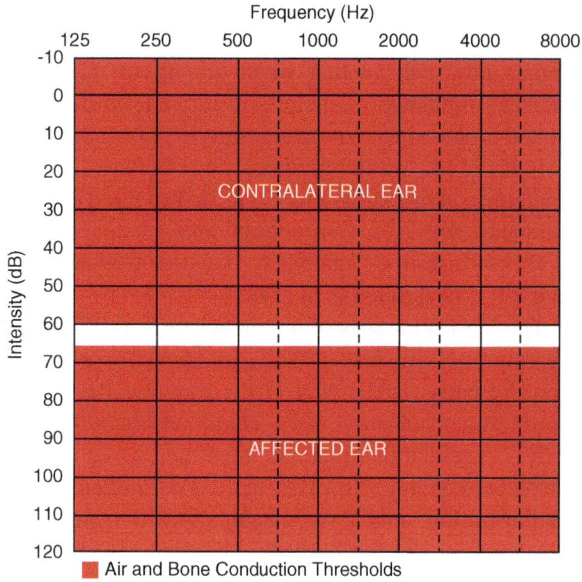


**Illustration 6.2** Audiogram showing the threshold levels considered for CI in SSD. Red shaded areas highlight the area where the thresholds must fall for the normal ear and the ear with the hearing impairment. The configuration can be any as long as they are in this area

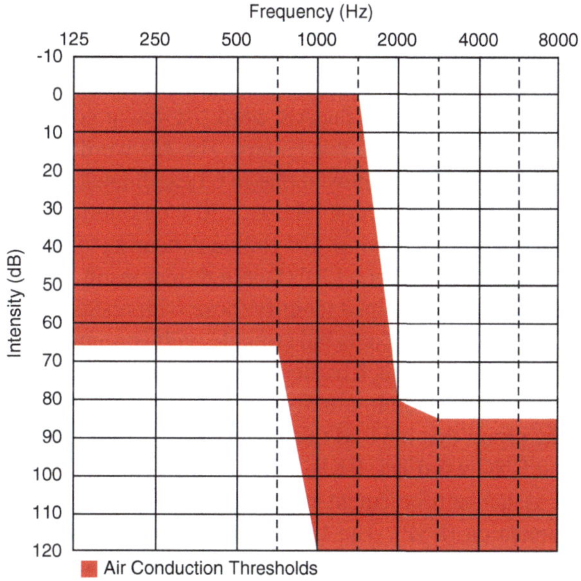


**Illustration 6.3** Audiogram showing the threshold levels considered for EAS in partial hearing loss. Red shaded area highlights the area where the thresholds must fall. The configuration can be any as long as they are in this area

As discussed earlier in the chapter, patients with partial hearing loss that demonstrate no benefit from acoustic hearing aids can be considered for a hybrid CI (EAS). The audiogram configuration consideration is shown in Illustration 6.3.

#### 6.3.2.2 Speech Perception

The importance of speech perception has grown in the recent years. Many professionals now believe that when aiming to improve speech understanding after cochlear implantation, the pre-operative level of speech understanding is the most critical prognostic factor to measure for CI candidacy [16] (Van der Straaten 2020).

In the USA, Minimum Speech Test Battery (MTSB) has been advocated for use in adults to assess suitability for a CI. The three leading CI manufacturers, Cochlear Americas, MED-EL Corporation, and Advanced Bionics LLC all recommend the MSTB for use in CI candidacy assessment in adults ([17] www.auditorypotential.com 2011, [18] Sphar et al. 2012).

The MSTB consists of a sentence test, AzBio Sentences (in quiet and in noise), Hearing in Noise Test (HINT), an adaptive speech-in-noise (SIN) test: Bamford–Kowal–Bench (BKB) SIN [19] (Etymotic Research 2005), and a monosyllabic word test: consonant-vowel nucleus consonant (CNC) word list.

It is excellent that there are identified speech perception lists that professionals are recommending. However, there is *a lot* of ambiguity in terms of variation in the administration of the tests, specifically with regard to test conditions, test materials, and definitions of 'best aided' conditions [16] (Van de Straaten 2020). The author states very firmly that this lack of uniformity is leading to variation in candidacy across the country regarding such important life-altering decisions such as implantation.

In the UK, the AB Word list is now the speech test of choice for adult CI candidacy determination [6] (2019 NICE). Vickers et al. [1] (2016) did a feasibility study in which they found the AB word list was a good test to assess perception and a useful addition to the test battery. The AB word list use was further backed up in a Welsh study. They showed that in CI candidates with a ski-slope hearing would fall outside the implantation criteria, <50% on Bamford–Kowal–Bench (BKB) sentence testing, despite having a significant hearing disability and limited benefit from acoustic amplification [20] (Doran & Jenkinson 2016). They concluded that the use of AB word list helped identify those with residual hearing that would traditionally be offered hearing aids but struggle with communication in real life situations.

Children are much harder to assess the same way, but an American group devised the Paediatric Minimum Speech Test Battery (PMSTB) in 2017 [21] (Uhler 2017). The group that devised this battery looked at various tests including open-set tests like CNC word list, BKB-SIN, and the paediatric AzBio; also closed-set tests such as visual reinforcement infant speech discrimination (VRISD) and Early Speech Perception (ESP). The Little Ears Auditory Skills Checklist is also included as a parental questionnaire. The goal is much the same as for the adults and that is to gauge the child's pre-implant speech and language levels and to pre-empt the benefit of CIs should the step be taken.

MED-EL Corporation has the Evaluation of Auditory Response to Speech (EARS) test battery aimed at the paediatric population. A similar concept to the PMSTB, it is made up of various open- and closed-set word tests. First put together in 1996 by a group of hearing professionals lead by Diane Allum-Mecklenfburg [22]. The first version had an open-set language specific sentence test but this was removed in 2002 and later the Common Object Toy Test (COT Test) was added [23] (Esser-Leyding & Anderson 2012). The EARS Test Battery has:

- Listening Progress Profile (LiP)
- Monosyllabic Trochee Polysyllabic (MTP) Word Test
- Monosyllable Closed-Set Test
- Tyler–Holstad Closed-Set Sentence Test
- Monosyllable Open-Set Test
- Glendonald Auditory Screening Procedure (GASP)
- Meaningful Auditory Integration Scale (MAIS) Questionnaire
- Meaningful Use Speech Scale (MUSS) Questionnaire
- Common Object Token (COT) Test

Once a child has been diagnosed with a hearing loss and the option of CI has been given, a common question parent have is that of speech development and language proficiency. It is important to have a tool that will reliably test the pre-implant level to first gauge the suitability of the CI and thereafter their likely development forecast. The EARS test battery fulfils the important goal of pre-operative assessment and a post-operative monitoring tool to track progress.

### 6.3.3 Medical Assessment

The ENT surgeon will assess the child's or adult's otological health status and the overall general medical integrity.

Otologically, a clinical exam of the outer ear, middle ear, and temporal bone from the scalp surface is looked at and ensured to be clear of infectious disease. Any structural abnormality is noted and added to the overall assessment.

The ENT will also test the facial nerve integrity by checking facial reflexes to ensure normal function. The vestibular function is assessed clinically also by checking the vestibular ocular reflex (VOR) and questioning balance in adults and motor development in children. If necessary, some services refer the adult patient for baseline vestibular function testing pre-implantation, however this is not yet a norm in most places globally.

It is also up to the medical professional to ensure that the correct vaccinations have been administered prior to implantation as it has been proven consistently that both paediatric and adult patients are at higher risk of acquiring *S. pneumoniae* meningitis [24] (Reefhuis et al. 2003). The finer details of the immunisation programme recommended for implantation care are beyond the scope of this chapter.

The medical profession should also consider the presence of syndromes and any other presenting disabilities. Many syndromes have hearing impairment as a symptom, but the presence and severity of other disabilities will also impact decisions to implant.

The medical assessment questions the overall health of the candidate including past medical issues and current medication if any.

The goal of the medical professional is to fully understand and assess the medical status of the patient and also judge the suitability for surgery.

### 6.3.4 Radiological Assessment

Pre-operative imaging is now a minimum pre-implant requirement and should be done for all potential candidates. Imaging of choice is Computed Tomography (CT) or Magnetic Resonance Imaging (MRI). The anatomical areas of interest are the inner ear, facial nerve, cochleovestibular nerve, brainstem, and brain [25] (Lee et al. 2020). The radiologist will look for:

- Patency of cochlear turns
- Ossification
- Hypoplasia or aplasia of the cochleovestibular nerve
- Narrow internal auditory meatus (IAM)
- Absence of bony cochlear nerve canal
- Cochlear malformations (e.g. Mondini dysplasia)
- Enlarged Vestibular Aqueduct

The result of the imaging will guide the surgeon to choose the side to implant and the size of the electrode required. This imaging also provides the surgeon with anatomical landmarks to be aware of during the surgery. More about radiology in cochlear implantation can be found in Chap. 5.

### 6.3.5 Psychological and Social Considerations

This section will just touch on the psychological and social aspects of the candidate. There was a time where developmental delay and additional needs were considered a contraindication for cochlear implantation. However, now it is universally accepted that development delay, cognitive delay, or additional needs are *not* an immediate exclusion factor.

Accepted that though there are large variations in outcome the overall is definite in the sense that there is broadened social interaction [26] (Corrales & Oghalai 2013), improved interaction, and less stress within the family ([27] Wiley et al. 2005 and [28] Oghalai et al. 2012). Each candidate must be assessed on their individual needs and suitability for implantation must be ascertained with thought also given to the degree of support from family network, school, and the candidate's own readiness to be implanted.

There is no standard questionnaire for this assessment and the psychological and social professional will need to evaluate the potential candidate based on the tools they consider optimal, however the need for this assessment is critical.

Other than the patients with additional needs, psychosocial assessment is needed on all CI candidates to see to the factors that may influence adjustment to and benefit from a CI.

If family support is lacking or there are behavioural issues this could be considered potential hinderances to CI success. A psychosocial assessment should be used to gauge the question of *expectations* from the patient and the family, and also the level of motivation and commitment to attend to an extended rehabilitation programme.

## 6.4 In Conclusion

In conclusion, it is fair to say that the conversation of candidacy is in the middle of some quick exchanges resulting in fast-paced changes to the approach to implantation and who gets considered. This chapter discussed the current major trends in candidacy from a global aspect and then looked more specifically at the current approach to the patient as an individual potential candidate.

Professionals in the hearing profession should ensure fair access to cochlear implantation. Once a potential candidate is identified, be it a child or adult, they should have all the areas of pre-operative assessment complete.

Though all countries have varied approaches to CI candidacy in general they are all *evolving* to include a much wider range of hearing impairments: partial hearing loss, AHL, and SSD being some of the main indications now firmly enveloped into this area.

The audiometric and speech perception tests are evolving rapidly and many places have adopted their own approach. There is still much more work needed to standardise the assessment approach to guarantee an equity of access to implants. This is an exciting phase in the world of CIs as technology continues to develop there will be more and more to learn about who and how to fit with this life-altering device.

## References

1. Vickers D, De Raeve L, Graham J. International survey of cochlear implant candidacy. Cochlear Implants Int. 2016;17(S1):36–41.
2. Summerfield AQ, Marshall DH. Cochlear implantation in the UK 1990–1994. HMSO; 1995.
3. Raine C, Vickers D. Worldwide picture for candidacy for cochlear implantation. ENT Audiol News. 2017;26(4). www.entandaudiologynews.com
4. Nice Guidelines Children and Adults for Cochlear Implantation. 2021. https://www.nice.org.uk/guidance/ta566
5. Consensus statement for the candidacy of Cochlear Implant on behalf of the British Cochlear Implant Candidacy Working Group. BCIG; 2017. https://www.cicandidacy.co.uk
6. NICE TA566. 2019. https://www.nice.org.uk/guidance/ta566
7. Carlson M, Sladen D, Gurgel R, Tombers N, Lohse C, Driscoll C. Survey of the American Neurotology Society on the Cochlear Implants Part 1: Candidacy assessment and expanding indications. Otolaryngol Neurotol. 2018;39(1):e12–9.
8. FDA. 2021. Cochlear implants. https://www.fda.gov/medical-devices/implants-and-prosthetics/cochlear-implants
9. National Institute of Deafness and Other Communication Disorders. 2021. Cochlear implants. https://www.nidcd.nih.gov/health/cochlear-implants\

10. Waltzman SB, Roland JT. Cochlear implantation in children younger than 12 months. Paediatrics. 2005;116(4):487–97.
11. Cosseti M, Roland JT. Cochlear Implantation in very young child: issues unique to under-1 population. Trends Amplification. 2010;14(1):46–57.
12. MED-EL. FDA Approves Cochlear Implants for SSD and Asymmetric Hearing Loss. MED-EL Press; 2019. https://s3.medel.com/downloadmanager/downloads/us_research/en-US/SSD+FDA+Approval+Press+Release_FINAL_7.22.19.pdf
13. Holcomb M, Smeal M. Paediatric Cochlear Implants: who is a candidate in 2020? Hear J. 2020;73(7):8–9.
14. Leigh JR, Moran M, Hollow R, Dowell R. Evidence-based guidelines for recommending cochlear implantation for postlingually deafened adults. Int J Audiol. 2016;55(Suppl 2):S3–8.
15. Zwolan TC, Schvartz-Leyzac KC, Pleasant T. Development of a 60/60 guideline for referring adults for a traditional cochlear implant candidacy evaluation. Otol Neurotol. 2020;41(7):895–900.
16. van der Straaten TFK, Burger AVM, Briaire JJ. The best preoperative measure to select post-lingually deafened candidates for cochlear implantation. Ear Hear. 2020.
17. Minimum Speech Test Battery (MTSB). 2011. http://www.auditorypotential.com/MSTB_Nav.html
18. Spahr AJ, Dorman MF, Litvak LM, et al. Development and validation of the AzBio sentence lists. Ear Hear. 2012;33(1):112–7.
19. BKB-SIN. Speech-in-Noise Test, Version 1.03 [audio CD]. Elk Grove Village, IL: Etymotic Research; 2005.
20. Doran M, Jenkinson L. Mono-syllabic word test score as a pre-operative assessment criterion for cochlear implant candidature in adults with acquired hearing loss. Cochlear Implants Int. 2016;17(Suppl 1):13–6.
21. Uhler K, Warner-Czyz AD, Gifford R. Pediatric minimum speech test battery. J Am Acad Audiol. 2017;28(3):232–47.
22. Allum D, Allum J, Baumgartner W, Brockmeier S, Dahm M, Egelierler B, Esser B, Gall V, Grosse G, Hildmann A, Ilchmann B, Kiefer J, Kühn H, Lautischer H, Leyrer M, Marchewka A, Moracchi A, Schürch N, Schneider A, Schorn K, Shehata-Dieler W, Vischer M, Winkler F. Multi-language international perceptual test battery for comparing performance of children in different countries: evaluation of auditory responses to speech (EARS). 3rd Eur Symp Pediatr Cochlear Implant, Hannover. 1996.
23. Esser-Leyding B, Anderson I. EARS®(Evaluation of Auditory Responses to Speech): an internationally validated assessment tool for children provided with cochlear implants. ORL. 2012;74:42–51.
24. Reefhuis J, Honein MA, Whitney CG, et al. Risk of bacterial meningitis in children with cochlear implants. N Engl J Med. 2003;349(5):435–45.
25. Lee K, Kutz JW, Issacson B. Indications for Cochlear Implants. 2020. www.emedicine.medscape.com
26. Corrales CE, Oghalai JS. Cochlear implant considerations in children with additional disabilities. Curr Otorhinolaryngol Rep. 2013;1(2):61–8. https://doi.org/10.1007/s40136-013-0011z.
27. Wiley S, Jahnke M, Meinzen-Derr J, Choo D. Perceived qualitative benefits of cochlear implants in children with multi-handicaps. Int J Pediatr Otorhinolaryngol. 2005;69(6):791–8. https://doi.org/10.1016/j.ijporl.2005.01.011.
28. Oghalai JS, Caudle SE, Bentley B, et al. Cognitive outcomes and familial stress after cochlear implantation in deaf children with and without developmental delays. Otol Neurotol. 2012;33(6):947–56. https://doi.org/10.1097/MAO.0b013e318259b72b.

# Prognostic Modelling and Machine Learning in Cochlear Implantation

7

Haroon Shakeel Saeed and Iain A. Bruce

## 7.1 Introduction

Cochlear Implantation (CI) has had a dramatic impact upon the lives of hundreds of thousands of profoundly deaf children and adults worldwide. It is arguably the biggest success story of a neural-prothesis translation into routine clinical healthcare [1]. As the field of CI continues to evolve, it is incumbent upon healthcare professionals and researchers to develop and clinically integrate novel efforts towards optimisation of both surgical and audiological outcomes. In this chapter, we focus on describing how precision medicine may be embraced and translated into clinical practice in the field of CI, to facilitate better candidate selection and outcomes.

Precision medicine is concerned with providing the *right treatment, for the right patient, at the right time*. Specifically, we will focus on two fundamentals of precision medicine: (1) harnessing *Prognosis Research* methodology to improve candidate selection and prognostic modelling in CI and (2) *Artificial intelligence (AI)* to optimise the use and benefit of patient data. Whilst both these disciplines share common ground, they represent important differences in the way that health data can be analysed. We aim to introduce the fundamentals of both these precision medicine disciplines and describe how they are impacting the future direction of CI research.

H. S. Saeed · I. A. Bruce (✉)
Paediatric ENT Department, Royal Manchester Children's Hospital, Manchester University NHS Foundation Trust, Manchester Academic Health Science Centre, Manchester, UK

Division of Infection, Immunity and Respiratory Medicine, Faculty of Biology, Medicine and Health, University of Manchester, Manchester, UK
e-mail: hsaeed@doctors.org.uk; Iain.Bruce@manchester.ac.uk



S. DeSaSouza (ed.), *Cochlear Implants*,
https://doi.org/10.1007/978-981-19-0452-3_7

## 7.2 Part 1: Prognosis Research and Prognostic Modelling

Prognosis research involves the selection of a patient group with a specific disease characteristic and deploying analytical methods in order to try and predict, or forecast, future outcomes. For example, in the broader field of medicine, this may be research that aims to predict mortality associated with cardiovascular disease based on an individual's routine biochemical measurements, or the ability to ascertain which specific disease biomarkers are pertinent to predicting 5-year survival in patients with head and neck cancer [2, 3]. As such, Prognosis research has wide applications across healthcare, and without it, clinicians would be prevented from informing individuals and their families about future health outcomes and from selecting and implementing the most effective and efficient policies for medical and surgical management [4]. Robust, evidence-based Prognosis research is fundamental to healthcare policy development and clinical decision making. Unfortunately, there is clear evidence that the correct concepts and methods involved in Prognosis research are seldom taught sufficiently to healthcare professionals, highlighting the need for an improved understanding of Prognosis research within all healthcare domains [5].

There is an unmet need to forecast hearing loss trajectory and timeframes for CI through robust Prognosis research. For example, in the field of CI, how can we predict when a child with progressive hearing loss will fall into the criteria for CI surgery? What are the pertinent clinical, genetic, and audiological features that may be important in determining hearing loss trajectory and subsequent need for early CI surgery in progressive congenital hearing loss? In adults with sensorineural hearing loss (SNHL), can we improve our ability to give an individual prognosis? For example, which adults will benefit from continued conservative management with conventional hearing aids? Without such understanding, our management of hearing loss is 'reactive' and largely reliant upon personal reports and 'best-guess' timeframes for auditory surveillance. As such, it is vital that clinical researchers embark on Prognosis research using a robust methodology, minimising the risk of their research falling short of providing accurate prediction outcomes.

The authors of this chapter conducted a Medline search for prognostic modelling or clinical prediction modelling in CI, and less than 10 pertinent studies were identified (since 2020). These studies are mainly related to predicting outcomes *after* CI surgery. The likely explanation for the paucity of robust studies in the field has been highlighted in a meta-analysis by Zhao et al.; namely insufficient evidence-based patient-related factors (known as *prognostic factors)* have been identified, collected and adequately reported within the literature [6]. The importance of identifying prognostic factors cannot be understated.

Within the United Kingdom (UK), a framework of publications has provided a blueprint for how Prognosis research (including prognostic modelling) should be conducted and are essential reading for researchers in the field of CI and hearing loss prognosis [7–9]. Taking this framework into consideration, it becomes immediately apparent that a Prognosis research fundamental should be to initially

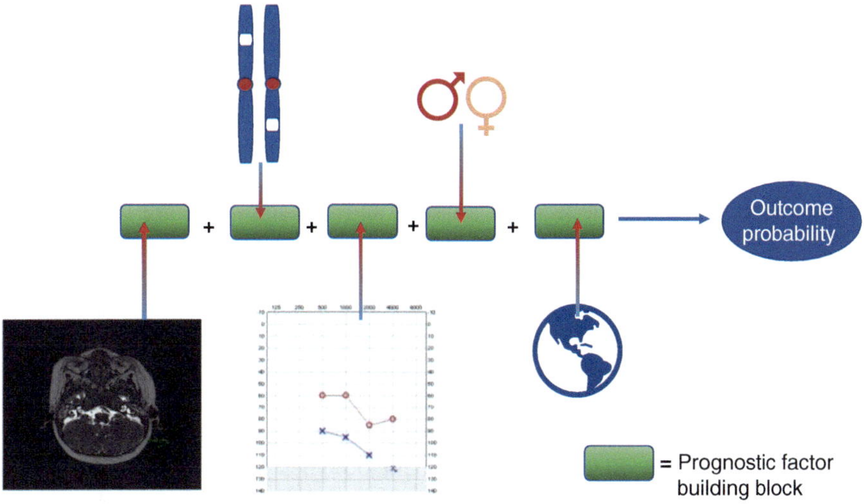


**Fig. 7.1** A schematic representing how individual prognostic factors can be combined in order to produce a prognostic model and predicted outcome. In this schematic, an example of outcome probability for hearing loss is produced by combining the individual example prognostic effects of radiological phenotype, genotype, audiological data, gender and geographical location/socio-economic status

characterise the individual *prognostic factors* that are important within the field of research. Prognostic factors are any clinical or biochemical measures that are present at a disease start point, which are associated with a clinical outcome (endpoint). By defining the key prognostic factors, researchers are essentially defining the building blocks that form a prognostic model (as multiple prognostic factors are combined to produce a prognostic model), see Fig. 7.1. It is extremely important to ensure that only scientifically robust prognostic factor building blocks are identified, either through undertaking a prognostic factor systematic review of the pertinent literature or by developing an adequately powered prospective study to explore prognostic factors. Failure to do this, will result in an inaccurate, clinically misleading prognostic model. The process of defining prognostic factors starts with an exploratory study of candidate prognostic factors (also termed as predictors). Within the field of hearing loss, an example of good practice is the UK *SeaShel* study [10]. The *SeaShel* study team has adhered to the tenets of prognostic factor research by undertaking a prospective study, defining their key patient inclusion criteria, ensuring an adequate sample size [11] for prediction model analysis, defining the primary outcome measures and ensuing an adequate data set and follow up period for time-to-event analysis. By using this methodology, it is expected the study will result in the development of a prognostic model for sudden sensorineural hearing loss (SSNHL). This would provide clinical benefits and could improve the ability of clinicians to identify those patients that would benefit from early CI.

The authors of this chapter have published a prognostic factor systematic review according to existing standards within the field of CI and hearing loss [12]. There are multiple benefits to undertaking a prognostic factor systematic review. It allows researchers within a given field to assess which candidate prognostic factors (if any) have been explored, whether the methodology used to explore the factors was adequate, and therefore whether the candidate prognostic factors are indeed confirmed to be clinical measures, which can be used in subsequent prognostic model construction [13]. By way of example, in our prognostic factor review, we aimed to ascertain which prognostic factors were relevant in progressive hearing loss associated with an enlarged vestibular aqueduct (EVA). This condition is associated with marked heterogeneity in hearing loss trajectory and the timing of CI surgery remains controversial [14, 15]. We have shown that potential exploratory prognostic factors include patient biomarkers (genotype and radiological morphology) as well as clinical parameters such as gender and frequency-specific hearing loss. Importantly, identifying prognostic factors within the literature provides a scaffold to build further prognostic model development, leading to optimised time frame for CI surgery in EVA on an individualised basis. A key methodological principle, which we found to be lacking in several papers exploring prognostic factors in hearing loss is the inclusion of multivariate regression analysis. This form of regression analysis is beneficial when identifying prognostic factors as it provides an objective way to analyse which individual candidate prognostic factor has the most prognostic effect when directly compared to other factors.

Once prognostic factors are identified, researchers in the field of CI and hearing loss have the building blocks for the development of a prognostic model. In order to progress to model development, there are several areas to consider. A detailed guide to prognostic model study development has been provided by Riley et al. [4], namely: (1) the research team should include a health data statistician capable of assisting with an adequate study design and applying a multivariate regression framework analysis to the data set in question, (2) the specific type of regression framework will vary depending upon the outcome the model wishes to predict; time-to-event outcomes and binary outcomes will utilise logistic regression and survival models, respectively, and (3) the prognostic model study should ideally be prospective and should use a high-quality data set with limited missing data and heterogeneity in prognostic factor measurements. Furthermore, researchers should strictly adhere to the *Transparent Reporting of a Multivariable Prediction Model for Individual Prognosis or Diagnosis* (TRIPOD) checklist and *Prediction Model Risk of Bias Assessment Tool* (PROBAST) when developing a prognostic model [5, 16]. Adhering to principles proposed by Riley et al. [5] will not only optimise the chances of publication of the research output but will give confidence to the research community and to key health policy stakeholders that the prognostic model should be utilised on the clinical frontline. The opinion of the authors of this chapter is that the unmet clinical need to improve prognostic model development in CI will be improved upon by researchers in the field adopting the principles of good Prognosis research highlighted in the above paragraphs.

This opinion is shared by Black et al., who aimed to systematically review the literature for known prognostic factors in CI outcome prediction, prior to the recent guidance provided in the PROGRESS papers [17]. Although their method of data extraction and synthesis from included papers differed from contemporary guidance, we can still highlight useful points from this systematic review. Despite obtaining a considerable body of initial papers, the majority of studies were lacking in appropriate case-control study design, with only 16/38 accounting for individual prognostic effects using an appropriate method of statistical analysis. Additionally, a plethora of heterogenous outcome measures hindered further meta-analysis. The study does however provide 'clues' for candidate prognostic factors the research community should further explore in well-structured confirmatory studies. These included age at implant, presence/absence of Connexin 26 mutation, history of meningitis and the presence of inner ear malformations.

So far, we have described the importance of developing studies that identify robust prognostic factor building blocks and then to utilise the framework set out by the PROGRESS papers to subsequently design and report upon clinical prediction models derived from the prognostic factors. Although there is a relative paucity of such studies in the CI literature it is important to discuss two important examples outlined below.

Artieres et al. have used multivariate analysis to explore age at implant as a candidate prognostic factor and provided evidence that early CI has a positive impact on post-surgical linguistic development [18]. Specifically, the authors identified and collected data on the possible candidate prognostic factors of age at implant, duration of CI use, age at hearing aid fitting, age at time of testing and pre-operative audiological thresholds. Importantly, the use of multivariate analysis allowed the study team to identify which of the candidate prognostic factors (if any) had an individual prognostic effect on speech perception, speech intelligibility and expressive and receptive language measures. Although this study was performed in 2009, the Prognosis research principles employed were sound. As a result, this study provides evidence to the research community that age at implant may have an independent prognostic effect on receptive language development. The logical progression would be for the research community to harness this prognostic factor and develop a confirmatory study. This would provide the stronger confidence to utilise age at implant in the construction of a clinical prognostic model for post-surgical language development.

Another useful example is provided by Han et al. [19]. In their study, the authors adopt the principles of prognosis research towards modelling auditory performance scores in children with cochlear nerve deficiency (a condition in which auditory outcomes after CI are highly variable). Han et al. focused on identifying candidate prognostic factors found within routine pre-implant imaging. The study provides evidence for radiological measurements that may predict post-CI Categories of Auditory Performance (CAP) scores in children with cochlear nerve deficiency. Specifically (through the use of multivariate regression modelling), 66% of variation in auditory performance scores could be predicted by the prognostic effects of pre-op auditory brainstem responses, and the ratio of the vestibulocochlear nerve to the facial nerve at the cerebellopontine angle.

Quality studies as described above give important examples of published Prognosis research within the CI literature. However, the overall paucity of studies emphasises that CI researchers have the opportunity to make better use of such an important research tool within our field. Prognosis research requires careful consideration if it is to provide clinically meaningful and robust guidance.

**Prognostic Modelling—Key Points**

- There is an unmet need to improve prognostic research relating to the hearing loss trajectory and optimal timeframe for CI surgery.
- Researchers should utilise the PROGRESS framework to improve Prognosis research.
- Identifying and challenging the role of individual prognostic factors within the research area of interest is a vital starting point—these are the building blocks for prognostic models.
- Prospective well-structured studies which adhere to the TRIPOD checklist and PROBAST will provide the most rigorous and robust clinical data.

## 7.3 Part 2: Machine Learning in Cochlear Implantation

Machine learning (ML) use has spread rapidly across almost all industry sectors, with a recent drive to harness its potential within healthcare through the development of novel collaborations between clinicians, health data scientists and policymakers [20]. ML is a subcategory of AI and involves the analysis of a data set using complex mathematical software algorithms. The algorithms learn from a set of training data. Uniquely, the training data results in the ML algorithm generating new, accurate conclusions without being pre-programmed to do so [21]. Different types of ML algorithms are applied to a data set depending upon the size of the data set, the complexity and the question that the researchers wish to answer.

The promise and excitement surrounding ML in healthcare are reflected by its ability to drive data-driven healthcare solutions and it is therefore predicted to generate billions of dollars towards the USA health economy within the next decade [22].

In the second part of the chapter, we focus on why ML can be successfully deployed as a precision medicine tool in the field of CI research and provide examples of recent studies. Broadly speaking, in *supervised machine learning (the* most *commonly used type of ML in the field of CI)*, medical images/data sets in the form of training data can be analysed initially by appropriate computerised ML algorithms. Importantly, within the training data set, salient features are highlighted to the algorithm, such that when new unseen data is presented to the algorithm, it selects the most important features to infer new information. The salient features presented to algorithm will depend upon the clinical question, for example, it may be specific patterns on images of the tympanic membrane if the algorithm is being used to automatically detect pathological changes to the tympanic membrane based on endoscopic images. The salient features may be specific genetic variants known to correlate with severe hearing loss, or they may be specific hearing loss thresholds known to correlate with poor auditory outcomes. The choice is driven by the outcome measure the research team would wish the ML algorithm to predict. New, unseen data is then introduced to the ML algorithm, allowing the system to apply what it has learnt from the training data to make meaningful predictions from the data in question. In *unsupervised machine learning*, the algorithm will detect patterns in data where the outcomes are unknown [1].

ML holds several potential advantages within the field of prognostic modelling and has become an attractive option as a clinical research tool. A particular advantage arises when dealing with 'big data'; extremely large numbers of patients (N) each with numerous parameters (P). In such cases, ML affords the ability to break away from traditional hypothesis-based NP research principles and work from the ground up, generating new hypotheses from the powerful analysis of large data set trends [23]. Therefore, by implementing ML in Prognosis research, there is potentially less constraint as to how complex data sets are analysed; fewer or no assumptions about the data are required, a multitude of prognostic factors can be included in an automated analysis, with resulting models having the ability to evolve, update and self-learn as the clinical landscape evolves.

ML can be used to aid in clinical prediction and forecasting health outcomes if applied successfully to a health data set. We consider ML prediction modelling and Prognosis research modelling to be 'two sides of the same coin' given that ultimately, they are both grounded in mathematical theory and when tested against each other can provide similar levels of predictive performance [24]. We, therefore, refer to them both as methodological frameworks within the same data science continuum (see Fig. 7.2). Where they differ is in their flexibility towards data, transparency/explanation pertaining to how predictions are derived, the personnel required

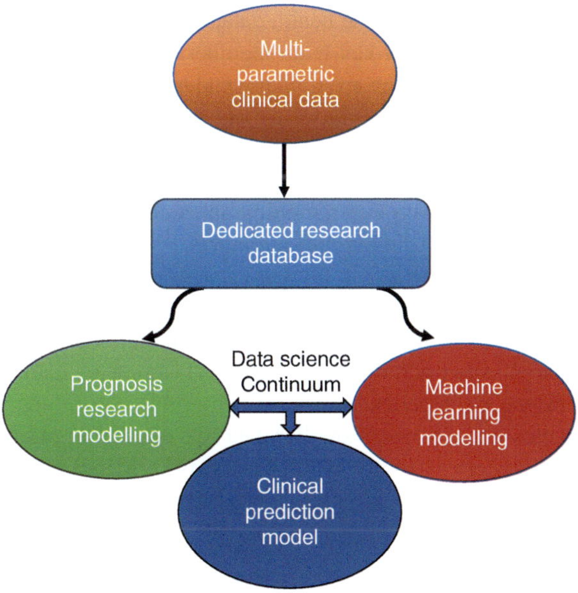


**Fig. 7.2** A schematic representing the data-science continuum. Multi-parametric clinical prognostic data should be housed on a suitable database for further analysis. Both Prognosis research and machine learning analytical methods can be used as part of a data science continuum to reach a viable clinical prediction/prognostic model

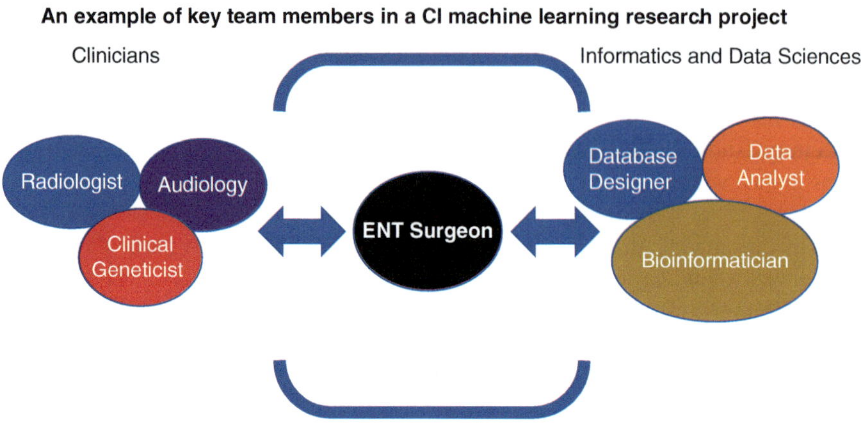


**Fig. 7.3** An example of a collaborative science team needed in order to initiate and implement a ML modelling study

for their implementation and the confidence/awareness of ML within the healthcare community [25–27].

If we briefly consider the personnel required to start a ML healthcare project, an efficient interaction within a collaborative science team is of fundamental importance. As depicted in Fig. 7.3, at the centre of such as team is often a healthcare professional with specific expertise within the field of research interest. For example, in the case of hearing loss CI candidacy/surgical outcome modelling, this may be a CI surgeon, audio-vestibular physician or clinical audiological scientist. Critical to this central role, is that the team member has approval to access pertinent healthcare data from both an ethical and an information governance standpoint. Without approved access to the health data, the other non-clinical team members are unable to progress. Other key team members are the database engineer and data analyst. Between them, they are fundamental to ensuring that the raw healthcare data is collated on an adequate platform that can facilitate the processes of data pre-processing and transformation. These processes are vital as they provide a way to manipulate the raw data set to account for the fact that routinely collected healthcare data is inherently 'messy' with multiple inaccuracies, episodes of missing data and varied ways to record similar measurements.

The data analyst is fundamental to guiding the clinical team as to which ML algorithms are best suited to their data. A detailed discussion of ML algorithms is beyond the scope of this chapter, but in general, powerful deep learning (artificial neural network) algorithms are best suited to data sets with greater than 3000 instances (or patients), whereas ensemble algorithms such as Random Forests are better suited towards smaller data sets consisting of hundreds of instances. Work is also underway to assess the capability of ML algorithms to make meaningful predictions based on smaller clinical data sets, which will be important in rare diseases [28].

Choice of the algorithm is also important when considering generalisability and ease of clinical translation; deep learning algorithms are referred to as 'black-boxes', that is to say the inner workings of the algorithm and how it reached its end prediction cannot easily be explained and therefore may not instil confidence in the clinical end user/health policymaker. In contrast to this, the aforementioned Random Forests may be less powerful, but base their predictions on amalgamating the outputs of multiple decision trees analysing the data in tandem. This is inherently more explainable and therefore more likely to meet the scrutiny and requirements of both patient and clinical policymakers. The final job of the data analyst is to assist with the interrogation of the pre-processed dataset through coding software. Here, exciting opportunities arise for clinicians to work closely with data analysts such that the nuances of the clinical data and how they should be analysed are not missed, whilst at the same time, accurate coding and algorithm interpretation can be completed in an optimal timeframe.

Other important members of the ML healthcare collaborative science team will vary depending on the data and expertise required. ML modelling within the field of congenital hearing loss, for example may require specialist genotype and radiological data to be captured and collated for second stage ML analysis. In such cases, other multidisciplinary clinical team members such as radiologists and clinical geneticists are necessary to ensure the optimal measurement and recording of potential biomarkers to record within the ML dataset.

Unsurprisingly, ML prognostic modelling within the field of CI is gaining momentum as a new focus for CI research. You et al. have recently analysed 39 studies in their systematic review with most studies published between 2015 and 2020 [29]. Four of the studies were concerned with prognostic modelling, namely audiological performance post-implantation. Biomarker data used to develop the ML models in these studies ranged from pre-operative MRI morphological data to pre-implant audiological data and disyllabic speech results. A mixture of ML algorithms was used (see Table 7.1) with outcome measures focusing on speech acquisition and quality of life improvement [30–33]. Subsequently, Crowson et al. have provided a good example of how big data and multiple predictors can be integrated for ML analysis using a combination of neural networks and ensemble ML algorithms [34]. These provided a prediction for both post-operative CI performance and pre-operative factors that influence performance based on multiparametric data sets from over 1000 CI users. Table 7.1 highlights that most CI ML modelling studies identified use smaller data sets (tens to hundreds of patients) as relatively smaller numbers of patients are available for analysis within CI clinical centres. These studies use ensemble techniques (e.g. Random Forests) to produce models with percentage predictive performance.

The challenge arises when smaller data set models are externally validated on unseen data. External validation of a model is a vital process, regardless if it has been developed through Prognosis research or ML. It is the process by which the model's predictive performance is assessed using high-quality clinical data that is completely external from the data set used in the model's development. This process allows researchers to test the effectiveness of the model in different healthcare

**Table 7.1** Examples of machine learning modelling studies. The majority of studies aim to model post-operative outcomes in CI patients and use ensemble algorithms suited to smaller data sets. Reporting on Algorithm is vital to promote transparency and confidence in reporting. Green cell = reporting deemed suitable based on current guidance, red cell = reporting lacking sufficient detail, orange cell = a moderate degree of reporting based on current guidance

| AUTHOR | OUTCOME MEASURE | MEASUREMENT TOOL/ predictors used | Machine Learning Algorithm(S) | N^O subjects | Main outcome(s) | Algorithm Reporting |
|---|---|---|---|---|---|---|
| Guerra-Jimenez et al | 1.Speech Recognition 2. Quality of Life | GBI & SQ | 1.Nearest neighbour, 2. Decision Tree | 29 CI recipients | Predictive variables for pre-operative GBI &SQ identified. | Percentage success rate only. No transparent reporting on linear regression. No multivariate analysis reported. |
| Ramos-Miguel et al | Disyllabic speech test performance | 24 pre-operative predictors | 1.Linear Regression, 2. Nearest neighbour | 60 bilaterally implanted patients | A pre-op disyllabic test result of < 70% is the most useful predictor for bilateral CI outcome. | Correlation index reported. Mean error and SD reported. |
| Tan et al | Effective language development 2 years post CI | Tool: CELF-P2 language performance tool. Predictor: Pre-implant cortical activation on MRI scan | 1.supervised support vector machine, 2. Semi-supervised support vector machine | 44 infants undergoing CI surgery | Left superior and middle temporal gyrus cortical mapping predicts language acquisition | Confidence intervals and AUC reported for model performance. Classification accuracy % reported |
| Feng et al | SRI-Q score post implant | Predictor: grey matter/white matter density on pre-op MRI. Tool: SRI-Q score 6 months post implant. | Support vector machine | 37 CI recipients | The presence of Brain areas unaffected by auditory deprivation are associated with better post op speech outcome. | Internal validation of algorithm reported. Spearman rank correlation reported |
| Crowson et al | HINT score | Predictors: 282 objective numerical & text measures | 1.neural network. 2. ensemble decision tree. | 1604 CI recipients | Audiometric variables, vestibular function, and subjective quality of life variables influenced post op performance | % prediction reported only. Explainability of model and performance not reported upon |
| Uhm et al | Siegel's criteria | Predictors: 35 variables clinical variables | 1.Decision tree. 2.Random Forest 3. Support Vector Machines 4.Absolute Shrinkage 5.Boosting | 244 patients undergoing treatment for sudden SNHL | Treatment delay, initial SNHL PTA (affected and non- affected ears), BMI and previous HL are predictors for recovery | Confidence intervals for the ROC-AUC are reported for model performance in addition to % recall and precision. |

*GBI* Glasgow Benefit Inventory, *SQ* specific questionnaire, *CI* cochlear implant, *SD* standard deviation, *HINT* hearing in noise, *SNHL* sensorineural hearing loss, *PTA* pure tone audiogram, *HL* hearing loss

settings and environments, for example in a different geographical location, in a different country and in different hospitals. Without the process of external validation, researchers are not able to assess whether or not an ML model derived from a relatively small data set overfits and performs badly outside the training data. It affords the opportunity for the research team to carefully consider how the ML model should be optimised and may require re-development and exposure to further training data. The complex and lengthy process of external validation may be a contributing factor as to why we are yet to see a CI ML prediction model fully integrated into clinical practice.

Despite the recent increase in ML, there are a limited number of studies that have directly aimed to use ML clinically to prognosticate hearing loss, whilst also reporting adequately upon prediction model performance [35, 36]. Park et al. and Uhm et al. have shown that Random Forest ML algorithms can be used to predict recovery in sudden sensorineural hearing loss (SSNHL) and in some cases outperform traditional multivariate regression techniques used in Prognosis research. Studies like this lay the foundation for researchers in the field of CI to adopt ML as a research tool in order to predict HL trajectory and possibly the time frames for CI surgery on an individualised basis.

Although the promise of ML as a future direction for CI research is evident, ML modelling studies across the medical landscape have scarcely penetrated the clinical 'frontline'. There are numerous reasons for this, including both public and clinician perceptions towards AI clinical solutions, the fact that ML modelling is still in its relative infancy, challenges faced when externally validating models and clinical interpretability of ML prediction models. The latter is an important area for researchers in CI and hearing loss ML modelling to consider. Just as we have recommended that in Prognosis research, prognostic models adhere strictly to the TRIPOD checklist and PROBAST tool during model development and reporting, the same principles should be implemented when developing ML prognostic models. Out of the selected studies identified in this chapter, only three out of seven studies were deemed to have robust model reporting (see Table 7.1). The current TRIPOD checklist and PROBAST tool are, however, designed for Prognosis research and therefore researchers in ML modelling may potentially find it incompatible to report on their ML models against such standards. This is emphasised by the fact that leaders in the field of Prognosis research in the UK are currently reviewing ML prognostic model studies and have a plan in place to evolve current tools and checklist to consider the increasing number of academic ML prognostic models emerging across healthcare [37]. They predict the realistic need to evolve the current TRIPOD checklist to 'TRIPOD-ML' in order to encourage improved ML prognostic model design and implementation.

**Machine learning modelling—key points**

- ML is a subcategory of AI, and ML prediction modelling in CI is a novel field of research.
- ML prediction modelling research requires an effective collaborative science team, including a clinician and data analyst.
- Single or multiple ML algorithms may be utilised to analyse a data set and the type of algorithm(s) chosen is dictated by the data set and outcome measure.
- ML prediction modelling has been used to predict audiological outcomes in CI, with few studies predicting hearing loss trajectory.
- Researchers should report upon ML models adhering to the TRIPOD checklist and PROBAST tool where possible, in order to increase the likelihood of adoption into routine practice.

## 7.4 Concluding Points

In this chapter, we have provided an overview of two 'state-of-the-art' research techniques that should be harnessed by researchers in the field of CI, in order to continually advance our understanding of both hearing loss modelling and clinical outcomes. Both Prognosis research modelling and Machine Learning form part of the same data science continuum and have the potential to take CI research in new and exciting directions. They require an effective interaction between clinicians, health statisticians, data analysts and database engineers from the offset. We emphasise the importance of strong prognostic factor studies/prognostic factor reviews prior to embarking upon a Prognostic modelling study and the need to report on Prognostic models using established guidelines. There is a paucity of Prognostic model studies within the field of CI. Such studies should be developed and based upon the principles of good Prognosis research outlined in Part 1. Machine Learning is an exciting new precision medicine tool in the field of CI modelling. There has been a steady increase in studies over the last 5 years, providing early evidence for the use of different ML algorithms to predict clinical outcomes after CI. The major challenge for researchers utilising ML is to ensure that models are reported upon in a transparent manner. Although this can be achieved to a degree by adhering to the same established guidelines provided in the field of Prognosis research, researchers utilising ML are faced with the unique challenges of making their algorithms explainable to both clinical and patient stakeholders, thus building trust and support for this novel precision medicine tool for adoption onto the clinical frontline. Current reporting tools and guidance are in a state of evolution in order to match the recent explosion of ML modelling across the medical research landscape. Researchers in the field of CI should keep abreast of such developments when constructing ML-based projects.

## Glossary

| Term | Definition |
|---|---|
| Artificial Intelligence (AI) | Artificial Intelligence (AI) is a broad field of science in which machines and computers are developed to perform tasks that would normally require human intelligence. |
| Big Data | Represents extremely large amounts of data that cannot be processed using traditional software or Internet-based platforms. It surpasses the traditionally used amount of storage, processing and analytical power.<br>Dash, S., Shakyawar, S.K., Sharma, M. *et al.* Big data in healthcare: management, analysis and future prospects. *J Big Data* **6,** 54 (2019) |
| Decision Tree | Decision trees are a type of ML algorithm used in data mining. Decision trees take multiple input variables (or features) and aim to predict the value of a target variable. The 'leaves' of the decision tree represent final outcomes or classifications and the 'branches' represent the decision direction (or flow) based upon the analysis of features on previous branches.<br>Lior Rokach and Oded Maimon. 2008. Data Mining with Decision Trees: Theory and Applications. World Scientific Publishing Co., Inc., USA. |
| Deep Learning | A subcategory of machine learning in which algorithm design is roughly based upon the biological structure and functionality of the brain. As such, deep learning algorithms consist of layers of nodes and connecting neurones in which complex data analyses occur. |
| Machine Learning | A subcategory of AI in which computer software algorithms automatically improve (or learn) from the experiences they have gained by analysing training data. This allows the algorithm to make inferences and predictions without being explicitly programmed to do so.<br>Claude Sammut and Geoffrey I. Webb. 2017. Encyclopedia of Machine Learning and Data Mining (2nd. ed.). Springer Publishing Company, Incorporated. |
| Overfitting | Overfitting describes the situation in which an algorithm or model is too familiar and customised to the training data, and so becomes unreliable at analysing and generating predictions based on new unseen data. |
| Precision medicine/ personalised medicine | The ability to target the right treatment (or healthcare intervention) to the right patient at the right time.<br>https://www.england.nhs.uk/healthcare-science/personalisedmedicine/ |
| Prognostic Factor | A prognostic factor is any variable that is associated with a subsequent outcome such as death or disability among people with a disease or health condition. They range widely from biomarkers, genotype to imaging features and lifestyle choices.<br>• Candidate prognostic factors are those that are initially derived from initial exploratory studies. They may or may not have an individual effect on prognosis and require further analysis to ascertain this.<br>• Confirmatory prognostic factors are those that have been derived from further confirmatory studies and have true, individual impact on disease prognosis.<br>Prognosis Research in healthcare: concepts, methods and impact. Riley D et al., 2019. Oxford University Press. ISBN-13: 9780198796619 |
| Random Forest | Random Forest ML algorithms use the outputs of multiple decision trees. This provides a way to enhance the final classification or prediction by utilising the mode or mean outputs from all the decision trees.<br>Link to book Hastie, Trevor; Tibshirani, Robert; Friedman, Jerome (2008). The Elements of Statistical Learning ($2^{nd}$ ed.). *Springer.* ISBN 0-387-95284-5. |

## References


1. Saeed HS, Stivaros SM, Saeed SR. The potential for machine learning to improve precision medicine in cochlear implantation. Cochlear Implants Int. 2019;20(5):229–30.
2. Hippisley-Cox J, Coupland C, Brindle P. Development and validation of QRISK3 risk prediction algorithms to estimate future risk of cardiovascular disease: prospective cohort study. http://www.bmj.com/
3. Johnson DE, Burtness B, Leemans CR, Lui VWY, Bauman JE, Grandis JR. Head and neck squamous cell carcinoma. Nat Rev Dis Primers. 2020;6.
4. Riley RD, van der Windt D, Croft P, Moons KGM. Prognosis research in healthcare: concepts, methods, and impact [Internet]. 2019. 354 p. https://global.oup.com/academic/product/prognosis-research-in-healthcare-9780198796619?cc=pt&lang=en&
5. Collins GS, Reitsma JB, Altman DG, Moons KGM. Transparent reporting of a multivariable prediction model for individual prognosis or diagnosis (TRIPOD): The TRIPOD Statement. BMC Med [Internet]. 2015;13(1):1. http://www.biomedcentral.com/1741-7015/13/1. Accessed 8 Jan 2021.
6. Zhao EE, Dornhoffer JR, Loftus C, Nguyen SA, Meyer TA, Dubno JR, et al. Association of patient-related factors with adult cochlear implant speech recognition outcomes: a meta-analysis. JAMA Otolaryngol Head Neck Surg [Internet]. 2020;146(7):613–620. https://jamanetwork.com/journals/jamaotolaryngology/fullarticle/2765789. Accessed 20 Jan 2021.
7. Hemingway H, Croft P, Perel P, Hayden JA, Abrams K, Timmis A, et al. Prognosis research strategy (PROGRESS) 1: a framework for researching clinical outcomes. BMJ. 2013;346(February):1–11.
8. Riley RD, Hayden JA, Steyerberg EW, Moons KGM, Abrams K, Kyzas PA, et al. Prognosis Research Strategy (PROGRESS) 2: prognostic factor research. PLoS Med [Internet]. 2013;10(2). http://www.progress-partnership. Accessed 16 Jan 2020.
9. Steyerberg EW, Moons KGM, Van Der Windt DA, Hayden JA, Perel P, Schroter S, et al. Guidelines and Guidance Prognosis Research Strategy (PROGRESS) 3: prognostic model research. http://www.progress-partnership.
10. Mandavia R, Hannink G, Nayeem Ahmed M, Premakumar Y, Shun Man Chu T, Blackshaw H, et al. Prognostic factors for outcomes of idiopathic sudden sensorineural hearing loss: protocol for the SeaSHeL national prospective cohort study. http://bmjopen.bmj.com/
11. Riley RD, Snell KI, Ensor J, Burke DL, Harrell Jr FE, Moons KG, et al. Minimum sample size for developing a multivariable prediction model: PART II – Binary and time-to-event outcomes. Stat Med [Internet]. 2019;38(7):1276–1296. http://doi.wiley.com/10.1002/sim.7992. Accessed 19 Jan 2021.
12. Saeed HS, Kenth J, Black G, Saeed SR, Stivaros S, Bruce IA. Hearing loss in enlarged vestibular aqueduct: a prognostic factor systematic review of the literature. Otol Neurotol. 2021;42(1):99–107.
13. Debray TPA, Damen JAAG, Snell KIE, Ensor J, Hooft L, Reitsma JB, et al. A guide to systematic review and meta-analysis of prediction model performance [Internet]. BMJ (Online). 2017;356:6460. https://doi.org/10.1136/bmj.i6460http://www.bmj.com/. Accessed 16 Jan 2020.
14. Gopen Q, Zhou G, Whittemore K, Kenna M. Enlarged vestibular aqueduct: review of controversial aspects. Laryngoscope [Internet]. 2011. http://doi.wiley.com/10.1002/lary.22083. Accessed 28 Nov 2019.
15. Hall AC, Kenway B, Sanli H, Birman CS. Cochlear implant outcomes in large vestibular aqueduct syndrome—should we provide cochlear implants earlier? Otol Neurotol. 2019;40(8):E769–73.
16. Wolff RF, Moons KGM, Riley RD, Whiting PF, Westwood M, Collins GS, et al. PROBAST: a tool to assess the risk of bias and applicability of prediction model studies. Ann Intern Med. 2019;170(1):51–8.

17. Black J, Hickson L, Black B, Perry C. Prognostic indicators in paediatric cochlear implant surgery: a systematic literature review. Cochlear Implants Int. 2011;12(2):67–93.
18. Artières F, Vieu A, Mondain M, Uziel A, Venail F. Impact of early cochlear implantation on the linguistic development of the deaf child. Otol Neurotol. 2009;30(6):736–42.
19. Han JJ, Suh M-W, Kyun Park M, Koo J-W, Lee JH, et al. A predictive model for cochlear implant outcome in children with cochlear nerve deficiency. https://doi.org/10.1038/s41598-018-37014-7. Accessed 19 Jan 2021.
20. Topol E. Preparing the healthcare workforce to deliver the digital future The Topol Review. An independent report on behalf of the Secretary of State for Health and Social Care. NHS. 2019;February:102.
21. Bur AM, Shew M, New J. State of the art review artificial intelligence for the otolaryngologist: a state of the art review. Otolaryngol Neck Surg [Internet]. 2019;160(4):603–11. http://otojournal.org
22. You E, Lin V, Mijovic T, Eskander A, Crowson MG. Artificial intelligence applications in otology: a state of the art review [Internet]. Otolaryngol Head Neck Surg (United States). 2020;163:1123–33. http://journals.sagepub.com/doi/10.1177/0194599820931804. Accessed 21 Jan 2021.
23. Yang S, Stansbury LG, Rock P, Scalea T, Hu PF. Linking big data and prediction strategies. Crit Care Med [Internet]. 2019;47(6):840–848. http://journals.lww.com/00003246-201906000-00014. Accessed 29 Jan 2021.
24. Li Y, Sperrin M, Ashcroft DM, Van Staa TP. Consistency of variety of machine learning and statistical models in predicting clinical risks of individual patients: longitudinal cohort study using cardiovascular disease as exemplar. BMJ. 2020;371:12–5.
25. Ribeiro MT, Singh S, Guestrin C. "Why should i trust you?" Explaining the predictions of any classifier. In: Proceedings of the ACM SIGKDD International Conference on Knowledge Discovery and Data Mining. New York, NY: Association for Computing Machinery; 2016. p. 1135–1144.
26. Black-box vs. white-box models – Towards Data Science.
27. Vollmer S, Mateen BA, Bohner G, Király FJ, Ghani R, Jonsson P, et al. Machine learning and artificial intelligence research for patient benefit: 20 critical questions on transparency, replicability, ethics, and effectiveness. BMJ. 2020;368:1–12.
28. Schaefer J, Lehne M, Schepers J, Prasser F, Thun S. The use of machine learning in rare diseases: a scoping review. Orphanet J Rare Dis. 2020;15
29. You E, Lin V, Mijovic T, Eskander A, Crowson MG. State of the art review artificial intelligence applications in otology: a state of the art review. Otolaryngol Neck Surg [Internet]. 2020;6:1123–1133. http://otojournal.org. Accessed 21 Jan 2021.
30. Guerra-JimÉnez G, De Miguel ÁR, González JCF, Andrea S, Barreiro B, Plasencia DP, et al. Cochlear implant evaluation: prognosis estimation by data mining system. J Int Adv Otol [Internet]. 2016;12(1):1–7. https://pubmed.ncbi.nlm.nih.gov/27340975/. Accessed 29 Jan 2021.
31. Ramos-Miguel A, Perez-Zaballos T, Perez D, Falconb JC, Ramosb A. Use of data mining to predict significant factors and benefits of bilateral cochlear implantation.
32. Tan L, Holland SK, Deshpande AK, Chen Y, Choo DI, Lu LJ. A semi-supervised Support Vector Machine model for predicting the language outcomes following cochlear implantation based on pre-implant brain <scp>fMRI</scp> imaging. Brain Behav [Internet]. 2015;5(12):1–25. https://onlinelibrary.wiley.com/doi/10.1002/brb3.391. Accessed 29 Jan 2021.
33. Feng G, Ingvalson EM, Grieco-Calub TM, Roberts MY, Ryan ME, Birmingham P, et al. Neural preservation underlies speech improvement from auditory deprivation in young cochlear implant recipients. Proc Natl Acad Sci U S A [Internet]. 2018;115(5):E1022–31. /pmc/articles/PMC5798370/?report=abstract. Accessed 29 Jan 2021.
34. Crowson MG, Dixon P, Mahmood R, Lee JW, Shipp D, Le T, et al. Predicting postoperative cochlear implant performance using supervised machine learning. Otol Neurotol. 2020;41(8):e1013–23.

35. Uhm T, Lee JE, Yi S, Choi SW, Oh SJ, Kong SK, et al. Predicting hearing recovery following treatment of idiopathic sudden sensorineural hearing loss with machine learning models. Am J Otolaryngol Head Neck Med Surg. 2021;42(2):102858.
36. Park KV, Oh KH, Jeong YJ, Rhee J, Han MS, Han SW, et al. Machine learning models for predicting hearing prognosis in unilateral idiopathic sudden sensorineural hearing loss. Clin Exp Otorhinolaryngol [Internet]. 2020;13(2):148–156. https://pubmed.ncbi.nlm.nih.gov/32156103/. Accessed 29 Jan 2021.
37. Andaur Navarro CL, Damen JAAG, Takada T, Nijman SWJ, Dhiman P, Ma J, et al. Protocol for a systematic review on the methodological and reporting quality of prediction model studies using machine learning techniques. BMJ Open [Internet]. 2020;10(11):38832. http://bmjopen.bmj.com/. Accessed 29 Jan 2021.

# Cochlear Implantation Using Posterior Tympanotomy and Cochleostomy

# 8

Jacques Magnan and Fathi Baki

The surgical procedure of cochlear implantation follows three main steps: the transmastoid approach, the posterior tympanotomy then the cochleostomy with the electrode insertion.

## 8.1 Retroauricular Transmastoid Approach

The extensive skin incisions proposed at the beginning of the Cochlear implant surgery have been definitively given up towards limited retro-auricular incisions with or without a superior extension. A restricted access "keyhole" cochlear Implant technique [1] is promoted with a progressively shortened incision to a 2-cm retroauricular flap.

The cortical bone of the mastoid process behind the ear canal, which can remain intact, is exposed. The Henlé's spine and the cribriform suprameatal angle or Mac Ewen's triangle are the landmarks to the initial drilling towards the antrum. The temporal line situated at the upper limit of the mastoid process is indicating the level of the middle fossa dura.

A bed to hold the electronic package of the implant is created by using a periosteal elevator in a superior and posterior direction. The inferior border of the implant should be roughly 5 cm from the Henlé's spine. Each implant has its own

**Supplementary Information** The online version contains supplementary material available at [https://doi.org/10.1007/978-981-19-0452-3_8].

J. Magnan (✉)
ORL, University of Aix-Marseille, Hopital Nord, Marseille, France

F. Baki
ORL, Alexandria Faculty of Medicine, Alexandria, Egypt


S. DeSaSouza (ed.), *Cochlear Implants*,
https://doi.org/10.1007/978-981-19-0452-3_8

specification as regards to create only a subperiosteal pocket or perform full bed drilled from the outer cortex.

The mastoidectomy is limited to a large antrotomy extended anteriorly towards the attic to expose the incus and inferiorly to thin the posterior canal wall. The mastoid tip is preserved to avoid interfering with the growing process in children.

Protecting the electrode can be ensured by keeping an overhang of the posterior and superior margin cortex and by its anchor through a tunnel or a groove.

## 8.2 Posterior Tympanotomy

Jansen in 1967 [2, 3] stated that the aim of the posterior tympanotomy is to create a direct access from the mastoid cavity to the tympanic cavity through the superior part of the bone of the posterior wall of the tympanic cavity: the facial recess (or Facial Recess approach). Prior to cochlear implantation in the early 1970s posterior tympanotomy was widely popularized in cholesteatoma treatment as a closed technique or intact canal wall technique. Posterior tympanotomy was the key factor of the surgical procedure to reach and to clean the retro-tympanum, the oval window and the round window areas without sacrificing the posterior bony ear canal wall. Such approach, following the longitudinal axis of the middle cavities, preserving the anatomical structures of the external and middle ears, offering a direct-transmastoid exposure to the round window and the basal turn of the cochlea, became the rational approach to insert the electrode array of cochlear implant devices. Nowadays, cochlear implant surgery is the most common indication of posterior tympanotomy.

### 8.2.1 Surgical Anatomy

**Surgical Anatomy of Retrotympanum**

- The tympanic posterior wall or mastoid wall "Tillaux" or intra tympanic facial wall "massif de Gellé" has a roughly vertical groove shape (Fig. 8.1) and is delimited:
  - Laterally by annulus tympanicus
  - Medially by the labyrinthine capsule
  - Inferiorly by the lower wall
  - Superiorly and medially by the fossa incudis (Fig. 8.2).
- The course of the second genu and of the upper part of the mastoid segment of the facial canal with the stapedial muscle delineate a vertical crest with the pyramidal eminence and two main sinuses on both sides (Figs. 8.3 and 8.4).
  - Lateral to the facial canal, the supra-pyramidal sinus (Sappey) is located between the annulus tympanicus and the facial canal. A thin bony bridge the cordal crest (Proctor), which does not correspond to the chorda tympani course, subdivides the sinus into two recesses:

    The superior is the facial recess [4] or tympanofacial recess [5].

    The inferior is the lateral tympanic sinus (Proctor).

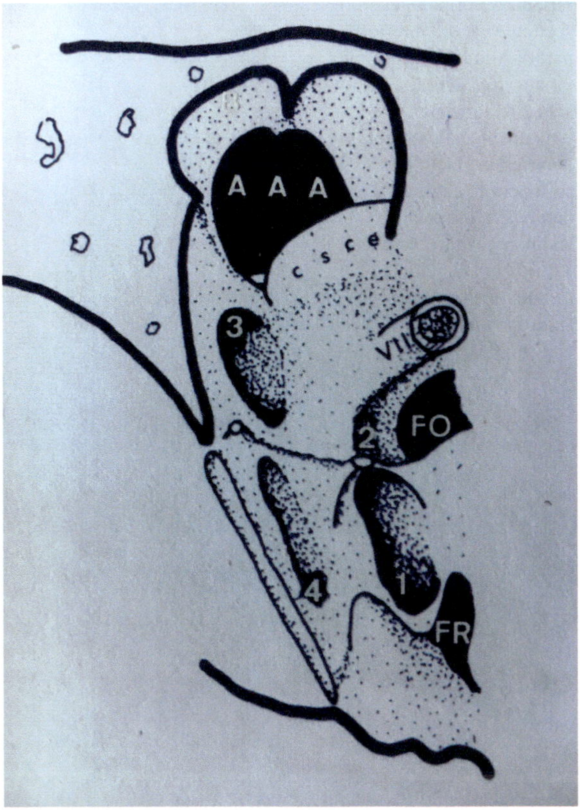


**Fig. 8.1** Retrotympanum schema: *AAA* Aditus Ad Antrum, *FO* Fenestrae Ovalis, *FR* Fenestrae rotundae, 1 Sinus tympani, 2 posterior sinus tympani, 3 Facial recess, 4 lateral tympanic sinus, A,B,C arrows level of the horizontal sections Figs. 8.2, 8.3, and 8.4

- Medial to the facial canal, this space is subdivided into two spaces:
  The superior is the posterior tympanic sinus.
  The inferior is the infra-pyramidal sinus (Huguier) or sinus tympani (Meckel and Steinbrugge). This is located between the facial canal and the labyrinthine capsule.

**Surgical Anatomy of Facial Recess (FR)**

- FR is a surgical rather than an anatomical space [6].
- FR Pneumatization: It varies from completely cellular to severe sclerosis and it is independent and not always related to general mastoid pneumatization (Fig. 8.5a, b).
- Posterior tympanotomy is a triangular opening between:
  - The chorda tympani and sulcus tympani laterally.
  - The facial nerve medial.
  - The chorda-facial angle inferiorly.
  - The incus bone buttress superiorly (forming the base of the triangle).

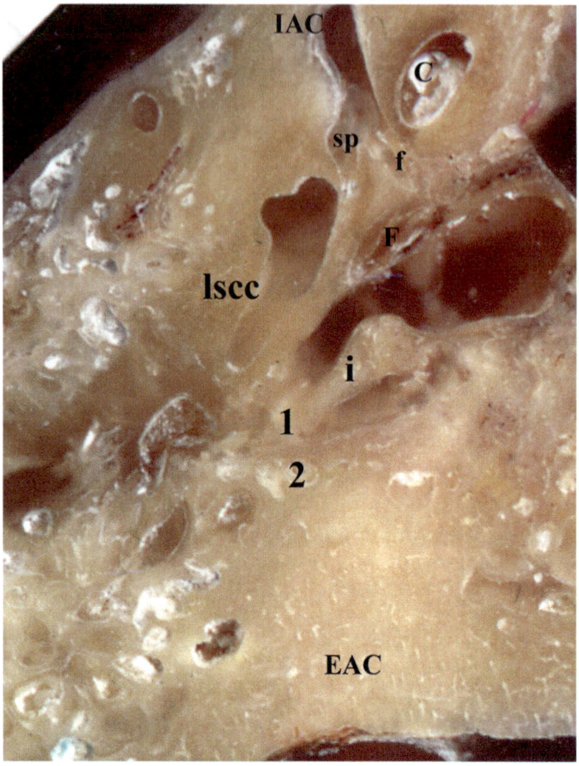


**Fig. 8.2** Horizontal section A: at the inferior part of Aditus Ad Antrum; *i* incus, *lscc* lateral semicircular canal, *F* tympanic facial nerve, *f* labyrinthine facial nerve, *sp* superior vestibular nerve, *IAC* internal auditory canal, *C* cochlea, *EAC* external auditory canal, 1 fossa incudis, 2 "antrum threshold"

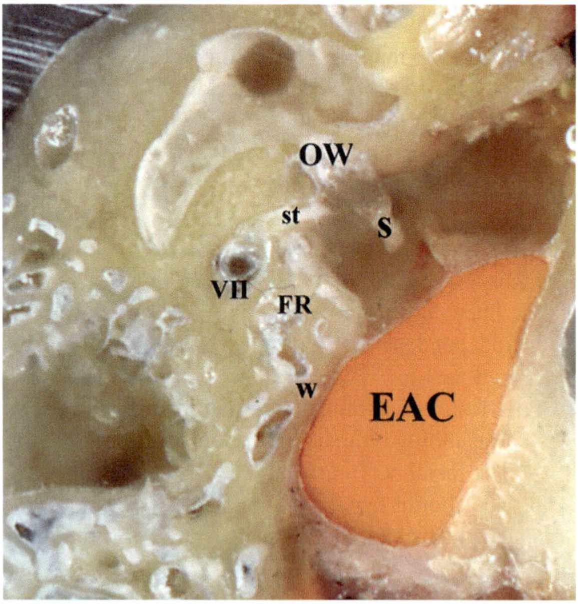


**Fig. 8.3** Horizontal section B at the Oval Window (OW); *VII* facial nerve, *st* stapedial tendon, *s* stapes, *w* cortical of the posterior canal wall, *FR* facial recess, *EAC* external auditory canal

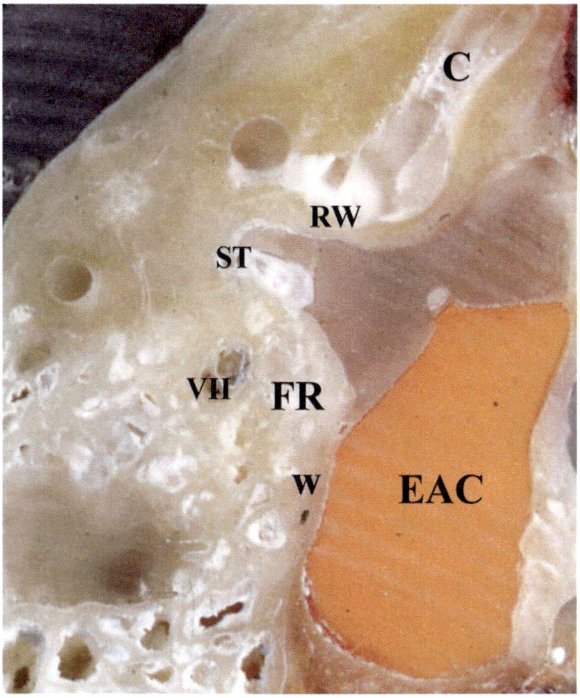


**Fig. 8.4** Horizontal section C at the Round Window (RW); *C* basal turn of cochlea, *VII* facial nerve, *w* cortical of the posterior canal wall, *FR* facial recess, *ST* sinus tympani, *EAC* external auditory canal

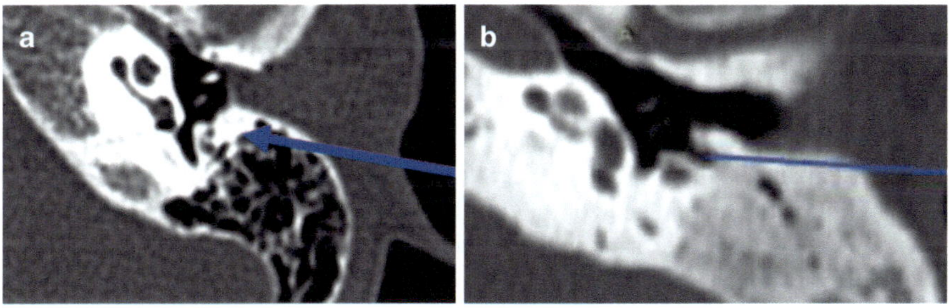


**Fig. 8.5** Correlation between pneumatization of FR and mastoid cellularity. (**a**) Left sclerosed facial recess (arrow) with a well pneumatized mastoid cavity. (**b**) Left cellular facial recess (arrow) with a sclerosed mastoid cavity

- The "antrum threshold" *Jako* [7, 8] corresponds to a bony buttress between the lateral semicircular canal and the ear canal wall after drilling and thinning the canal wall with enlargement of aditus ad antrum. The "antrum threshold" or the incus buttress, which is created by the surgeon, defines the surgical base of the posterior tympanotomy (Figs. 8.2 and 8.6).
- The facial nerve is the medial limit of facial recess. The top to bottom course of the vertical portion of the facial canal within the tympanic posterior wall intersects the obliquity of sulcus tympani at a variable level of the round window

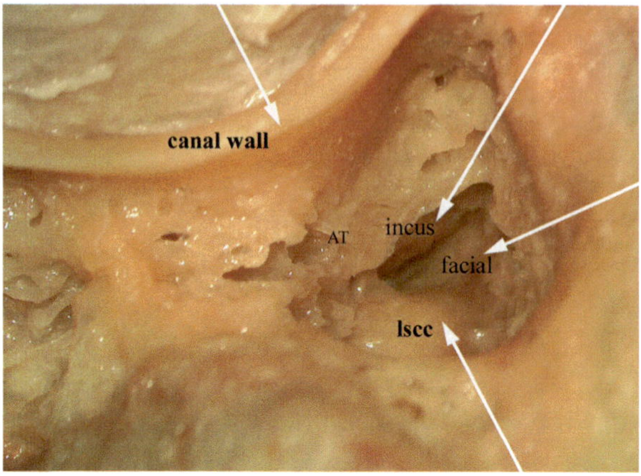


**Fig. 8.6** Antrotomy extended anteriorly with posterior atticotomy or superior tympanotomy to visualize the incus and to create the "antrum threshold" (AT)

(Broca) which define the triangular size of the posterior tympanotomy and the exposure of the round window niche (RWN).

- FR width:
  - It is adult size at birth [9].
  - It is 3–4 mm at the level of the oval window, 2–3 mm, at the level of the round window. There is no significant difference between adults and children [10].

**Surgical Anatomy of Facial Nerve**

- Whatever the indications, we must have an intimate knowledge of the intratemporal facial nerve course. Sheehy [11] stated that "The facial nerve was placed in the ear to serve as a guide, not as a hindrance. If one is afraid of the facial nerve, then he or she should not be doing any type of ear surgery. There are no exceptions."
- The tympanic segment of facial nerve (10–12 mm) extends from the geniculate ganglion to the second genu of the facial nerve. It passes posteriorly and laterally along the medial wall of the tympanic cavity, perpendicular to the long axis of the petrous bone [12]. Here it lies above the oval window and below the bulge of the lateral semi-circular canal. The mastoid segment of the facial nerve (13–15 mm) extends from the second genu to the stylomastoid foramen. Here the nerve assumes a vertical position, dropping downward in relation to the posterior wall of the tympanic cavity and the anterior wall of the mastoid to exit at the base of the skull through the stylomastoid foramen [13].
- The mastoid segment of facial nerve is protected by a perineural sheet, which progressively becomes thicker closed to the stylomastoid foramen.
- Iatrogenic injury of the facial nerve should not be acceptable in any middle ear surgery and obviously in cochlear implantation. The use of facial monitoring does not compensate for the lack of anatomical knowledge.

### 8.2.2 Surgical Technique

The drilling technique towards and through the facial recess can be used along two routes (Tos) [14]:

A. *Lateral route and opening of posterior tympanotomy from up to down*

The landmark is the incus (Figs. 8.6, 8.7, and 8.8).

The drilling is a continuation of the thinning of the bony canal wall lateral to the short process of incus (Fig. 8.7a) using a very small (0.5 mm) cutting or diamond burr, or just inferior to the fossa incudis with a 1 or 1.5 mm diamond burr and as a result preservation of bone buttress along the incus (Fig. 8.7b). The chorda is located

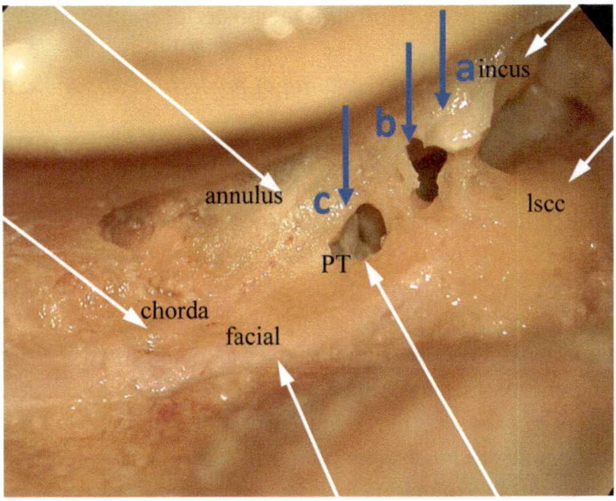


**Fig. 8.7** Posterior tympanotomy (PT): drilling from up to down; (a) arrow lateral to the incus; (b) arrow below the fossa incudis; (c) arrow closed to chorda and annulus at a distance from the facial nerve

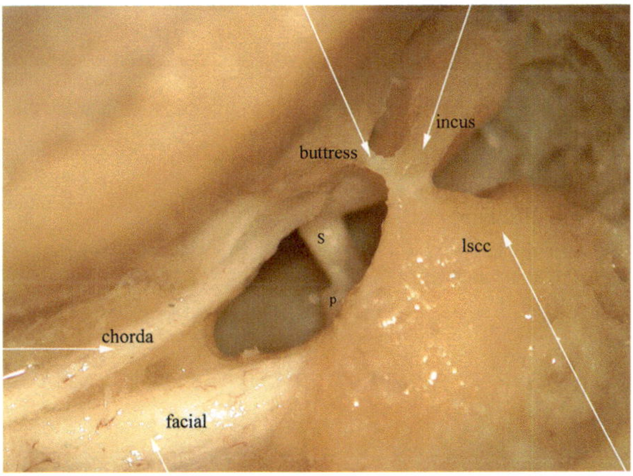


**Fig. 8.8** Posterior tympanotomy is done, a small bony bridge (buttress) individualized the drilling lateral to the short process of the incus and the drilling following the axis of the long process of the incus, *p* pyramidal eminence, *s* stapes

inferiorly. Outside the chorda canal, the chorda tympani runs toward the long process of the incus. By continued thinning the bony canal the opening of the posterior tympanotomy occurs at its upper part where the second genu of facial is distant (Fig. 8.7c). This opening is commonly performed through a well-pneumatized or spongy bone in children. The long process of the incus can be seen, and the drilling follows its axis and exposed the chorda tympani which is the lateral limit of the posterior tympanotomy, then the incus–stapes joint and stapedial tendon will be visualized. Continuing with diamond burr, a gradual extension of the drilling progressively enlarged the posterior tympanotomy medially towards the facial nerve and inferiorly toward the chorda-facial angle (Fig. 8.8). In order to see as much as possible, the round window the mastoid segment of the facial can be carefully unroofed on its lateral and anterior aspects, which becomes the definitive medial limit of the posterior tympanotomy.

This route looks safer regarding the facial nerve but the price to be safe is to get a limited approach through the posterior tympanotomy.

B. *Medial route and opening of posterior tympanotomy from down to up*

The landmark is the mastoid segment of the facial nerve (Figs. 8.9 and 8.10).

The thinning of the posterior canal wall until the level of the short process is continued at the level of the mastoid process using a finishing burr around 3–4 mm in diameter (a cutting burr is risky, a diamond burr stop bleeding and all structures are white). The drilling is performed parallel to the course of the facial nerve until some bleeding signals the fallopian canal and the proximity of the nerve. The chorda tympani is slightly superficial to the facial and often the first exposed and followed until the chorda-facial angle. With a diamond burr the course of the whitish mastoid segment of the facial nerve is clearly individualized but not necessarily unroofed. Then, a large posterior tympanotomy is safely performed between the chorda-facial nerve angle preserving an incus bone buttress at its upper part (Figs. 8.9, 8.11, and 8.12).

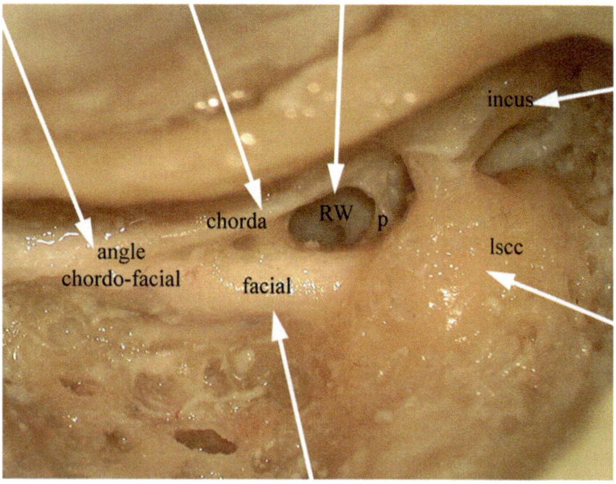


**Fig. 8.9** Posterior tympanotomy with mastoid segment of facial nerve as landmark, the incus buttress preserved the incus without limitation of the visualization of the round window (RW), *p* pyramidal eminence

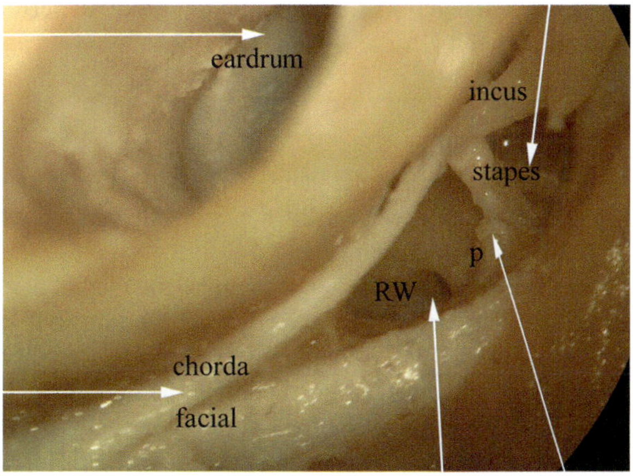


**Fig. 8.10** Posterior tympanotomy enlarged superiorly to expose round window (RW), stapes, incus, *p* pyramidal eminence

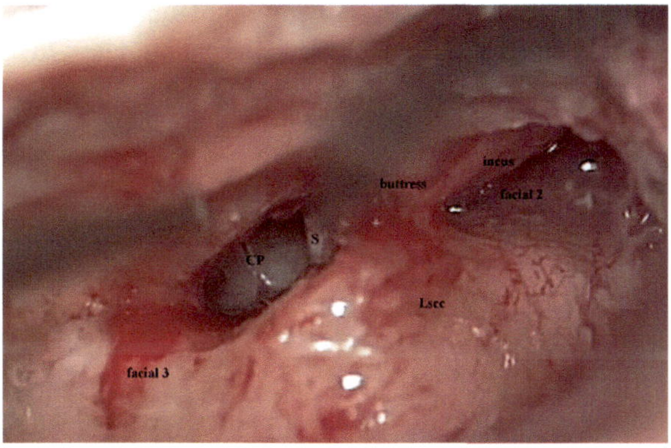


**Fig. 8.11** Surgical view of a left posterior tympanotomy showing the cochlear promontory (CP) and the superior limit of the round window; *s* stapes

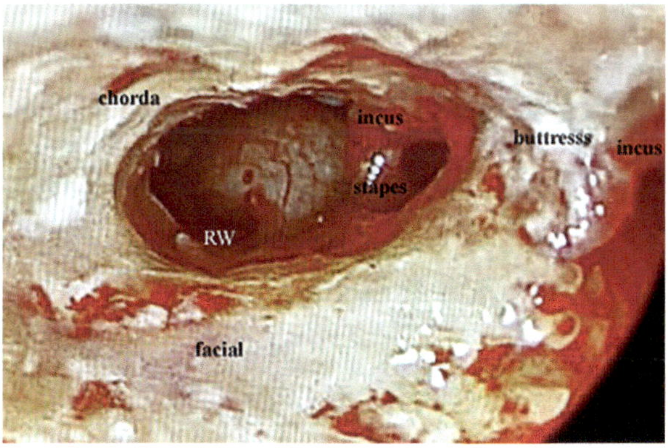


**Fig. 8.12** Endoscopic panoramic view through the posterior tympanotomy towards the cochlear promontory to visualize the round window (RW)

The author used and recommended such a procedure because finally in all cases we must know the exact location of the facial nerve and it is much better to immediately and completely solve this question. It is a basic principle in surgery to first identify the dangerous structure and therefore, to perform a safe surgery for patient and the surgeon [15].

**Tips and Tricks**

- During Drilling:
  - Avoids touching the incus, especially in hearing preservation surgery.
  - Near facial nerve works in parallel strokes with abundant irrigation. No pressure should be applied.
  - Care should be taken not to injure the medial part of the facial nerve either by the blind end of the burr or by the rotating shaft.
- Visibility of RWN through posterior tympanotomy can be improved by:
  - Turning the patient head making the line of sight perpendicular to FR.
  - Removal of incus buttress is rarely needed.
  - Sacrifice of chorda tympani could help for inferior extended posterior tympanotomy.
  - Drilling of the lateral bony lip of sinus tympani medial to facial canal. Care should be taken not to induce heating injury to the facial nerve.
  - Applying the combined approach to identify the RWN through the external ear canal should be used only in some rare cases of congenital inner ear anomaly.
- Subtotal petrosectomy would be the last aggressive resort facing uncommon situation as cochlear implantation in ossified cochlea and in chronic otitis cases

## 8.3 Cochleostomy

Cochlear implantation started initially with round window insertion. Then there was a shift to promontory cochleostomy to afford insertion of multi-electrode array. Since atraumatic insertion can be achieved directly through or enlarged round window, preserving the intracochlear structures [16] there was a shift back towards round window insertion.

The cochleostomy provides the surgical approach when the round window approach is not feasible due to the size of the posterior tympanotomy or due to unfavourable anatomy and/or pathology round window and/or basal cochlear turn.

### 8.3.1 Surgical Anatomy

**The Round window area Anatomy:**

- The RWN on the posterior surface of the promontory facing the retro-tympanum is a well-defined cavity but extremely variable in size and shape (Proctor) [17].
- The walls of the RWN consist of the tegmen superiorly, the anterior pillar (Postis Anterior) and the posterior pillar (Postis Posterior) (Fig. 8.13).
- Inferiorly only a very thin bony shell remains from the developing cartilage bar. In the middle of this inferior wall a stick-shaped bony elevation extending in the niche, the fustis, indicates the former cartilage bar [18].

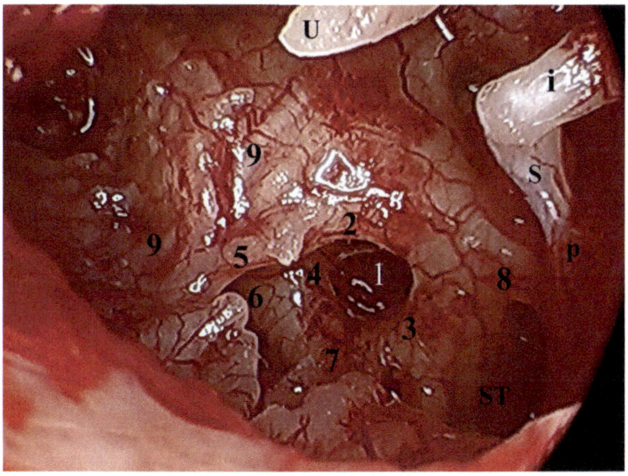


**Fig. 8.13** Left round window niche and cochlear promontory (*courtesy Dr. Sreeram Murthy*). 1) round window membrane, 2) tegmen of the round window niche, 3) postis posterior, 4) postis anterior, 5) sustentaculum promontori, 6) tunnel of the promontory, 7) fustis, 8) ponticulus, 9) Jacobson nerve, *u* umbo, *p* pyramidal eminence, *ST* sinus tympani, *i* incus

- Different parts of the RWN grow at different rate and at different time resulting in variable phenotypes of RWN anatomy [19] giving rise to significant variability in the overall size and shape of the RWN [20].
- The Round Window membrane (RWm) is conical in shape with a horizontal portion, located postero-superiorly, and a vertical part, situated antero-inferiorly with a ratio of size of 3:4 [21].
- An incomplete mucous membrane referred to as pseudo-membrane may persist at the entrance of the RWN. Occasionally, it can be ossified leading to the appearance of an absent RWN [19].
- The variable morphology of the round window, of the bony overhang and of the hook curved basal region of the cochlear tube does not offer a clear indication for the most appropriate route to the scala tympani without offending the spiral lamina from the scala vestibuli.
- Rarely the round window may be missing due to abnormal development or due to obliteration by an otosclerotic focus.

**Anatomy of Basal part of the cochlea**

- The basal or noncoiled part of the cochlea is 5–6 mm includes the round window and it lies medial to the posterior half of the promontory.
- The cochlear tube is divided internally into two semi-cylinders by a partition wall formed by the osseous spiral lamina medially, the secondary spiral lamina laterally and the basilar membrane in between. Externally such a partition is not visible and there is no clear definition for the surgical anatomy of the cochlear promontory confined below and behind the RWN (Fig. 8.14).
- The round window is the main landmark for the correct positioning of the cochleostomy towards the scala tympani [22].
- Variation in cochlear morphology is not just in size, shape and the coiling geometry but also in the internal anatomy of the cochlea [23]. Some degrees of malformation in cochlear anatomy are estimated around 20% [24].

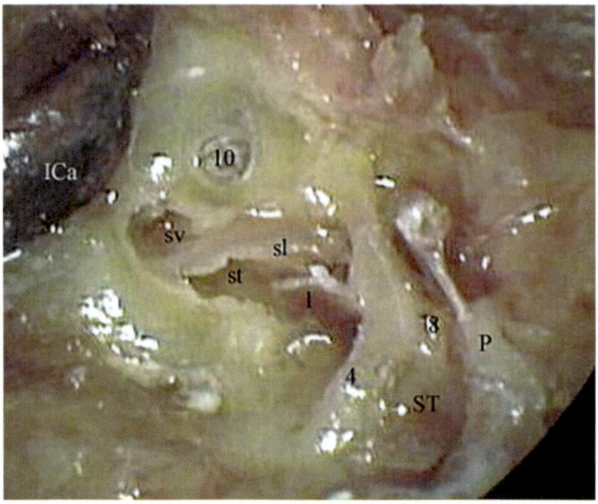


**Fig. 8.14** Anatomical dissection with drilling of the tegmen of the round window, of the postis anterior and the basal part of the cochlea to visualize the spiral lamina (sl). 1 round window membrane, 4 postis posterior, 8 ponticulus, 10 second turn of cochlea, *p* pyramidal eminence, *st* scala tympani, *sv* scala vestibuli, *ST* sinus tympani, *ICa* internal carotid artery

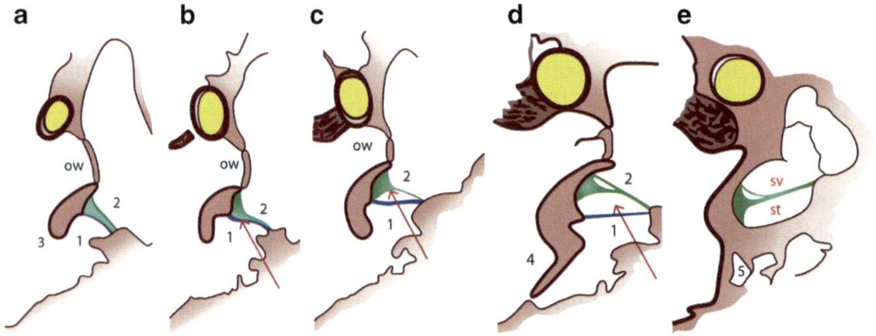


**Fig. 8.15** Drawings of vertical cuts, every 0.3 mm, at the level of round window niche to see the relationships between the round window membrane (blue) (1) and the lamina spiral (green) (2) from the ptosis posterior (**a**) of the round window to the anterior margin (**e**) of the oval window (OW), the distance between (**a**) and (**e**) is 1.8 mm (Scenario from Wolff D., Bellucci R., Eggston A. Surgical and microscopic anatomy of the temporal bone Hafner New York, 1971), 3: tegmen of round window, 4: sustentaculum promontory, 5: tunnel of the promontory, arrow the scala tympani (st), *sv* scala vestibuli

**The hook region:**

- It is the most basal part of the basal turn of cochlea.
- This is where the osseous spiral lamina; basilar membrane and spiral ligament merge [25].
- Anterior to the RWm the diameter of the scala tympani is more than 2 mm then decreases posteriorly with the angle formed by the obliquity of the RWm and the insertion of the spiral lamina.
- The posterior margin and the superior edge of the RWm correspond to the initial and horizontal part of the spiral lamina (Fig. 8.15).
- Knowledge of the anatomy of the hook region will avoid damage of structures important to preserve residual hearing during cochlear implant surgery [26].

**Crista Fenestra and Crista Semilunaris**

The literature showed great confusion about the use of terms of crista fenestra and crista semilunaris. They have been used interchangeably to designate either:

- The inferior bony wall of the RWN which is a very small thin bony shell where the round window membrane is attached inferiorly.
- or
- A small bony crest in the inferior wall of the scala tympani just at its entrance near the cochlear aqueduct [18]. Baki et al. [27] have suggested to term it as crista of scala tympani and restrict the term of crista fenestra to the anterior-Inferior bony margin of RWN to avoid any confusion of terminology.

## 8.3.2 Imaging Assessment

Multiple studies have been attempted to use CT scan assessment to predict possible difficulty in visualization of the round window. If RWN is not visible through posterior tympanotomy an additional measure would be needed either to increase exposure of RWN or to perform a promontory cochleostomy. The visibility of RWN and RWm can be detected on imaging by any of the following methods:

- Kashio et al. method [28] where it assesses a line parallel to external auditory canal and passing through mastoid segment of FN in relation to RWM. This line was classified as passing:
  - Posterior to RWM (Fig. 8.16a): Predicting Good visibility of RWN.
  - Anterior to RWM (Fig. 8.16b): Predicting Poor visibility of RWN.
- Lloyd et al. method [29] by measuring the angle of the basal turn of cochlea in relation to mid-sagittal plane in axial CT scans. The bigger this angle is the less the visibility of the RWN would be expected during surgery. This angle gets smaller with age which might explain why cochlear implantation is more difficult in paediatric population.

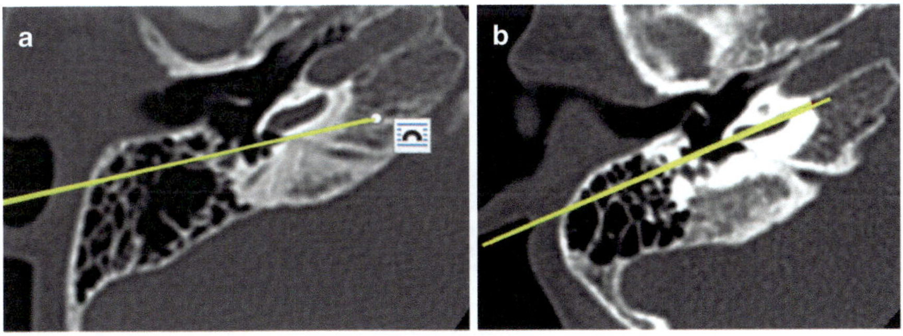


**Fig. 8.16** Kashio's method for RWN visibility: (**a**) Right ear—Kashio's line posterior to round window predicting good visibility of RWN. (**b**) Right ear—Kashio's line anterior of the round window predicting low visibility

- Hasaballah and Hamdy method [30] by measuring the distance between RWN and facial nerve. They have suggested that the bigger this distance is the better the visibility.
- Pendem et al. method [31] by measuring the distance between oval window and round window. They concluded that the smaller the distance is the more visible the RWN would be because it would be more superior within the posterior tympanotomy opening.
- Elzayat et al. [32] method by commenting on shape of the round window and describing C-shaped as visible RWm (Fig. 8.17) and O-shaped as barely visible RWm (Fig. 8.18). However, these authors commented on single cut.
- Park et al. method [33] by studying four consecutive cuts in axial section for a more reliable result. Identification of three or more cuts where the RWm is completely covered by bony niche (O-shaped) was a predictor of low or no visibility of RWm whereas identification of three or more cuts where the RWm is not covered by bony niche (C-shaped) was a predictor of good visibility of RWm.
- Galal et al. [34] method by measuring the RWN depth using the coronal cut with the deepest RWN and simply measured distance in mm from the free edge to the first point of RWm (Fig. 8.21). A cut-off point was detected:
  - More than 1.43 mm having low or no visibility of RWm (Fig. 8.19a).
  - Less than 1.43 mm having good visibility of RWm (Fig. 8.19b).

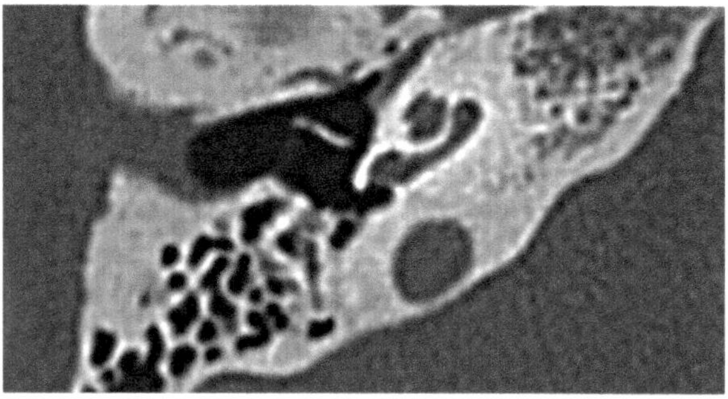

**Fig. 8.17** Elzayat's method: Axial view showing C-shaped RWN predicting a good visibility of RWm

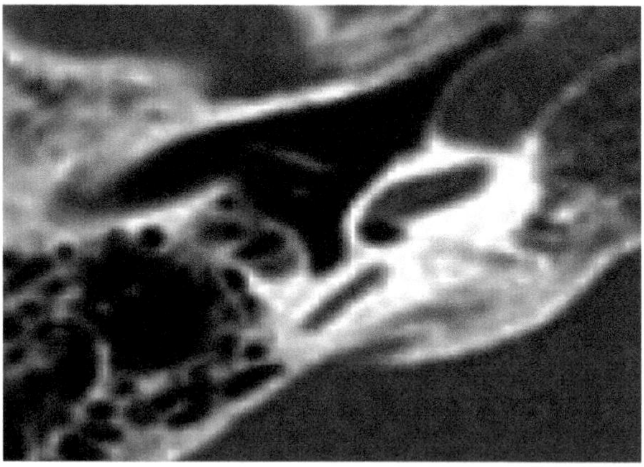

**Fig. 8.18** Elzayat's method: Axial view showing O-shaped RWN predicting an invisible or barely visible RWm

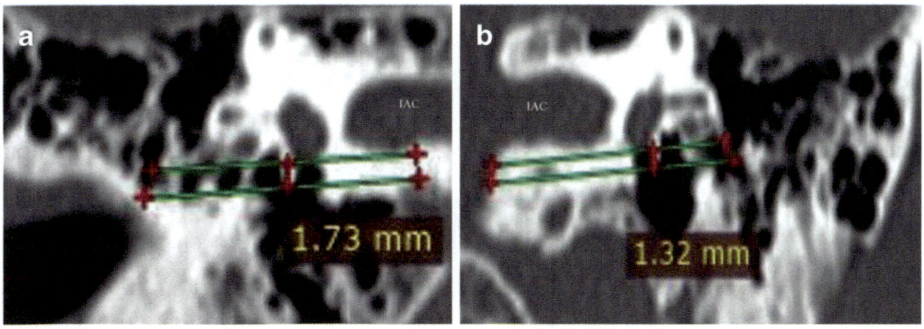


**Fig. 8.19** Galal's method RWN depth on left coronal CT scan showing: (**a**) RWN depth measurement of 1.73 mm with low visibility of RWN. (**b**) RWN measurement of 1.32 mm with good visibility of RWN (*IAC* internal auditory canal)

### 8.3.3 Surgical Technique

Promontory Cochleostomy is usually performed either when the surgeon prefers it over round window approach or when exposition of the round window membrane through the posterior tympanotomy is not possible. When RWN is partially visible but the electrode cannot be inserted through the round window, the surgeon has to move to cochleostomy.

According to their relation to the round window; different *sites* for cochleostomy were proposed:

- *Anteroinferior cochleostomy* (*AICO*) [35, 36]: This is the most accepted placements in promontory to ensure appropriate insertion of electrodes in the scala tympani. It entails drilling at the lateral corner of the round window at a point immediately in front of the inferior lip of the round window niche keeping a small rim of bone between the cochleostomy and the margin of the round window membrane (Fig. 8.20). Antero-inferior cochleostomy was suggested to provide a straighter course for the array and a place for insertion away from the hook region. Yet, although damage to the spiral lamina was less, it still existed.
- *Inferior cochleostomy* (*ICO*): A more inferior cochleostomy further decreases risk of damage to the hook region, nevertheless, it risks injury to the cochlear aqueduct and common modiolar vein which represents a major drainage for cochlea [25]. Consequently, its injury would affect cochlear physiology and compromise hearing preservation [37]. Additionally, inferior cochleostomy needs an extended posterior tympanotomy and skeletonization of the facial nerve [38]. Also, it can lead to under promontory wrong track [20].
- *In between AICO et ICO* [39]: In such limited space, the risk of misinterpretation of the site is high and the choice of selected cochleostomy placement is inter-surgeon variability [40].
- *RW marginal cochleostomy*: Drilling the anterior-inferior lip of the RWN until the annulus of the RWm is visualized, then drilling a 1 or 2 mm more antero-

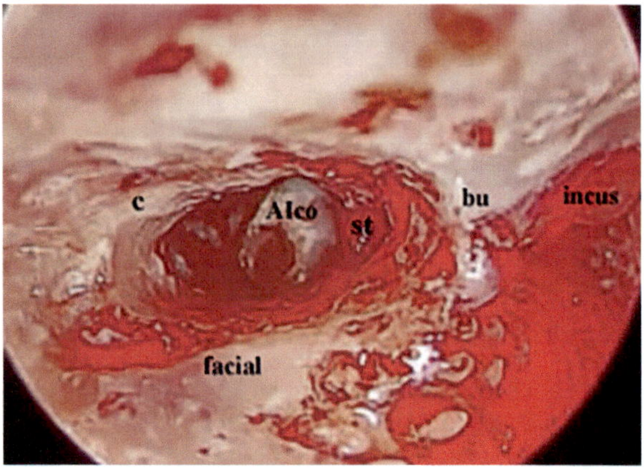


**Fig. 8.20** Anterior-Inferior cochleostomy (AIco) 1 mm in diameter through the posterior tympanotomy. The round window is not visible

inferior. Roland [37] called this a RW marginal cochleostomy because it is formed partially by inferior annulus of round window and partially by the bony extension of the RWN. This same technique was described also as the enlarged round window approach.

- *Anterior cochleostomy* (*ACO*) *and Anterosuperior cochleostomy* (*ASCO*)*:* Must be avoided regarding the risk of scala vestibuli opening and scalar dislocation. Anterior cochleostomy has been proven to be constantly damaging the hook region. Drilling a too superior cochleostomy leading to seeing a whitish not a bluish or greyish hue means that this is the spiral ligament about to be injured [25].

According to their relation to oval window, the following sites for cochleostomy were proposed:

- Scala Vestibuli Insertion: In cases of ossified scala tympani of the basal turn of the cochlea, cochleostomy is performed just anterio-inferior to the oval window. It is to be noted that insertion of electrode in scala vestibuli have the potential risk for causing balance problem.
- Middle Turn Cochleostomy: In cases of completely ossified basal turn of the cochlea, cochleostomy is performed 2.5 mm anterior to the oval window and 1 mm below cochleariformis process to insert the electrode in the middle turn.
- Scala Tympani Insertion: In cases where RWN is not visible even with extended posterior tympanotomy; cochleostomy is performed 2.5–3 mm below the anterior crus of the foot plate of the oval window.

To ensure Hearing Preservation Surgery the following *technique* for cochleostomy was proposed

- Use low speed drilling.
- Drill through the posterior tympanotomy a bony shell of the promontory covering the cochlea using a diamond burr (1 mm). The size of the cochleostomy will

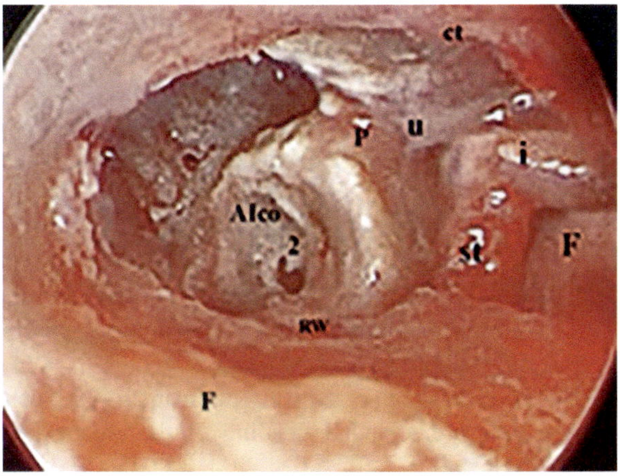


**Fig. 8.21** Endoscopic view (*courtesy Dr. Elaini Sherif*). Anterior Inferior cochleostomy (AIco) 1 mm in diameter, the periosteum is opened (2). RW is the localization of the barely visible round window even with endoscope, *P* promontory, *u* umbo, *ct* chorda tympani

depend on the device selected ranging between 0.6 and 1.2 mm in diameter. Drilling should respect the cochlear endosteum preventing bone debris produced or blood from entering the scala tympani.

- The scala tympany endosteum is opened with a sharp needle for reducing to a minimum the leak of perilymphatic fluid (Fig. 8.21). Healon can be instilled just before opening the endosteum to reduce the entrance of bone dust or blood in scala tympani.
- Despite the surgeons' best efforts, the burr frequently tears and perforates the cochlear endosteum because the drilling channel bottom has the same convex cup shape as the burr [41]. Consequently, the exposition of an enough area that matches the diameter of electrodes without damaging the endosteum is a challenging task [42].
- Once the cochlea is opened Intracochlear suctioning is prohibited or kept to minimum.
- If crista semilunaris is present it should be removed to allow proper insertion of the electrode without deflection towards the modiolus. Its removal is suggested by using curettes and hooks not drills to decrease heat, bone dust with potential future fibrosis and inflammation within the scalar lumen.

To respect *Soft Surgery Concept* proposed by Lenhardt [43], the following associated procedures should be undertaken:

*Before Opening of Cochlea*

- Administer high dose steroid to decrease inflammatory reaction.
- Avoid bone dust and blood entrance in scala tympani by:
  - Perform Cochleostomy after finishing all other bony drilling procedures.
  - Aggressive control of bleeding and using cottonoids with epinephrine over the promontory.

- Avoid acoustic trauma by:
  - Preventing contact of the drill with the ossicular chain.
  - Use of low speed drilling of the RWN.
- At this stage, it is highly recommended that the surgical team change their gloves to manipulate the device and introduce the electrode array.

*Atraumatic Insertion of Electrode*

- The direction for insertion should be superior to inferior and posterior to anterior.
- The slowest rate with the least interruptions possible (preferably non-stop) for insertion should be exerted.
- The insertion is progressively performed with "gentle gestures" without excessive pressure to avoid bending of the electrode or/and intracochlear trauma (Fig. 8.22).
- Design of electrode is a crucial factor in hearing preservation. Use electrode shorter than 24 mm [44] with depth of insertion 360–400 degrees at maximum [45].
- The type of the electrode could affect the decision and preference of RWm versus cochleostomy insertion:
  - Perimodiolar electrodes are nearly always best inserted through a bony cochleostomy.
  - Straight delicate electrodes are appropriate for RWm insertions [46].

*After Insertion of Electrode*

- The full inserted electrode array into the cochlea closed the cochleostomy (Fig. 8.23). The sealing is reinforced by inserting small pieces of temporalis muscle or periosteum between the edges of the cochleostomy and the electrode, but without over packing.

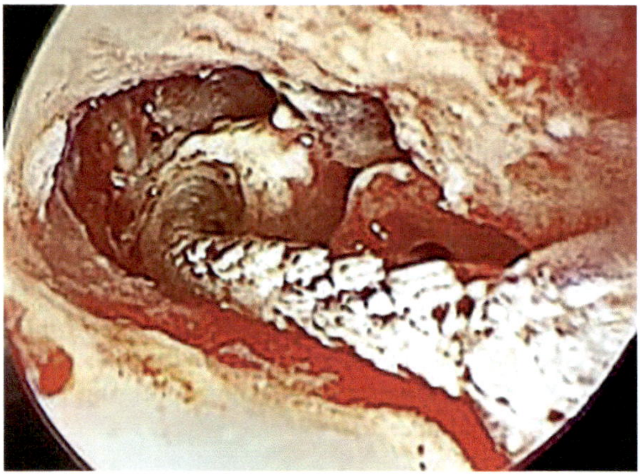

**Fig. 8.22** Insertion of the electrode array through the cochleostomy

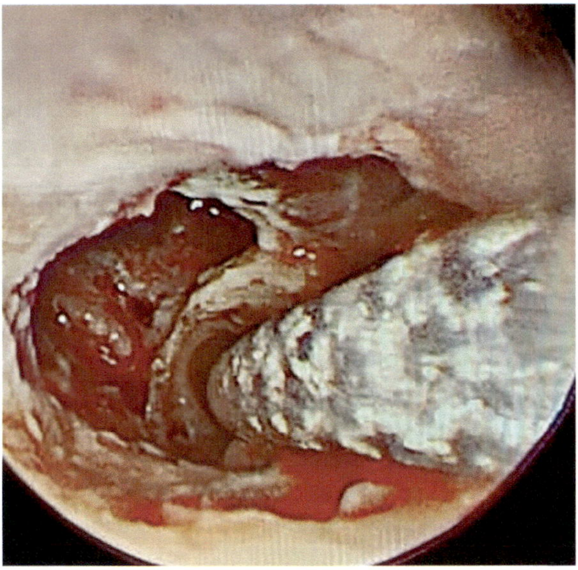

**Fig. 8.23** Full electrode insertion requires additional sealing to close the cochleostomy

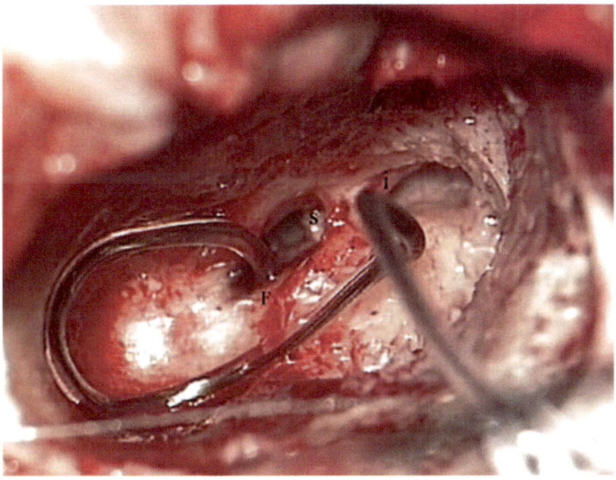

**Fig. 8.24** After electrode insertion, the cable of the electrode array must be not let in contact with the facial nerve (F), *s* stapes, *i* incus

- A thicker “stopper” on the electrode can be used to plug the cochleostomy in case of Gusher.
- At the level of the posterior tympanotomy the cable of the electrode is sealed off the facial nerve with periosteum (Fig. 8.24).
- The surgery ends with the fixation of the electronic device on the skull within the delineated bed with bony well stich or simply screws under the temporal muscle following the specific characteristics of the selected cochlear implant.

## 8.4 Future Developments

Further refinements and developments are currently in process to improve the outcome of cochlear implant surgery. The following is an enumeration of some of these aspects:

- The research may provide more knowledge about optimal cochleostomy and trajectory pathways for electrode insertion using new imaging techniques such as micro-CT and synchroton radiation [16].
- Laser cochleostomy using the $CO_2$ Laser to achieve clean cuts on bone and precisely approximated the endosteum surface or using the holmium YAG laser to reopen the basal turn for ossified cochlea have been reported [47].
- An Optical Coherence Tomography (OCT) system for the detection of the bone—endosteum—perilymph structures could solve the key problem hindering the clinical application of laser cochleostomy [41].
- Cochlear implantation using a robot-assisted insertion to offer a safe and reliable insertion of electrode array and to reduce the scalar translocation rate are already used in a few centres [48]. Robot device drilling a tunnel through the mastoid to the facial recess and round window is being experimented.
- Another aspect of research for hearing preservation is the development of intracochlear drug delivery [49].

Continuous efforts to perfect the techniques and the equipment are based on the desire to minimize the inner trauma and to preserve residual hearing, and the final word is never written [48] (Video 8.1).

## References

1. Black B. Keyhole cochlear implantation: current status. Otol Neurotol. 2011;32:1459–63.
2. Jansen C. Posteriore Tympanotomie : Zugang zum Mittelohr mit Erhaltung des Aussenren Gehorgangsi Arch. Ohr Nas U Kehlk-Heils. 1967;188:558.
3. Jansen C. The combined approach for tympanoplasty. J Laryngol. 1968;82:779–93.
4. Anson B, Donaldson J. Surgical anatomy of the temporal bone and ear. Philadelphia: W.B. Saunders; 1973.
5. Amjad A, Starke J, Scheer A. Tympanofacial recess in human ear. Arch Otolaryngol. 1968;88:131.
6. Eby TL, Nadol JB. Postnatal growth of the human temporal bone. Implications for cochlear implants in children. Ann Otol Rhinol Laryngol. 1986;95(4 Pt 1):356–64.
7. Jako G. The posterior bony ear canal and the antrum threshold angle in conservative middle ear surgery. Laryngoscope. 1966;76:1260.
8. Jako G. The posterior route to middle ear: posterior tympanotomy. Laryngoscope. 1967;77:306–16.
9. Bielamowicz S, Coker N, Jenkins H, et al. Surgical dimensions of the facial recess in adults and children. Arch Otolaryngol Head Neck Surg. 1988;114:534–7.
10. Eby T. Development of the facial recess: implications for cochlear implantation. Laryngoscope. 1996;106(Suppl 80):1–7.

11. Sheehy J, Patterson M. Intact canal wall tympanoplasty with mastoidectomy. A review of eight years' experience. Laryngoscope. 1967;77:1502–42.
12. Nager G, Proctor B. The facial canal: normal anatomy, variations and anomalies. II. Anatomical variations and anomalies involving the facial canal. Ann Otol Rhinol Laryngol Suppl. 1982;97:45–61.
13. Maru N, Cheita A, Mogoanta C, et al. Intratemporal course of the facial nerve: morphological, topographic and morphometric features. Rom J Morphol Embryol. 2010;51:243–8.
14. Tos M. Manual of middle ear surgery: mastoid surgery. Stuttgart: G. Thieme Verlag; 1995.
15. Mansour S, Magnan J, Haidar H, et al. Comprehensive and clinical anatomy of the middle ear. Heidelberg: Springer; 2013.
16. Schart-Moren N. The human cochlea and cochlear implantation. Uppsala: Acta Universitatis Upsaliensis; 2018.
17. Proctor B. Surgical anatomy of the ear and temporal bone. Stuttgart: G. Thieme Verlag; 1989.
18. Angeli J, Enio T, Setoguttic E, et al. The crista fenestra and its impact on the surgical approach to the scala tympani during cochlear implantation. Audiol Neurotol. 2017;22:50–5.
19. Toth M, Alpar A, Patonay L, et al. Development and surgical anatomy of the round window niche. Ann Anat. 2006;188:93–101.
20. Marchioni D, Alicandri-Ciufelli M, Pothier D, et al. The round window region and contiguous areas: endoscopic anatomy and surgical implications. Eur Arch Otorhinolaryngol. 2015;272:1103–12.
21. Okuno H, Sando I. Anatomy of the round window. A histopathological study with a graphic reconstruction method. Acta Otolaryngol. 1988;106:55–63.
22. Finley C, Holden T, Holden K, et al. Role of the electrode placement as a contributor to variability in cochlear implant outcomes. Otol Neurotol. 2008;29:920–8.
23. Erixon E, Hogstrop H, Wadin K, et al. Variational anatomy of human cochlea: implication for cochlear implantation. Otol Neurotol. 2009;30:14–22.
24. Sennaroglu L, Bajin M. Classification and current management of inner ear malformations. Balkan Med J. 2017;34:397–411.
25. Atturo F, Barbara M, Rask-Andersen H. On the anatomy of the 'hook' region of the human cochlea and how it relates to cochlear implantation. Audiol Neurootol. 2014;19:378–85.
26. Stidham KR, Roberson JB Jr. Cochlear hook anatomy: evaluation of the spatial relationship of the basal cochlear duct to middle ear landmarks. Acta Otolaryngol. 1999;119:773–7.
27. Baki F, Shewel Y, Eshomi M, Mehanna A. Cadaveric study of crista fenestra: revisited. J Int Adv Otol. (in press)
28. Kashio A, Sakamoto T, Kakigi A, et al. Predicting round window niche visibility via facial recess using high-resolution computed tomography. Otol Neurotol. 2015;36:18–23.
29. Lloyd S, Kasbekar A, Kenway B, et al. Developmental changes in cochlear orientation–implications for cochlear implantation. Otol Neurotol. 2010;31:902–7.
30. Hasaballah M, Hamdy T. Evaluation of facial nerve course, posterior tympanotomy width and visibility of round window in patient with cochlear implantation Egypt. J Otolaryngol. 2014;30:317–21.
31. Pendem S, Rangasami R, Arunachalam RK, et al. HRCT correlation with round window identification during cochlear implantation in children. J Clin Imaging SCI. 2014;4:70.
32. Elzayat S, Mandour M, Lotfy R, et al. Predicting round window visibility during cochlear implantation using HRCT. J Int Adv Otol. 2018;14:15–7.
33. Park E, Amoodi H, Kuthubutheen J, et al. Predictors of round window accessibility for adult cochlear implantation based on pre-operative CT scan: a prospective observational study. J Otolaryngol Head Neck Surg. 2015;44:20–6.
34. Galal A. Clinico-radiological classification of round window accessibility for cochlear implantation. Ph.D. Thesis, Alexandria University, Faculty of Medicine. 2019, p. 113.
35. Adunka O, Buchman C. Scala tympani cochleostomy: results of a survey. Laryngoscope. 2007;117:2187–94.
36. Adunka O, Radeloff A, Gstoettner W, et al. Scala tympani cochleostomy: topography and histology. Laryngoscope. 2007;117:2195–200.

37. Roland PS, Wright CG, Isaacson B. Cochlear implant electrode insertion: the round window revisited. Laryngoscope. 2007;117:1397–402.
38. Briggs R, Tykocinski M, Xu J, et al. Comparison of round window and cochleostomy approaches with a prototype hearing preservation electrode. Audiol Neurootol. 2006;11(Suppl 1):42–8.
39. Badr A, Shabana Y, Mokbel K, et al. Atraumatic scala tympani cochleostomy; resolution of the dilemma. J Int Adv Otol. 2018;14:190–6.
40. Torres R, Kazmitchef G, Bernardeschi D, et al. Variability of the mental representation of the cochlea anatomy during cochlear implantation. Eur Arch Otorhinolaryngol. 2016;273:2009–18.
41. Roland P, Wright C. Surgical aspects of cochlear implantation: mechanical insertion trauma. Adv Oto-Rhino-Laryngol. 2006;64:11–30.
42. Zhang Y, Pfeiffer T, Weller M, et al. Optical coherence tomography guided laser cochleostomy. BioMed Res Int. 2014;Article ID 251814, 10 p.
43. Lenhardt E. Intracochlear placement of cochlear implant electrodes in soft surgery technique. HNO. 1993;7:356–9.
44. Friedland D, Runge-Samuelson C. Soft cochlear implantation: rationale for the surgical approach. Trends Amplif. 2009;13(2):124–38.
45. Talbot K, Hartley D. Combined electro-acoustic stimulation: a beneficial union? Clin Otolaryngol. 2008;33:536–45.
46. Lenarz T, Stover T, Buechner A, et al. Temporal bone results and hearing preservation with a new straight electrode. Audiol Neurootol. 2006;11(Suppl 1):34–41.
47. Jovanovic S. Lasers in otology. In: Huttenbrink K, editor. Lasers in otorhinolaryngology. Stuttgart: G. Thieme Verlag; 2005. p. 21–52.
48. Daoudi H, Lahlou G, Torres R, et al. Robot-assisted cochlear electrode array insertion in adults: a comparative study with manual insertion. Otol Neurotol. 2020;10:1092.
49. Ibrahim H, Helbig S, Bossard D, et al. Surgical trauma after sequential insertion of intracochlear catheters and electrode arrays. Otol Neurotol. 2011;32:1444–7.

# Cochlear Implant Surgery Using the Veria Technique

# 9

Trifon Kiratzidis

## 9.1 History and Evolution of the Technique

I started cochlear implantations at the Veria General Hospital, where the first Cochlear Implant Center of Greece was organized, in September 1993. Initially I was using the classic mastoidectomy and posterior tympanotomy technique proposed by W. House [1]. At that time, the knowledge about the surgical anatomy of the cochlea was limited to the oval window niche from the stapes surgery, or to the experience from the destructive surgery of the trans-labyrinthine approach to the cerebelo-pontine angle. Though there was a huge amount of knowledge on the fine structure of the cochlea, there was only a limited knowledge about the variabilities in size, exact position, and changes in relation to the neighboring structures.

Two years later, in 1995, operating the left ear of a 45-year-old lady, I came across a strange condition. I could not locate the basal turn of the cochlea through the posterior tympanotomy, even though I had extended it posteriorly and inferiorly. I could only see the incudostapedial joint, the head of stapes and the beginning of the crura.

The middle ear seemed to be completely empty, and the cochlea seemed to be missing.

Spending much time trying and thinking and keeping in mind that the cochlea was there on the CT scan, I decided to switch to the endaural approach to see directly what was going on.

**Supplementary Information** The online version contains supplementary material available at [https://doi.org/10.1007/978-981-19-0452-3_9].

T. Kiratzidis (✉)
Euromedica Cochlear Implant Center, Thessaloniki, Greece

Veria Medical Center, Veria, Greece
e-mail: trifonk@otenet.gr


S. DeSaSouza (ed.), *Cochlear Implants*,
https://doi.org/10.1007/978-981-19-0452-3_9

Through the endaural view, everything was clear. The middle ear cavity was exceptionally large as the promontory was flat or empty. The oval window and the medial part of the stapedial crura were hidden behind the facial canal and so was the round window niche. The whole cochlea seemed to have been rotated backwards around the longitudinal axis of the oval window niche. Under the direct endaural vision the basal turn of the cochlea, though rotated, could be safely identified and the exact point for the cochleostomy could be defined. So, I performed the cochleostomy through the endaural approach and completed the operation successfully.

After this painful experience I decided to modify my surgical approach to an extended endaural approach with double flap opening. First, I was directly entering the middle ear with a small endaural incision, identifying the basal turn of the cochlea, defining the point for the cochleostomy, and making the cochleostomy through the canal. Then inspect the patency of the cochleostomy and temporary sealing the cochleostomy with fascia or gel-foam.

If everything was fine only then I was proceeding to the rest of the operation: extension of the incision, preparation of the skin flaps, mastoidectomy and posterior tympanotomy, drilling of the implant bed and implantation.

I was using this complicated but safe technique for a period. The mastoidectomy was becoming smaller and smaller by time, and the posterior tympanotomy finally was limited to a small opening, enough to pass the active electrode.

In 1997, having accumulated all this experience, I decided to abandon the mastoidectomy and the posterior tympanotomy. I replaced them with a simple tunnel, large enough only to pass the active electrode.

Initially I was drilling a small hole, 3 mm wide to accept the shaft of the burr, and 5–6 mm deep, behind the spine of Henle close to the canal, leaving an eggshell-thick plate of the bone. From the bottom of this well, at a point corresponding to 10 h in the right ear and to 2 h in the left, with a cutting burr of 1.6 mm, I was drilling a tunnel through the posterior bony canal wall, towards the upper part of the facial recess trying to push the chorda tympani, and that was the end of the drilling. (Fig. 9.1).

For 2 years, I was doing this exceptionally fine drilling that was extremely easy for me and proved to be very safe. I presented this technique in several meetings

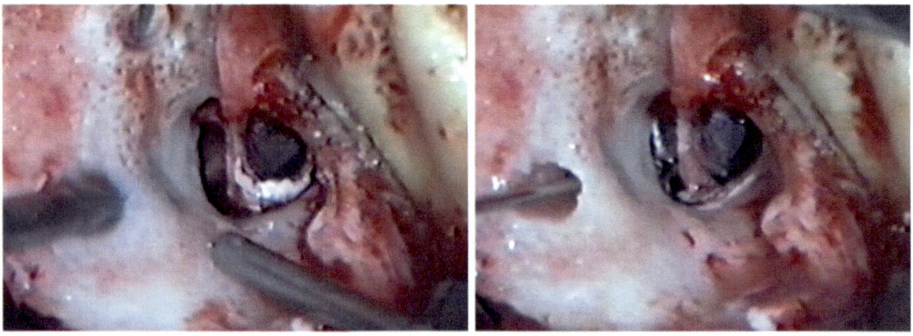

**Fig. 9.1** Free hand drilling of direct tunnel

trying to explain why it was easy and safe, but it remained very scary for the other surgeons who criticized it as a "blind" one and dangerous for the facial nerve.

In 1999 I presented the technique in the APSCI congress in Seoul, where my presentation was selected by the faculty to be included in the published volume by Karger in the Advanced Otorhinolaryngology, in 2000.

In 1999, after the Seoul meeting, I was motivated by my friend clinical engineer Alexei Iltcenko who told me by word: "Trifon, why don't you make a device, not everybody can do what you are doing".

So, I designed and built a special perforator with a guide along the drill-bit, allowing to drill in a precisely controlled depth and direction on the bone, making the drilling of a direct tunnel simple and safe, even at hands of beginners in the field of cochlear implantation (Fig. 9.2). The development of this perforator was mentioned in the publication of 2000.

At the same time, I designed a special electrode forceps for safe handling of the active electrode in the middle ear (Fig. 9.3). This was a left curved fine crocodile forceps, properly treated to be atraumatic for the electrode. This is suitable for use in both ears for the right-handed surgeon.

## 9.2 The Technique

The technique has been updated up to now regarding certain steps, like skin incision, cochleostomy or round window insertion, which are all possible and simple.

The trans meatal approach is used. That offers a wide visibility and accessibility to the middle ear structures. The incision can be made either endaural or postauricular. The endaural incision offers a wider visibility and accessibility to the middle ear structures than the proposed postauricular with intact canal skin. Therefore, cases with any particular problem such as cochlear obliteration or malformation, should be handled with the endaural incision.

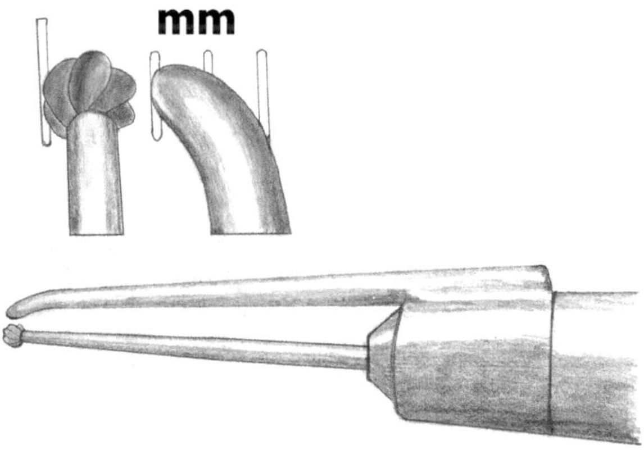


**Fig. 9.2** Veria perforator safety drilling device

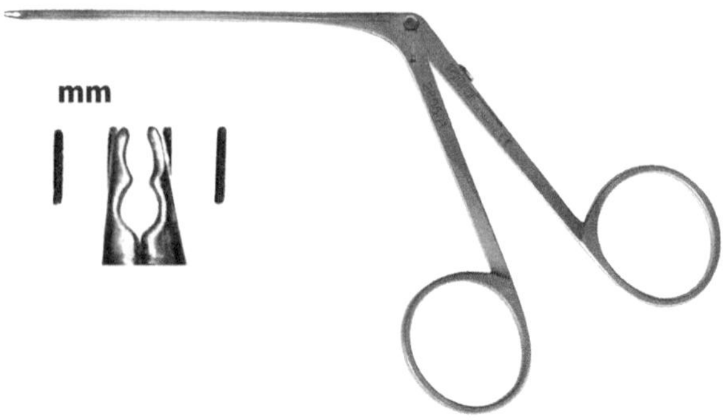


**Fig. 9.3** Safety electrode forceps

### 9.2.1 Steps of the Operation

**Step 1a: Endaural Incision**

I start with a typical small endaural incision, starting at 12 h intra canal and extending between tragus and helix. The incision is extended superio-posteriorly around the auricle sufficiently enough to expose the temporal line and the mastoid cortex (Fig. 9.4). The tympanomeatal flap is created and the middle ear cavity exposed. We prefer to make the circular incision of the canal skin quite deep, 5 mm from the annulus, creating a small thin tympanomeatal flap, which then can be rolled over the anterior part of the tympanic membrane, leaving the canal completely free of any tissue.

**Step 1b: Postauricular Incision**

It is a reverse S for the right side (Fig. 9.5) and an S for the left, with the upper part turned posteriorly. The skin is then elevated to the fascial—periosteal plane and retracted posteriorly. A circular incision is made on the periosteum down to bone at the posterior rim of the meatus and the meatal skin of the posterior wall is elevated anteriorly without incision till the anulus, and the middle ear is opened (Fig. 9.6). Then a second incision is done on the periosteum from the inferior part or the meatal rim posteriorly for about 2.5 cm and then turned up, creating a superiorly base periosteal flap, that is elevated upwards like a tongue, and kept superiorly by a suture (Fig. 9.7).

**Step 2: Inspection of the Middle Ear Anatomy**

By a small atticotomy, if required, the incudo-stapedial joint and the facial canal are exposed and inspected to rule out any irregularities. The round window niche and basal turn of the cochlea are safely identified. Contrary to the limited exposure through the posterior tympanotomy, the wide exposure of the intra-meatal approach makes the identification of the basal turn of the cochlea and the point of the cochleostomy safe. That prevents any surgical failure with misplaced electrode or incomplete surgery, where the cochlea was not properly identified through the posterior tympanotomy. We have seen and successfully revised a considerable number of unpublished such cases, using the trans-meatal approach. During this stage we mark

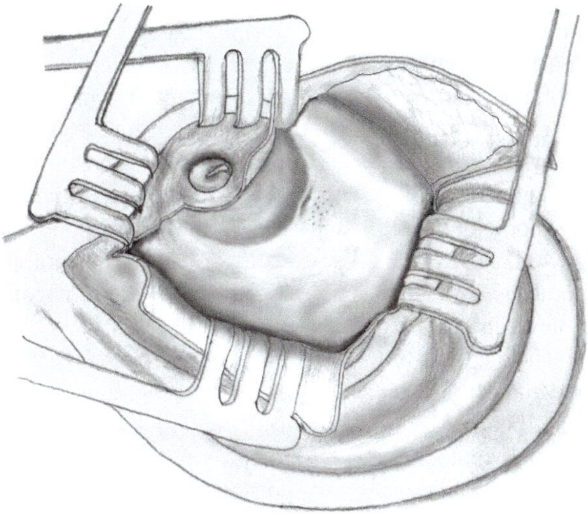

**Fig. 9.4** Trans-canal approach with endural incision

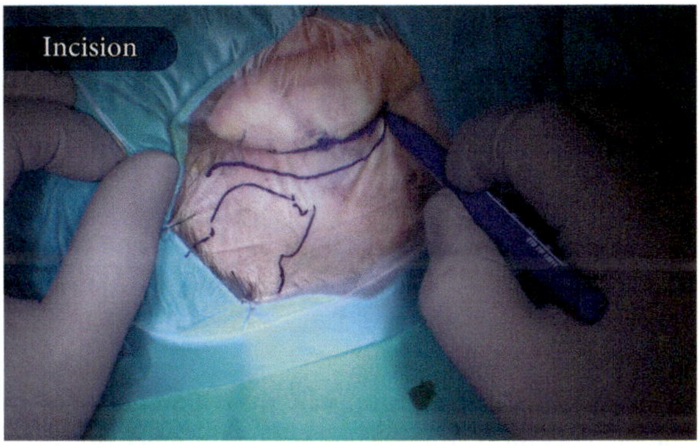


**Fig. 9.5** Postauricular incision

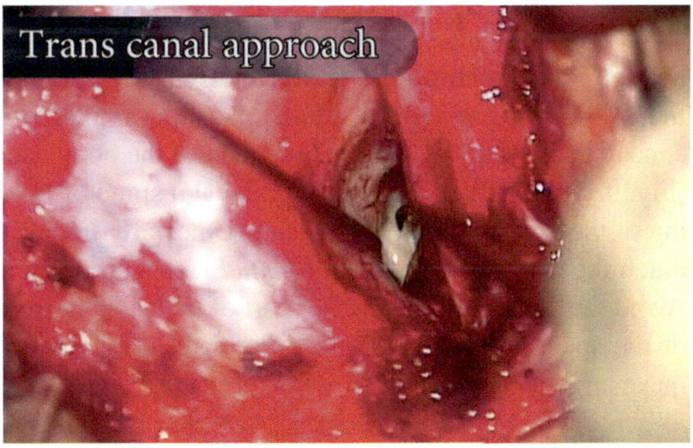


**Fig. 9.6** Trans-canal approach with postauricular incision intact canal skin

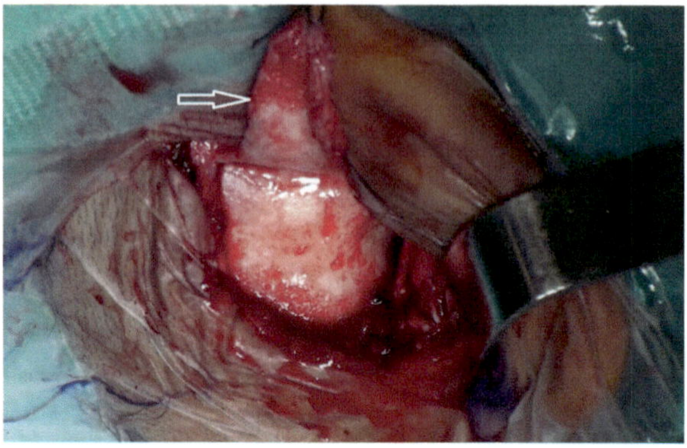

**Fig. 9.7** Postauricular incision. Superiorly based periosteal flap (Tongue flap)

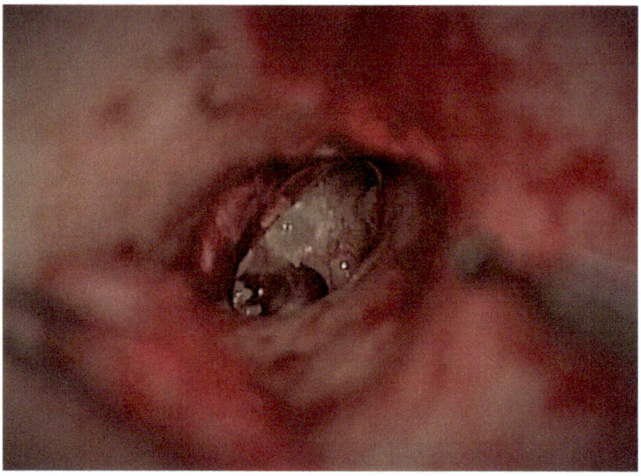

**Fig. 9.8** Marking of the cochleostomy

the point of the cochleostomy by initializing the drilling of it with a 1 mm diamond bur, but not completing it (Fig. 9.8). This mark is useful landmark during drilling the direct tunnel. In case we prefer to use the round window insertion this mark is replaced by drilling of the rim of the round window niche (Fig. 9.9).

**Step 3: Straightening the Posterior Bony Canal Wall**

In some cases, particularly adults, the superio-posterior bony canal wall presents a concavity. By drilling out the outer rim of the bony canal posteriorly and superiorly (Fig. 9.10), together with the suprameatal spine of Henle if necessary, a straightening of the wall is achieved, which is especially important because it facilitates very much the drilling of the *direct tunnel* (see step 6) by use of the special perforator. Avoid the drilling of the medial part of the canal because this will support the guide of the special perforator during the drilling of the direct channel. If you need to make an atticotomy make it with curette.

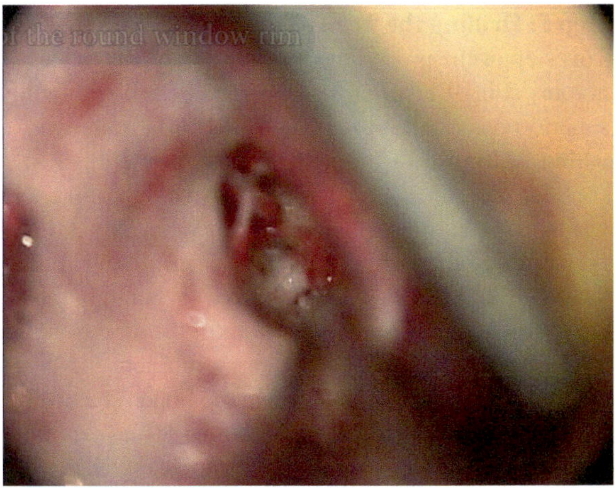


**Fig. 9.9** Drilling out the rim of the round window niche, preparing for electrode insertion

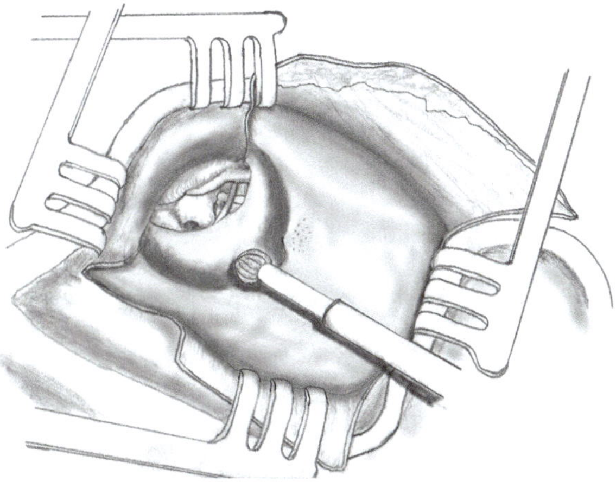

**Fig. 9.10** Straightening the posterior canal wall

**Step 4: Drilling the Suprameatal Hollow**

Using a 5-mm cutting burr, we drill a round hollow 8–10 mm wide and 5–6 mm deep (Fig. 9.11), starting on the cribriform area and drilling up to the temporal line superiorly, and adjacent to the superio-posterior rim of the bony canal wall anteriorly, leaving only a thin bony plate between the canal and the hollow. We take care to drill in such a way to leave a considerable overhang in the cortical rim of the hollow. This suprameatal hollow has been designed to accommodate any final excess of the active electrode, which is rolled in the hollow and kept in place spontaneously under the overhang rim by springing. Besides, it was proved to be useful in other aspects: (1) it facilitates the drilling of the *direct tunnel* by shortening the distance to be drilled and by allowing better control of the perforator, and (2) it ensures the continuous irrigation by being saline filled during drilling.

**Step 5: Drilling the Trans-Wall Direct Tunnel**

This step of the procedure is replacing the mastoidectomy and the posterior tympanotomy (Fig. 9.12). For the creation of the direct tunnel, we use the thickness of the superio-posterior bony canal wall itself (trans-wall), by drilling very accurately within it, by use of the special perforator (Fig. 9.2). This is a simple device that contains a cutting burr paired with a straight guide. The cutting burr used initially was 1.6 mm carbite but later was replaced by a 1.4 mm one. The tip of the guide is very close to the burr allowing the drilling to be only 0.5 mm under the surface of the bone. Apart from controlling very accurately the depth of the drilling, the guide also permits a very efficient control of the direction of the drilling, since it is always visible in the canal, showing every moment the position and the direction of the drilling burr, which is hidden into the bone. The drilling of the direct tunnel starts at the uppermost point of the bottom of the *suprameatal hollow* adjacent to the superio-posterior bony wall of the canal (Fig. 9.12). This corresponds to 10.00 h for

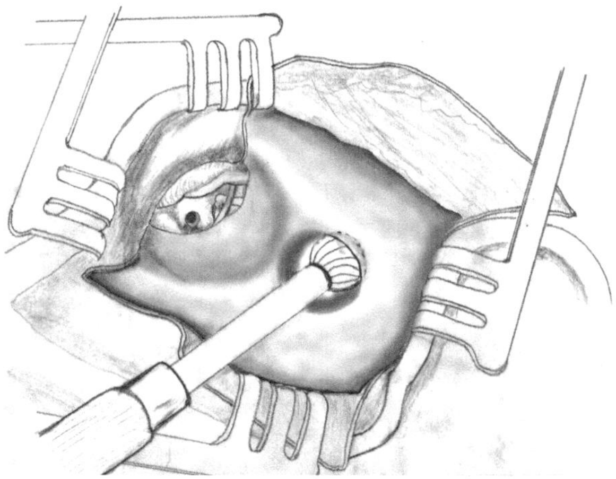

**Fig. 9.11** Drilling of the suprameatal hollow

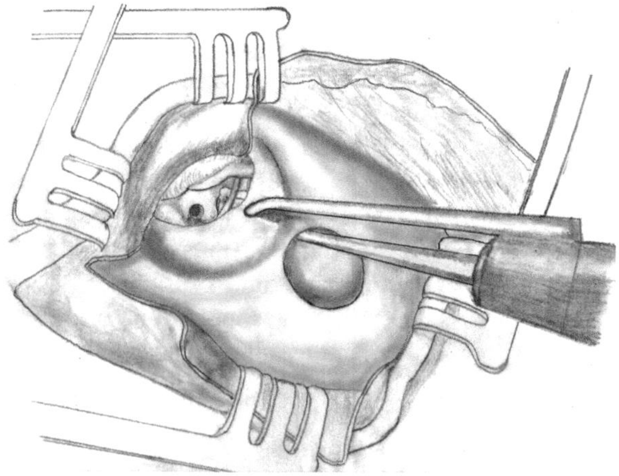

**Fig. 9.12** Drilling the direct tunnel

the right ear and 2.00 h for the left ear. The suprameatal hollow is saline filled and the drilling is done with a low speed, no more than 5000 rpm, in a push–pull movement of the drill to allow continuous irrigation of the tip of the drilling burr. For the direction of the drilling, we follow a straight line from the point of the start towards the marking of the cochleostomy we did previously or towards the anterior rim of the round window. If the point of exit of the chorda tympani is above this line, we then drill higher to this point to avoid damage of the nerve. When the burr enters the middle ear, the direct tunnel has been completed and the perforator is removed from inside out with the drill running. Using a fine suction tip on a syringe, any bone dust is washed out from the tunnel and the middle ear, and besides the potency of the tunnel is controlled. The direct tunnel is sufficiently large for any electrode array, but it can be further enlarged if necessary, by drilling sidewise superiorly with the perforator. Thus, it was possible, in several ossified cochlea cases, to use the double array implant (split electrode), passing two electrode arrays through the direct tunnel.

*Highlights* of the drilling of the direct tunnel are:

1. *Direction:* From the uppermost point of the superio-posterior canal wall to the cochleostomy. This oblique direction is very important for two reasons: (a) to create a tunnel almost parallel to the long process of the incus, approaching the basal turn of the cochlea at a very closed angle, and (b) it moves the line of the drilling higher from the point of exit of the chorda tympani increasing safety for this nerve.
2. *Depth of drilling:* Mst superficially, preserving 0.5 mm of thickness of the cortex. This is achieved by the special perforator and makes the cover of the canal eggshell thick, which is almost transparent. This superficial drilling combined with the width of the tunnel (1.4 mm) makes the total depth of the drilling less than 2 mm, meaning that the tunnel is drilled through the thickness of the canal bone. This is very important for the safety of the facial nerve, since is embryologically impossible and there has never been reported any irregularity where the nerve is growing into the canal wall.
3. In case there is any dehiscence of the bony cover of the tunnel, this can be closed with bone dust.
4. The existence of a sufficient space for a safe drilling of the direct tunnel can always be predicted preoperatively on the HRCT scans [2]. This, in combination with the inspection of the middle ear and facial nerve anatomy during operation, could rule out any facial nerve irregularities, preventing the application of this technique in such cases. In our series we did not come across any such cases.

**Step 6a: Cochleostomy**

We continue the drilling of the cochleostomy on the marked point that we did previously, through the canal with a 1-mm diamond burr, drilling exactly over the anterior rim of the round window niche, creating a 1.2-mm opening of the scala tympani. After the opening has been created, the outer posterior rim is drilled out and then by drilling from inside out, the inner anterior rim is removed. In this way the created tunnel of the cochleostomy has an oblique direction from posterio-superior to anterio-inferior, facilitating the insertion of the electrode into the scala tympani without pressing on the modiolus.

Highlights for the cochleostomy are: (1) Drilling is done with a low speed, in a smooth circular motion of the burr, trying rather to skeletonize (blue lining) the scala tympani before entering it, than perforating it directly by direct drilling. (2) Care is taken so that an outflow of perilymph is possible (patient's head down). The flow of the perilymph prevents the bone dust to enter in the scala tympani (may cause ossification), and the air bubbles (affects the impedance of the electrodes making early fitting difficult) and also prevents contamination. (3) After opening the scala tympani the trimming of the rim is done by inside-out drilling. The timing of the cochleostomy may change according to the preference of the surgeon and may be done initially when handling questionable cases, regarding patency of the cochlea. In that case there is early identification of the degree of difficulty, permitting proper planning of the procedure. In cases where the choice is quitting the procedure, the surgical trauma and time would be minimal.

**Step 6b**

*Round window* opening may be used alternatively. In that case the anterior and superior rim of the round window niche is trimmed out until the secondary membrane is visualized. The final opening is done with a Rosen needle at the time of electrode insertion (Fig. 9.13). In case there is any suspicion about the potency of the cochlea from the preoperative CT and MRI study [2], the round window insertion should not be considered an option.

**Step 7: Alignment of the Direct Tunnel to the Cochleostomy**

This step is optional but when done it facilitates the insertion of the electrode into the scala tympani without touching the modiolus at all. It is performed using a 1.2 mm diamond burr with a conically thinned rod (Fig. 9.14). This burr is inserted running into the direct tunnel with a push-pull movement, under irrigation, and polishes the tunnel. After that it is directed to the cochleostomy in an attempt to be

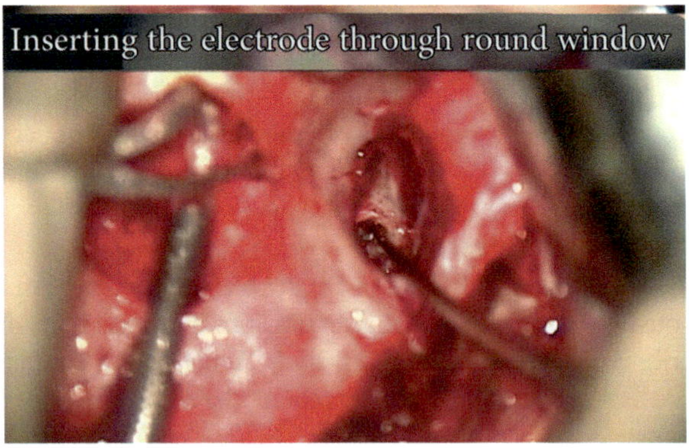


**Fig. 9.13** Puncturing the secondary membrane for insertion of the electrode through round window

inserted into it. Some final polishing of the cochleostomy is sometimes necessary to achieve this.

**Step 8a: Extension of the Incision and Preparing of the Flaps**

When the endaural incision is used, this is extended superio-posteriorly on a curved line without cutting the fascial layer (Fig. 9.15). The skin with the auricle is elevated inferiorly, creating the *inferiorly based skin flap*. A lower incision of the fascial-periosteal layer close to the tip of the mastoid permits the elevation of the fascia-muscle-periosteum superiorly, creating the *superiorly based flap* offering free area for drilling the bed for the implant electronics. From the posterio-superior part of the incision, an elevator is inserted subperiosteally, and a sub-periosteal pocket is created for accepting the coil of the implant.

**Fig. 9.14** Aligning the direct tunnel to cochleostomy

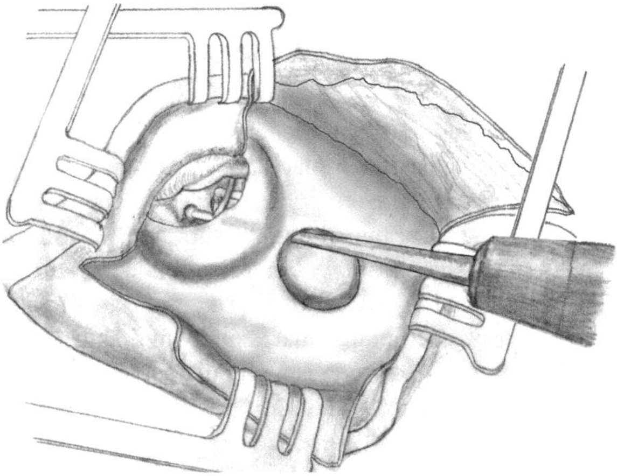

**Fig. 9.15** Endaural incision. Extension superio-posteriorly

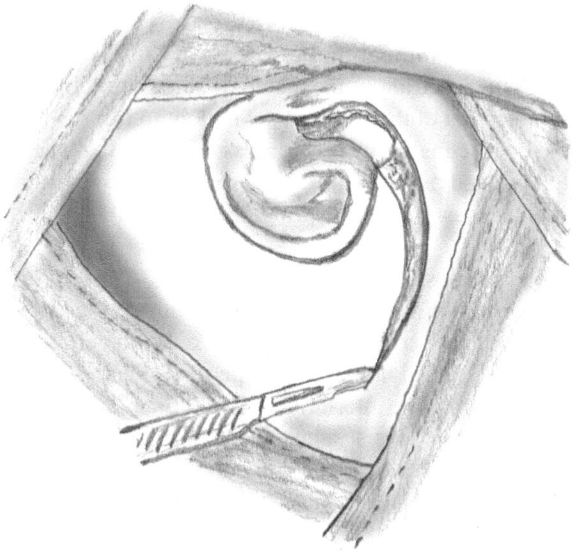

**Step 8b**

*When the postauricular incision* is used, after elevating the superiorly based periosteal flap (the tongue flap as mentioned in the step 2b), an elevator is inserted subperiosteally, and a sub-periosteal pocket is created for accepting the coil of the implant. Then the flap is retracted backwards to allow space for drilling the bed for the implant electronics.

**Step 9: Creating the Bed and Fixing Device**

The drilling of the device bed is done at a distance from the canal to leave sufficient space for the speech processor. A grove is drilled from the lower point of the bed towards the suprameatal hollow. At the very last few millimeters, the grove may become a closed tunnel. In this connecting grove and tunnel will run the active electrode of the device, entering the suprameatal hollow and from there into the direct tunnel, to be inserted into the cochlea. The device is fixed in place with 3-0 Vicryl or Prolene tie-down suture, passed through several holes drilled around the implant bed. Any other way of fixation may be used, even a tight periosteal pocket only.

**Step 10: Insertion of the Electrodes**

After fixing the device in place, the reference electrode, if available, is placed subperiosteally under the temporal muscle. The active electrode is passed through the connecting grove or tunnel into the suprameatal hollow and advanced into the direct tunnel. By pushing from within the suprameatal hollow the electrode is advanced in the direct tunnel and from there it is inserted straight into the cochleostomy or the round window membrane (that is punctured with a needle) and into the basal turn of the cochlea. The electrode is manipulated very gently, initially with the fingers and then using the special claw and the specially designed safety electrode forceps (Fig. 9.3), which can be used in cases where manipulation of the electrode within the middle ear is required. The cochleostomy or the round window opening is sealed with a piece of connective tissue pushed around the electrode.

**Step 11: Manipulating the Excess of the Electrode**

After the insertion of the electrode into the cochlea has been completed, its excess is pulled out of the suprameatal hollow so that the first part after the device lies into the connecting grove. The excess then is rolled very gently with a soft anatomical forceps and pushed with a finger under the overhang into the hollow. It stays there spontaneously fixed by springing (Fig. 9.16).

**Step 12: Closing**

*Endaural Incision:* First the tympanomeatal flap is put back in place very precisely and the inner part of the canal is packed with gel-foam soaked in antibiotic. Then the superiorly based fascia-muscle-periosteal flap is sutured in place with a few stitches of 3-0 Vicryl. The inferiorly based skin-and-auricle flap is then put back in place and sutured in two layers, subcutaneous with 3-0 Vicryl and skin with running suture of 4-0 Prolene. Then we go endaurally and we put the posterior flap of the canal skin in place precisely, and the canal is fully packed with gel-foam. The cavum conchae

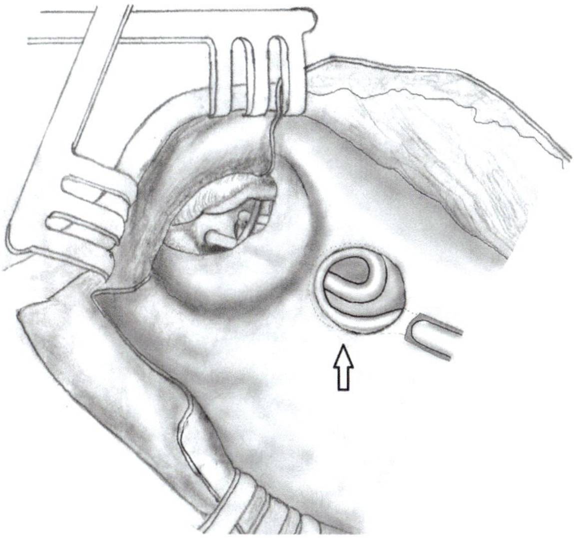

**Fig. 9.16** Accomodation of the excess electrode in the superficial hollow

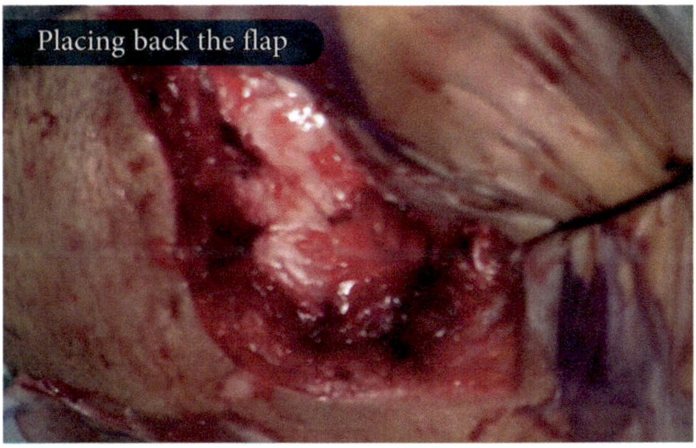


**Fig. 9.17** Tongue flap in place fixing and isolating implant

is packed with an absorbing cotton pad and the head, after the necessary electrophysiologic measurements, is properly bandaged.

*Postauricular Iicision:* First the tongue-like periosteal flap is sutured in place inferiorly and posteriorly isolating the device and the electrodes completely from the skin (Fig. 9.17). Then the postauricular incision is sutured in layers and the canal skin is pushed back to the canal wall and packed with gel-foam. The cavum conchae is packed with an absorbing cotton pad and the head, after the necessary electrophysiologic measurements, is properly bandaged.

*Immediate Switch On:* After the measurements and before the bandaging, an antenna coil with a short cable is put in a glove finger and fixed on the implant coil magnet by a piece of adhesive tape (Fig. 9.18). Then the head is properly bandaged, with the cable extended upwards out of the bandage, and the speech processor is attached to the coil cable (Fig. 9.19). The fitting of the speech processor is defined

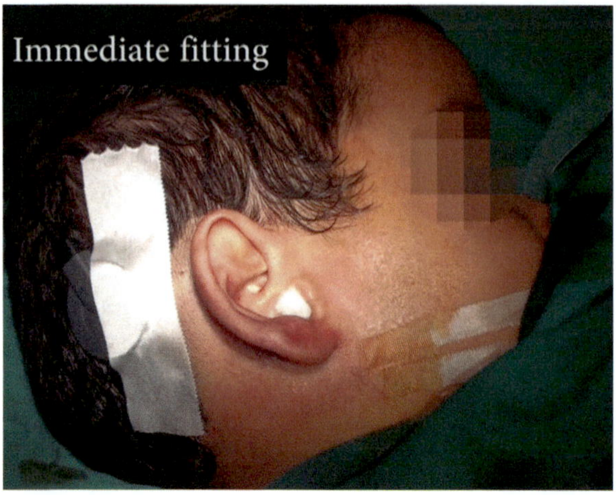


**Fig. 9.18** Antenna coil in place for immediate switch-on

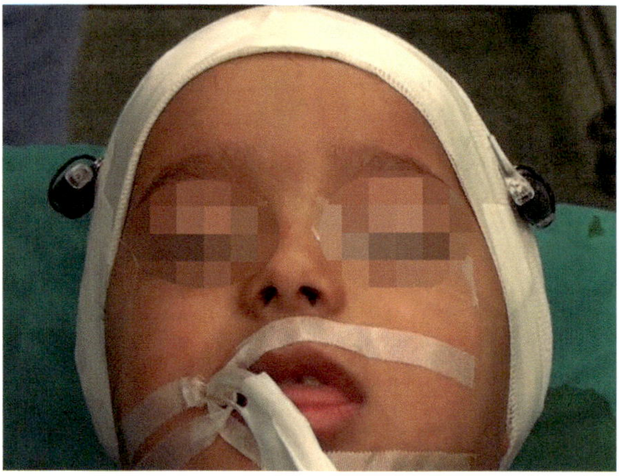

**Fig. 9.19** Speech processors attached and switched-on

by the results of the measurements and some values above and below are given for adaptation.

*Postoperative Situation:* The postoperative situation in the temporal bone is demonstrated in Fig. 9.20a–d. The electrode is running in the direct tunnel, which is very superficial (a). The electrode excess is nicely accommodated in the suprameatal hollow (b). The deep electrode insertion of a Med-El standard electrode is clearly demonstrated, with the first contact at the apex (c). The facial canal is at a safe distance from the direct tunnel (d). The middle ear, the additus and mastoid air-cell system are entirely unaffected from the surgery and they maintain their normal anatomy and function. Not any resection of healthy bone was necessary. No scar tissue and no foreign body material lies in the mastoid. Normal growth of the temporal and mastoid bone is not affected in small children.

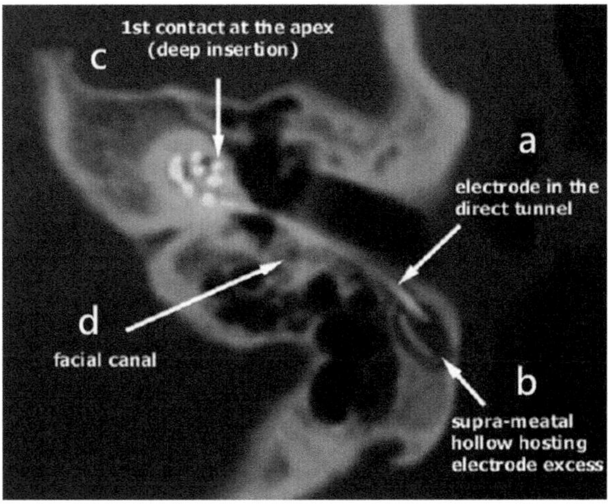


**Fig. 9.20** Post-operative situation. Details in the text

## 9.3 Patients and Results

Greece is a small country with a population about 10 million people. When we started in 1993 with the classic technique of mastoidectomy and posterior tympanotomy, the number of cochlear implantations was small. I started using the newly evolved technique in 1997 and in the period 1997–1998 we presented 24 cases [3], with 16 primary operations, and 8 revisions already, cases which I was invited to revise them abroad. In three of these revision cases, there was a misplaced electrode and five remained unfinished because the electrode could not be inserted, either because of partial obliteration of the cochlea or because the cochlea could not be found during primary operation. All of them were unpublished cases.

From 1999 to 2002, we cooperated with the University Clinic of Thessaloniki (Prof. T. Iliades) and the University Clinic of Munich (Prof. W. Arnold), and in 2002 we presented 101 cases [4, 5], in which we included the initial 24 cases. In this series, 78 cases were primary cases, but the revision cases increased to 23, 18 of which were surgical failures from the classic technique and 5 were device failures. The patients aged 2.5–75 years. From the surgical failures, in 13 cases a misplaced electrode was found, in 5 cases the implantation was not completed. In four of them, the cochlea was not found through the posterior tympanotomy. In one case a major vessel was opened during primary operation, and the middle ear was packed to control bleeding. Of the five device failure cases, two were revisions for broken device (Med-El) due to head trauma. In one case there was an electrode failure in a 10-year-old girl (Med-El) 3 years after implantation, where the electrode was palpable, lying under the postauricular skin and the child liked to play continuously with it by palpating it. Since then, I never leave an electrode free on the surface of the bone, no matter if it is under the periosteum, but I always drill a groove or tunnel, or both, to place it in there. In one case there was a coil failure (Nucleus) due to bending of the device inside a cyst protruding on the head. The contraction from the chronic infection of the fibrous encapsulation, distorted and bent the implant. The formed cyst was suppurated. In one case (Clarion) there was a broken electrode at the point of the junction with the shaft.

We were able to successfully implant or re-implant all the cases of this series, using the Med-EI devices. The follow-up range was from 6 months to 7 years.

***Complications*** In a malformation case (U.C. Munich) the electrode was inserted retrograde in the vestibule and from there into the superior semicircular canal. This case was revised 4 weeks later, and the electrode was properly inserted in the scala tympani. In another case (Veria CI center), there was a thick skin flap, which was corrected 3 months later under local anesthesia. In 5 out of the 13 revisions with the misplaced electrodes (42.7%), the initial device got damaged, and it had to be replaced. The implants were switched on 2–10 days postoperatively and they all functioned well.

In 2001 I moved from Veria General Hospital to the private sector and now I am the head of the Cochlear Implant Center of "Euromedica General Hospital", Thessaloniki, Greece.

In the period 2001–2020 I have performed 356 cochlear implantations on 257 patients, using the Veria technique. The 62.2% were children (158) below 14 years old. It is interesting that the percentage of the children increased year by year. In the first 5 years it was 37.0%, and then it went up to 77.5%. Bilateral implantation had 77 patients, 71 children and 6 adults. The percentage of bilateral implantations in the total cohort was 30.3%, but in the children's cohort the percentage was 48.7%.

Also, the age of the children was reduced. The first 5 years the average age was 3.84 years and then it went down to 2.8 years.

I implanted a variety of cases, normal cochleae, ossified, congenital malformations, and made many revisions correcting failure cases from the classic technique. The results, regarding the major complications, are like the previously mentioned series, and I can summarize them shortly: Not any facial palsy, not any misplaced electrode, not any incomplete or abandoned surgery, not any extrusion, not any suppuration not any flap necrosis. One- or two-days hospitalization, switch-on intraoperatively.

## 9.4 The Impact of the Veria Technique and the Veria Variants

When I did my first trans-meatal cochlear implantation in 1995, I did not feel very comfortable, despite the good result. I had been operating a lady for hours, opening the ear from posteriorly and then anteriorly, producing a lot of trauma. I thought all this was because of my limited experience in the field, though I was an experienced ear surgeon.

It took me some years to realize what exactly I had achieved. I found out that by using the trans-meatal approach I was able to handle puzzled cases. I was doing

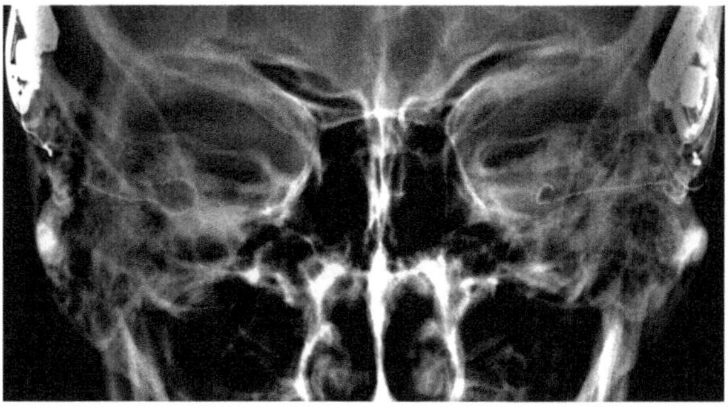

**Fig. 9.21** Congenital malformation operated with the Veria technique

easily multiple cochleostomies in cochlear ossifications, succeeding full insertion in many cases. I was also implanting congenital anomalies like Mondini's and common cavities (Fig. 9.21) through a thars-meatal cochleostomy. All those achievements were transferred by the clinical engineers to their company and soon I started to receive invitations to travel and handle such cases in other hospitals abroad or revise failure cases, most of them unpublished, and some of them failures of very able and famous surgeons.

Then I realized that there was not a problem of the surgeons but a problem of the technique they were using. This was apparent also to many other surgeons.

After my technique was published in 2000 [2], other authors presented similar "trans-canal" or "trans-meatal" cochlear implantations, producing several variants of the Veria technique.

I will mention the first three of them, with whom we cooperated and formed a group and organized many meetings under the auspice of Med-El company, the "International Conferences on Alternative Approaches for Hearing Implants", from 2001 till 2007, which many surgeons attended from all over the world.

1. Prof. Rudolf Häusler from Bern, Switzerland, presented the "Epicanal Technique" [5]. He used the trans-canal approach for the cochleostomy and he drilled a groove on the posterior canal wall where he "buried" the electrode and fixed it with bone cement (Fig. 9.22).
2. Prof. Jona Kronenberg, from Tel Aviv, Israel, presented the "Supra Meatal Approach (SMA)" [6]. He transferred the electrode tunnel at the roof of the canal wall, drilling with free hand, guiding to the Prussak's space. The electrode was inserted in the middle ear from above, between the malleus handle and the long process of the incus and entered the cochleostomy which was performed further anteriorly on the basal turn of the cochlea (Fig. 9.23).
3. Prof. Klaus Boeheim, from Saint Poelten, Austria, presented the "Trans Epitympanic Approach" [7, 8]. He used again the trans-canal approach and made an opening to the epitympanum, drilling through the cribriform plate and above and lateral to the incus to create the pathway for the active electrode, avoiding the use of the special perforator, as well as the criticism of the "blind" technique (Fig. 9.24).

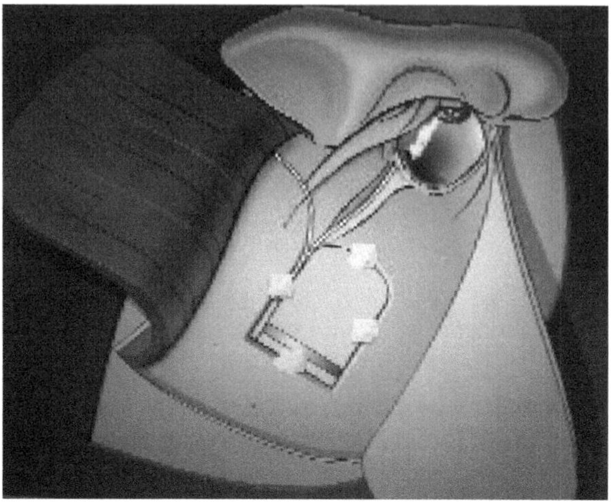

**Fig. 9.22** Pericanal technique by Rudolf Häusler

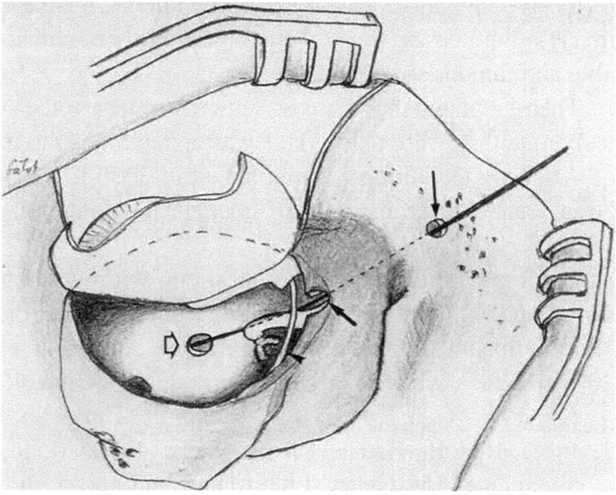

**Fig. 9.23** Suprameatal approach (SMA) by Jona Kronenberg

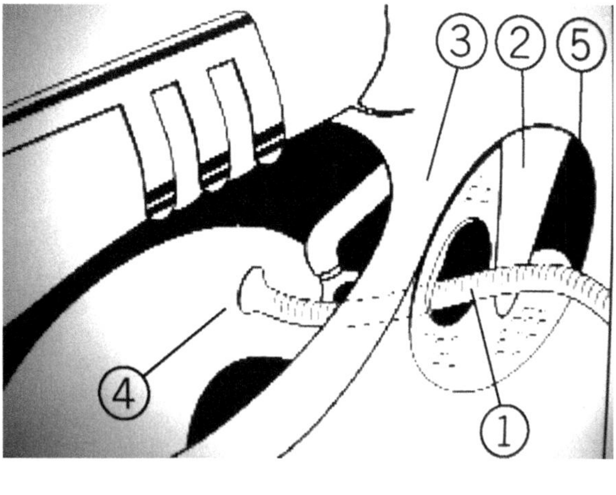


**Fig. 9.24** Trans-epitympanic approach by Klaus Boeheim

I was also invited to several Clinics abroad, besides surgeries, to organize workshops. Apart from the Balkan vicinity and central Europe, I visited many CI centers in Turkey, Russia, the Middle East countries, and Pakistan, and India.

The largest group of Veria surgeons was organized in India, where the Veria technique has become a movement and over 60 surgeons are using the technique, producing publications with large number of cases. Frequently workshops are organized, and newcomers, traditional users of the classic technique, continuously are joining the group. Also, the special Veria perforator was manufactured in India and became available there.

## 9.5 Discussion

In the late 1990s it was the first time after more than two decades, since the mastoidectomy and posterior tympanotomy technique was introduced by William House [1] in cochlear implantations, when someone dared to talk about another technique, better than that. It was the time when the "golden standard" was in doubt.

To tell the historical trough William House was a pioneer in cochlear implantations, and I could say, a patriarch in the field, and not only. He proposed the posterior tympanotomy as the ideal technique for cochlear implantation at that time. The father of posterior tympanotomy, Claus Jansen, introduced the posterior tympanotomy in late 1950s [9] to eradicate cholesteatomas without radical mastoidectomy, using the combined approach tympanoplasty. Claus Jansen's clinic was not related to a University, but he organized in Gummersbach, Germany, yearly workshops of temporal bone to teach the posterior tympanotomy during the 1960s and 1970s (mentioned by Sade [10]).

When William House proposed the posterior tympanotomy for cochlear implantations, all the knowledge about the surgical anatomy of the cochlea, its variabilities in size, position, and relations with the neighboring structures we have today, was missing. Therefore, he could not expect that there would be certain cases for which posterior tympanotomy would not the perfect technique. Furthermore, when House started, certain conditions like small children, residual hearing, ossifications, and malformations, were contraindications for cochlear implantation, which nowadays are not. And posterior tympanotomy, generally nowadays, is not the perfect technique for all those cases, but Intra meatal technique is [2, 11, 12].

Initially my technique was criticized in the meetings as a "blind" one and dangerous for the facial nerve. But the criticism was more theoretical, since those who criticized it, had no personal experience from the technique but only imagination. They were speaking in a religious way, they would not listen scientific evidence. Jona Kronenberg told me in a personal communication that in the year 2001–2002 some magazines rejected his paper with the comment "bad surgery". But by time the results from thousands of cases showed absolutely the opposite.

Prof. J.M. Hans from India reported over 1400 cases with no complications [11].

Recent comparative studies showed that the intra meatal techniques in general are without risks. Moreover, they recognized that "these alternative techniques should be employed when anatomical constraints require nontraditional approaches" [11–13]. Now they are discussing about what I discovered in 1995: that the classic technique was not suitable for all cases.

*What I have always advised to posterior tympanotomy lovers is this: When you are facing any difficulty, or you are in any doubt with your cochlear implant surgery, just switch to the endaural approach and you will solve the problem and complete the operation with success.*

## 9.6 Conclusions

The "Veria technique" for cochlear implantation is a non-mastoidectomy technique using the endomeatal approach for the cochleostomy and the trans-canal wall approach for the electrode. It is an effective tool to improve surgical results in cochlear implantations because it provides certain advantages: (1) It is simple, and the learning curve is fast. (2) It is safe for the facial nerve. (3) It produces minimal trauma and therefore (a) the healing is faster and (b) the hospitalization time and the postoperative complications are reduced. (4) It is a suitable method for difficult cases because it offers a wide visibility and accessibility to the middle ear structures, and therefore it (a) reduces the surgical failures and (b) reduces revision operations and consequently reduces cost (the risk factor for the device to be damaged during revision was 41.7% in our series). (5) It is a suitable method for infants and small children, where the mastoid may not have been yet sufficiently developed, as no mastoidectomy and posterior tympanotomy is needed and furthermore, it leaves the anatomy, the physiology, and the growth of the temporal bone unaffected.

*In conclusion, the Veria technique opened a way for considering that time has come to think of something new and something better in cochlear implant surgery. And the new way is the Veria technique, or any variant using the same approach, the trans-canal approach for cochlear implantation. It is the future.*

And one more comment: competent surgeons should avoid the fear of any criticism by people without experience and use the Veria perforator with confidence. It is the safest way to avoid any complications from the facial nerve.

It proved to be a real facial nerve protector.

## References

1. House WF. Cochlear implants. Ann Otol Rhinol Laryngol. 1976;85(Suppl 27):1–93.
2. Jain R, et al. A clinico-radiological study: Veria technique of cochlear implant—a study of 50 cases. Indian J Otolaryngol Head Neck Surg. https://doi.org/10.1007/s12070-019-01633-x
3. Kiratzidis T. 'Veria operation': Cochlear implantation without a mastoidectomy and a posterior tympanotomy. A new technique. In: Kim CS, Chang SO, Lim D, editors. Updates in cochlear implantation, vol. 115. Basel: Karger; 2000. p. 283–5.
4. Kiratzidis T, Arnold W, Iliades T. Veria operation updated I. The trans-canal wall cochlear implantation. ORL. 2002;64:406–12.

5. Kiratzidis T, Iliades T, Arnold W. Veria operation II. Surgical results from 101 cases. ORL. 2002;64:413–6.
6. Häusler R. Cochlear implantation without mastoidectomy: the pericanal electrode insertion technique. Acta Oto-Laryngologica. 2002;122:715–9.
7. Kronenberg J, Mirigov L, Dagan T. Suprameatal approach: new surgical approach for cochlear implantation. J Laryngol Otol. 2001;115:283–5.
8. Nahler A, Böheim K. „Kombinierter Epitympanaler – Transmeataler Zugang bei Cochleaimplantation" 47. Österreichischer HNO-Kongreß 2003.
9. Jansen C. Colesteatoma in children. 1st International meeting of the Politzer Society, February 1978.
10. Sade J. Remarks on the conception, birth and history of the Politzer Society. Politzer Society Newsletter Issue 4, February 2010.
11. Hans JM, Prasad R. Cochlear implant surgery by the Veria technique: how and why? Experience from 1400 cases. Indian J Otolaryngol Head Neck Surg. 2015;67(2):107–9.
12. Freni F, Gazia F, et al. Endomeatal approach versus posterior tympanotomy. Int J Environ Res Public Health. 2020;17(12)
13. Zeitler DM, Balkany TJ. Alternative approaches to cochlear implantation. Oper Tech Otolaryngol Head Neck Surg. 2010;21(4):248–53.

# Cochlear Implantation Through the Round Window Approach

# 10

Mario Sanna, Anna Lisa Giannuzzi, and Antonio Caruso

## 10.1 Surgical Technique

*Four types of skin incisions* are used (Fig. 10.1) for CI surgery:

- Normal retroauricular incision.
- Wide C-shaped retroauricular incision: it creates a wound over the implant (that is not favorable) but is useful in well-aerated mastoids and subtotal petrosectomy.
- Lazy S incision: it properly covers the receiver-stimulator area.
- Minimal access incision: two incisions are often required (for getting access to the mastoid and middle ear).

The purpose is to avoid the array extrusion creating adequate coverage of the receiver-stimulator.

The skin incision should be situated anterior-inferior to the site of the receiver-stimulator and not crossing it, in order to cover the receiver-stimulator with skin and temporal muscle.

The musculoperiosteal flap must cover the implant and electrode arrays. Some surgeons create alternating flaps in relation to the skin incision, so as to get the best coverage and protection of the implant [1] (Figs. 10.2 and 10.3).

It is not necessary to create a wide mastoidectomy, especially when no pathology is present and it is better to leave an internal rim of cortical bone along the cavity to hold the electrode array. Visualization of the landmarks (horizontal, tympanic part

**Supplementary Information** The online version contains supplementary material available at [https://doi.org/10.1007/978-981-19-0452-3_10].

M. Sanna (✉) · A. L. Giannuzzi · A. Caruso
Otology and Skull Base Unit, Gruppo Otologico Piacenza, Piacenza, Italy
e-mail: mario.sanna@gruppootologico.com


S. DeSaSouza (ed.), *Cochlear Implants*,
https://doi.org/10.1007/978-981-19-0452-3_10

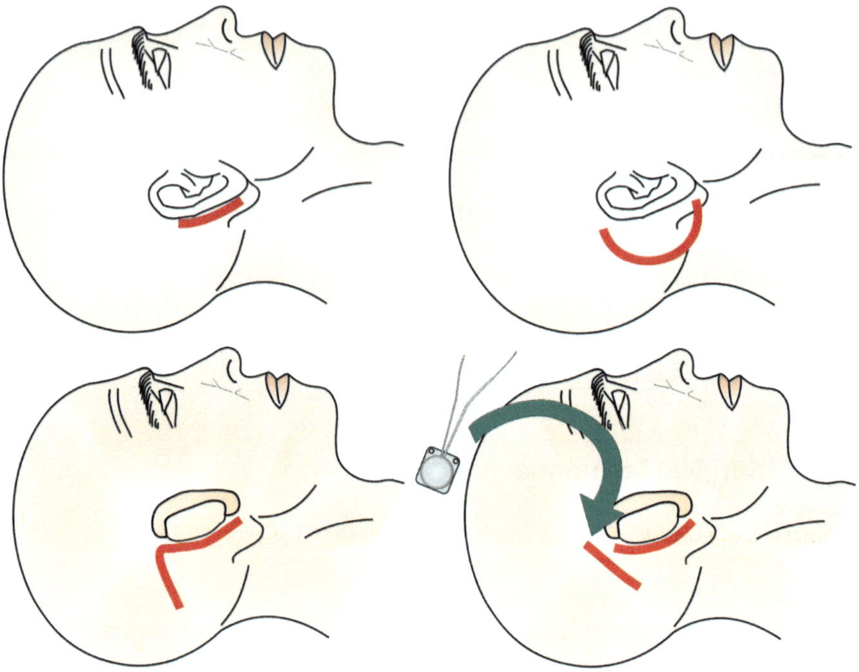

**Fig. 10.1** Skin incisions

**Fig. 10.2** Exposure of mastoid

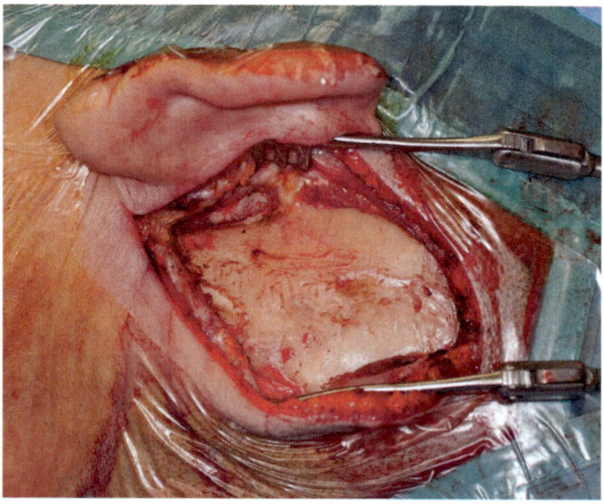

of the facial nerve, the short process of the incus, the lateral semicircular canal, and sometimes also the digastric ridge) helps assessing the position of third segment of the facial nerve and the posterior tympanotomy. The posterior tympanotomy should be wide enough to expose the cochlea and round window niche.

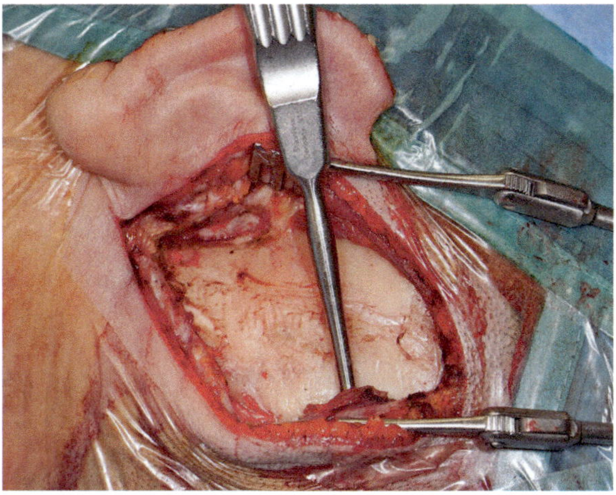

**Fig. 10.3** A pocket for the implant

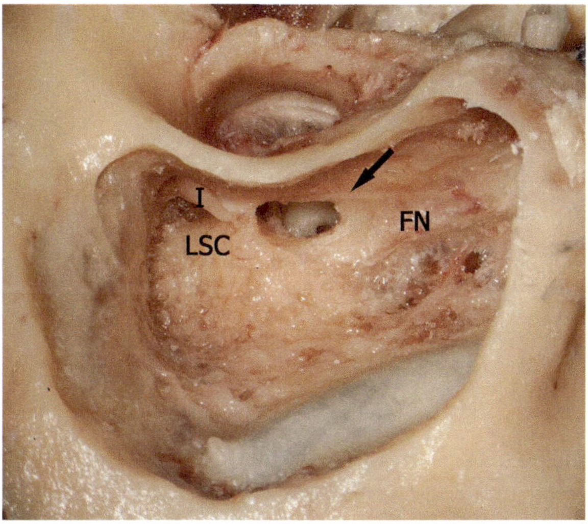


**Fig. 10.4** The posterior tympanotomy. *FN* facial nerve, *I* incus, *LSC* lateral semicircular canal, *arrow* chorda tympani

The tympanic annulus is lateral to the chorda tympani (Fig. 10.4), therefore, during drilling anteriorly and laterally, care must be taken not to damage it. In order to protect the short process of the incus, the buttress can be left.

The round window niche can be more or less visible through the posterior tympanotomy or hidden by a superior extension of the pneumatization of the hypotympanum (Fig. 10.5).

The round window niche is usually covered by a bony lip superiorly and a bony lip inferiorly. Moreover, a pseudomembrane can be present and cover the niche. The two bony lips need to be removed to visualize properly the round window. In particular, the superior overhang should be removed to enable the surgeon to reach the scala tympani at the correct axial line for insertion that is from a posterior-superior toward anterior-inferior direction (Figs. 10.6, 10.7, and 10.8).

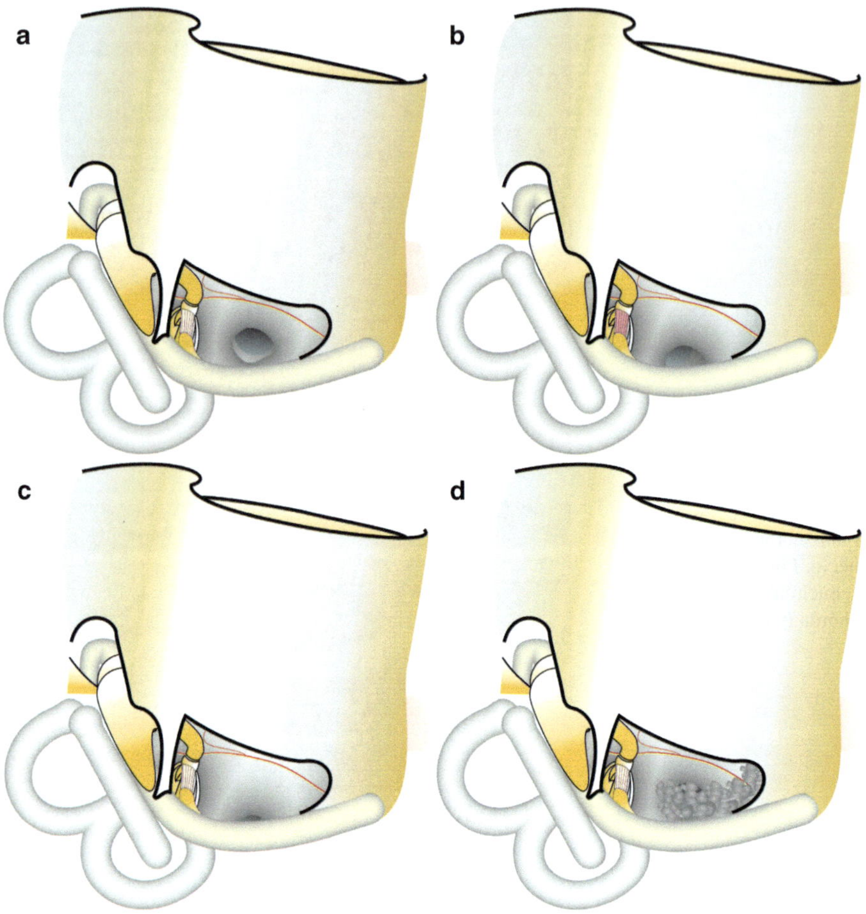

**Fig. 10.5** Different degrees of visibility of the round window niche (**a**, **b**, **c**) and superior extension of hypotympanic pneumatization (**d**)

Drilling the bony lips increases visibility and enlarges the access to the round window, with a correct angle of insertion [2, 3].

For some implants, a receiver-stimulator bed has to be drilled out (Fig. 10.9), while others require to be fixated with screws (Fig. 10.10).

Fixation of the implant is advisable because in case of MRI the execution of the examination is safer.

We create two small bony canals, superior and inferior of the receiver bed and use a non-resorbable tie-down suture for fixation of the implant. In children, the skull is thinner and instead of bony canals, we tight suturing of the temporal muscle over the implant. Moreover, the implant can be fixated by drilling a canal from the receiver to the mastoid cavity for the arrays, both fixing the implant and protecting the most vulnerable part of the electrode.

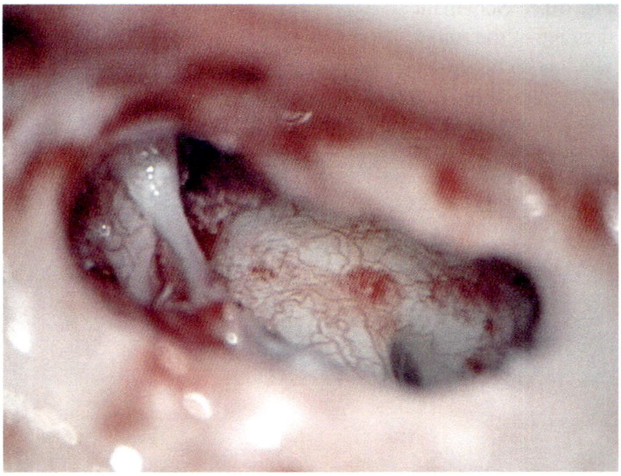

**Fig. 10.6** The round window niche with superior bony lip still present

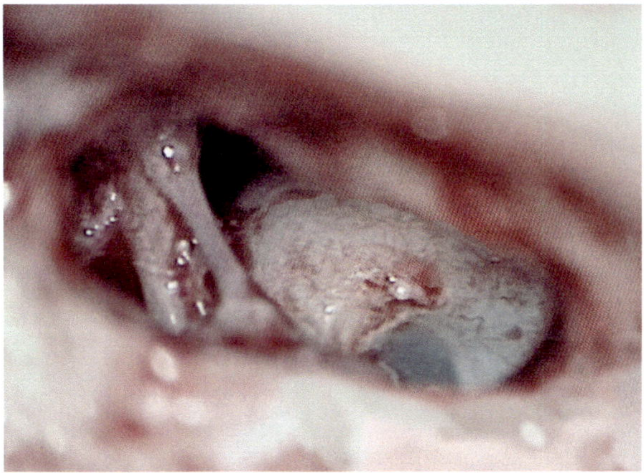

**Fig. 10.7** Round window view

The array should be inserted slowly avoiding intracochlear trauma or misplacement.

In case of precurved implant, an "advanced-off stylet" technique should be used: insertion of the first part of the array while the last part is gently pushed off the stylet, while the stylet is kept in a stable position.

In case of resistance, the array should be drawn back slightly, and the procedure has to be repeated.

The round window insertion has several significant advantages if compared to the standard cochleostomy because the round window directly leads into the scala tympani. Using the RWI we avoid to drill into the cochlea preventing that bone powder enters the scala tympani [4]. Moreover, with this technique, the basilar membrane is longer of 2 mm for electrode stimulation. We can use the secondary membrane for a better sealing around the electrodes; thus, the incidence of postoperative labyrinthitis and perilymph fistula might be reduced [3].

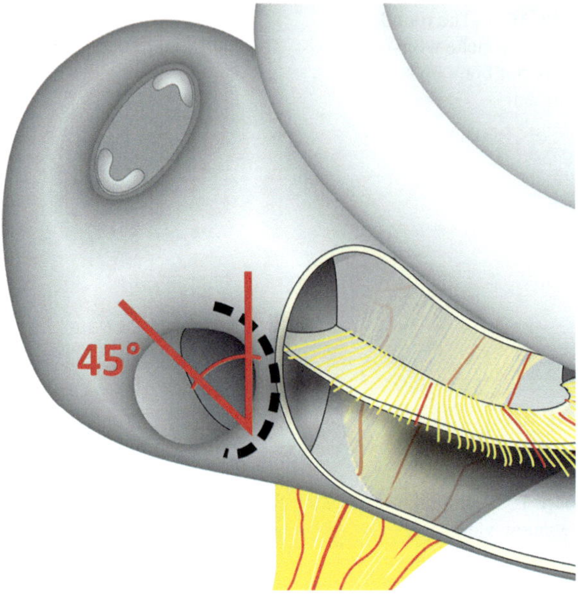


**Fig. 10.8** Schematic drawing of the round window niche showing the angulation of the round window membrane

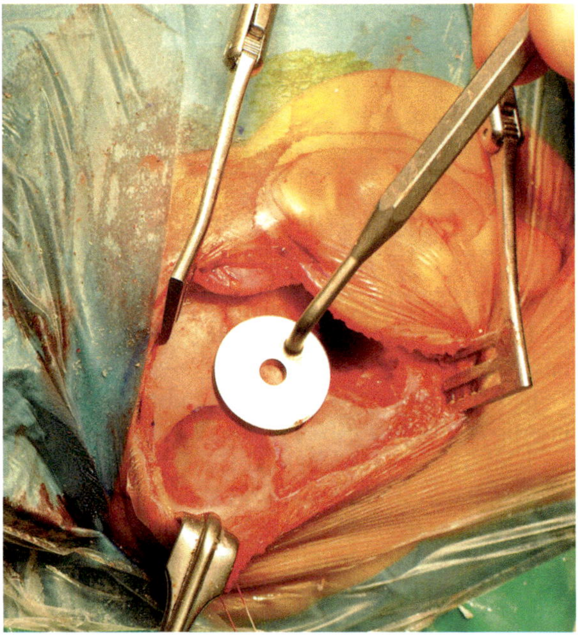

**Fig. 10.9** Receiver bony bed for the Advanced Bionics device

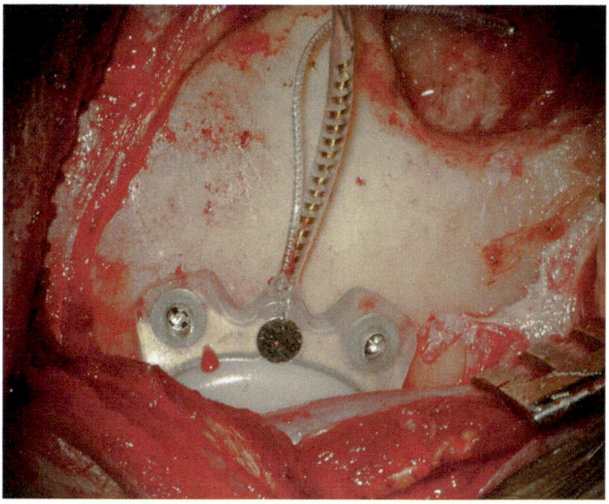

**Fig. 10.10** Fixation of the Oticon implant with screw

Some surgeons choose the cochleostomy, especially when the round window niche is posterior and difficult to be visualized. In our opinion, through a wide posterior tympanotomy, is always possible to reach the niche.

## References


1. Adunka OF, Pillsbury HC, Buchman CA. Minimizing intracochlear trauma during cochlear implantation. Adv Otorhinolaryngol. 2010;67:96–107. https://doi.org/10.1159/000262601. Epub 2009.
2. Briggs RJ, Tykocinski M, Xu J, et al. Comparison of round window and cochleostmy approaches with a prototype hearing preservation electrode. Audiol Neurotol. 2006;11(Suppl 1):42–8.
3. Roland SP, Wright CG, Isaacson B. Cochlear implant electrode insertion: the round window revisited. Laryngoscope. 2007;117:1397–401.
4. Pau HW, Just T, Bornitz M, et al. Noise exposure of the inner ear during drilling a cochleostomy for the cochlear implantation. Laryngoscope. 2007;117:535–40.


## *Suggested Reading*


Mcrackan TR, Bauschard M, Hatch JL, et al. Meta-analysis of quality-of-life improvement after cochlear implantation and associations with speech recognition abilities. Laryngoscope. 2018;128:982–90.

Jiam NT, Jiradejvong P, Pearl MS, et al. The effect of round window vs cochleostomy surgical approaches on cochlear implant electrode position: a flat-panel computed tomography study. JAMA Otolaryngol Head Neck Surg. 2016;1142:873–80.

# Classification and Management of Inner Ear Malformations

11

Levent Sennaroglu

## 11.1 Introduction

Inner ear malformations (IEM) represent approximately 20% of congenital hearing loss cases based on radiology [1, 2]. Majority of these patients have bilateral severe to profound hearing loss and are candidates for cochlear implantation. Those cases with severe malformations may require modifications during the surgical approach for implant placement. Decision-making between cochlear implantation (CI) and auditory brainstem implantation (ABI) may also be challenging in some cases of IEMs.

There are certain challenges in the management of IEMs:

- Choosing the correct implantation method; CI vs. ABI
- Cerebrospinal fluid gusher and risk for meningitis
- Facial nerve anomalies
- Choosing the right surgical approach and the type of electrode
- Timing of surgery

Classification of IEMs is based on differences in cochlear anatomy in various malformations. With this classification, cochlear anomalies with similar appearance are grouped together. They demonstrate similar clinical findings and treatment options. This may not represent the functional outcome with CI, which is closely related to the situation of the cochlear nerve. If there is cochlear nerve deficiency, this will have a negative influence on the audiological and speech and language developmental after implantation. Therefore, during preoperative decision-making for choosing the method of implantation, three factors should be considered: classification of IEMs, situation of the cochlear nerve and preoperative audiological

L. Sennaroglu (✉)
Department of Otolaryngology, Hacettepe University, Ankara, Turkey



S. DeSaSouza (ed.), *Cochlear Implants*,
https://doi.org/10.1007/978-981-19-0452-3_11

findings. Only in this way, a clinician may have a better estimate of the audiological outcome in a given IEM. This is very important during preoperative counseling of the family.

ABI can be used in children with severe IEMs. Patients with incomplete partition type II and III and large vestibular aqueduct almost always have cochlear and cochlear nerve development and therefore, ABI is not indicated in their (re)habilitation. In the consensus paper, Sennaroglu et al. [3] divided the ABI indications in IEMs into two groups:

A. *Definite Indications:*
   1. Complete labyrinthine aplasia (Michel aplasia)
   2. Rudimentary Otocyst
   3. Cochlear aplasia
   4. Cochlear nerve aplasia
   5. Cochlear aperture aplasia

B. *Probable Indications:*
   1. Hypoplastic cochlea with hypoplastic cochlear aperture
   2. Common cavity and incomplete partition type I cases where cochlear nerve is apparently missing.
   3. Common cavity and incomplete partition type I cases if the cochlear nerve is present: even if the nerve is present, the distribution of the neural tissue in the abnormal cochlea is unpredictable, and ABI may be indicated in such cases if CI fails to elicit an auditory sensation.
   4. The presence of an unbranched cochleovestibular nerve (CVN) is a challenge in these cases. In this situation, it is not possible to determine the amount of cochlear fibers traveling in the CVN. If there is a suspicion, a cochlear implant can be used in the first instance, and ABI can be reserved for the patients in whom there is insufficient progress with CI.
   5. The hypoplastic cochlear nerve: the cochlear nerve is less than 50% of the usual size of the cochlear nerve or less than the diameter of the facial nerve. Radiology of these patients should be carefully reviewed with an experienced neuroradiologist. If sufficient amount of neural tissue cannot be followed into the cochlear space, an ABI may be indicated.

In this chapter, characteristics of individual malformations together with treatment options are presented.

## 11.2 Inner Ear Malformations

According to present literature [4, 5], IEMs are classified into eight distinct groups:

**1. Complete Labyrinthine Aplasia (Michel Deformity)**

Complete Labyrinthine aplasia (CLA) is the absence of the cochlea, vestibule, semicircular canals, vestibular and cochlear aqueducts (Fig. 11.1). Middle ear

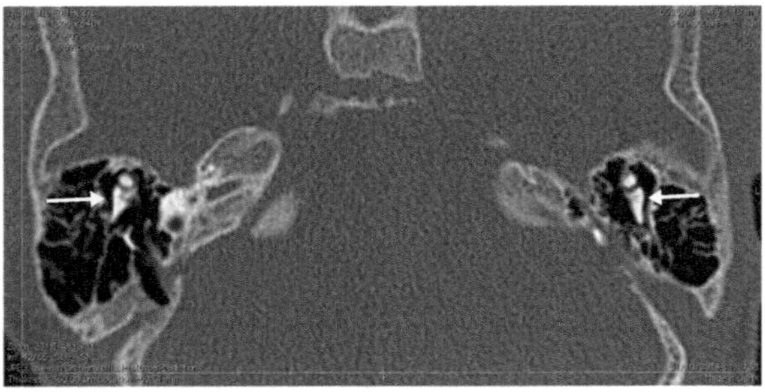

**Fig. 11.1** Complete Labyrinthine aplasia, where cochlea, vestibule, semicircular canals, vestibular and cochlear aqueducts are absent. Middle ear ossicles are present on both sides (white arrows)

ossicles are present in spite of severe inner ear developmental abnormality. The petrous bone may be hypoplastic, whereas the otic capsule may be hypoplastic or aplastic [4, 6]. In the majority of patients, the internal auditory canal (IAC) consists only of the facial canal, and the labyrinthine, tympanic and mastoid segments of the facial nerve can be identified in the temporal bone. In some patients, however, it may not be possible to observe the facial canal in the temporal bone in spite of normal facial functions.

According to radiological findings [4], three subgroups of CLA are present:

(a) *CLA with Hypoplastic or Aplastic Petrous Bone*

Petrous bone is hypoplastic or aplastic in this subgroup of CLA. Middle ear may be located adjacent to posterior fossa.

(b) *CLA Without Otic Capsule*

Here the development of the petrous bone is normal, but the otic capsule is hypoplastic or aplastic.

(c) *CLA with Otic Capsule*

In this subgroup of CLA, the development of the petrous bone and the otic capsule is normal. Labyrinthine segment of the facial canal can be seen in its normal location. This finding demonstrates that otic capsule formation is essential for the facial canal to obtain its normal position.

**Audiological Findings**

Audiological examination reveals no response at all. It is also possible to have profound sensorineural hearing loss (SNHL) at 125, 250 and 500 Hz at the upper limits of the audiometer. The latter finding demonstrates it has to be interpreted as a vibrotactile sensation rather than true hearing. This finding can also be observed in cases with a rudimentary otocyst and cochlear aplasia.

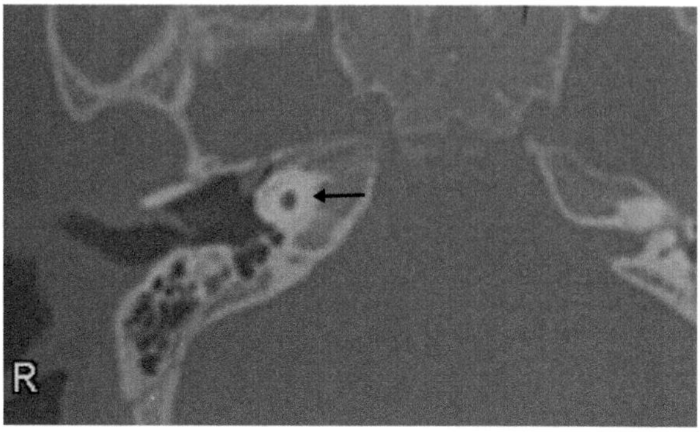


**Fig. 11.2** A rudimentary otocyst with incomplete millimetric representations of the otic capsule (round or ovoid in shape) without an IAC (black arrow)

**Management**

As there is no inner ear development, cochlear implant (CI) surgery is not possible in these children. Auditory brainstem implantation (ABI) is the only surgical option for hearing habilitation, as discussed in the first Consensus Meeting on ABI in Children [3].

2. **Rudimentary Otocyst**

A rudimentary otocyst is added to the classification in 2013, and it is defined as incomplete millimetric representations of the otic capsule (round or ovoid in shape) without an IAC (Fig. 11.2). Parts of the semicircular canals may accompany rudimentary otocyst. This anomaly is between a CLA and common cavity. In CLA (Michel deformity), there is no inner ear development, while in common cavity (CC), there is an ovoid or round cystic space instead of a separate cochlea and vestibule. The CC communicates with the brainstem via the nerves in the IAC. The rudimentary otocyst is a few millimeters in size without the formation of an IAC.

**Audiological Findings**

Findings are similar to CLA and in general there is no response at all. It is also possible to have profound loss on low frequency as a result of vibrotactile stimulation.

**Management**

Rudimentary otocyst has no connection with the brainstem. In addition, it is too small to have meaningful cochlear fibers inside. Therefore, it is a contraindication to CI surgery. Rudimentary otocyst is also a definite indication for ABI.

3. **Cochlear Aplasia**

Cochlear aplasia is described as the absence of the cochlea. Vestibule and semicircular canals are in their normal anatomic location; at the posterolateral part of IAC. The accompanying vestibular system may be normal or it may have an enlarged vestibule [7]. The labyrinthine segment of the facial nerve is anteriorly displaced and usually occupies the normal location of the cochlea (Fig. 11.3).

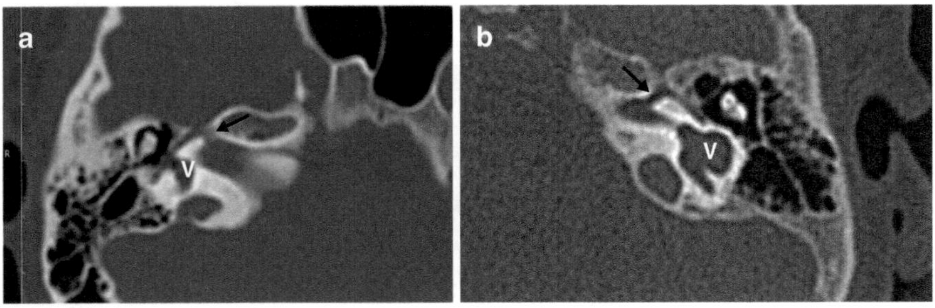


**Fig. 11.3** (**a**) Cochlear aplasia with normal labyrinth. Vestibule (V) and semicircular canals are normally developed and located. Labyrinthine segment of the facial nerve is anteriorly dislocated to the usual location of the cochlea (black arrow). (**b**) Cochlear aplasia with a dilated vestibule. IAC is located in its usual position, and the dilated vestibule is at the posterior lateral part of IAC

There are two subgroups according to accompanying vestibular system:

(a) *Cochlear Aplasia with Normal Labyrinth* (Fig. 11.3a): vestibule and semicircular canals are normally developed.
(b) *Cochlear Aplasia with a Dilated Vestibule (CADV)* (Fig. 11.3b): vestibule and semicircular canals show dilatation. It is very important to differentiate CADV from a common cavity (CC) deformity. In CADV, IAC is normally developed, and dilated vestibule occupies normal location at the posterolateral part of the fundus. In CC, however, IAC is usually posteriorly directed and opens into the center of CC. In CC cochlear implantation can be done if hearing response is obtained during audiological evaluation and if cochleovestibular nerve (CVN) is present. *In CADV, CI surgery is contraindicated.* However, in some patients, it may be very difficult to distinguish between CADV and CC. As in every CI candidate, during preoperative evaluation for implantation, audiological findings should be considered in choosing the right method of implantation.

Cochlear aplasia with normal labyrinth is usually symmetric. Similar appearance is present in different individuals, suggesting a genetic etiology. In CADV, however, asymmetric development may be present; pathology may be due to genetic or environmental factors.

**Audiological Findings**

As mentioned in previous anomalies, they usually have no response in audiological evaluation. They may also demonstrate profound hearing loss on low frequency, which should be accepted as vibrotactile stimulation.

**Management**

As there is no cochlea, CA is a definite indication for ABI [3].

**4. Common Cavity**

A common cavity (CC) is defined as a single chamber (ovoid or round in shape) representing the cochlea and vestibule (Fig. 11.4). Theoretically, this structure has

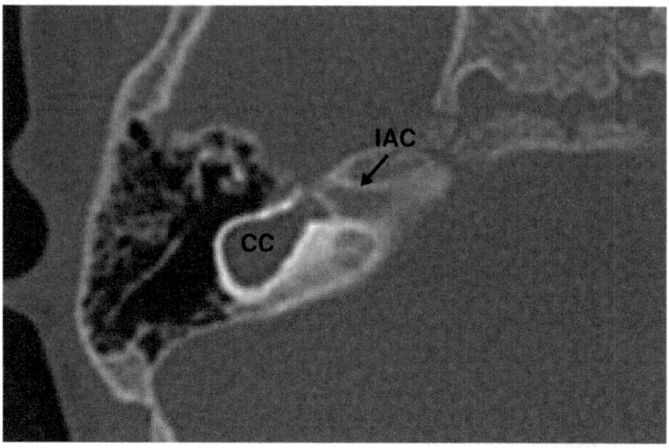


**Fig. 11.4** A common cavity (CC) consisting of a single ovoid chamber representing the cochlea and vestibule. IAC comes and opens into the center of CC (Black arrow)

cochlear and vestibular neural structures. There may be accompanying semicircular canals (SCC) or their rudimentary parts. IAC usually enters the cavity at its center. Cases with vestibular dilatation are occasionally termed as "vestibular common cavity;" however, this is not a correct term.

It is very important to differentiate common cavity from cochlear aplasia with dilated vestibule [1]. *Cochlear aplasia with dilated vestibule* (CADV) (Fig. 11.3b) has a dilated vestibule and semicircular canals at the posterolateral part of the IAC fundus, which is their usual location. External outline resembles the normal labyrinth. The enlarged vestibule is at its expected location. The accompanying SCCs may be enlarged or normal. A *common cavity (CC)* (Fig. 11.4), on the other hand, is an ovoid or round structure. SCCs or their rudimentary parts may accompany a CC. The IAC usually enters the cavity at its center. The location of a CC may be anterior but usually posterior to the normal location of the labyrinth. It is very important to differentiate these malformations from each other, because cochlear implantation in a CC may result in acoustic stimulation, whereas in CAVD, no functional stimulation will occur with CI. In spite of this, it may sometimes be difficult to differentiate between the two malformations.

The nerve entering the CC is common cochleovestibular nerve (CVN). It contains cochlear and vestibular nerve fibers, however, with the present radiological investigations, it is not possible to determine the percentage of cochlear fibers within the CVN. CVN has to be demonstrated by 3 Tesla MRI in candidates undergoing evaluation for CI candidacy. Audiological evaluation is very important to determine if hearing is present in CC, which indirectly gives an estimate of the cochlear fibers within the CVN. If a behavioral audiometric response or language development is present with hearing aid use, it can be assumed that a meaningful population of cochlear fibers exists and the patient may benefit from a CI. If the CVN cannot be demonstrated with MRI or there is a narrow or long IAC, where the presence of cochlear fibers is questionable, an ABI may be a better option. As the postoperative hearing cannot be accurately predicted before CI surgery, it is advisable to counsel the family that contralateral ABI may be necessary in case of limited language development with CI. In the first consensus meeting, these cases are grouped as "Possible Indications for an ABI" [3]. This decision should be done as early as possible.

**Audiological Findings**
These patients usually have profound hearing loss.

**Management**

- *Transmastoid Labyrinthotomy*: It is described by McElveen [8]. It is advisable to use a straight (non-modiolar hugging) electrode. This will have a position on the periphery of the CC with better contact with the neural tissue. A precurved electrode will stay in the center of the cavity and have the contacts located medially and may not stimulate the periphery of the CC efficiently. As a result, it is not advisable to use a precurved electrode in CC. As the size of common cavity shows variation, it is important to estimate the length of the electrode before surgery. The length of the electrode can be calculated using the formula $2\pi r$, where r is the radius of CC [1].
- *Double Labyrinthotomy*: It is described by Beltrame et al. [9]. Two labyrinthotomy openings are created in the area of lateral semicircular canal, separated by 3–4 mm. The tip of the electrode is caught in the second hole. In this way, the tip of the electrode is prevented from going into IAC. They also described a special electrode for common cavity. This electrode has an inactive tip that is caught by a hook through another hole. The terminal nonactive part of the electrode array ends with a small ball, which is needed to hook the electrode array. This nonactive part of the implant is pushed into the superior labyrinthotomy until it is seen and hooked using a 0.5 mm hook through the inferior labyrinthotomy. Then the two arms are advanced together to position the array along the inner wall of the cavity through the inferior labyrinthotomy.
- If hearing and language development is insufficient with CI use, ABI is indicated on the contralateral side (possible ABI indication). This will allow bilateral stimulation.
- If CVN is absent or no IAC is present, ABI is the only option in the first place.
- Patients with CC require bilateral implantation. If CVN is present on both sides, bilateral CI is the preferred method of implantation.
- In case of asymmetric development, patients with CC obtain the best outcome with bimodal stimulation of CI and ABI in our patient series [10]. CI is applied to the side with better-developed CVN and better audiological response; ABI is used in the side with hypoplastic CVN without any behavioral response during audiological evaluation with insert earphones.

**Cochlear Hypoplasia and Incomplete Partitions**
These are more developed groups of IEMs; there is a clear differentiation into a cochlea and vestibule. Cochlear hypoplasia is the group where the size of the cochlea is less than normal. Incomplete partition is the largest group of IEMs where the cochlear size is similar to normal.

## 5. Cochlear Hypoplasia

In this deformity, there is a clear differentiation between cochlea and vestibule. In cochlear hypoplasia (CH) external dimensions are less than those of a normal cochlea with various internal architecture deformities. In smaller cochlea, it is usually difficult to count the number of turns with CT and/or MRI. But the definition "cochlea with 1.5 turns" should be used for hypoplasia (particularly type III), rather than for IP-II cochlea. Measurements are very important for differentiating CH-III from normal cochlea and CH-II from IP-I and our recent study shows that this can be done very easily by measuring the length of the basal turn of the cochlea [11]. If the length of the basal turn is less than 7.5 mm, the cochlea is classified as hypoplastic. The only exception is CH-IV, which has a normal basal turn but can easily identified by hypoplastic middle and apical turns. Four different types of cochlear hypoplasia have been defined [4].

**Types of cochlear hypoplasia**

(a) *CH-I (Bud-Like Cochlea)*: The cochlea is like a small bud, round or ovoid in shape, arising from the IAC (Fig. 11.5a). Internal architecture is severely deformed; no modiolus or interscalar septa can be identified.

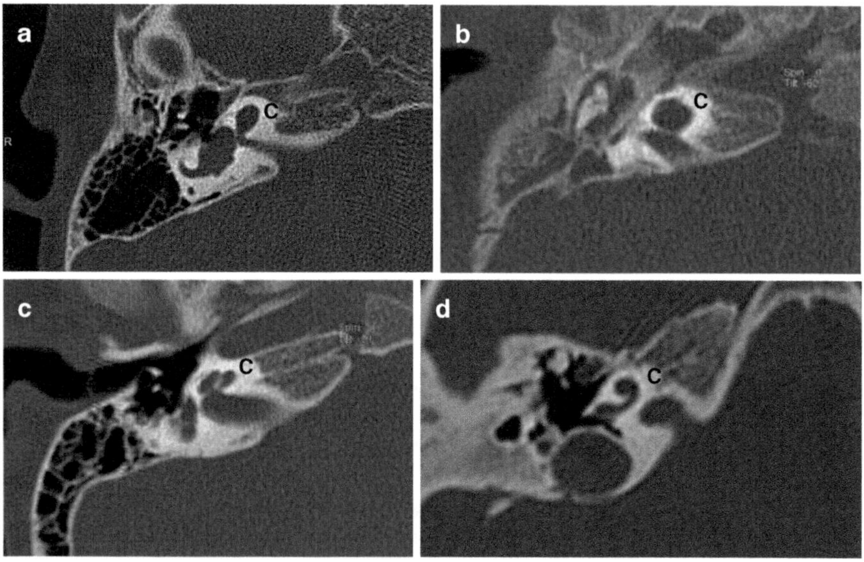


**Fig. 11.5** (**a**) CH-I (Bud-like cochlea): Ovoid shaped bud-like cochlea (C) arising from the IAC. (**b**) CH-II (Cystic hypoplastic cochlea): Small cystic cochlea (C) with defective modiolus and interscalar septa. (**c**) CH-III (Cochlea with less than two turns): The cochlea (C) has a short modiolus (black arrow) and the overall length of the interscalar septa is reduced, resulting in fewer turns. (**d**) CH-IV (Cochlea with hypoplastic middle and apical turns): Cochlea (C) with basal turn, which is nearly normal in size and appearance, however, the middle and apical turns are severely hypoplastic

(b) *CH-II (Cystic Hypoplastic Cochlea):* Small cochlea has defective modiolus and interscalar septa, but its external architecture is similar to normal cochlea (Fig. 11.5b). Fundus may be defective, resulting in a connection between cochlea and the IAC. As a result, gusher and unintentional entry of the CI electrode into IAC is possible. The vestibular aqueduct may be enlarged, and the vestibule may be dilated.
(c) *CH-III (Cochlea with Less Than Two Turns):* The cochlea has a short modiolus and the overall length of the interscalar septa is reduced, resulting in fewer turns (i.e., less than two turns). The internal (modiolus, interscalar septa) and external architecture are similar to that of a normal cochlea, but the dimensions are smaller and number of turns are fewer (Fig. 11.5c). The vestibule is usually hypoplastic. Semicircular canals are hypoplastic or aplastic. The cochlear aperture may be hypoplastic or aplastic.
(d) *CH-IV (Cochlea with Hypoplastic Middle and Apical Turns)*: Basal turn is nearly normal in size and appearance; however, the middle and apical turns are severely hypoplastic and located anterior and medially rather than in their normal central position (Fig. 11.5d). The labyrinthine segment of the facial nerve is characteristically located anterior-superior to the cochlea rather than in its usual location [12].

**Audiological Findings**

There is no characteristic audiological configuration in CH. Patients will present with a range of thresholds on audiometric testing. Decision-making about the best habilitation options may be difficult, particularly in patients with a hypoplastic cochlear nerve. Patients with mild to moderate hearing loss can be habilitated with hearing aids and have near normal to normal language development. The majority of cochlear hypoplasia patients have severe to profound hearing loss where a CI would be a reasonable option, if they have a cochlear nerve.

Some patients have cochlear aperture aplasia with cochlear nerve aplasia and thus, an ABI would be the best hearing habilitative option. Other patients with cochlear hypoplasia have hypoplastic cochlear nerves. The best option in these cases is to use CI in the side with response during audiological evaluation with insert earphones or the side that is more suitable to CI surgery. If there is limited hearing and language development, an ABI should be considered for the contralateral side.

Facial nerve abnormality is most frequently seen in cochlear hypoplasia [13]. The tympanic segment may be inferiorly dislocated lying on the oval window or promontory. This is usually due to associated semicircular abnormalities. This may cause difficulty during cochlear implantation and it is suggested to evaluate axial and coronal CT scans carefully before surgery in regard to facial nerve anomaly in patients with cochlear hypoplasia. In addition, facial nerve stimulator must be used during CI surgery in all cases of cochlear hypoplasia.

Some cases of hypoplasia (particularly hypoplasia type IV) may have mixed hearing loss in which the conductive component is due to stapedial fixation.

**Management**

(a) *Stapedotomy*: Cases with conductive or mixed type of hearing loss: these patients may benefit from stapedotomy. This can be done in childhood if the family is motivated and can result in enhanced oral language development. If the hearing loss is mixed, they may need a hearing aid after stapedotomy. It is very important to have all vaccinations before stapedotomy.

(b) *Cochlear Implantation*: A transmastoid facial recess approach can be used in the majority of these patients. During surgery, facial nerve malposition is to be expected because of associated semicircular abnormalities. Particularly important is the lateral semicircular canal; if it is underdeveloped, the facial nerve may be in an unusual location. Facial nerve may lie on the round window or promontory.

If the cochlea is hypoplastic, the promontory may not have the usual protuberance, and it may be difficult to identify the hypoplastic cochlea and the necessary landmarks (such as round window) for cochlear implantation through the facial recess. In these situations, an additional transcanal approach may be necessary to provide better access to the hypoplastic cochlea.

*Electrode Choice*: As the cochlea is smaller than normal, the length and cross-sectional area of the cochlear duct are smaller when compared to that of a normal cochlea. Thinner and shorter electrodes should therefore be used. A standard electrode may be too long for the cochlea, and it may not be possible to obtain a full insertion.

CH-II has the possibility of CSF leakage. A short electrode with a stopper type silicon ring may be used along with other measures for managing a CSF gusher. Because of the possibility that a full insertion may not be obtained, we developed a shorter version of the electrode (19 mm) with a cork-type silicon stopper (FORM 19) which is useful for cochlear implantation in a hypoplastic cochlea (particularly CH-II) [14].

It should be noted that the anatomy is particularly distorted in CH-I. Even though CI can be successfully placed into a hypoplastic cochlea, limited language development is expected. During the initial consent, the family should be informed that ABI surgery will most likely be required on the contralateral side in the future.

(c) *ABI*: ABI is indicated for patients with aplastic cochlear aperture and cochlear nerve aplasia. As indicated before, if the child does not demonstrate significant improvement with CI, ABI should be considered as soon as possible on the contralateral side.

(d) If there are extremely hypoplastic cochlear nerves, the possibility of obtaining good outcome with CI is low. Therefore, *CI and ABI surgery* can be done simultaneously in selective cases [15]. This is done to avoid the loss of valuable time until ABI surgery if the chance of benefit from CI surgery is low. Simultaneous CI and ABI surgery has been performed on six patients in our department.

## 6. Incomplete Partition of the Cochlea

Incomplete partition anomalies represent a group of cochlear malformations, where there is a clear differentiation between cochlea and vestibule, with normal external dimensions of the cochlea. The difference between them comes from various internal architecture defects. Incomplete partitions constitute 39.5% of inner ear malformations, according to the database of Hacettepe University Department of Otolaryngology. There are three different types of incomplete partition groups according to the defect in the modiolus and the interscalar septa.

### Types of Incomplete Partition Groups

(a) *Incomplete Partition Type I (IP-I)*

This type of incomplete partition (IP) anomaly was defined and named as "*cystic cochleovestibular malformation*" in 2002 by Sennaroglu and Saatci [16]. These represent approximately 11.5% of inner ear malformations. Cochlea can be clearly differentiated from vestibule. External dimensions (height and length) of an IP-I cochlea are similar to normal cases [17]. Cochlea is located in its usual location in the anterolateral part of the fundus of the IAC and lacks the entire modiolus and interscalar septa (Fig. 11.6), giving the appearance of an empty cystic structure. Cochlea is accompanied by an enlarged, dilated vestibule. Vestibular aqueduct enlargement is very rarely seen. There may be a defect between the IAC and the cochlea due to developmental abnormality of the cochlear aperture, and the absence of the modiolus and CSF may completely fill the cochlea.

IP-I anomaly is due to endosteal developmental anomaly [4]. This is most probably the reason for defective stapes footplate. If there is a histological defect between IAC and cochlea, CSF may fill the cochlea. This can easily lead to recurrent meningitis in IP-I patients even prior to their CI surgery or in their non-operated ear. There is a cystic structure in the stapes footplate which is easily infected during an attack of otitis media. This is very characteristic for IP-I. Spontaneous CSF fistula and recurrent meningitis can be seen, although less frequently in cochlear CH-II. This is because both IP-I and CH-II have endosteal developmental anomaly leading to defective footplate development [4]. It is interesting to note that IP-III cases always

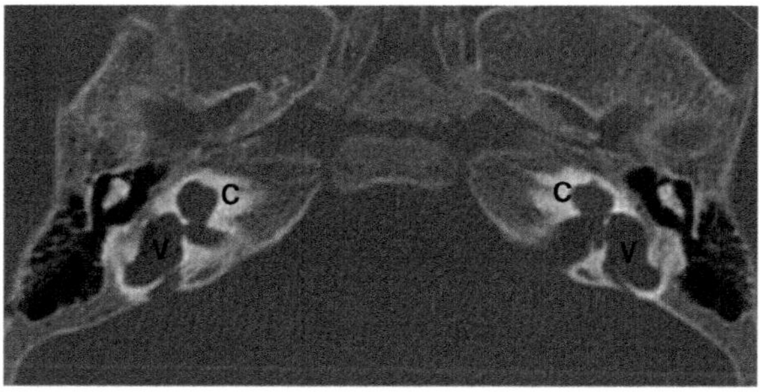


**Fig. 11.6** IP-I anomaly consisting of a cochlea (C) that lacks the entire modiolus and interscalar septa, giving the appearance of an empty cystic structure accompanied by an enlarged and dilated vestibule (V)

have a high-volume CSF gusher during CI surgery but meningitis is very rarely reported in these patients [7, 18]. This is most likely due to the fact that the stapes footplate is normally developed, because in IP-III, pathology is in the outer two layers of the otic capsule and endosteum is normal. Therefore, a defect in the footplate in IP-III is very unlikely. Our recent study demonstrated that stapes footplate fistula is also frequently encountered in the images of common cavity deformity, but because the fundus defect is less likely in CC, they do not cause meningitis as often as in IP-I [19].

*All patients with IP-I and recurrent meningitis who have normal tympanic membranes but fluid filling the middle ear and mastoid should have an exploration of the middle ear with special attention to the stapes footplate* [19]. Endaural incision is preferred in these cases. During exploration a cyst coming from a defect at the stapes footplate is usually discovered. After excising the cyst, a defect at the oval window was observed, and CSF gusher is encountered. The defect is plugged with fascia in a dumbbell fashion. It is also very important to keep stapes suprastructure and the ossicles intact in order to stabilize the fascia in place.

**Management**

- Majority of IP-I patients have severe to profound SNHL. They are almost always candidates for CI.

  Size of the cochlea is normal. Therefore, straight electrode about 25 mm is preferred. Precurved electrodes should not be used; if there is a leak, it shows that there is a defect in the modiolus, and the electrode may be displaced into the IAC. FORM 24 is developed for these cases [14]. The length is 24 mm, which makes a full turn around the basal turn. In IP-I anomaly there is 50% chance of CSF gusher. The conical stopper of FORM24 is used to stop CSF leakage around electrode. It is passed through a 2 × 2 mm fascia, and they are inserted together. Silicon stopper pushes and stabilizes the fascia into the cochleostomy. It also keeps it in place.

  In case of gusher, it is most important to stop the CSF leakage from the cochleostomy. *The surgeon should not leave operation room without controlling the leakage.* After controlling the leakage, subtotal petrosectomy can be done as an additional measure. The benefit of subtotal petrosectomy in cochlear implantation is to seal the middle ear space from the nasal passage. But if the leakage is not controlled and continues around the electrode, it is not correct to rely on subtotal petrosectomy to avoid complications. Most important principle is to stop the leakage from the cochleostomy completely.
- CN may be aplastic in some cases with IP-I, making CI a contraindication. Therefore, an ABI is indicated in IP-I patients with aplastic CN. Eight patients with IP-I and an aplastic CN have received ABI in our department.
- As in CC, an ABI may be indicated on the contralateral side in case of insufficient progress with CI as a possible indication for ABI [3].

(b) *Incomplete Partition Type II (IP-II)*

In IP-II, the apical part of the modiolus is defective (Fig. 11.7). This anomaly was originally described by Carlo Mondini and together with a minimally dilated vestibule and an enlarged vestibular aqueduct (EVA) (Fig. 11.7) constitute the triad of the *Mondini deformity*. The term "Mondini" should be used only if the above-mentioned triad of malformations is present [1, 16, 18, 20]. The apical part of the modiolus and the corresponding interscalar septa are defective, giving the apex of the cochlea a cystic appearance due to the confluence of middle and apical turns. The external dimensions of the cochlea (height and diameter) are similar to that seen in normal cases [17]. Therefore, it is not correct to define this anomaly as a cochlea with 1.5 turns [17]. The term "cochlea with 1.5 turns" should be used only for cochlear hypoplasia. IP-II constitutes 25% of IEMs in our database.

Sennaroglu L [4] in his recent study on histopathology demonstrated that modiolar defects may be due to high CSF pressure transmission into the inner ear as a result of EVA. He hypothesized that an enlarged endolymphatic sac and duct occurs as a result of genetic abnormality and widened aqueduct then transmits high CSF pressure into the inner ear. This results in a mild dilatation in the walls of the vestibule. Depending on the severity and timing of the insult, the pathology may stay at this stage and cause EVA only, or with the transmission of CSF pressure into the cochlea, it may cause a spectrum of anomalies ranging from scala vestibuli dilatation, scala communis, superior (cystic apex), partial, subtotal and in some cases complete modiolar defects [4]. The high pressure in the SV causes bulging of the ISS upwards. This is a constant finding in all cases, showing that cochlear pathology may be the result of high pressure in the SV and that it happened during the developmental phase, otherwise high pressure would have fractured the osseous spiral lamina [21]. If there is higher pressure, it is natural to expect more destruction at the upper and possibly the lower part of the modiolus. During CI surgery in IP-II, pulsation observed at the round window is due to the third window defect of EVA transmitting CSF pressure into the cochlea. CSF oozing and gusher sometimes observed in CI surgery in IP-II are due to modiolar defects occurring as a result of high CSF pressure transmission [22].

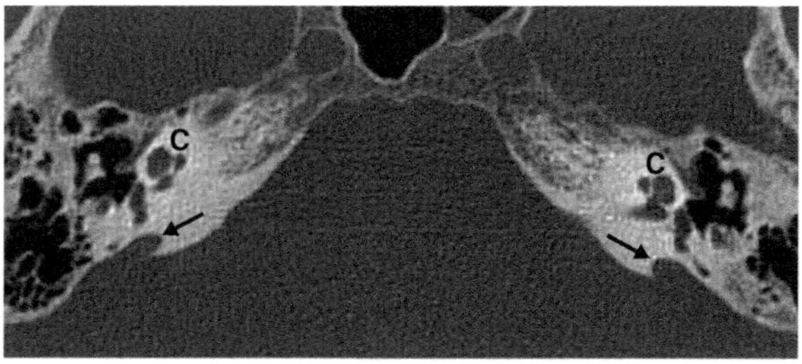


**Fig. 11.7** IP-II cochlea (C) with defective modiolus resulting in cystic apex and enlarged vestibular aqueduct (black arrows)

**Audiological Findings**

These patients do not have a characteristic hearing level, as their audiometric threshold testing varies from normal to profound. The hearing loss can be symmetric or asymmetric, but it is usually progressive. It is also possible to have sudden SNHL. Patients with IP-II usually have an air-bone gap, particularly at low frequencies. This may be due to a "third window" effect from the EVA. Tympanometry is normal in the absence of otitis media and acoustic reflexes are generally present.

**Management**

It has been observed that some cases with IP-II were born with completely normal hearing. They usually show fluctuations and progressive hearing loss, they become candidates for hearing aid.

Usually the progression in hearing loss continues, ultimately creating a need for CI at some point in their life. High pulsating CSF pressure may be responsible for the progression of hearing loss. A role for head trauma has been suggested, and these patients are advised to wear helmets when playing sports and avoiding contact sports completely. In our department, we have also implanted IP-II cases at the age of 1, who have profound SNHL since birth. As basal part of the modiolus is normal all kinds of electrodes can be used during surgery. Six of the 93 patients with IP-II had severe gusher during CI surgery [22]. Oozing is also common in these patients. Therefore, electrode with silicon stopper is advisable in IP-II. FORM 24 makes one full turn around the basal turn and controls CSF leakage around the electrode efficiently.

Stapedotomy is contraindicated in these cases as air-bone gap is most probably due to the third window effect of EVA.

As all cases of IP-II have cochlear nerve, ABI is *never* indicated in IP-II.

(c) *Incomplete Partition Type III (IP-III)*

Incomplete partition type III (IP-III) is the type of anomaly seen exclusively in X-linked deafness, which was described by Nance et al. [23] for the first time in 1971. Cochlea has interscalar septa, but the modiolus is completely absent (Fig. 11.8)

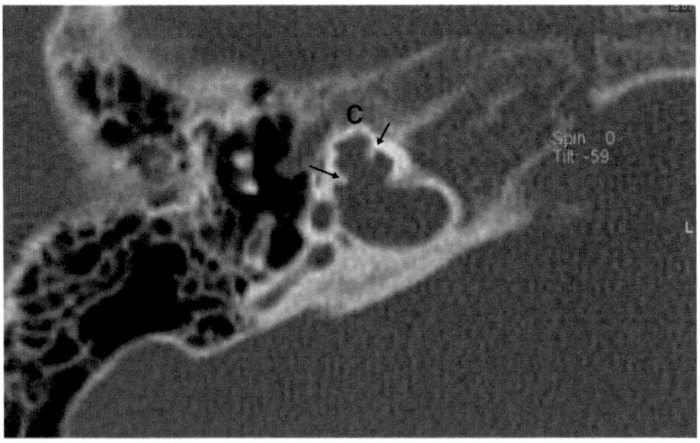


**Fig. 11.8** IP-III cochlea (C) with interscalar septa (black arrows) and absent modiolus

[1]. Phelps et al. [24] described some of the HRCT findings associated with this condition, and this characteristic deformity was included under the category of incomplete partition deformities for the first time by Sennaroglu et al. in 2006 [25]. IP-III constitutes 2.9% of the IEMs in the database in Hacettepe University Department of Otolaryngology. Therefore, they are the rarest form of incomplete partitions.

Sennaroglu L [4] recently described the possible pathophysiology of IP-III. In IP-III cochlear otic capsule around the membranous labyrinth is thinner when compared to that in a normal cochlea. HRCT demonstrates that in IP-III, the otic capsule around the cochlea is thin and follows the outline of the membranous labyrinth as if it is formed by a thick endosteal layer. Instead of the usual three layers, probably the second and third layers are either absent or very thin. Innermost endosteal layer appears to be thickened without enchondral and outer periosteal layers.

Phelps et al. [24] reported that there is a bulbous IAC, incomplete separation of the coils of the cochlea from the IAC. Talbot and Wilson [26] later added that the modiolus is absent, and there is a more medial origin of the vestibular aqueduct with varying degrees of dilatation. Sennaroglu L [27] reported that in this deformity the interscalar septa are present but the modiolus is completely absent. This gives the cochlea a characteristic appearance. From an earlier study, the external dimensions of the cochlea (height and diameter) were found to be similar to the normal cochlea [25], therefore, it is appropriate to include IP-III under the incomplete partition anomalies. In addition, labyrinthine segment of the facial nerve is located almost above the cochlea instead of making a gentle curve around the basal turn on axial sections [27]. The *labyrinthine segment of the facial nerve* is the most superior structure in the temporal bone. Thin otic capsule around cochlea and labyrinth, consisting of only a thick endosteal layer, may be responsible for this. Tympanic and mastoid segments appear to be in their normal position.

**Audiological Findings**

In IP-III there may be mixed type HL or profound SNHL. Conductive component may be due to thin otic capsule and stapes fixation. Because of high risk of gusher and further SNHL, *stapes surgery is contraindicated in IP-III.*

**Management**

Mixed hearing loss gives the impression of stapedial fixation. *Stapedotomy results in severe gusher and further SNHL, and thus, it should be avoided.*

- *Hearing Aids*: Patients with moderate to severe mixed or SNHL can be managed with hearing aids.
- *Cochlear Implantation*: Patients with severe HL are candidates for CI. Because of the absent modiolous and large defect at the cochlear base, all patients with IP-III have severe gusher during CI surgery, and there is a very high chance of electrode misplacement into IAC. Precurved electrodes have more chance to migrate into IAC. Because of this, *precurved electrodes should be avoided in IP-III. The position of the electrode should be checked intraoperatively in all*

*cases of IP-III*. FORM 24 electrodes make one full turn around the cochlear base and also control CSF leakage around the electrode. If the interscalar septa are thick, they reduce intracochlear volume, and a long electrode may be misdirected into IAC. In such a case, FORM 19 is advisable. Digisonic Classic and Digisonic Evo electrodes (Oticon) also have a silicon stopper which might be useful for controlling gusher, but they are longer than FORM electrodes, and they might go into the IAC. Spontaneous CSF fistula through the stapes footplate and recurrent meningitis is never experienced in Hacettepe University in a case of IP-III in spite of high-volume CSF leak during CI surgery. This is most probably due to normal or thickened footplate due to normal endosteal development in IP-III.

- All IP-III cases have well-developed cochlear nerves. Therefore, ABI is *not* indicated in this group of incomplete partitions.

## 7. Enlarged Vestibular Aqueduct (EVA)

Enlarged Vestibular Aqueduct (EVA) indicates the presence of an enlarged vestibular aqueduct (i.e., the midpoint between posterior labyrinth and operculum is larger than 1.5 mm) in the presence of a normal cochlea, vestibule, and semicircular canals. Difference between EVA and IP-II is that cochlea and vestibule are completely normal on HRCT and MRI in EVA.

Sennaroglu L [4] indicated before that EVA is due to a genetic defect. It appears to be responsible for the transmission of CSF pressure into the inner ear causing progressive or sudden SNHL [4]. Certain characteristics of audiological findings are a result of a third window phenomenon.

We have recently added the vertical dimension to the definition as well [5]. Classically EVA is described when the midpoint between posterior labyrinth and operculum is larger than 1.5 mm on axial sections. We have observed that EVA can be followed in a number of successive axial images. It may therefore, not be correct to evaluate EVA only on axial sections. We have to take vertical dimension of EVA into account as well. More correct definition of EVA may be "vertical and axial width larger than 1.5 mm on the midpoint between labyrinth and operculum."

Audiological presentation and management are similar to that of IP-II.

## 8. Cochlear Aperture Abnormalities

The cochlear aperture (CA), cochlear fossette, or bony cochlear nerve canal transmits the cochlear nerve from the cochlea to IAC. This can be visualized in the mid-modiolar view as well as coronal sections on HRCT (Fig. 11.9a).

The cochlear aperture is considered hypoplastic (Fig. 11.9b) if the width is less than 1.4 mm [28]. The CA is considered to be aplastic when the canal is completely replaced by bone, or there is no canal on mid-modiolar view (Fig. 11.9c).

CA abnormalities may be accompanied by a narrow IAC on HRCT. The IAC is considered narrow if the width of the midpoint of the IAC is smaller than 2.5 mm. Narrow IAC can accompany other malformations or with a normal cochlea. In cases

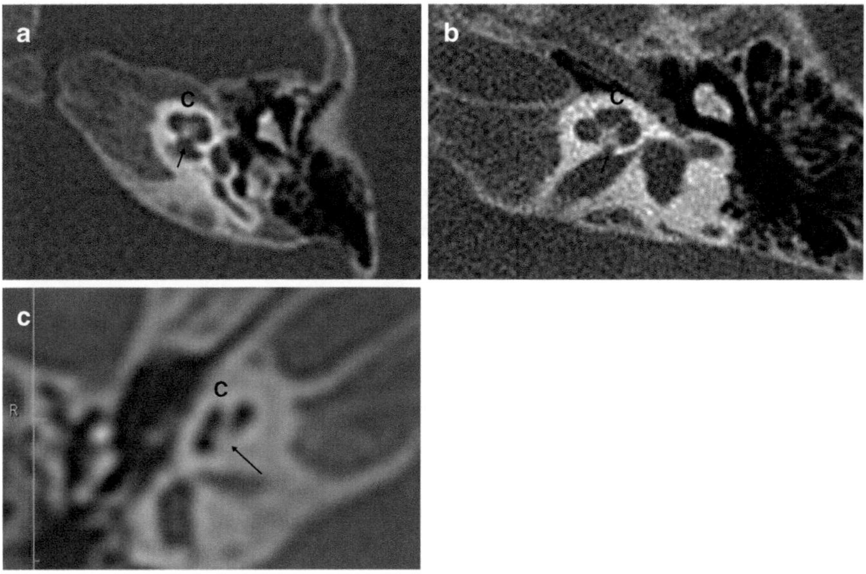

**Fig. 11.9** Cochlear aperture. (**a**) Normal, (**b**) Hypoplastic, (**c**) Aplastic (C—cochlea, black arrow—cochlear aperture)

of narrow IAC, MRI should be obtained to demonstrate if CN is normal, aplastic, or hypoplastic. Axial and sagittal oblique high T2 weighted images (i.e. CISS, Fiesta, etc.) images are necessary for this purpose. It is very important to obtain direct sagittal oblique images rather than reformats [29]. In CN aplasia, no nerve can be identified in the anterior inferior part of the IAC.

On axial section, CN is followed until modiolus. On sagittal oblique MR sections, four distinct nerves can be visualized in the IAC. CA aplasia is typically accompanied by cochlear nerve aplasia. CN may be hypoplastic or aplastic when CA is hypoplastic. CA hypoplasia and aplasia can also be observed in a normal cochlea.

**Audiological Findings**

Severe to profound SNHL is usually present. As the cochlea is normal, otoacoustic emissions (OAE) may be present and the child may pass newborn hearing screening if automated ABR is not used in the diagnosis. Their hearing loss is typically discovered later on in childhood based on the family's concerns of lack of sound awareness and language development. If the newborn screening protocol involves OAE and automated ABR, this malformation can be diagnosed during infancy. Diagnostic audiological evaluation will reveal profound hearing loss.

**Management**

Hearing aids usually do not provide sufficient amplification in patients with CA hypoplasia and aplasia. In patients with bilateral hypoplastic CA with hypoplastic cochlear nerve, hearing aid trial is necessary. If this does not provide adequate functional hearing, these patients usually become candidates for CI. The family should be counseled that if CI does not provide sufficient hearing in terms of auditory perception, contralateral ABI may be necessary to achieve improved audiologic and language outcomes.

In CA aplasia, ABI is indicated as a first-line therapy. In patients with extremely hypoplastic CN best outcome is obtained by bimodal stimulation with CI on the better audiologically profile side and ABI on the side with no response during behavioral audiological evaluation.

**Audiological Outcome IEMs:**
Ozkan et al. [30] recently reported the audiological outcome of CI in 274 patients with different inner ear malformations. Among the IEMs, the EVA group had a higher score in the closed-set test than CI users with no IEM. EVA is a congenital anomaly with a progressive sensorineural hearing loss. In the beginning, their hearing may be normal, but it deteriorates with time. It was thought that children with EVA suffer from hearing loss at the peri- or postlingual period rather than the prelingual period. Children with EVA scored better than children with IP-II because of the modiolar defect that makes the outcome slightly worse. Scores of children with EVA, IP-II, and IP-III were comparable to those of children without IEM; this is because a good-sized cochlear nerve always accompanies these IEMs. ABI surgery is never indicated in EVA, IP-II, and IP-III.

The outcome of CI is worse in more complex IEMs such as IP-I, common cavity and cochlear hypoplasia. These latter subgroups definitely need bilateral implantation. If cochlear nerve is present, bilateral CI is necessary as unilateral implantation is usually not sufficient for the development of language. If the cochlear or cochleovestibular nerve is absent, contralateral ABI is the treatment choice for these complex IEMs.

There is a controversy regarding the type of implant to be used in the treatment of patients with hypoplastic CN [31]. Occasionally it is possible to obtain good hearing and language development in certain cases with hypoplastic CN. Majority of the reports indicate insufficient or no hearing, and limited language development with CI [31].

Sennaroglu et al. [10] reported the long-term results of ABI in pediatric patients with severe IEMs. Majority of the patients were in CAP 5 category. Among 35 children, 29 had closed-set discrimination and 12 developed open set discrimination above 50%. In the second consensus meeting, similar findings were reported [29]. Therefore, it was concluded that bilateral stimulation should be done in cases of complex IEM's.

Batuk et al. [32] recently reported the audiological outcome in IEM's with hypoplastic cochlear nerve. Hearing thresholds only with CI and only with ABI did not reveal significant difference, and however, auditory perception scores improved with bimodal stimulation. Children with CN deficiency showed better performance with CI and contralateral ABI combined. Depending on the audiological and radiological results, bimodal stimulation should be advised for children with CN deficiency.

## 11.3 Conclusion

Inner Ear Malformations is a special group of patients. Unfortunately, until recent years the term "Mondini" has been used to describe many different anomalies. There are variety of IEMs and they all present in a different way. As can be seen easily each group has different characteristics in terms of presentation, radiology, hearing, and surgical findings. Proper classification is very important in the management of IEMs. If the anomaly is correctly classified, appropriate treatment can be decided more correctly. Finally, proper classification also will create a common language around the world, where clinicians can understand each other better.

## References


1. Sennaroglu L. Cochlear implantation in inner ear malformations–a review article. Cochlear Implants Int. 2010;11(1):4–41.
2. Lemmerling MM, et al. Normal modiolus: CT appearance in patients with a large vestibular aqueduct. Radiology. 1997;204(1):213–9.
3. Sennaroglu L, et al. Auditory brainstem implantation in children and non-neurofibromatosis type 2 patients: a consensus statement. Otol Neurotol. 2011;32(2):187–91.
4. Sennaroglu L. Histopathology of inner ear malformations: do we have enough evidence to explain pathophysiology? Cochlear Implants Int. 2016;17(1):3–20.
5. Sennaroglu L, Bajin MD. Classification and current management of inner ear malformations. Balkan Med J. 2017;34(5):397–411.
6. Ozgen B, et al. Complete labyrinthine aplasia: clinical and radiologic findings with review of the literature. AJNR Am J Neuroradiol. 2009;30(4):774–80.
7. Sennaroglu L. Cochlear implantation in inner ear malformations–a review article. Cochlear Implants Int. 2009;
8. McElveen JT Jr, et al. Cochlear implantation in common cavity malformations using a transmastoid labyrinthotomy approach. Laryngoscope. 1997;107(8):1032–6.
9. Beltrame MA, et al. Double posterior labyrinthotomy technique: results in three Med-El patients with common cavity. Otol Neurotol. 2005;26(2):177–82.
10. Sennaroglu L, et al. Long-term results of ABI in children with severe inner ear malformations. Otol Neurotol. 2016;37(7):865–72.
11. Pamuk G, et al. Radiological measurement of cochlear dimensions in cochlear hypoplasia and its effect on cochlear implant selection. J Laryngol Otol. 2021:1–7.
12. Sennaroglu L, et al. Cochlear hypoplasia type four with anteriorly displaced facial nerve canal. Otol Neurotol. 2016;37(10):e407–9.
13. Sennaroglu L, Tahir E. A novel classification: anomalous routes of the facial nerve in relation to inner ear malformations. Laryngoscope. 2020;
14. Sennaroglu L, Atay G, Bajin MD. A new cochlear implant electrode with a "cork"-type stopper for inner ear malformations. Auris Nasus Larynx. 2014;41(4):331–6.
15. Sennaroglu L, et al. Simultaneous cochlear and auditory brainstem implantation in children with severe inner ear malformations: initial surgical and audiological results. Otol Neurotol. 2020;41(5):625–30.

16. Sennaroglu L, Saatci I. A new classification for cochleovestibular malformations. Laryngoscope. 2002;112(12):2230–41.
17. Sennaroglu L, Saatci I. Unpartitioned versus incompletely partitioned cochleae: radiologic differentiation. Otol Neurotol. 2004;25(4):520–9. discussion 529.
18. Phelps PD, King A, Michaels L. Cochlear dysplasia and meningitis. Am J Otol. 1994;15(4):551–7.
19. Sennaroglu L, Bajin MD. Management of stapes footplate fistula in inner ear malformations. Int J Pediatr Otorhinolaryngol. 2021;140:110525.
20. Lo WW. What is a 'Mondini' and what difference does a name make? Am J Neuroradiol. 1999;20(8):1442–4.
21. Sennaroglu L. Another evidence for pressure transfer mechanism in incomplete partition two anomaly via enlarged vestibular aqueduct. Cochlear Implants Int. 2018;19(6):355–7.
22. Bajin MD, et al. The association between modiolar base anomalies and intraoperative cerebrospinal fluid leakage in patients with incomplete partition type-II anomaly: a classification system and presentation of 73 cases. Otol Neurotol. 2018;39(7):e538–42.
23. Nance WE, et al. X-linked mixed deafness with congenital fixation of the stapedial footplate and perilymphatic gusher. Birth Defects Orig Artic Ser. 1971;7(4):64–9.
24. Phelps PD, et al. X-linked deafness, stapes gushers and a distinctive defect of the inner ear. Neuroradiology. 1991;33(4):326–30.
25. Sennaroglu L, Sarac S, Ergin T. Surgical results of cochlear implantation in malformed cochlea. Otol Neurotol. 2006;27(5):615–23.
26. Talbot JM, Wilson DF. Computed tomographic diagnosis of X-linked congenital mixed deafness, fixation of the stapedial footplate, and perilymphatic gusher. Am J Otol. 1994;15(2):177–82.
27. Sennaroglu L. Special article: incomplete partition type III. In: Naito Y, editor. Pediatric ear diseases diagnostic imaging atlas and case reports. Karger; 2013. p. 106–8.
28. Wilkins A, et al. Frequent association of cochlear nerve canal stenosis with pediatric sensorineural hearing loss. Arch Otolaryngol–Head Neck Surg. 2012;138(4):383–8.
29. Sennaroglu L, et al. Consensus statement: long-term results of ABI in children with complex inner ear malformations and decision making between CI and ABI. Cochlear Implants Int. 2016;17(4):163–71.
30. Ozkan HB, et al. Audiological performance in children with inner ear malformations before and after cochlear implantation: a cohort study of 274 patients. Clin Otolaryngol. 2021;46(1):154–60.
31. Sennaroglu L, Atay G. Auditory brainstem implantation in children. Curr Otorhinolaryngol Rep. 2013;1:80–91.
32. Batuk MO, et al. Bimodal stimulation in children with inner ear malformation: one side cochlear implant and contralateral auditory brainstem implant. Clin Otolaryngol. 2020;45(2):231–8.

# Bilateral Cochlear Implants 12

Joachim Mueller

## 12.1 Introduction

Hearing has two main functions: speech understanding (which is the basis for human communication) and acoustic source localization (as part of spacial hearing as part of warning function, for example). For children hearing is essential to acquire spoken language skills. A critical task for the central auditory pathways is to process the auditory information sent by the two ears to the brain, the segregation and localization of auditory objects constitute an essential means of separating target signals from noise and competing sources. People with normal hearing naturally benefit from hearing in both ears, often without being aware of it. Many everyday listening situations can only be coped if the human being has the ability to hear binaurally thanks to the fact being equipped with two independent ears. Paired hearing organs are also widespread in the animal world; apparently, since primeval times, hearing with both ears has offered greater chances for successful survival [1]. In fact, the various tasks to be mastered in every day listening situations can only be mastered with two ears.

*The fact that both ears are necessary for sound localization seems self-evident to us today, but it is considered proven knowledge through experiments by the physiologist Ernst Heinrich Weber (1795–1858): "Weber held two clocks that could be distinguished by their ticking, to the ears. The test subjects were able to tell exactly which clock was ticking on which ear." This was remarkable, because "at the beginning of the 19th century there was still a philosophical prejudice that sounds had no spatial expansion and that they could therefore not be located with sensory organs like objective objects"* [2].

J. Mueller (✉)
Department of Otorhinolaryngology, Head & Neck Surgery, Ludwig-Maximilians-University (LMU) Munich, Munich, Germany
e-mail: joachim.mueller@med.uni-muenchen.de



S. DeSaSouza (ed.), *Cochlear Implants*,
https://doi.org/10.1007/978-981-19-0452-3_12

The best-known example of this is the localization of a sound source. However, binaural hearing plays not only an important role for sound localization, but also contributes to many other listening tasks, such as the separation of sound sources, the suppression of sound discoloration and a better understanding of speech in background noise. Appropriate hearing quality, better speech understanding in noise, directional hearing, source separation and spatial hearing can only be achieved with two ears.

**Brief Historical Excursus:**
*It is said, that already William House at the end of the 1970s* [3] *had a speculating vision, that bilateral Cochlear Implants (CI's) could bring improvements for the patients being treated. However, in clinical routine, as a rule, CI's were supplied monaurally, often far into the beginning of this millennium In the period before 1995, an occasional conducted bilateral Cochlear Implantation usually was done to improve unsatisfactory hearing performance on the first side by offering a CI to the opposite ear, the implantation of second side was more considered to be a technology upgrade than a "bilateral implant." Instead of exchanging an older or poorly functioning CI system, for example, the opposite side was implanted. Viewed retrospectively, this approach is understandable, especially against the background of the speech understanding that was achievable with the CI's representing "state of the art" at that time, which appears very limited from our today's perspective; binaural hearing with CI was not an issue back then. Certainly, the knowledge on speech coding gained by comparing different systems contributed to the further development of speech coding strategies and cochlear implants in general. Interestingly, sporadic reported, individual, mainly electrophysiological results already suggested that electrical stimuli applied in both cochleae can be processed together, even if the bilateral stimulation did not result in measurable improvements in speech understanding* [4]. *The first results in the early 1990s with a bilaterally implanted patient were not very encouraging with respect to an improvement in speech comprehension* [5, 6]. *A fusion of the auditory impression stimulated by both implants was achieved, but there were no relevant improvements in speech understanding* [5]. *The approach of improving hearing by means of bilateral cochlear implant treatment was initially not pursued further after these not encouraging results* [7]. *In 1996 it was possible for our group for the first time ever to improve speech comprehension in quiet and in noise just 4 weeks after the initial adjustment in a bilaterally implanted patient and to restore the ability to hear directionally* [8]. *Possibly the "fast speech coding strategy" already implemented in the CI systems used at that time (MED-EL Combi 40), namely the CIS strategy published by B. Wilson* [9] *in 1991, contributed to the favorable results compared to the results mentioned above (note: the CIS strategy as an example of a "fast stimulation strategy" was also discussed controversially at the time). After the first results were confirmed in adults, children have been given binaural cochlear implants since 1998. The results, which were convincing at an early stage, were presented to a broad scientific public in 1999 as a registered discussion note in the hope that these sustainable improvements would also be made available to children in greater*

*numbers as soon as possible* [10]. *Even though it was initially not clear in the end, whether and how much children would benefit from the second implant, when implanting the first children, it seemed plausible and highly likely to us, after the encouraging results in adults and in analogy to hearing aid care, to assume that binaural hearing is beneficial for the auditory language development and the general development of the children, especially in view that animal experiments also demonstrate the neuroprotective effect of electrical stimulation on the auditory nerve* [11] *and the maturation of the auditory pathway. Luckily, the objections and arguments against bilateral CI's, which were quite violent and aggressive presented in discussions within the scientific community at the time, esp. that one had to keep an eye out for later upcoming technologies and preserve one ear for the future, were not confirmed and did not bear up examination, as we can easily see retrospectively from today.*

For bilaterally (= on two sides, on both sides) implanted postlingually deaf adults, it could be shown that they benefit from hearing with two CI's in the same way and take advantage of the same effects like normal hearing subjects from hearing with two ears or like hearing aid wearers from two hearing aids. CI patients with bilateral CI's benefit from head shadow effect, squelch effect and from binaural summation and redundancy effects. In addition, when implanting both ears, the better ear is always implanted.

The physical-acoustic *head shadow* is immediately available to every listener effect and does not have to be learned [12], the prerequisite is that the person hears bilaterally or is provided with hearing aids/implants on both sides. The head shadow effect describes the improvement in speech understanding when a background noise comes from a lateral direction and at the same time speech reaches the ear or CI facing away from the noise side and shadowed against the noise by the head either from the front or from the side. This is also the case if, for example, when a sound source is moved from one side to the other, so that the ear that hears through the cochlear implant is sealed off from an interfering sound source by the head (shadow). The acoustic shadow reduces the background noise level on the isolated ear, which leads to an improved signal-to-noise ratio and thus to improved speech understanding.

*The squelch effect*, based on neurophysiologically comparative processing of the signals of both auditory pathways, describes the advantages of binaural noise suppression, which result from spatially separated noise and signal sources for the CI wearer by adding a CI on the side of the noise source. Squelch effect describes the ability of the auditory system to combine the information from both ears centrally and segregate the speech from the noise by the differences in sound between both ears.

*Binaural summation* summarizes the effects and advantages that arise from the fact that both cochlear implants deliver signals to the auditory pathway via both sides. On the one hand, the information given on both ears are redundant but also complement each other. Additionally, binaural hearing increases a loudness perception., which cannot be compensated by increasing the volume on one side. The double sound processing leads to stronger excitation patterns, which above all results in an increased loudness perception of speech [12].

*Related to this aspects, Lawson & Wilson et al. have conducted interesting experiments. They have broken down the spectrum into narrow spectral ranges in a comb-like manner by filtering the speech signal and assigned it to different transmission channels. With every second channel of the first CI they stimulated the auditory nerve on one side and with the remaining channels the second Ci on the other side. As a result, they transmitted the spectral subranges to the left and right CI in such a way that they interlocked the information so that they presented the complete signal to both ears. Surprisingly, the test subjects' brain was able to combine the information that was split up on both sides and process it in a meaningful way* [1, 13, 14]. *If two cochleae show different damage patterns, which is likely to be the case, it is to be expected that CI patients will benefit from the redundant signals of two completely fitted CI's even more than people with normal hearing* [15]. *Lawson's experiment also proves that in bilateral cochlear implant surgery, an electrode placed exactly symmetrically on the sides with exactly tonotopically assigned stimulation contacts is probably not absolutely necessary in order to generate many advantages for the patient.*

Bilateral CI users can benefit from the same effects when hearing with two CI's as people with normal hearing benefit from when hearing with two earsand the second CI fills the gaps that the first leaves behind

## 12.2 Results of Bilateral Cochlear Implants in Adults

Exemplarily for many papers that could confirm the sustainable improvements in speech understanding, our results of an early study are given: All of our sequentially implanted adult subjects reported benefit from bilateral stimulation. Speech scores for all subjects were higher with bilateral than with unilateral stimulation. The average score across subjects for sentence understanding in noise was 31.1 percentage points higher with both cochlear implants compared with the cochlear implant ipsilateral to the noise, and 10.7 percentage points higher with both cochlear implants compared with the cochlear implant contralateral to the noise. The average score for recognition of monosyllabic words in a standard German test was 18.7 percentage points higher with both cochlear implants than with one cochlear implant. All of these differences in average scores were significant at the 5% level.

Also, postlingually deafened adult patients with short duration of deafness who received their implants simultaneously showed a significant beneficial effect of bilateral CIs on speech understanding of the bilateral condition compared to the left or right ear only. The improvement obtained using CNC word tests in quiet in the bilateral condition was significant and consistent over the better unilateral condition during the first year of bilateral implant use. Similar to binaural summation, the head shadow effect was evident after only 6 months. The squelch effect was not reliably observed after 6 months, but the longitudinal design of the study allowed for the analysis of auditory development in adults. The squelch effect then was consistently present for most subjects at the 1-year measurement interval, indicating a development of binaural processing skills even in adult CI users [16].

Interestingly, these improvements are not limited to "Western" languages that use intonation to express or stress grammatical structures (just like in German, where for example, the voice is raised at the end of a question). For tonal languages in where the pitch course can determine the meaning of the word, the language understanding improved through the bilateral CI's too [17].

In tonal languages, such as Chinese, which knows four different tones and a neutral tone, the pitch of a vowel is crucial in order to distinguish between different independent words. Every change in tone is accompanied by a change in the meaning of a word.

Example:

- First tone (constant high): mā 媽 «mother»
- Second tone (rising): má 麻 «hemp»
- Third tone (falling-rising): mǎ 馬 «horse»
- Fourth tone (falling): mà 罵 «insulting»

In tonal languages, the tone is an integral part of the word—and there are words with completely different meanings that only differ in the tone. This is why there is no way in these languages to use the tone for grammatical purposes. (Source: Art History Institute of the University of Zurich/Department of Art History of East Asia/Daniel Schneiter, Jorrit Britschgi & Harald Kraemer via www.eastasianarthistory.com/index.php?nid=170) [18]

Bilateral Cochlar Implantation leads to better Speech Understanding in Quiet and in Noise

The discussions on how the improvements after bilateral implantation can and finally should be measured and recorded on the one hand side and the scientific striving for a fundamental understanding of how binaural hearing works with CI's, on the other hand, are reflected in different experimental set-ups that were used in numerous studies that contribute to our current knowledge on binaural hearing with Cis. They aim—both to demonstrate the benefits, to answer fundamental questions, but also to address interesting detailes. Schleich et al., e.g., used an adaptive sentence test and were able to show improvements in a larger group of bilateral CI wearers through a significant head shadow effect of 6.8 dB as well as the squelch effect (0.9 dB) and summation effects (2.1 dB); both also significantly different in the comparison of bilateral to unilateral CI use [19]. The head shadow effect is the largest and dominant effect; it also sets in quickly [16, 20].

The squelch effect is more difficult to measure. Litowsky [21], for example, was able to detect it only in a few test subjects. Apparently, it takes a certain before it is availabe for bilateral CI wearers. After bilateral cochlear implantation with a shorter interval in between the two surgeries, it only takes a few months for the head shadow effect and summation effects to be measurable, while the squelch effect, as a sign of binaural processing in the auditory pathway, can be measured, if so, much later, often after a year or even later [16]. The binaural processing of electrically applied stimuli in the auditory pathway itself evidently needs a certain amount of time in order to develop, even in adult CI wearers who have been deaf for a short time and who have had acoustic hearing experience. The neurophysiological effects of binaural hearing are therefore not immediately available when the electrical hearing begins.

As Steffens explains, for acoustic hearing, some effects of binaural hearing must first be acquired by training of the neurons involved on the basis of adequate stimuli that stimulate the auditory pathway and auditory cortex (area of hearing processing in the cerebral cortex) and thereby trigger specific neuron connections. Like in children with normal hearing, where they develop within the first few years of life [12].

Bilateral CIs enable "binaural hearing":

CI wearers benefit from the same effects as those with normal hearing if they are provided with both sides: head shadow effect, squelch effect, binaural summation and redundancy effects

## 12.3 (Re) Restoration of Directional and Spatial Hearing After Bilateral CI Treatment in Adults

An essential achievement of binaural hearing is to convey spatial auditory impression of the environment and spatial hearing, in the general, i.e., to enable directional hearing and distance hearing.

Bilaterally with Cis supplied, postlingually deaf patients gain, or better regain, the ability for lateralization and localization with two cis. The mean localization error was, for example, 16.6° with bilateral CIs compared to an error of 53.7° with unilateral CI use, which corresponds to chance level [22]. In doing so, the CI wearers had access to both interaural level and interaural time differences (envelope ITD) of the stimuli offered [23].

Another possibility to get a picture of bilateral ci users abilities to localize is, as Senn investigated, to determine the minimal audible angle between two neighboring sound sources. This alternative measure for spatial hearing, the minimum audible angle (MAA) test, determines the smallest angular separation perceived by the ci wearer when the two sounds come from distinct sources. MAA is an excellent measure that is consistent and reliable in discriminating left/right task. Bilateral CI wearers discriminated almost as well as normal hearing control persons. This so-called directional difference threshold (Minimum Audible Angle, MAA) in the horizontal plane was found to be 3–8° for bilateral CI wearers and thus almost reached the accuracy of normal-hearing control persons, who came to a resolution of 1–4° [15].

Bilaterally with Cis supplied, postlingually deaf patients gain, or better regain, the ability for lateralization and localization with two cis.

## 12.4 Results of Bilateral Cochlear Implants for Children

Children with bilateral CIs benefit from hearing improvements similar and at least as adults and beyond. Children who were implanted on both sides showed better speech understanding with two Cis, both in quiet and in noise [24–26]. In addition, bilateral cochlear implantation seems to have a positive effect on general hearing and language development [25].

After initially hesitant acceptance of the new care offer and often lengthy and laborious procedures to obtain a reimbursement declaration from the health insurers, the children implanted in the early days of bilateral CI care in the mid-1990s inevitably resulted in a rapidly growing population, and enormously contributing patient population, that show the advantages of bilateral cochlear implants similar to the results observed from adults or even more but the above mentioned factors resulted in a ultimately quite heterogeneous. Although the improvements in language comprehension were quickly apparent, new questions arose:

- What parameters, not just medical ones, may influence the results?
- Are there biologically important time windows for the supply?
- How should the time interval between the two operations be selected?
- What influence does have the age at first or second implantation?
- Which aspects have to be considered during fitting and rehabilitation?

Bilaterally cared for children benefit in the same way as adults from binaural hearing and beyond: Many bilaterally cared for children acquire language faster than only one-sided children and have a larger vocabulary after a defined time window

The vast majority of children and adolescents enjoy a good to very good gain from the second implant, even if there was a longer time interval between the two operations [27]. In Strom et al. for example, speech understanding 12 and 24 months after implantation was significantly greater with both CIs compared to both the first and second CI, with a shorter interval between the two operations contributing to higher speech understanding with the second CI [26]. It was not possible to determine a defined time interval after which the second CI no longer had a positive effect in the examined patient collective [26]. Rare individual observations that described that individual children do not benefit from the second ci or did not show any significant improvement or maybe disliked to wear the ci or took the second CI off, are explained by the fact that these children were typically older when they were first implanted (from today's perspective) and/or were implanted on the second side at an older age, having a not stimulated, deaf ear from birth without residual hearing or a hearing aid period when being implanted later on the second side [27]. A long interval between the two operations led to poor speech understanding on the second side and to an increased risk that some children use second CI only to a limited extent, even if a head shadow effect (noise from the opposite side of the second CI) was detectable [28]. The increasing willingness to accept the advantages of bilateral ci care, which were already visible after a short time after introduction of this therapeutic approach led, together with the parallel ongoing development to implant children earlier and no longer only with complete deafness but also with residual hearing, to a steadily growing Patient group: Young children increasingly received their first CI in the first year of life, sometimes even from the fourth month of their life and quickly followed or even simultaneously received the second CI, so that they received bilateral CIs before the second babble phase. Bilateral Cis implanted and activated before the second babble phase should ideally be aimed at in our opinion from a physiological developmental point of view. The integration of the second implant and the possibilities of using binaural information develop more quickly in younger children and in children who were treated with a short time interval between the two implantations (see e.g., [9, 24, 26, 28, 29]). Older children and those with a longer interval between the two operations benefit as well in many aspects, but require special training in order to "train" the hearing performance of the second ear. Early observations from rehabilitation facilities caring for children with bilateral care already suggested that the time interval between the two implantations could influence binaural hearing performance [25].

In everyday situations, too, the parents observed positive changes in the children's hearing behavior within 24 months of receiving the second side for speech intelligibility, directional hearing and hearing quality, which were recorded with questionnaires. As expected, the changes observed were gradually dependent on the age of the implantation, the interval between both operations and the duration of the bilateral hearing experience [30]. Subsequent studies examined aspects of bilateral CI fitting and possible influencing factors in sequentially implanted patients in more detail. For children, early implantation has proven to be beneficial for communication behavior when entering school (speech understanding in quiet and in noise for words and sentences, language status and language production). Dettmann et al., for example, worked out on a patient collective of 403 Australian children who were implanted in three centers between 1990 and 2014 using regression analysis that, in addition to cognitive abilities, early implantation has a favorable prognostic effect on hearing and language development [31]; Likewise, with Strom-Roum or Ona Bo

Wie, for example, a short time interval between the two operations was found to be advantageous [9, 26]. An early implantation and a short interval between the two operations is also a positive predictive factor for good speech understanding with the second implant [26].

Children who are implanted early (i.e., between the ages of 5 and 18 months) develop their language skills and their language skills faster than would be expected according to their listening age; After 8 months, the LittleEARS test score largely corresponded to that of age-appropriate, normal-hearing children. 12–48 months after implantation, 81% of the bilaterally treated children had receptive language skills in the age-appropriate normal range, while 57% had expressive skills in the age-appropriate normal range within the normal range between 1 and 4 years of age [9]. Of particular significance is the observation that children who received their implants within the first 12 months of life achieve expressive and receptive language skills within the normal range faster than the group implanted after age 1. This suggests that very early implantation may be able to close the gap between the performance of children with bilateral CIs and normal hearing children even faster than was previously thought.

Since "learning to hear" is, so to say, evolving fluently and taking place gradually in developmental phases over a longer period of time, adequate stimuli have to be present for and act on the auditory pathway in biologically correct time windows in order to initiate further maturation and development processes. As known from animal experience, early acoustic experience is essential for central processing, i.e., to develop directional hearing [32]. It appears plausible to assume that there is probably a time window given by biological framework conditions in which the bilateral cochlear implantation should take place in order to achieve the best possible result.

If the language performances of the children at the age of 6 years were compared between children who were implanted between 5–11 months and 12–29 months at the time of surgery, the receptive vocabulary at the 6-year estimation revealed a significant negative correlation between the age at the time of the first CI and receptive vocabulary. The data suggest that a 1-year delay in surgery, on average, caused a delay of 1.3 years delay in receptive vocabulary at 6 years of age. The study concluded that fitting CI before a child's first birthday was crucial for spoken language development at 6 years of age. Infants who received their implants before 9 months of age had an even more age-typical language profile. The medical risks associated with CI surgery under 9 months were no greater than for children who were older when they had CI surgery [33].

Early implantation of the first side, followed by rapid bilateral treatment with a short interval between the two operations, or simultaneous operation is advisable

Electrophysiological longitudinal studies in which Sharma et al. found fundamental differences in the morphology of CAEPs (cortical auditory evoked potential)

in children who were bilaterally implanted early (children younger than 3.5 years) compared to late (older than 7 years) children, the authors lead to the conclusion that, in accordance with animal models, there are relatively short sensitive phases for the development of the auditory pathway [34]. A correlation of the electrophysiological findings with speech comprehension of the children examined is not discussed. Nevertheless, Sharma's investigations can be interpreted as an additional argument in favor of early and bilateral implantation with a short interval; they are consistent with the clinically oriented studies already mentioned.

## 12.5 Directional and Spatial Hearing After Bilateral CIs in Children

One of the most exciting aspects and scientifically extremely interesting was to observe whether children with bilateral Cis can develop spatial and directional hearing abilities. As part of her dissertation, C. Edelmann followed the first 13 bilaterally implanted children over a period of 3 years. It turned out that spatial hearing developed at different speeds in this heterogeneous group of children. On average, it took 1½ years to develop a sense of spatial hearing. Over the course of 3 years, the children not only developed the ability to hear where a sound is coming from, but with increasing frequency in using both CIs, the errors of judgment where a sound comes from decreased. The results can be interpreted in a way that the children not only gained the ability to locate a sound source in a three-dimensional acoustic environment, but also over time acquired the ability to localize more precisely. A follow-up examination after 5 years of this patient group confirmed this assumption [35].

Spatial hearing is of immense importance for growing children. It allows to separate important from unimportant sound sources, helps to locate warning noises and helps to orientate themselves acoustically in traffic. More recent publications by Ruth Litowsky et al., who systematically examined the localization skills in children, also confirm that children with two CIs can localize better than children after only unilateral implantation or bimodal care, which combines a CI on one side with a hearing aid on the other. The localization skills develop gradually [36], similar to normal-hearing children, in whom spatial hearing is relatively well developed by the age of 5 [36]. For example, bilaterally implanted children who were implanted on the second side before the age of 3 develop localization skills, while children of the same age who are cared for on one side do not develop these skills. Here, too, the early treatment seems to have a positive effect: children who were implanted up to 14 months of age showed localization capabilities after an average of 10 months of wearing bilateral CIs [21, 36, 37]. Providing care for both sides as early as possible accelerates the development of directional hearing, e.g., if the second side was supplied before the fourth birthday [38]. In comparison to and in line with animal models, where early bilateral acoustic stimulation of the auditory pathway is necessary to develop complex interconnections of inhibitory and excitatory influences to detect interaural time differences (such interaural time differences (ITDs) are encoded in the auditory brain stem) as the main cue to localize low-frequency sound in the azimuth [32], an early bilateral supply seems entirely plausible. Even if there are further relationships between the localization accuracy and the age at the first implantation or the interval between the two surgeries have not yet been worked out.

## 12.6 Listening Effort and General Development of Children

The various efforts that the hearing impaired subjects have to make in communication situations are often underestimated by hearing people. In addition to increased stress in difficult listening situations, psychological tension and increased concentration effort, hearing impaired feel burdened by the uncertainty as to whether they have understood correctly what they had "the impression to have heard." CI patients with bilateral care report reduced listening effort: they can concentrate longer in listening situations, and they report that hearing is less strenuous and less tiring. These descriptions, which are difficult to measure, but easily to understand and believable, can be better evaluated by nonlinguistic visual response-time task than by speech intelligibility tests [4]. Questionnaires are also a suitable instrument for self-assessment of everyday listening situations [30, 39].

Hughes and Galvin were able to objectify changes in listening effort for the first time. Their investigations showed that, on the one hand, the listening effort was less for young adult bilateral CI wearers than for unilaterally implanted patients [40] and, on the other hand, the listening effort of the cochlear implantees, when using bilateral CIs corresponded to the listening effort of the normal hearing group, when the two groups were achieving similar speech perception scores. Also Schnabl et al. concluded on the basis of a study based on questionnaires that a second CI can reduce listening effort [29, 39, 41].

Children given bilateral ci care show more rapid language development and acquire a greater vocabulary than children given unilaterally CIs after a defined, comparable period of time, for example, at age 8 years. Vocabulary and language acquisition are influenced by multiple factors, but in addition to family background, upbringing, educational background and education at home, which had also an influence, 50–60% of the variance was explained by the type of CI provision (unilateral or bilateral) [42].

Bilateral Cochlear Implantation reduces listening effort and has a positive effect on language development

## 12.7 Simultaneous or Sequential Surgery

The question of whether a sequential or simultaneous CI supply is more advantageous is internationally discussed controversially. It should not be answered too dogmatically but tailored to the individual case. In this complex multi-layer discussion, for both, the children and adults, a variety of different but individual aspects have to be considered: the amount of residual hearing, asymmetry of hearing, vestibular function, age and weight in babies, concomitant diseases, individual medical aspects (e.g., duration of anesthesia in small children, blood loss; surgical technique, logistics in OR ...). but also the knowledge about critical periods of the development and maturation processes of hearing, especially the sensitive phases of binaural hearing [35, 43] as well as rehabilitation aspects (training effort for the second side ...) should be taken into account in the decision-making, preferred in the individual context. Occasionally or sometimes, depending on the region and country, more weighted, economic arguments to support simultaneous surgery at reduced costs are brought into the discussion [44].

Experience to date has shown that both simultaneously and sequentially implanted patients benefit from binaural hearing. On the basis of general neurophysiological considerations, one should assume that binaural hearing develops faster and that both ears develop more evenly when children are implanted simultaneously. However, the experience of almost 25 years now shows that children with consecutive implantations also benefit from the bilateral CI restoration. A sequential implantation does not appear to be necessarily disadvantageous according to the available experience, however, the therapeutic rehabilitation measures in the case of sequential implantation with a longer interval between the two operations may have to be tailored to the individual circumstances.

Simultaneous treatment in the case of complete deafness would suggest that both ears would be treated in one operation and under anesthesia and that both auditory tracts would be stimulated at the same time. However, since nowadays, as mentioned, increasingly younger children who are implanted often no longer have to be completely deaf in order to receive a CI and therefore usually a certain residual hearing is present, there are reservations that claim that a child can be simultaneous on both sides Care goes through a phase of complete deafness until speech processor activation is definitely worth considering and an argument in favor of sequential care with a short interval. Even if a hearing aid can just be used to convey a noise detection that is not sufficient for speech development, in the case of sequential supply via an opposite ear supplied with hearing aids, an acoustic sensory channel remains open until the CI is activated. Once the CI has been adjusted and accepted, the implantation of the second side will usually follow quickly, usually after 3–6 months. At the latest, when a child takes off the hearing aid because it obviously no longer provides any benefit, the second side is due. Determining this point in time is certainly a demanding pediatric audiological task, above all in the knowledge of the advantages of rapid bilateral care, but also in the knowledge that the children could suffer disadvantages by waiting too long.

In the case of decision-making for a sequential or simultaneous procedure, the surgical risks of a longer intervention with bilateral simultaneous implantation must be weighed against the aspects of a sequential procedure or a short-term sequential implantation. Maybe a simultaneous initial fitting may possibly represent a sensible compromise. Considerations and discussions on this aspect are enriched by the recently introduced notifications about an early first fitting, which takes place a few days after the operation instead of 4–6 weeks and wound healing has been completed [2].

Even in the case of a primarily planned simultaneous CI surgery, after implantation of the first side, it is important to consider whether the procedure can be continued as planned or whether it is less risky to continue the procedure sequentially. 22% of the interventions planned as a simultaneous procedure, for example, were not conducted as originally planned but continued sequentially for various intraoperative reasons [3].

## 12.8 Optimal Timing for Bilateral Cochlear Implantation?

From clinical experience and knowledge about the maturation of the auditory system, we can assume that the earlier a child is adequately provided with hearing aids and or with CIs, and starts to "hear" (with both ears/CIs), the better the two devices can be coordinated and the complex interacting interconnections between left and right input to the auditory pathways and the auditory cortex and start to evolve. Ci surgery is possible in some specialized centers from around the fourth month of the child's life onwards with a weight of approx. 5.5 kg.

In the meantime, however, the "soft" described and not exactly sharp defined time windows for development as described above ("as early as possible supply of the first side" and "as quickly as possible in succession" or "simultaneously") has been made more concrete, however, an exact time window after which a CI supply of the second side seems not to work, has not yet been found or worked out (as also explicitly stated [26]). For clinical routine, the assumption that ideally the first side can be supplied between the 4th and 12th month of life and the second side quickly afterwards, i.e., within a few months, is emerging as a practically useful ideal (see also [9, 24, 26, 45]).

## 12.9 Bilateral CI Treatment After Meningitis: The Danger of Delay—An Aim for Rapid, Possibly Simultaneous CI Treatment on Both Sides

There is no doubt that swift action is required after meningitis, because of the threat of obliteration in both cochleae and the subsequently resulting risk of not being able to place the electrode into the cochlear lumen (either scala tympani or vestibuli) during surgery. A rapid bilateral simultaneous supply should be aimed for, if there are no serious medical contraindications. The implantation should be done quickly and not be delayed too long, as partial or severe obliteration can be observed within a few weeks after infection (own observation: almost complete obliteration after 4 weeks!), having in mind that there is a lack of reliable data on the time window for the development of an obliteration. Audiological checks, CT, and MRI at short intervals can be helpful in recognizing the first signs of ossification, which may be visible first in the horizontal semicircular canal, and not missing the right time for the operation [31, 37, 46].

## 12.10 Are There Any Contraindications to Bilateral Care?

First of all, as part of the medical preexaminations and complete presurgical diagnostic investigations, the anatomical and physiological status and the given situation are checked for each side individually. If, for example, a asymmetrical hearing is found that allows the beneficial combination of hearing aid on the one side and a cochlear implant on the other, the benefits of Hearing aid should be critically examined and, if necessary, sequential surgery for bilateral CIs should be sought, as soon as the hearing aid is no longer useful. If the cochlea or the auditory nerve is missing on one side, the treatment will naturally be limited to a unilateral Cochlear implantation. Even with unilateral malformations and anatomically and morphologically normal cochlea on the opposite side, it can make sense to limit oneself to unilateral CI treatment.

In the case of asymmetrical biological conditions, including also the vestibular system, with a vestibular deficiency or loss on one side, as from time to time found in older adults, a carefully weighing up the advantages bilateral Cis and risks of a complete bilateral vestibular loss is advisable.

Older children and adolescents should have the second implant after being involved in the decision-making process; if they show the necessary intellectual maturity and understanding that such decision owns, they should become part of the decision-making process, and they should accept in particular the subsequent training that may be required for the second side—these children usually cannot expect the second ear immediately as good as the first implanted ear after years of habilitation I fit was not stimulated with a hearing aid for example. A young person's unwillingness in general to wear a second implant should be taken seriously into consideration. Sometimes in older children decision-making may require careful paving and guiding of the child's decision and acceptance.

If the vestibular function is unilaterally extinguished, the risk of impairment of the remaining vestibular function as a result of a rare, sometimes to observe complication after surgery and the resulting consequences must be weighed against the gain and advantages of the expected bilateral hearing. Modern electrodes, originally developed for hearing-preserving cochlear implantation in combination with round window access to scala tympani further reduce this risk of vestibular damage.

The question of bilateral cochlear implant care is probably difficult to answer for older patients with concomitant diseases and possibly increased risks of surgery and anesthesia. The operation itself, certainly thanks to the advances in modern anesthesia management, is not afflicted with increased complication rates [47, 48]. Those who want bilateral care to improve their situation and who have paid into the social security system for many years should receive care. The surgery for the second side can probably not be withheld, especially if they are prepared to take the risks after detailed counseling and the expected benefits. Inadequately compensated hearing loss in old age has far-reaching consequences and can be associated with a decline in cognitive functions; this can be prevented by early and adequate compensation of the hearing loss, as Mosnier et al. were able to show. The rehabilitation of hearing ability, including also (bilateral) CI treatment, has a positive influence on the maintenance of cognitive functions and also has a positive influence on the quality of life [48, 49].

## 12.11 Socio-economic Framework: Ethical, Economic, and Legal Considerations

Bilateral Cis are recommended whenever medically indicated and affordable within the framework of local social and reimbursement systems. Withholding significant opportunities to improve the hearing situation of deaf children for reasons of economy to save money should be refused from a medical point of view. However the situation may vary in different areas of the world, but in many countries, bilateral Cis have meanwhile been accepted as standard care.

*According to the Ottawa Declaration, every child has "a natural right to life and the right to access appropriate facilities for promoting health, preventing and treating diseases and restoring health. Physicians and other health care providers have an obligation to recognize and support these rights and to work hard to provide the medical equipment and human resources to defend and enforce these rights. In Article 24 of the United Nations Convention on the Rights of the Child of November 20, 1989, the contracting states recognize the child's right to the highest attainable health and to use facilities for the treatment of diseases and for the restoration of health" [http://www.bundesaerztekammer.de/patienten/patientenrechte/recht-des-kindes-auf-gesundheitliche-versorgung/].*

Given the limited number of cochlear implantations that are carried out in Germany, it does not appear ethically justifiable to withhold the proven and essential hearing improvements from affected children [50], especially if one considers the amount of money, which is available in the system. The benefits that can be achieved through bilateral care go far beyond the costs of implantation if the path to better hearing and thus the opportunities for vocational training and integration and participation, including in the labor market, can be paved for children. From an economic point of view, it certainly makes more sense to keep working patients able to continue working through bilateral implantation (and thus also as taxpayers and contributors to health insurance and social security systems) than to retire them at the expense of the social security systems [50].

Fortunately, nowadays, costs for bilateral Cis are usually taken over by the moneygivers in Germany, and almost all of the European Union (EU) countries, the USA and Canada, had agreed to reimburse the cost of bilateral CI treatment. The previously numerous legal disputes we had in Germany between those persons being affected and their health insurance companies, which often lasted for years, have nowadays decreased significantly. In the beginning of the era of bilateral CIs, as a young doctor, it was almost unimaginable for me that a patient would have to sue his insurance company in order to get right, but patients had to do so, And indeed, in the majority of cases the courts ruled in their favor based on the background of the social legislation in Germany and Europe. Lawyer B. Kochs has reported on legal backgrounds and commented in public on legal questions of bilateral CI supply in several articles, including in the German self-helping group journal "Schnecke." Patients are entitled according to the social legislation for disability compensation (as complete as possible). The goal to be strived for is the situation of non-disabled people, i.e., the best possible compensation, also for the lost sense of hearing, is supported by law.107 of the 108 proceedings conducted by himself were concluded with positive results for the affected persons, in one case, the parents did not want to continue the proceedings—before a final decision–for personal reasons [45]. These early cases taken to court from 1997 onwards lead to precedence cases and finally to a general coverage of most second CIs by the health insurance before the year 2005. This was a major contribution to reimburse bilateral CIs aside of medical arguments.

Although the healthcare system is in great shape in the Western world, there is a space for improvement in the rest of the world, and more specifically, an immense potential lays in allowing the bilateral hearing to every single patient in need, and in advancing the necessary reimbursement systems which currently obstruct this.

## 12.12 Outlook

Further development of speech coding strategies, implant technology or the mapping of, e.g., the sound-influencing properties of the auricle have the potential to enable further improvements. Further improvements are also conceivable in the future through improved coding of specific parameters that are important for binaural hearing, such as improved ITD coding [51, 52].

And perhaps in the not too distant future, hearing without visible external components will also be possible for bilateral CI wearers, if one considers the latest developments and the first implantations of the TICI ("totally implantable cochlear implant"), the fully implantable CI, which took place in November 2020 in Munich CI within a feasibility study.

**Conclusion**

CI patients implanted in both ears with Cis using modern speech coding strategies benefit significantly from improved hearing and increased quality of life.

Like people with normal hearing, they benefit from bilateral hearing because

1. The two cochlear implant systems interact and complement each other and.
2. This enables beneficial bilateral hearing in the first place.
3. The person implanted on both sides now has always a "closer ear" to a signal source on each side.
4. The signal/noise ratio is more favorable at the "closer ear."
5. Interfering noises are generally less obscuring
6. Two CI's enable directional hearing and thus.
7. "Spatial hearing" becomes possible with binaural CI supply.
8. Bilateral implanted persons have always the better ear implanted and thus.
9. The second CI can fill in the "gaps" left by the first CI may.

## References


1. Steinle C. Messung der Sprachverständlichkeit mit dem HSM-Satztest bei ein- und beidohrigem Abhören. Dissertation Universität Würzburg, Medizinische Fakultät 2008 urn:nbn:de:bvb:20-opus-3349225.
2. Hagr A, Garadat SN, Al-Momani M, Alsabellha RM, Almuhawas FA. Feasibility of one-day activation in cochlear implant recipients. Int J Audiol. 2015;54(5):323–8.
3. Holland JF, Galvin KL, Briggs RJ. Planned simultaneous bilateral cochlear implant operations: how often do children receive only one implant? Int J Pediatr Otorhinolaryngol. 2012;76(3):396–9.
4. Pals C, Sarampalis A, Baskent D. Listening effort with cochlear implant simulations. J Speech Lang Hear Res. 2013;56(4):1075–84. Epub 2012 Dec 28.
5. van Hoesel RJM, Tong YC, Hollow RD, Clark GM. Psychophysical and speech perception studies: a case report on a binaural cochlear implant subject. J Acoust Soc Am. 1993;94:3178–89.
6. Tyler RS, Dunn CC, Witt SA, Preece JP. Update on bilateral cochlear implantation. Curr Opin Otolaryngol Head Neck Surg. 2003;11(5):388–93.
7. Wilson BS. pers. Mitteilung, Wullstein Symposium 2001, Würzburg.
8. Müller J. Erste Ergebnisse der Bilateralen Cochlear Imjplant Versorgung. Eur Arch Oto Rhino Laryngol. 1998;255:38.
9. Wie OB. Language development in children after receiving bilateral cochlear implants between 5 and 18 months. Int J Pediatr Otorhinolaryngol. 2010;74(11):1258–66. https://doi.org/10.1016/j.ijporl.2010.07.026. Epub 2010 Aug 25.
10. Müller J. Angemeldete Diskussionsbemerkung. Aachen: Dt HNO-Kongress; 1999.
11. Leake PA, Hradek GT, Snyder RL. Chronic electrical stimulation by a cochlear implant promotes survival of spiral ganglion neurons after neonatal deafness. J Comp Neurol. 1999;412(4):543–62.
12. Steffens T. Bilaterale CI Versorgung heute. In: Ernst A, Battmer R, Todt I, editors. Cochlear Implant heute. Heidelberg: Springer Medizin Verlag. ISBN 978-3-540-88235-0.
13. Lawson D, Wilson B, Zerbi M, Finley C. Speech processors for auditory prostheses. Fourth Quarterly Progress Report, July 1 through September 31, 1999, NIH Project N01-DC-8-2105, Research Triangle Institute; 1999. http://www.rti.org/reports/capr/N01-DC-8-2105QPR04.pdf
14. Lawson D, Wolford R, Brill St, Schatzer R, Wilson B. Speech processors for auditory prostheses. Twelfth Quarterly Progress Report, July 1 through September 31, 1999, NIH Project N01-DC-8-2105, Research Triangle Institute; 1999. http://www.rti.org/reports/capr/N01-DC-8-2105QPR12.pdf
15. Senn P, Kompis M, Vischer M, Haeusler R. Minimum audible angle, just noticeable interaural differences and speech intelligibility with bilateral cochlear implants using clinical speech processors. Audiol Neurootol. 2005;10(6):342–52.
16. Buss E, Pillsbury H, Buchman C, Pillsbury C, Clark M, Haynes D, Labadie R, Amberg S, Roland P, Kruger P, Novak M, Wirth J, Black J, Peters R, Lake J, Wackym P, Firszt J, Wilson B, Lawson D, Schatzer R, D'Haese P, Barco A. Multicenter U.S. bilateral MED-EL cochlear implantation study: speech perception over the first year of use. Ear Hear. 2008;29(1):20–32.
17. Au DK, Hui Y, Wei WI. Superiority of bilateral cochlear implantation over unilateral cochlear implantation in tone discrimination in Chinese patients. Am J Otolaryngol. 2003;24(1):19–23. PMID: 12579478.
18. Schneiter D, Britschgi J, Kraemer H. Kunsthistorisches Institut der Universität Zürich / Abteilung Kunstgeschichte Ostasiens über. www.eastasianarthistory.com/index.php?nid=170
19. Schleich P, Nopp P, D'Haese P. Head shadow, squelch and summation effects in bilateral users of the MED-EL COMBI 40/40+ cochlear implant. Ear & Hearing. 2004;25:197–204.
20. Litovsky RY, Parkinson A, Arcaroli J, Peters R, Lake J, Johnstone P, Yu G. Bilateral cochlear implants in adults and children. Arch Otolaryngol Head Neck Surg. 2004;130(5):648–55.
21. Litovsky RY, Johnstone PM, Godar S, Agrawal S, Parkinson A, Peters R, Lake J. Bilateral cochlear implants in children: localization acuity measured with minimum audible angle. Ear Hear. 2006;27(1):43–59.

22. Nopp P, Schleich P, D'Haese P. Sound localization in bilateral users of MED-EL COMBI 40/40+ cochlear implants. Ear Hear. 2004;25(3):205–14.
23. Schoen F, Mueller J, Helms J, Nopp P. Sound localization and sensitivity to interaural cues in bilateral users of the MED-EL COMBI 40/40+cochlear implant system. Otol Neurotol. 2005;26(3):429–37.
24. Gordon KA, Papsin BC. Benefits of short interimplant delays in children receiving bilateral cochlear implants. Otol Neurotol. 2009;30(3):319–31. https://doi.org/10.1097/MAO.0b013e31819a8f4c.
25. Kühn-Inacker H, Shehata-Dieler W, Müller J, Helms J. Bilateral cochlear implants: a way to optimize auditory perception abilities in deaf children? Int J Pediatric Otorhinolaryngol. 2004;68:1257–66.
26. Strom-Roum H, Laurent C, Wie OB. Comparison of bilateral and unilateral cochlear implants in children with sequential surgery. Int J Pediatr Otorhinolaryngol. 2011;2011
27. Vischer M, Senn P, Kompis M, Häusler R, Caversaccio M. Predictive factors for the performance of the second cochlear implant in sequentially bilateral implanted children, adolescent and adults. Cochlear Implants Int. 2012;12(Suppl 1):S127–9.
28. Myhrum M, Strøm-Roum H, Heldahl MG, Rødvik AK, Eksveen B, Landsvik B, Rasmussen K, Tvete OE. Sequential bilateral cochlear implantation in children: outcome of the second implant and long-term use. Ear Hear. 2016; [Epub ahead of print].
29. Steel MM, Papsin BC, Gordon KA, Steel MM, Papsin BC, Gordon KA. Binaural fusion and listening effort in children who use bilateral cochlear implants: a psychoacoustic and pupillometric study. PLoS One. 2015;10(2):e0117611. https://doi.org/10.1371/journal.pone.0117611. eCollection 2015.
30. Galvin KL, Mok M. Everyday listening performance of children before and after receiving a second cochlear implant: results using the parent version of the speech, spatial, and qualities of hearing scale. Ear Hear. 2016;37(1):93–102.
31. Dettman SJ, Dowell RC, Choo D, Arnott W, Abrahams Y, Davis A, Dornan D, Leigh J, Constantinescu G, Cowan R, Briggs RJ. Long-term communication outcomes for children receiving cochlear implants younger than 12 months: a multicenter study. Otol Neurotol. 2016;37(2):e82–95. https://doi.org/10.1097/MAO.0000000000000915.
32. Seidl AH, Grothe B. Development of sound localization mechanisms in the mongolian gerbil is shaped by early acoustic experience. J Neurophysiol. 2005;94(2):1028–36. https://doi.org/10.1152/jn.01143.2004.
33. Karltorp E, Eklof M, Ostlund E, et al. Cochlear implants before 9 months of age led to more natural spoken language development without increased surgical risks. Acta Paediatr. 2020;109(2):332–41.
34. Sharma A, Dorman MF, Kral A. The influence of a sensitive period on central auditory development in children with unilateral and bilateral cochlear implants. Hear Res. 2005;203(1–2):134–43.
35. Kühn H, Schön F, Edelmann K, Brill S, Müller J. The development of lateralization abilities in children with bilateral cochlear implants. ORL J Otorhinolaryngol Relat Spec. 2013;75(2):55–67. https://doi.org/10.1159/000347193. Epub 2013 May 16.10.
36. Litovsky RY, Johnstone PM, Godar SP. Benefits of bilateral cochlear implants and/or hearing aids in children. Int J Audiol. 2006;45(Suppl 1):S78–91.
37. Litovsky RY, Gordon K. Bilateral cochlear implants in children: effects of auditory experience and deprivation on auditory perception. Hear Res. 2016. pii: S0378-5955(15)30200-8. https://doi.org/10.1016/j.heares.2016.01.003. [Epub ahead of print].
38. Asp F, Eskilsson G, Berninger E. Horizontal sound localization in children with bilateral cochlear implants: effects of auditory experience and age at implantation. Otol Neurotol. 2011;
39. Schnabl J, Bumann B, Rehbein M, Müller O, Seidler H, Wolf-Magele A, Sprinzl G, Windfuhr J, Weichbold V. Listening effort with cochlear implants: unilateral versus bilateral use. HNO. 2015;63(8):546–51.

40. Hughes KC, Galvin KL. Measuring listening effort expended by adolescents and young adults with unilateral or bilateral cochlear implants or normal hearing. Cochlear Implants Int. 2013;14(3):121–9.
41. Steel MM, Papsin BC, Gordon KA, Steel MM, Papsin BC, Gordon KA. Correction: Binaural fusion and listening effort in children who use bilateral cochlear implants: a psychoacoustic and pupillometric study. PLoS One. 2015;10(10):e0141945. https://doi.org/10.1371/journal.pone.01419.
42. Sarant JZ, Harris DC, Bennet LA. Academic outcomes for school-aged children with severe-profound hearing loss and early unilateral and bilateral cochlear implants. J Speech Lang Hear Res. 2015;58(3):1017–32. https://doi.org/10.1044/2015_JSLHR-H-14-0075.
43. Grieco-Calub TM, Litovsky RY. Spatial acuity in 2-to-3-year-old children with normal acoustic hearing, unilateral cochlear implants, and bilateral cochlear implants. Ear Hear. 2012;33(5):561–72. https://doi.org/10.1097/AUD.0b013e31824c7801.
44. Merdad M, Wolter NE, Cushing SL, Gordon KA, Papsin BC. Surgical efficiency in bilateral cochlear implantation: a cost analysis. Cochlear Implants Int. 2014;15(1):43–7. https://doi.org/10.1179/1754762813Y.0000000042. Epub 2013 Nov 25.
45. Jacobs E, Langereis MC, Frijns JH, Free RH, Goedegebure A, Smits C, Stokroos RJ, Ariens-Meijer SA, Mylanus EA, Vermeulen AM. Benefits of simultaneous bilateral cochlear implantation on verbal reasoning skills in prelingually deaf children. Res Dev Disabil. 2016;58:104–13. Epub 2016 Sep 5.
46. Aschendorff A, Klenzner T, Laszig R. Deafness after bacterial meningitis: an emergency for early imaging and cochlear implant surgery. Otolaryngol Head Neck Surg. 2005;133(6):995–6.
47. Sterkers O, Mosnier I, Ambert-Dahan E, Herelle-Dupuy E, Bozorg-Grayeli A, Bouccara D. Cochlear implants in elderly people: preliminary results. Acta Otolaryngol Suppl. 2004;552:64–7.
48. Wong DJ, Moran M, O'Leary SJ. Outcomes after cochlear implantation in the very elderly. Otol Neurotol. 2016;37(1):46–51.
49. Mosnier I, Bebear JP, Marx M, Fraysse B, Truy E, Lina-Granade G, Mondain M, Sterkers-Artières F, Bordure P, Robier A, Godey B, Meyer B, Frachet B, Poncet-Wallet C, Bouccara D, Sterkers O. Improvement of cognitive function after cochlear implantation in elderly patients. JAMA Otolaryngol Head Neck Surg. 2015;141(5):442–50. https://doi.org/10.1001/jamaoto.2015.129.
50. Helms J, Muller J, Schon F, Brill S. Cochlea-Implantation: Ergebnisse und Kosten, eine Ubersicht. Laryngorhinootologie. 2003;82(12):821–5.
51. Egger K, Majdak P, Laback B. Channel interaction and current level affect across-electrode integration of interaural time differences in bilateral cochlear-implant listeners. J Assoc Res Otolaryngol. 2016;17(1):55–67. https://doi.org/10.1007/s10162-015-0542-8. Epub 2015 Sep 16.
52. Wimmer W, Weder S, Caversaccio M, Kompis M. Speech intelligibility in noise with a pinna effect imitating cochlear implant processor. Otol Neurotol. 2016;37(1):19–23.

## *Suggested Reading*

Bauer PW, Sharma A, Martin K, Dorman M. Central auditory development in children with bilateral cochlear implants. Arch Otolaryngol Head Neck Surg. 2006;132(10):1133–6.
Blauert J. Räumliches Hören. Stuttgart: S. Hirzel Verlag; 1974.
Dodds A, Tyszkiewicz E, Ramsden R. Cochlear implantation after bacterial meningitis: the dangers of delay. Arch Dis Child. 1997;76(2):139–40.
Hellbrück J. Hören. Physiologie, Psychologie und Pathologie. Göttingen: Hogrefe Verlag; 1993.
House WF, Berliner KI, Eisenberg LS. Present status and future directions of the Ear Research Institute cochlear implant program. Acta Otolaryngol. 1979;87(3–4):176–84.

Kochs B. Entwicklung bei der Durchsetzung des Anspruchs auf beidseitige Implantation. Schnecke 49_S42-80.qxd 22.07.2005 15:52 Seite 62.

Konkle D, Schwartz D. Binaural amplication: a paradox. In: Bess FN, Freeman BA, Sinclair S, editors. Amplication in education. Washington, DC: Alexander Graham Bell Association for the Deaf; 1981. p. 342–57.

Lammers MJ, Lenarz T, van Zanten GA, Grolman W, Buechner A. Sound localization abilities of unilateral hybrid cochlear implant users with bilateral low-frequency hearing. Otol Neurotol. 2014;35(8):1433–9. https://doi.org/10.1097/MAO.0000000000000433.

Laszig R, Aschendorff A, Stecker M, Müller-Deile J, Maune S, Dillier N, Weber B, Hey M, Begall K, Lenarz T, Battmer RD, Bohm M, Steffens T, Strutz J, Linder T, Probst R, Allum J, Westhofen M, Doering W. Benefits of bilateral electrical stimulation with the nucleus cochlear implant in adults: 6-month postoperative results. Otol Neurotol. 2004;25:958–68.

Laszig R, Aschendorff A, Schipper J, Klenzner T. Aktuelle Entwicklung zum Kochleaimplantat. HNO. 2004;52(4):357–62.

Merkus P, van Furth AM, Goverts ST, Suèr M, Smits CF, Smit C. Postmeningitis deafness in young children: action warranted before obliteration of the cochlea. Ned Tijdschr Geneeskd. 2007;151(22):1209–13.

Müller J, Schön F, Helms J. Speech understanding in quiet and noise in bilateral users of the MED-EL COMBI 40/40+ cochlear implant system. Ear-Hear. 2002;23(3):198–206.

Müller J. Wiederherstellende Verfahren bei gestörtem Hören: Die apparative Versorgung der Schwerhörigkeit: Cochlea Implantate und Hirnstammimplantate Aktuelle Entwicklungen der letzten 10 Jahre. Laryngorhinootologie. 2005;84(Suppl 1):60–9.

Noble W. Assessing binaural hearing: results using the speech, spatial and qualities of hearing scale. J Am Acad Audiol. 2010;21(9):568–74.

Offeciers E, Morera C, Muller J, Huarte A, Shallop J, Cavalle L. International consensus on bilateral cochlear implants and bimodal stimulation. Acta Otolaryngol. 2005;125(9):918–9.

Pelizzone M, Kasper A, Montandon P. Binaural interaction in a cochlear implant patient. Hear Res. 1990;48(3):287–90.

Schön F, Müller J, Helms J. Speech reception thresholds obtained in a symmetrical four-loudspeaker arrangement from bilateral users of MED-EL cochlear implants. Otol Neurotol. 2002;23(5):710–4.

Wilson BS, Finley CC, Lawson DT, Wolford RD, Eddington DK, Rabinowitz WM. Better speech recognition with cochlear implants. Nature. 1991;352(6332):236–8.

Winkler F, Schön F, Peklo L, Müller J, Feinen C, Helms J. Würzburger Fragebogen zur Hörqualitat bei CI-Kindern (WH-CIK). The Wurzburg questionnaire for assessing the quality of hearing in CI-children (WHCIK). Laryngorhinootologie. 2002;81(3):211–6.

Zheng Y, Godar SP, Litovsky RY. Development of sound localization strategies in children with bilateral cochlear implants. PLoS One. 2015;10(8):e0135790. https://doi.org/10.1371/journal.pone.0135790. eCollection 2015. PMID: 26288142.

Dhanasingh A, Hochmair I. Thirty years of translational research behind MED-EL. Acta Oto Laryngologica. 2021;141(Suppl 1):i-cxcvi. https://doi.org/10.1080/00016489.2021.1918399.

# Subtotal Petrosectomy and Cochlear Implantation

# 13

Mario Sanna, Gianluca Piras, and Lorenzo Lauda

## 13.1 Introduction

Patient eligibility for cochlear implantation has dramatically expanded in the last decades due to ongoing technological progress and increasing accessibility. Alongside this development, otologists are faced with a growing class of patients for which classical posterior tympanotomy (PT) may be technically challenging or at high risk for complications, such as in chronic otitis media (COM), previous open mastoidectomy and inner ear malformations (IEM).

The abovementioned conditions have been addressed through various surgical techniques, out of which subtotal petrosectomy (STP) has stood out in time as an efficient and reliable procedure [1–19]. This practice warrants multiple benefits including eradication of middle ear/mastoid disease, safe/stable environment for cochlear implantation, wide surgical exposure, accurate identification of anatomical landmarks, enhanced array stability, optimal management of intraoperative adverse findings (i.e., cerebrospinal fluid (CSF) leaks or meningo-encephalic herniations (MEH)), eliminates the need for lifelong cavity care. The main principles of the surgical technique are secure double-blind sac closure of the external auditory canal (EAC), extensive drill of all mastoid cell tracts, comprehensive removal of the tympanomastoid disease and mucosa, occlusion of the eustachian tube (ET), and obliteration of remnant mastoid cavity.

**Supplementary Information** The online version contains supplementary material available at [https://doi.org/10.1007/978-981-19-0452-3_13].

M. Sanna (✉) · G. Piras · L. Lauda
Gruppo Otologico and Mario Sanna Foundation, Piacenza-Rome, Italy
e-mail: mario.sanna@gruppootologico.com


S. DeSaSouza (ed.), *Cochlear Implants*,
https://doi.org/10.1007/978-981-19-0452-3_13

Published results concerning STP with cochlear implant (CI) insertion are encouraging. So, the validity and widespread acceptance of this method as current standard practice, as well as clear indications have been established [3, 7, 8, 17].

The main indications for STP with Cochlear Implantation are:

- COM/Cholesteatoma/Osteoradionecrosis of the temporal bone
- Presence of a radical cavity/canal wall down technique
- Cochlear ossification/obliteration
- Inner ear malformations (IEM)
- Fracture of the temporal bone with otic capsule involvement
- Revision cases
- Unfavorable anatomical conditions for posterior tympanotomy

## 13.2 Subtotal Petrosectomy with Cochlear Implantation: Surgical Anatomy (Figs. 13.1, 13.2, 13.3, 13.4, 13.5, 13.6, 13.7, 13.8, 13.9, and 13.10)

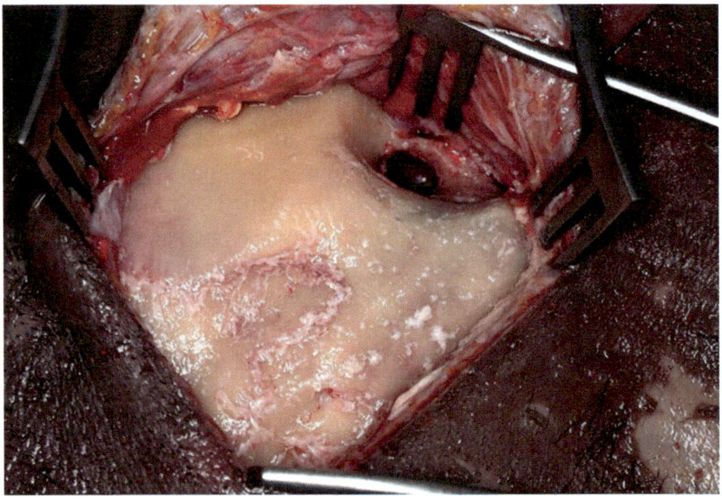

**Fig. 13.1** Skin incision, musculo-periosteal flap. Right ear. A wide retroauricular incision along the hairline gives best access, the pinna and subcutaneous tissue should be reflected anteriorly for the work on the blind sac closure

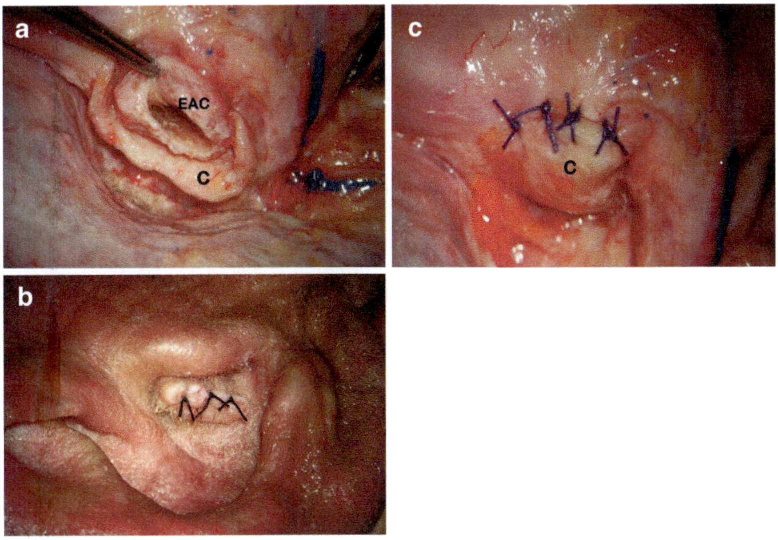


**Fig. 13.2** (**a**–**c**) Blind sac closure of the EAC. (**a**) In the plane beneath the pedicled flap, the skin and cartilage (*C*) of the external auditory canal (*EAC*) are transected. Anteriorly a clamp could be passed underneath the subcutaneous tissue anterior from the tragal cartilage for protection of the vascular capsule of the parotid gland and branches of the facial nerve. More lateral transection of the skin and cartilage of the external ear canal give less risk to the parotid capsula and facial nerve branches. The skin of the lateral part of the external canal is elevated from the cartilage for the length of 1 cm and is subsequently everted. (**b**) The skin edges, now on the outside, are sutured with resorbable vicryl 4.0 sutures. (**c**) The second layer consisting of subcutaneous tissue or tragal cartilage is folded back and sutured to the anterior rim of the remaining cartilage (*C*)

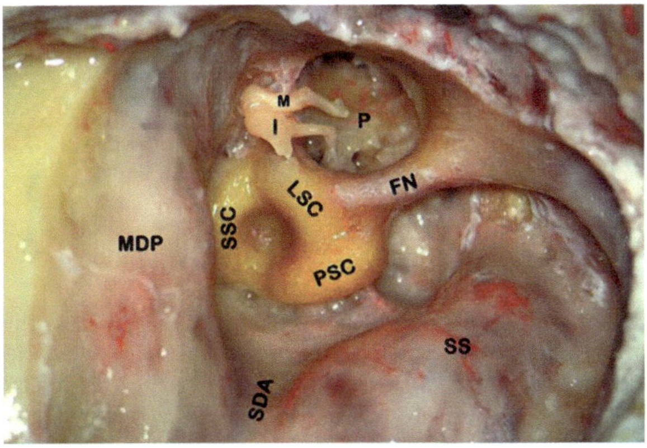


**Fig. 13.3** Canal wall down mastoidectomy. The external auditory canal (EAC) skin is elevated from the EAC up to the level of the annulus. The lateral part of the skin is removed. The more medial part is removed in a later stage together with the tympanic membrane, annulus, and ossicles. After mobilizing the subcutaneous tissue and temporalis muscle a canal wall down mastoidectomy can be performed, removing as many pneumatized cells as possible. Some surgeons also remove the mastoid tip. Abbreviations: *MDP* middle fossa dura plate, *SS* sigmoid sinus, *SDA* sinodural angle, *SSC* superior semicircular canal, *PSC* posterior semicircular canal, *LSC* lateral semicircular canal, *FN* facial nerve, *I* incus, *M* malleus, *P* promontory

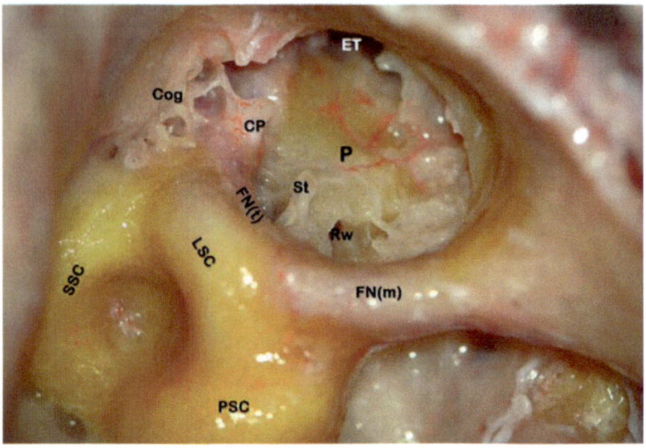


**Fig. 13.4** Removal of the skin of the medial portion of the external ear canal with annulus, malleus, and incus. The medial remnant of the skin of the EAC with the annulus is now elevated. The incudo-stapedial joint is separated. Skin, annulus, and tympanic membrane with malleus and incus can be removed en-block to lower the risk of leaving some skin behind. Abbreviations: *LSC* lateral semicircular canal, *SSC* superior semicircular canal, *PSC* posterior semicircular canal, *FN(t)* tympanic segment of the facial nerve, *FN(m)* mastoid segment of the facial nerve, *P* promontory, *M* malleus, *I* incus. *St* stapes, *RW* round window, *P* promontory, *ET* Eustachian tube, *CP* cochleariform process

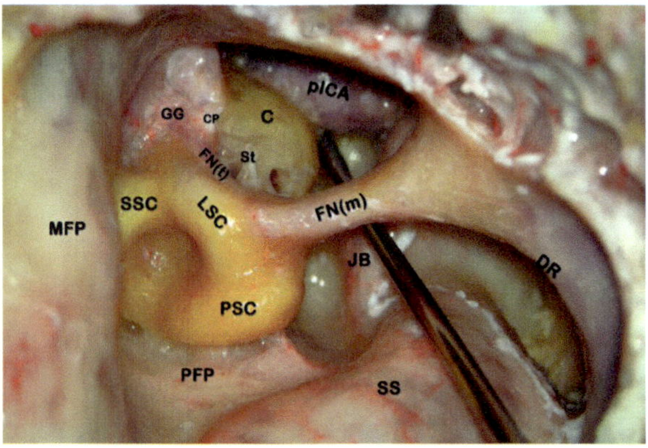


**Fig. 13.5** Removal of subfacial, infralabyrinthine, and pericarotid air cells. This step is not performed in case of Cochlear Implantation, but is useful to remark the boundaries of the subtotal petrosectomy, as described by Fisch [20]. Abbreviations: *LSC* lateral semicircular canal, *PSC* posterior semicircular canal, *SSC* superior semicircular canal, *FN(t)* tympanic segment of the facial nerve, *FN(m)* mastoid segment of the facial nerve, *GG* geniculate ganglion, *C* cochlea, *St* stapes, *CP* cochleariform process, *pICA* petrous internal carotid artery, *SS* sigmoid sinus, *DR* digastric ridge, *JB* jugular bulb

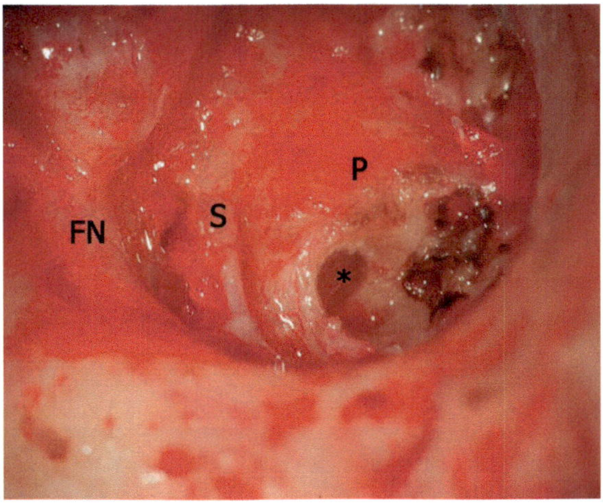


**Fig. 13.6** Exposure of the round window. Surgical view, right ear. Comparable to normal cochlear implantation the round window niche is widened by removing the superior and anterior-inferior overhangs by drilling. Abbreviations: *S* stapes, *FN* tympanic portion of the facial nerve, *P* promontory; *Asterisk* round window membrane

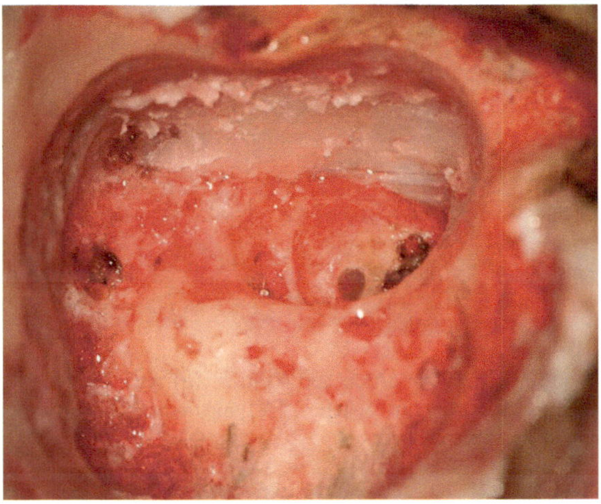

**Fig. 13.7** Closure of the Eustachian tube. The Eustachian tube is sealed with periosteum and bone wax

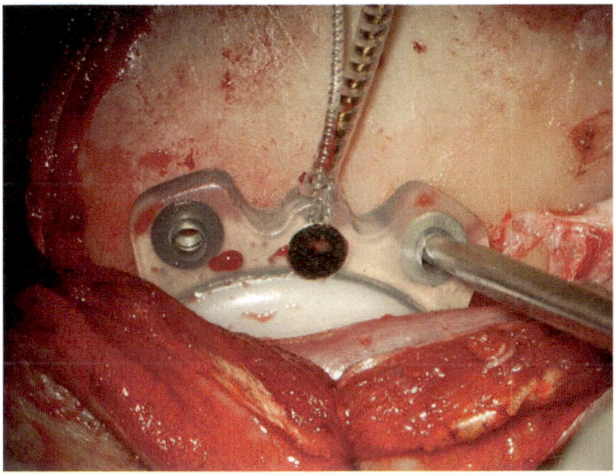

**Fig. 13.8** Implant fixation. Depending on the type of CI a receiver well is drilled or just a pocket underneath the temporalis muscle is created. In this case, a pocket underneath the temporalis muscle is created and the CI is fixated with screws

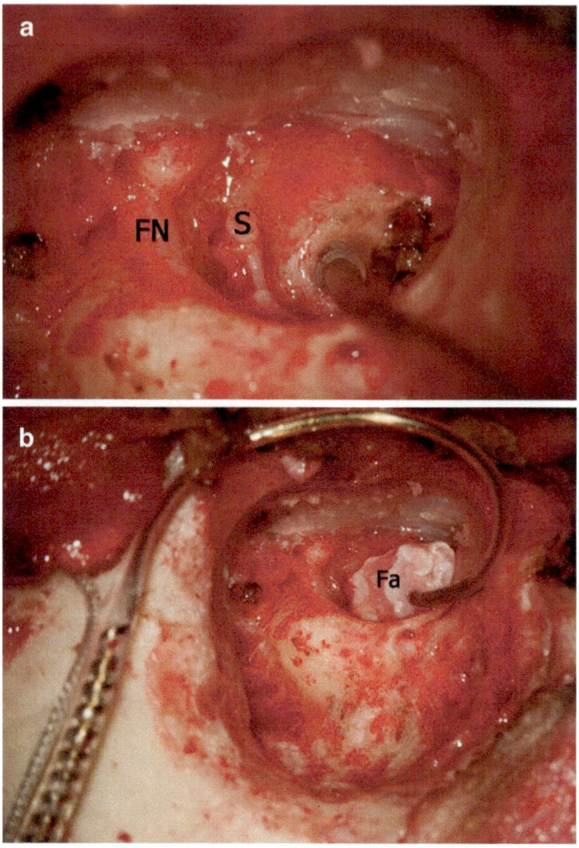


**Fig. 13.9** Array insertion and fixation. (**a**) Array insertion through the round window is performed. Abbreviations: *S* stapes, *FN* tympanic. (**b**) The array is fixated with fascia (*Fa*) in the round window cochleostomy

**Fig. 13.10** Obliteration of the cavity with fat. The cavity is filled with abdominal fat (*F*) marinated in an antibiotic solution (yellow color)

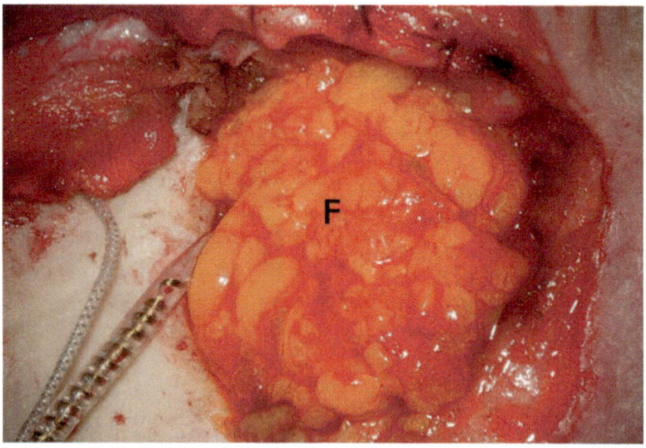

## 13.3 Indications

### 13.3.1 COM/Cholesteatoma/Osteoradionecrosis of the Temporal Bone

The most important risk of cochlear implantation in case of COM is represented by a returning infection leading to either labyrinthitis or meningitis or leading to extrusion of the CI. This can be either extrusion of the electrode array out of the cochlea or through the tympanic membrane, or breakdown of the retroauricular skin covering the receiver-stimulator [12–15]. Also the fact that the CI might be introduced through a contaminated field during a single-stage procedure has to be considered. In chronic suppurative otitis media tympanoplasty in the same procedure or in a staged procedure is the alternative option, however with the remaining risk of recurrence of disease [12–18]. In case of recurrence of disease revision surgery in the presence of a CI is always a challenge with a significant risk of accidentally sacrificing the implant during the procedure. Sparing the CI during the revision procedure while at the same time performing radical surgery with removal of all pathology is challenging, if not impossible. On the contrary, a staged procedure means postponing the cochlear implantation, which is not always favorable.

In case of cholesteatoma, a simultaneous cochlear implantation through an STP can be performed only when a total removal of the disease and matrix is secured. In case of doubt about radicality, a staged procedure with cochlear implantation after 6–12 months is recommended. However, it has to be considered that a recurrence of cholesteatoma is possible even after 12 months. So, a radiological follow-up is necessary due to the risk of residual cholesteatoma in the obliterated cavity.

In both types of pathology (COM with/without cholesteatoma), an STP gives higher chances of radical removal of the disease and avoids further infection of the cavity due to exclusion of the middle ear space [16, 18].

An atelectatic middle ear is common in COM and may lead to the development of cholesteatoma. Therefore, an STP should be preferred in these cases and in general for patients with an impaired ET function (i.e., cleft palate) [19, 21].

In case of osteoradionecrosis, the blood supply to the temporal bone is compromised with resulting necrotizing bone. This pathology can be treated with local debridement, local antibiotics, hyperbaric oxygen and sometimes surgical removal of bone sequesters. Due to the radiation after tonsillar, nasopharyngeal, or parotid tumors, the cochlear function could decrease over time [22], resulting in a bilateral hearing loss. Management of these cases can be challenging but an ear without any infection and rehabilitated with a CI is possible [23].

### 13.3.2 Presence of a Radical Cavity/Canal Wall Down Technique

Early attempts to insert the CI in a radical cavity/canal wall down procedure resulted in a high rate of complications, mainly extrusion of the array through the very thin epithelial lining of the cavity [10, 12, 18, 24]. Also, cavities are in direct contact with the external environment and can easily and repeatedly become infected. These patients usually need cleaning of the cavity once or twice a year and this procedure can lead to damage of the epithelial lining with a potential risk for the implant. Infections of the cavity give are at risk of developing labyrinthitis and meningitis and of implant extrusion (Figs. 13.11, 13.12, 13.13, 13.14, 13.15, 13.16, 13.17, 13.18, and 13.19).

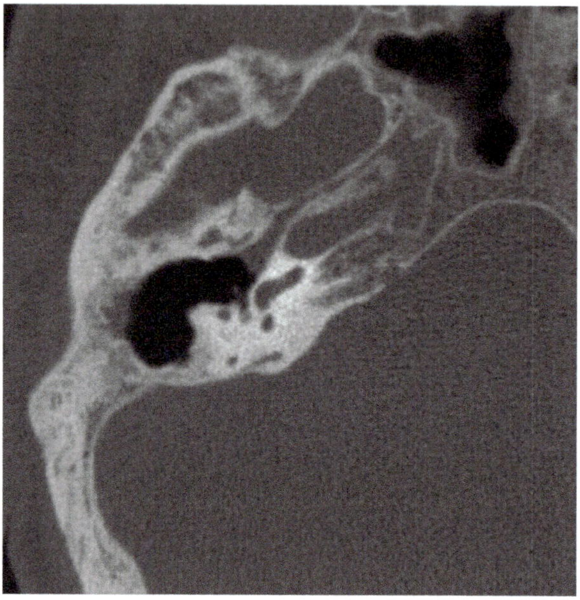

**Fig. 13.11** **Case 1.** This case represents an example of STP combined with CI in a previous radical cavity. A 70-year-old man underwent a right radical tympanoplasty with anacusis 17 years before our last clinical consultation. On the other side, he had residual hearing with minimal benefit from a hearing aid. On CT scan there were no signs of cochlear ossification

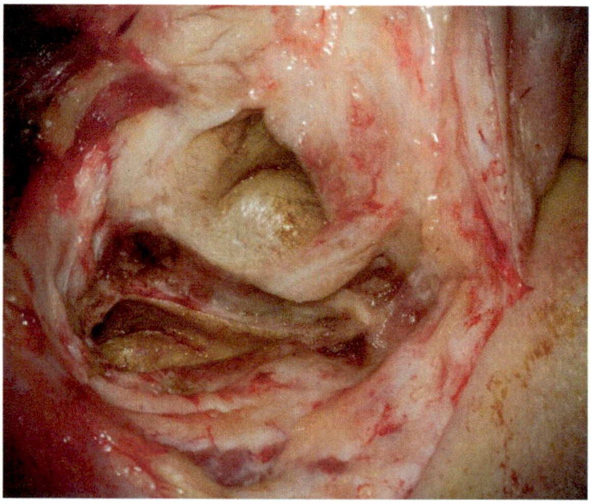

**Fig. 13.12** **Case 1.** Transection of the EAC of the previously enlarged meatus

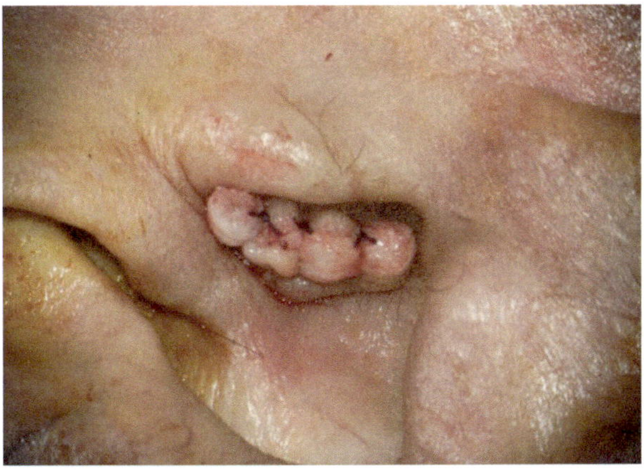

**Fig. 13.13** **Case 1.** The skin is everted and sutured using resorbable material

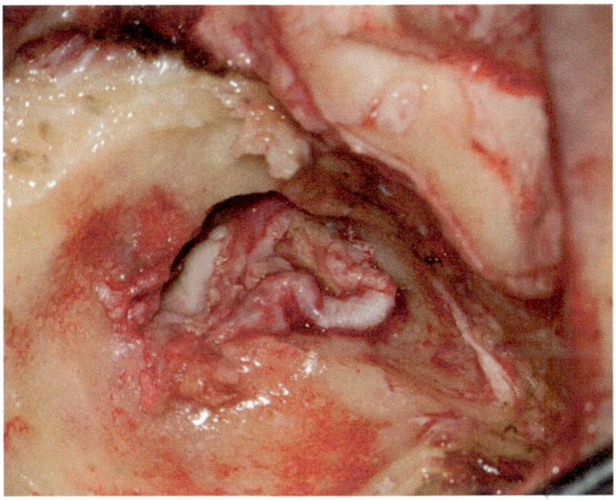

**Fig. 13.14** **Case 1.** The skin lining of the cavity has to be removed meticulously. This is to prevent entrapment of skin that can develop into cholesteatoma once the cavity is closed off

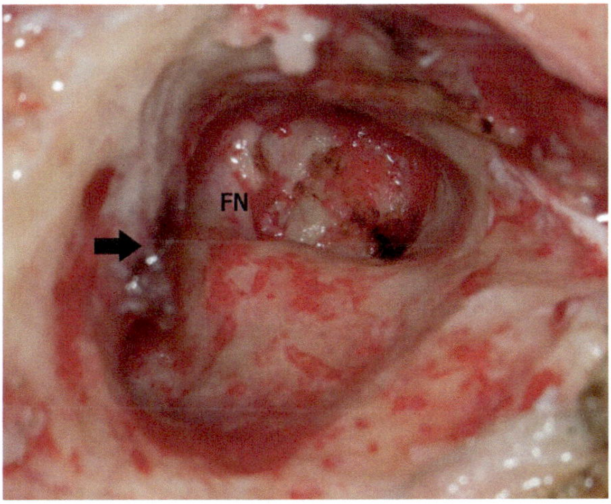


**Fig. 13.15** **Case 1.** Removal of the skin and tympanic membrane with the ossicles has been completed. Abbreviations: *FN* facial nerve, *arrow* meningo-encephalic herniation

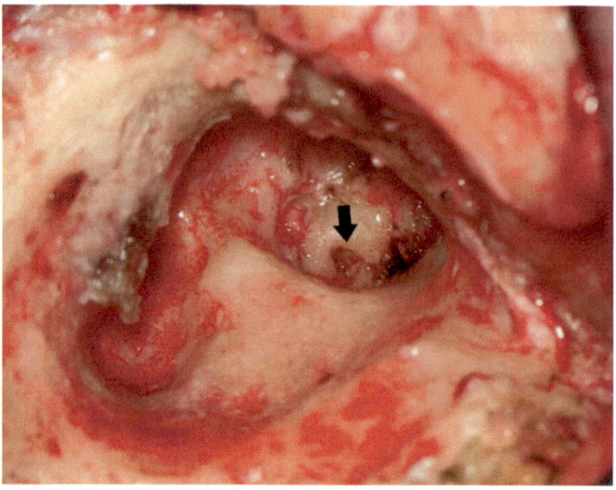

**Fig. 13.16** **Case 1.** The area of the RW niche (*arrow*) is cleaned

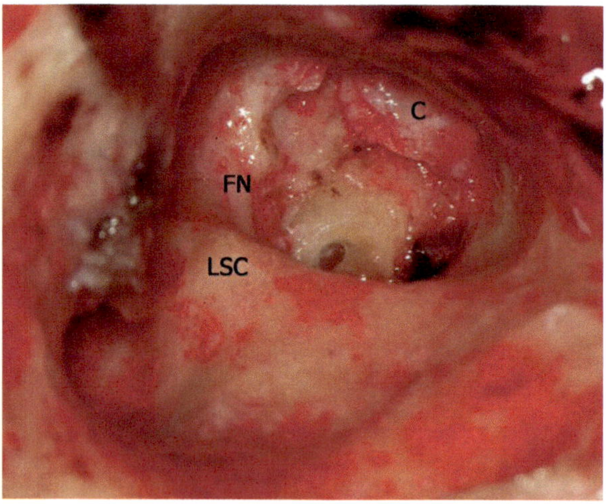


**Fig. 13.17** **Case 1.** The bony borders of the RW niche are drilled, allowing visualization and exposure of the RW membrane. Then, the ET is obliterated with cartilage and periosteum (*C*) to exclude the cavity from the nasopharynx. Abbreviation: *FN* facial nerve, *LSC* lateral semicircular canal

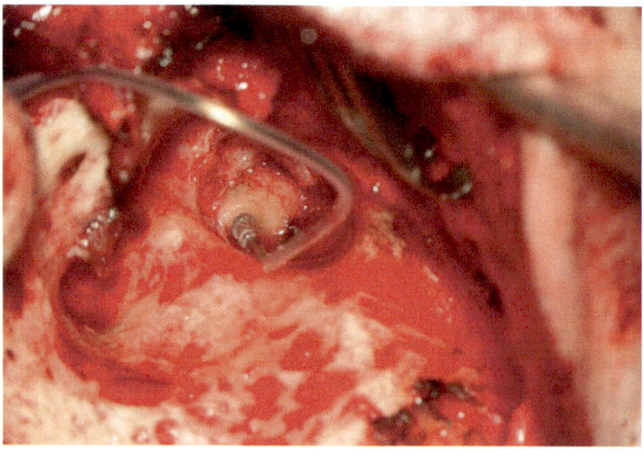

**Fig. 13.18** **Case 1.** After implant fixation, a full array insertion has been accomplished

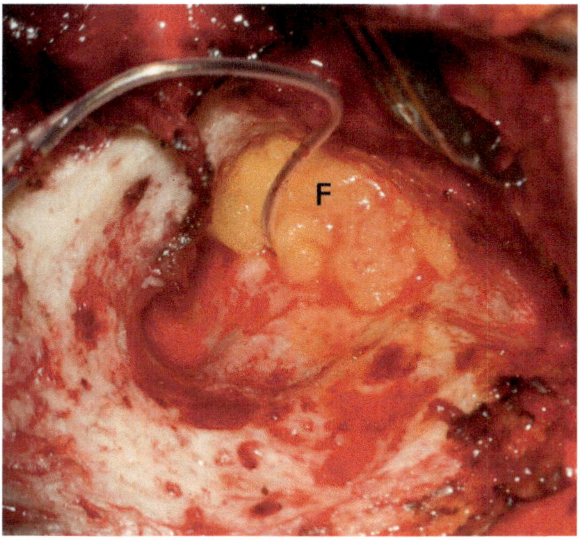


**Fig. 13.19** **Case 1.** After electrophysiologic tests, the cavity is obliterated with abdominal fat (*F*)

### 13.3.3 Cochlear Ossification/Obliteration

A partially or totally obliterated cochlea can be present as a result of [25–27]:

- Bacterial meningitis
- Autoimmune inner ear disease
- Fracture of the labyrinth/intracochlear hemorrhage/labyrinthitis
- COM or cavity infection
- Loss of labyrinthine blood supply (i.e., after translabyrinthine surgery)
- Otosclerosis

In presence of cochlear ossification cochlear implantation through a drill-out procedure of the cochlea would be the first step in hearing rehabilitation, because cochlear implantation is expected to give better hearing results than ABI [25]. Theoretically the drill-out procedure may be performed through a PT approach. However, this may result in a demanding and dangerous situation, because the narrow approach does not permit a complete control of all the anatomical landmarks. A dangerous complication of a drill-out procedure through a PT approach could be damage of the carotid artery, which is located in close relationship with the most anterior part of the basal and middle turns of the cochlea. STP offers an unobstructed view of all middle ear anatomy, with identification of additional structures such as the carotid artery and jugular bulb, when required. Unfortunately, not all attempts of a drill-out procedure lead to a successful implantation as the cochlear lumen cannot always be found. In case the drill-out procedure fails, surgical conversion to an auditory brainstem implant (ABI) can be done during the same procedure [27] (Figs. 13.20, 13.21, 13.22, 13.23, 13.24, and 13.25).

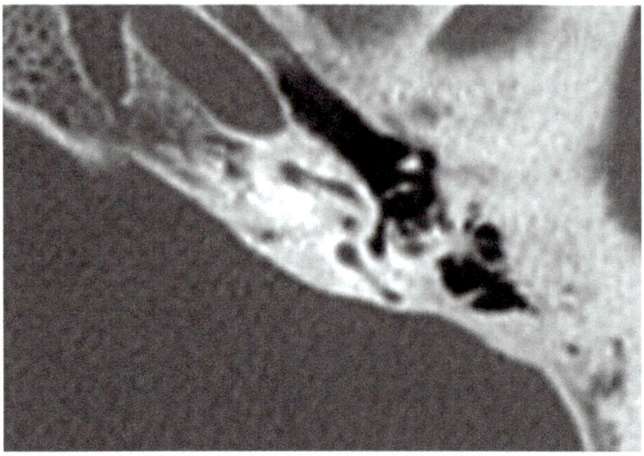

**Fig. 13.20 Case 2.** Case of basal turn ossification with patent scala vestibuli in a patient with advanced otosclerosis

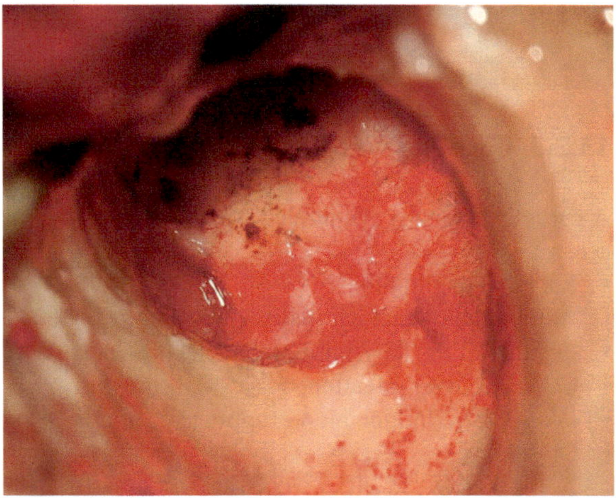

**Fig. 13.21 Case 2.** RW area is under view after removal of the canal wall, the eardrum and the remaining ossicles. Also the soft tissue in the middle ear is removed and the drill-out procedure is started, using with the oval window and RW as landmarks

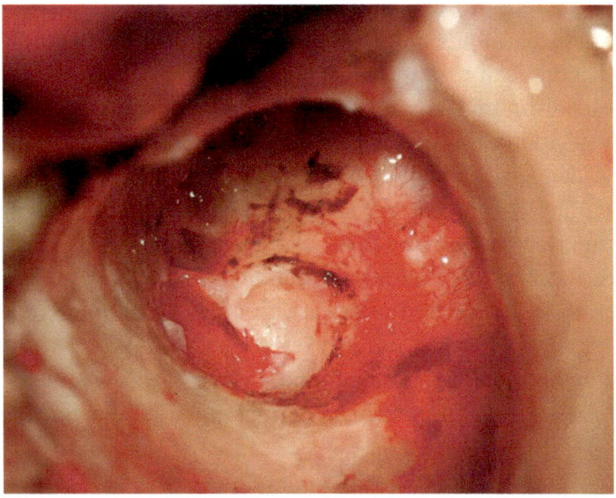

**Fig. 13.22 Case 2.** The drill-out procedure is started. As expected, no lumen is visible in the scala tympani area

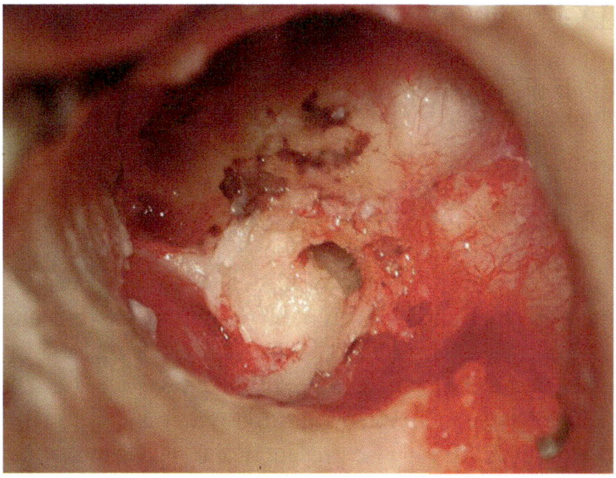

**Fig. 13.23** **Case 2.** The scala vestibuli opening is enlarged

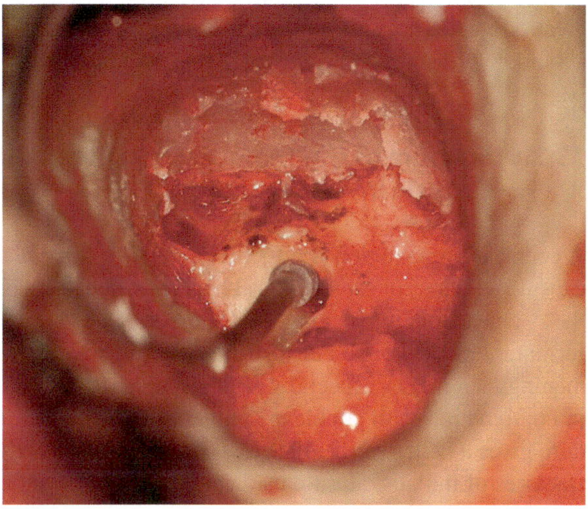

**Fig. 13.24** **Case 2.** A full implantation through the scala vestibuli is completed. Neural response measurements confirmed a functional implant and a correct placement of the array. The ET is closed and the cavity obliterated with fat at the end of the procedure

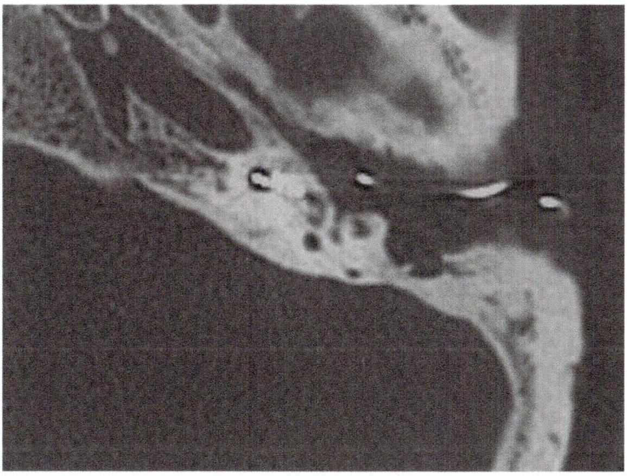

**Fig. 13.25** **Case 2.** Postoperative CT scan shows the more anterior position of the array within the basal turn according to the scala vestibuli position

### 13.3.4 Inner Ear Malformations

There are three reasons to perform cochlear implantation using the STP technique in IEM.

First, there is the need to identify the available landmarks; aberrances of middle ear structures like the RW niche and facial nerve can be present. Second, the possibility of an intraoperative CSF leak/gusher is higher in IEM. In literature up to 45% of the CI cases with various kinds of malformations resulted in a CSF leakage during surgery [28–30]. The CSF leak/gusher is better controlled by obliteration of the ET orifice and removal of all peritubal cells, closure of the EAC and obliteration of the cavity. Third, in IEM the risk of developing meningitis during lifespan is higher than in the normal population, even without CI surgery [28]. In some IEM (especially in incomplete partition type I and type III) a cystic structure filled with perilymph/CSF may be present at the oval window niche, with the bony footplate being incomplete [28, 31] .

Therefore, in case of a common cavity malformation the introduction of a straight electrode via a transmastoid translabyrintotomy technique combined with an STP should be preferred [32].

### 13.3.5 Fracture of the Temporal Bone with Otic Capsule Involvement

A cochlear implantation is possible in severe trauma leading to a fracture of the otic capsule with loss of sensorineural hearing when the cochlear nerve is still intact and the cochlear lumen patent [33–35]. Fractures of the otic capsule do not heal with formation of new bone but just by a fibrous bonding. Therefore, a lifelong risk of meningitis remains, especially after a standard CI approach [36]. In these cases STP in combination with cochlear implantation is mandatory. Additionally, this procedure gives a better surgical access and exposure of the fractured temporal bone. As fractures of the otic capsule can lead to cochlear ossification, urgent evaluation for a cochlear implantation is necessary (Figs. 13.26, 13.27, and 13.28).

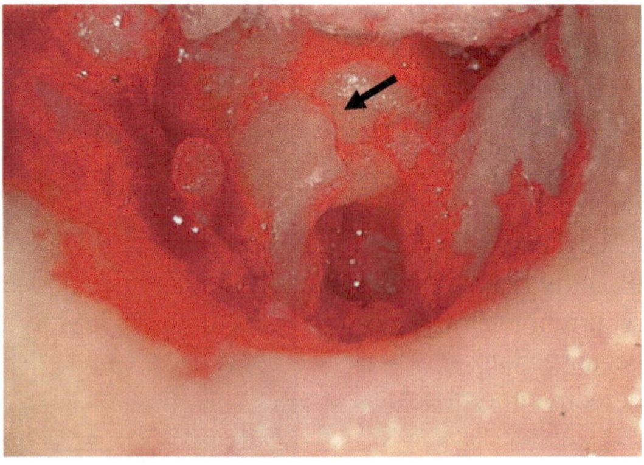

**Fig. 13.26** Case 3. Patient with otic capsule fracture (*arrow*). This case underwent previous ABI implantation with no hearing results. Preoperative CT scan showed a patent cochlea. So, a cochlear implantation through an STP was performed with satisfying results

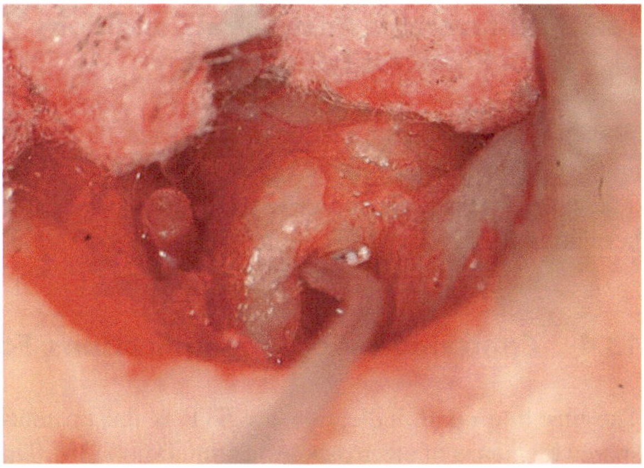

**Fig. 13.27** **Case 3.** Full array insertion

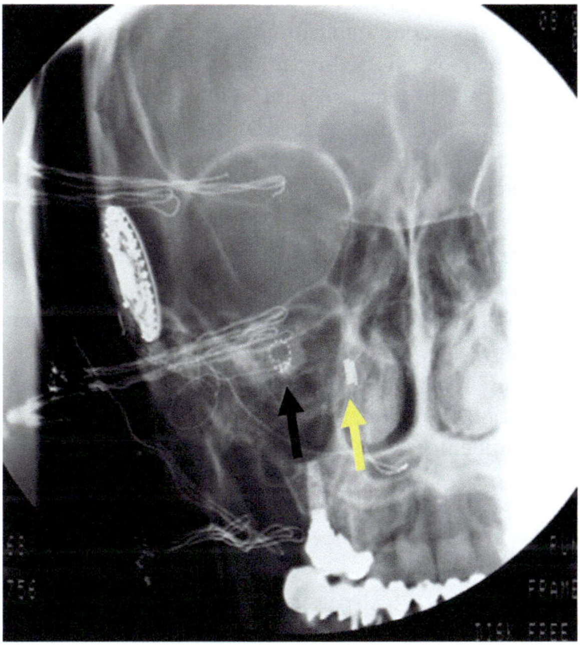

**Fig. 13.28** **Case 3.** Postoperative X-ray shows the presence of both the CI (*black arrow*) and the ABI (*yellow arrow*)

### 13.3.6 Revision Cases

In case of multiple surgeries with failed array insertion, an STP should be performed to increase the surgical view of all the middle ear landmarks and facilitate an eventual drill-out procedure.

### 13.3.7 Unfavorable Anatomical Conditions for Posterior Tympanotomy

A standard cochlear implantation could not be easy to perform in cases with an anteriorly positioned sigmoid sinus or other anatomical limitations. Additionally, an STP would be the preferred approach for a CI in case of dural or meningo-encephalic herniation [8, 37].

## 13.4 Contraindications, Complications, Follow-Up

The absolute contraindication for STP is the presence of residual hearing to be spared by means of electroacoustic stimulation [38]. This technique requires a wider speech processor with an intrameatal (acoustic) hearing aid. Therefore, an open EAC is mandatory for the acoustic part of this stimulation.

A relative contraindication is the presence of active purulent infection of the middle ear or cavity, in particular in case of multi-resistant microorganisms or tuberculosis. In such condition, a first stage STP with total eradication of the infection under antibiotic coverage has to be performed. After 3 to 6 months, when there is no sign of infection, the obliterated cavity can be re-opened and the cochlear implantation performed.

Risks specifically ascribed to the STP approach are infection of the abdominal fat, breakdown of the blind sac closure and entrapment of cholesteatoma in the closed cavity (‘entrapped cholesteatoma’). Additional risks are related to the abdominal wound, as infection or subcutaneous hematoma.

Follow-up with CT scan at 1, 3, 5, and 10 years postoperatively is mandatory. The presence of a CI limits the use of magnetic resonance imaging in the postoperative period. However, the abdominal fat in the surgical cavity creates an ideal interface for identification of residual/recurrent cholesteatoma on CT scan [1, 39].

## References


1. Sanna M, Free R, Merkus P, et al. Surgery for cochlear and other auditory implants. Stuttgart: Georg Thieme Verlag; 2016.
2. Casserly P, Friedland PL, Atlas MD. The role of subtotal petrosectomy in cochlear implantation. J Laryngol Otol. 2016;130:S35–40.
3. Polo R, Del Mar MM, Arístegui M, et al. Subtotal petrosectomy for cochlear implantation: lessons learned after 110 cases. Ann Otol Rhinol Laryngol. 2016;125:485–94.
4. Barañano CF, Kopelovich JC, Dunn CC, Gantz BJ, Hansen MR. Subtotal petrosectomy and mastoid obliteration in adult and pediatric cochlear implant recipients. Otol Neurotol. 2013;34(9):1656–9.
5. Szymański M, Ataide A, Linder T. The use of subtotal petrosectomy in cochlear implant candidates with chronic otitis media. Eur Arch Otorhinolaryngol. 2016;273:363–70.
6. Postelmans JTF, Stokroos RJ, Linmans JJ, Kremer B. Cochlear implantations in patients with chronic otitis media: 7-years’ experience in Maastricht. Eur Arch Otorhinolaryngol. 2009;266:1159–65.

7. Bernardeschi D, Nguyen Y, Smail M, et al. Middle ear and mastoid obliteration for cochlear implant in adults: indications and anatomical results. Otol Neurotol. 2015;36:604–9.
8. Free RH, Falcioni M, Di Trapani G, Giannuzzi AL, Russo A, Sanna M. The role of subtotal petrosectomy in cochlear implant surgery—a report of 32 cases and review on indications. Otol Neurotol. 2013;34:1033–40.
9. Altuna X, García L, Martínez Z, Pinedo MF. The role of subtotal petrosectomy in cochlear implant recipients. Eur Arch Otorhinolaryngol. 2017;274:4149.
10. Issing PR, Schonermark MP, Winkelmann S, et al. Cochlear implantation in patients with chronic otitis: indications for subtotal petrosectomy and obliteration of the middle ear. Skull Base. 1998;3:127–31.
11. Gray RF, Irving RM. Cochlear implants in chronic suppurative otitis media. Am J Otol. 1995;16:682–6.
12. Leung R, Briggs RJS. Indications for and outcomes of mastoid obliteration in cochlear implantation. Otol Neurotol. 2007;28:330–4.
13. Vincenti V, Pasanisi E, Bacciu A, Bacciu S. Long-term results of external auditory canal closure and mastoid obliteration in cochlear implantation after radical mastoidectomy: a clinical and radiological study. Eur Arch Otolaryngol. 2014;27:2127–30.
14. Kim CS, Chang SO, Lee HJ, et al. Cochlear implantation in patients with a history of chronic otitis media. Acta Otolaryngol. 2004;124:1033–8.
15. Incesulu A, Kocaturk S, Vural M. Cochlear implantation in chronic otitis media. J Laryngol Otol. 2004;118:3–7.
16. Sanna M, Dispenza F, Flanagan S, De Stefano A, Falcioni M. Management of chronic otitis by middle ear obliteration with blind sac closure of the external auditory canal. Otol Neurotol. 2008;29:19–22.
17. Prasad SC, Roustan V, Piras G, Caruso A, Lauda L, Sanna M. Subtotal petrosectomy: surgical technique, indications, outcomes, and comprehensive review of literature. Laryngoscope. 2017;127:2833–42.
18. Vashishth A, Fulcheri A, Prasad SC, Dandinarasaiah M, Caruso A, Sanna M. Cochlear implantation in chronic otitis media with cholesteatoma and open cavities: long-term surgical outcomes. Otol Neurotol. 2018;39:45–53.
19. Cohen NL, Hoffman R. Complications of cochlear implant surgery in adults and children. Ann Otol Rhinol Laryngol. 1991;100:708–11.
20. Fisch U, Mattox D. Microsurgery of the skull base. Stuttgart: Georg Thieme Verlag; 1988.
21. Roehm PC, Gantz BJ. Cochlear implant explantation as a sequel of severe chronic otitis media: case report and review of the literature. Otol Neurotol. 2006;27:332–6.
22. van der Putten L, de Bree R, Plukker JT, Langendijk JA, Smits C, Burlage FR, Leemans CR. Permanent unilateral hearing loss after radiotherapy for parotid gland tumors. Head Neck. 2006;28(10):902–8.
23. Adunka OF, Buchman CA. Cochlear implantation in the irradiated temporal bone. J Laryngol Otol. 2007;121(1):83–6.
24. Pasanisi E, Vincenti V, Bacciu A, Guida M, Berghenti T. Cochlear implantation in radical mastoidectomy cavities. Otolaryngol Head Neck Surg. 2002;127:432–6.
25. Vashishth A, Fulcheri A, Prasad SC, Bassi M, Rossi G, Caruso A, Sanna M. Cochlear implantation in cochlear ossification: retrospective review of etiologies, surgical considerations, and auditory outcomes. Otol Neurotol. 2018;39:17–28.
26. Vashishth A, Fulcheri A, Rossi G, Prasad SC, Caruso A, Sanna M. Cochlear implantation in otosclerosis: surgical and auditory outcomes with a brief on facial nerve stimulation. Otol Neurotol. 2017;38:e345–53.
27. Sanna M, Khrais T, Guida M, Falcioni M. Auditory brainstem implant in a child with severely ossified cochlea. Laryngoscope. 2006;116:1700–3.
28. Sennaroglu L. Cochlear implantation in inner ear malformations – a review article. Cochlear Implants Int. 2010;11(1):4–41.

29. Farhood Z, Nguyen SA, Miller SC, Holcomb MA, Meyer TA, Rizk HG. Cochlear implantation in inner ear malformations: systematic review of speech perception outcomes and intraoperative findings. 2017;156:783–93.
30. Isaiah A, Lee D, Lenes-Voit F, et al. Clinical outcomes following cochlear implantation in children with inner ear anomalies. Int J Pediatr Otorhinolaryngol. 2017;93:1–6.
31. Ehmer DR Jr, Booth T, Kutz JW Jr, Roland PS. Radiographic diagnosis of trans-stapedial cerebrospinal fluid fistula. Otolaryngol Head Neck Surg. 2010;142(5):694–8.
32. McElveen JT, Carrasco VN, Miyamoto RT, Linthicum FH. Cochlear implantation in common cavity malformations using a transmastoid labryinthotomy approach. Laryngescope. 1997;107:1032–6.
33. Khwaja S, Mawman D, Nichani J, Bruce I, Green K, Lloyd S. Cochlear implantation in patients profoundly deafened after head injury. Otol Neurotol. 2012;33:1328–32.
34. Serin GM, Derinsu U, Sarı M, et al. Cochlear implantation in patients with 470 bilateral cochlear trauma. Am J Otolaryngol. 2010;31:350–5.
35. Medina M, Di Lella F, Di Trapani G, et al. Cochlear implantation versus auditory brainstem implantation in bilateral total deafness after head trauma: personal experience and review of the literature. Otol Neurotol. 2014;35:260–70.
36. Sudhoff H, Linthicum FH. Temporal bone fracture and latent meningitis: temporal bone histopathology – study of the month. Otol Neurotol. 2003;24:521–2.
37. Feenstra L, Sanna M, Zini C, Gamoletti R, Delogu P. Surgical treatment of brain herniation into the middle ear and mastoid. Am J Otolaryngol. 1985;4:311–3.
38. Von Ilberg CA, Baumann U, Kiefer J, Tillein J, Adunka OF. Electric-acoustic stimulation of the auditory system: a review of the first decade. Audiol Neurootol. 2011;16:1–30.
39. De Foer B, Vercruysse JP, Pouillon M, et al. Value of high-resolution computed tomography and magnetic resonance imaging in the detection of residual cholesteatomas in primary bony obliterated mastoids. Am J Otolaryngol. 2007;28:230–4.

# 14 Cochlear Implants for Single-Sided Deafness

Emily Kay-Rivest, J. Thomas Roland Jr, and David R. Friedmann

## 14.1 Introduction

Single-sided deafness (SSD) refers to a severe to profound sensorineural hearing loss (SNHL) in one ear, with normal or close to normal hearing in the other ear. A more precise definition was provided in 2015, during a round table panel discussion focusing on asymmetric hearing loss interventions [1]. They defined SSD as a severe to profound loss in the poorer ear, with a pure-tone average (PTA) of 30 dB HL or above in the better ear [1]. Asymmetric hearing loss (AHL) was defined as severe to profound loss in the poorer ear, with a threshold above 30 dB HL but less than or equal to 60 dB HL in the better hearing ear. The PTA was calculated using four frequencies (0.5, 1, 2 and 4 kHz). These definitions were proposed in order to promote uniformity in reporting of results.

Currently, the rehabilitation options available to those with SSD include a contralateral routing of signal hearing aid (CROS-HA), a bone conduction device (BCD) and a cochlear implant (CI). A cochlear implant is the intervention best suited to restore aspects of binaural hearing, with the potential benefits of better speech understanding in quiet and in noise, improved sound localization, improved quality of life, and possible tinnitus suppression [2–9].

This chapter will describe the prevalence and etiologies of SSD and then focus on the current literature regarding candidacy criteria and outcomes of cochlear implants in adults and children with SSD.

E. Kay-Rivest · J. T. Roland Jr · D. R. Friedmann (✉)
Department of Otolaryngology—Head and Neck Surgery, Division of Otology and Neurotology, New York University, New York, NY, USA
e-mail: David.friedmann@nyulangone.org


S. DeSaSouza (ed.), *Cochlear Implants*,
https://doi.org/10.1007/978-981-19-0452-3_14

## 14.2 Prevalence of Single-Sided Deafness

The prevalence of SSD is not clear from available literature. This is due to several confounding factors, including the lack of a consistent definition used in reporting. Recently, Golub et al. reviewed data from the US National Health and Nutrition Examination Study (NHANES) [10]. This database provides air conduction thresholds of individuals over the age of 18. With this information, Golub and his colleagues estimated that the prevalence of unilateral hearing loss (worse ear above or equal to 41 dB HL) was 1.5%. It can therefore be assumed that the rates of SSD in adults are likely to be much lower than 1%.

The prevalence of unilateral hearing loss at birth and in school-aged children is estimated at 0.3% and 3%, respectively [11]. However, as in many reports, this encompasses all unilateral hearing loss, ranging from mild to profound. A report by Ross et al. highlighted this variability by evaluating the NHANES data but using different definitions and criteria for unilateral hearing loss. Just changing the frequencies used to calculate the PTA had a significant effect on the prevalence [12]. Unfortunately, many of the epidemiological studies evaluating pediatric unilateral hearing loss do not further stratify based on severity [11], and therefore the exact prevalence of SSD in children is unknown.

## 14.3 Etiology of Single-Sided Deafness

Among adults, the most common cause of acquired SSD is still idiopathic. Usami et al. reported on the various etiologies of SSD among a total of 527 patients at their center between 2006 and 2016, in a cohort of both children and adults [13]. Among congenitally or early-onset deafened children, the most common cause of SSD was cochlear nerve deficiency (43.7% of patients), followed by cytomegalovirus (CMV) infection, mumps infection, anomalies of the inner ear and auditory neuropathy spectrum disorder (ANSD). Meningitis and head trauma were rare causes of unilateral hearing loss. Pollaers et al. also demonstrated a high rate of absent cochlear nerves in their cohort of SSD patients [14]. On the other hand, among post-lingually deafened individuals, SSD was idiopathic in more than half (54.6%) of their group, and other causes included otitis media (6.4%), cholesteatoma (6.4%) and tumors of the cerebellopontine angle (5.2%). Rare etiologies included head trauma, mumps, and vasculitis. With the advent of universal hearing screening (UHS), the distribution of etiologic factors has changed [15], with more children being diagnosed with congenital hearing loss, as it can be accurately detected at birth rather than later in life where it may be classified as idiopathic.

## 14.4 Benefits of Binaural Hearing

Having two normal-hearing ears has several advantages. Numerous reports have outlined that speech discrimination in noise is impaired in patients with unilateral hearing, even with lesser degrees of hearing loss [6]. Three main mechanisms contribute to enhanced auditory perception with binaural input: binaural squelch, binaural summation and the head shadow effect. Binaural squelch is a central processing phenomenon that allows for modulation in the signal-to-noise ratio of the incoming sound [16]. In simplistic terms, one can imagine a specific signal of interest arriving from one location and additional noise arriving from another. Both the signal of interest, as well as the noise, will arrive at each ear at a slightly different time and a slightly different intensity. With two functional ears, these signals are processed centrally and our brain separates the signal of interest from the background noise, increasing the signal-to-noise ratio. Binaural summation refers to the fact that sound received from both ears is greater in amplitude than the same signal received by only one ear [16]. This increase in perceptual loudness is thought to improve speech intelligibility in noisy environments. Furthermore, in order to know where the sound is coming from, two different cues are used: interaural time difference and interaural intensity difference. The one ear closer to the sound source and therefore receives the sound slightly earlier and at a different amplitude and allows the brain to use these interaural differences to localize sound. This is caused by the head shadow effect, where sound is attenuated by the head itself, though this particular issue can be overcome by routing of sound to the hearing ear in cases without two functioning ears.

## 14.5 Candidacy Evaluation for CI in SSD

At our institution, preparation for cochlear implantation in SSD patients involves several steps. First, we perform an unaided audiogram (both air and bone conduction), tympanometry, speech perception in quiet using consonant-nucleus-consonant (CNC words) and AzBio sentences at 60 dB HL. Next, hearing in background noise with various signal-to-noise ratios (SNR) is also evaluated with either the Bamford-Kowal-Bench Sentence-In-Noise (BKB-SIN) or adaptive Hearing in Noise Test (HINT). The BKB-SIN evaluates sentence recognition in noise with varied presentation in 3-dB steps at fixed signal-to-noise ratios. We obtain a speech reception threshold (SRT) where the patient can repeat key words 50% of the time. A lower numerical score indicates better performance. The test is performed in three different conditions using a speaker array: (1) speech front/noise front, (2) speech front/noise right and finally, (3) speech front/noise left. It is also possible to simulate these configurations using Direct Connect software. Sound localization can be assessed in a room with multiple speakers spanning −90 to 90 degrees on a horizontal plane. Sound bursts are emitted from one speaker, and the listener is asked to identify where the sound came from. Root-mean-squared (RMS) error is used as a marker of success, where a lower rate of error equates to better performance. Sound localization can also be assessed with the Direct Connect system, which uses "virtual locations." A summary of our institutional protocol for cochlear implantation in SSD patients can be found in Table 14.1.

**Table 14.1** Institutional protocol for cochlear implantation in SSD

| |
|---|
| Pure-tone air and bone conduction thresholds |
| Immittance measures including tympanometry, acoustic reflexes and otoacoustic emissions |
| MRI or CT imaging confirmation of a cochlea and cochlear nerve and to detect inner ear malformations or evidence of ossification |
| Speech reception thresholds and speech discrimination where age appropriate (CNC, HINT) |
| Adaptive HINT is also done with sound field using CROS amplification and/or the BAHA soft band |
| Localization testing |
| Vertigo and tinnitus questionnaires are included in evaluation |
| All post-implantation testing is performed using a manufacturer-specific direct connect system or insert phones |

## 14.6 Cochlear Implants for Single-Sided Deafness in Adults

### 14.6.1 Which Adults with Single-Sided Deafness Should Be Implanted?

Identifying appropriate candidates in the SSD population can be difficult. Some adults with congenital SSD and others who have a progressive or sudden loss adapt very well to SSD and elect not to undergo any intervention. This decision-making is quite different than in a pediatric scenario. Adults with SSD that seek rehabilitation may elect for a CI for a variety of reasons, including difficulty hearing in noisy environments or the desire for better sound localization. The decision can be influenced by someone's daily demands, such as their profession, for example. Another motivation might be intractable tinnitus, which is discussed below. Another indication may be impending decline of the better hearing ear. One example of this scenario would be a patient with a vestibular schwannoma or other retrocochlear pathology on the better or only hearing ear. In this situation, pre-emptive cochlear implantation on the deaf ear may have several advantages. The first is the assurance that there is a back-up in case of sudden loss in the better hearing ear, avoiding a period of being "off-line" when this occurs. The other is to avoid prolonging the duration of deafness in the worse ear, in the case that the threatened ear may not be amenable to cochlear implantation, as this is an important predictor of a successful outcome [9]. Another important indication for adult cochlear implantation in the context of SSD would be related to late-stage unilateral Menière's disease, where the vertigo is intractable despite all medical therapies and the hearing is poor. In these situations, undergoing a labyrinthectomy with simultaneous cochlear implantation may be life-changing by ablating the vestibular input and improving hearing [17, 18].

### 14.6.2 Outcomes of Cochlear Implants in Adults with SSD

**Improved Hearing in Quiet and in Noise**

There are a number of reports which have considered outcomes in these populations. Galvin et al. evaluated ten patients who underwent cochlear implantation for

SSD. They found a mean improvement of CNC word recognition of 66.8%, 76%, and 84%, respectively, at 1, 3, and 6 months postoperatively in the CI ear. They also noted that HINT sentence recognition improved by 36.4%, 40.7%, and 51.1% in that same timeframe [2]. Finally, they evaluated speech understanding in noise using SRT, which they defined as the signal-to-noise ratio needed to produce 50% correct recognition of words in sentences. They noted the SRT for HINT sentences with binaural listening was −4.2 dB. In our own cohort of 10 adult patients with SSD, we used BKB-SIN testing. Our results demonstrated that noise presented to the SSD/CI ear from the front led to significantly decreased signal-to-noise ratio, with an average reduction of 2.0 dB SNR in nine patients [9]. When the noise was presented to the better hearing ear, the signal-to-noise ratio decreased even more significantly (reduction of 4.6 dB). Zeitler et al. evaluated 23 patients (17 adults) who underwent cochlear implantation for SSD [19]. They showed significant improvements in word and sentence scores, although scores did not reach the levels of improvement seen in patients with bilateral hearing loss. They report that normal-hearing individuals likely rely more heavily on their better ear, which could prevent maximal improvement in their implanted ear.

**Improved Sound Localization**

Arndt et al. performed a prospective study on 11 patients with SSD, focusing on sound localization. First, they assessed sound localization scores of patients under in three conditions: (1) normal hearing (NH) alone, (2) CROS and NH and (3) bone conduction hearing aid and NH condition. Following this first series of testing, all patients subsequently underwent cochlear implantation. Sound localization results from before and after CI were compared. There was significantly better sound localization scores in the CI with NH condition, as well as speech comprehension [20]. These findings have since been replicated in other series [4, 19, 21, 22]. Interestingly, in our own cohort of 10 adult patients, no significant difference in sound localization was noted 1 year postoperatively [9].

**Tinnitus Suppression**

Tinnitus suppression is a known benefit reported by many after cochlear implantation and was the main motivation for some of the first patients implanted in Europe with this pattern of hearing loss [23]. The hypothesized mechanism is the restoration of sensory input to the brain after initial hearing loss. Van de Heyning et al. reviewed 21 adult patients with profound hearing loss in the ear to be implanted as well as severe intractable tinnitus that did not respond to medical and psychological therapy. These subjects received cochlear implants, and a significant reduction in the tinnitus loudness was noted in 95% of participants [23]. They also found a significant improvement of scores on the Tinnitus Questionnaire. Similar findings have been confirmed by other groups [24, 25].

**Improve Quality of Life**

In addition to the improvements in spatial hearing and tinnitus suppression, there is evidence that treating SSD with cochlear implantation improves patients' quality of life as per the Speech, Spatial and Qualities of Hearing Scale (SSQ) and other

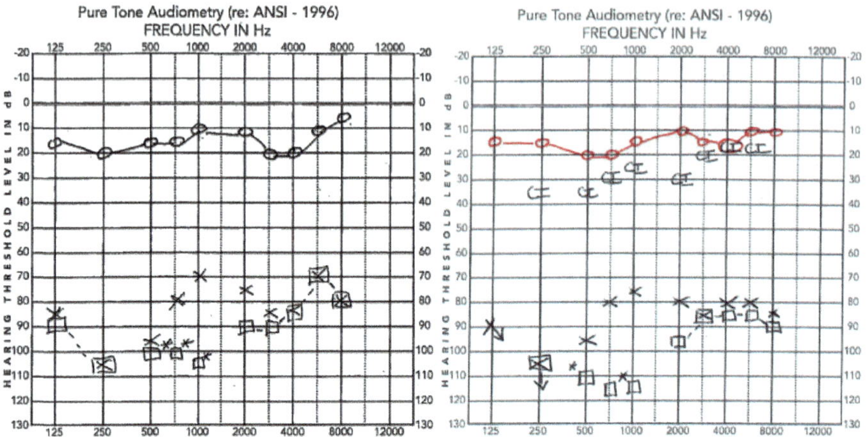


**Fig. 14.1** Audiograms before and after cochlear implantation in patient with SSD

**Table 14.2** Speech perception scores post-implantation in a patient with left SSD

| CNC words | Right* | Left cochlear implant | Bilateral |
|---|---|---|---|
| Words | 100% | 78% | 100% |
| Phonemes | 100% | 89% | 100% |
| Adaptive BKB-SIN (noise front/speech front) | −3.0 dB | 6.5 dB | −3.0 dB |
| Adaptive BKB-SIN (noise left/speech front) | −6.5 dB | 8.5 dB | −7.0 dB |
| Adaptive BKB-SIN (noise right/speech front) | −2.5 dB | −2.0 dB | −5.5 dB |

*Normal hearing ear

quality of life questionnaires [6, 22]. We recently assessed the quality of life in our cohort of 32 SSD CI patients in both disease-specific and general quality of life, which is currently under peer review for publication.

Figure 14.1 shows two audiograms, before and after cochlear implantation, in a 35-year-old man with SSD following mechanical ventilation and prolonged hospitalization for a respiratory viral infection. Shown here are his pre- and postoperative audiograms. Table 14.2 shows his speech perception scores post-implantation, with materials presented at 60 dBA and varied SNR for noise conditions.

## 14.7 Cochlear Implants for Single-Sided Deafness in Children

### 14.7.1 Why Implant Children with SSD?

Children with SSD, or any unilateral hearing loss may be difficult to identify early in life without ear-specific testing given that they are likely to develop normal speech and not be in environments for a number of years where a deficit in localization is likely to be noticed. This has improved with UHS, but either because of inaccurate testing or progressive losses, some go undetected until later in life. Over the course of the 1980s and 1990s, several studies highlighted educational and behavioral disadvantages in children with SSD compared to normal-hearing children. Children with SSD may be at risk of worse performance on auditory skills testing, despite having one functional ear [26]. Furthermore, sound localization scores in children with SSD were significantly poorer than normal-hearing children [11]. Challenges faced by children with SSD include speech understanding in noise [27], sound localization [28], and diminished quality of life [27]. Not only this, it has been postulated that SSD in children leads to an increased "listening effort," which results in more cognitive exhaustion and may inhibit learning [29].

Work in this area highlighted the importance of identifying unilaterally deaf children early in life [30]. He performed a survey of parents who had children with SSD and found that 35% failed at least one grade in school, and another 13% required other resources in school. Teachers described children with unilateral hearing loss as having difficulty with peers, lower confidence, more dependence on their teachers and increased withdrawn behaviors.

A landmark report by Lieu et al. involved a case-control study of children 6–12 years of age with unilateral hearing loss [31]. Seventy-four children were compared to their normal-hearing siblings. Scores on the oral portion of the Oral and Written Language Scales (OWLS) were the main outcome measure. Despite having one functional ear, children with unilateral hearing loss scored significantly worse than their siblings on the OWLs. This study highlighted the importance of recognizing and appropriately treating children with single-sided deafness. Similar findings have emerged throughout the literature [27, 28, 32].

Providing children with SSD cochlear implants presents an opportunity to restore aspects of binaural hearing benefits and thus improve sound localization and speech understanding in noise. As with bilateral hearing loss, the sooner the intervention, the less likely the child is to encounter cognitive and behavioral challenges. Still, a large number of children with SSD develop normal speech and language and succeed academically. Knowing which children are most susceptible to poor school performance would be useful to guide counseling and treatment. To date, only a small number of risk factors for educational impairment have been identified, and these include early age of hearing loss onset. Not surprisingly, the severity of the SNHL also plays a role as a risk factor, as do other underlying disabilities.

### 14.7.2 Which Children with Single-Sided Deafness Should Be Implanted and When?

Patients with cochlear nerve deficiency are usually discouraged from undergoing a CI for SSD. As mentioned earlier, it is believed that up to 50% of cases of severe to profound unilateral congenital hearing loss patients have a deficient cochlear nerve. This highlights the importance of careful review of the preoperative MRI. Although the presence of a narrow bony cochlear nerve canal may be predictive on a CT, an MRI is best for assessing SSD candidacy, especially if no auditory thresholds were detected in that ear during the evaluation. For families of children considering cochlear implantation, we advocate for neuro-imaging in the process for at least two distinct reasons. For children where cochlear nerve aplasia is apparent, we can avoid the emotional and financial cost of completing a cochlear implant evaluation for someone who is not a candidate. Secondly, imaging allows determination regarding the status of the contralateral ear. For example, both an enlarged vestibular aqueduct (EVA) and congenital cytomegalovirus (cCMV) may begin as unilateral disease and progress to bilateral. Among our own patients, two children with EVA had a decline in their hearing during the course of their follow-up. In fact, the knowledge of a contralateral susceptibility may prompt more expedient intervention, in order to avoid a bilateral deafness. These children represent a unique group who should be closely monitored and in whom cochlear implantation may be more strongly considered.

Knowing when to implant children with SSD remains a challenge. In the series from our center, the best performers were those implanted before the age of 4 years. This finding was also noted by Arndt et al., who reported a trend towards better outcomes in children with shorter durations of deafness [33].

### 14.7.3 Outcomes of Cochlear Implants in Children with SSD

Benchetrit et al. published a systematic review and meta-analysis evaluating the outcomes of CI for children with SSD [34]. They reviewed 12 studies encompassing 119 children with SSD. In terms of audiologic outcomes, they found that 79.6% of children experienced improved speech perception in noise with their cochlear implant. For speech perception in quiet, 81% of children showed improvement. Furthermore, among six studies, sound localization was also determined to be significantly improved. They were able to evaluate device usage time in 101 children and found that 74.3% used their device regularly. The nonusers were significantly older at the time of implantation and had longer durations of deafness. There was evidence that lack of improvement was often associated with congenital SSD as well as patients implanted over the age of 4. Finally, they looked at patient-reported outcomes, which once again demonstrated that acquired SSD and shorter duration of deafness was associated with improved quality of life.

A retrospective cohort study in two tertiary care cochlear implant centers evaluated children between the ages of 1.5 and 15 years old with SSD [35]. Among a group of nine patients, they found significant benefits in speech outcomes after cochlear implantation. They also noted high rates of device use. The only patient in their cohort who did not show benefit was congenitally unilaterally deaf and was implanted at age 9. The remaining four congenitally deaf children in their series had a mean duration of deafness of 6.5 years and had significant benefit post-implantation.

Our group retrospectively reviewed 14 pediatric patients implanted for SSD [8]. The cohort had a mean duration of deafness of 3 years, although it ranged from 0.6 to 7 years. The mean improvement for word recognition scores in the CI-only condition was 49.3%. We did not find a worsening in speech performance with the cochlear implant in the binaural condition.

Overall, in children with unilateral SNHL, underlying etiology should be investigated, including consideration of CMV testing, as well as ophthalmologic assessment. An MRI should be obtained early in the process if a cochlear implant is being considered. Amplification should be implemented early on, and early intervention programs should be initiated. No matter the treatment strategy pursued, these children require close follow-up for progression or worsening of the contralateral ear.

## 14.8 Conclusion

Both children and adults may greatly benefit from cochlear implants in the context of SSD. Cochlear implants for unilaterally deaf patients may provide improved hearing in noise, better sound localization, decreased tinnitus and improved quality of life. In children, specifically, further research is needed to understand the maximal duration of deafness that will lead to successful outcomes, as well as to delineate risk factors that can better predict which patients will have more difficulties associated with their SSD.

## References

1. Vincent C, Arndt S, Firszt JB, Fraysse B, Kitterick PT, Papsin BC, et al. Identification and evaluation of cochlear implant candidates with asymmetrical hearing loss. Audiol Neurootol. 2015;20(Suppl 1):87–9.
2. Galvin JJ III, Fu QJ, Wilkinson EP, Mills D, Hagan SC, Lupo JE, et al. Benefits of cochlear implantation for single-sided deafness: data from the House Clinic-University of Southern California-University of California, Los Angeles Clinical Trial. Ear Hear. 2019;40(4):766–81.
3. Welsh LW, Welsh JJ, Rosen LF, Dragonette JE. Functional impairments due to unilateral deafness. Ann Otol Rhinol Laryngol. 2004;113(12):987–93.
4. Slattery WH III, Middlebrooks JC. Monaural sound localization: acute versus chronic unilateral impairment. Hear Res. 1994;75(1–2):38–46.
5. Iwasaki S, Sano H, Nishio S, Takumi Y, Okamoto M, Usami S, et al. Hearing handicap in adults with unilateral deafness and bilateral hearing loss. Otol Neurotol. 2013;34(4):644–9.
6. Wie OB, Pripp AH, Tvete O. Unilateral deafness in adults: effects on communication and social interaction. Ann Otol Rhinol Laryngol. 2010;119(11):772–81.
7. Vermeire K, Van de Heyning P. Binaural hearing after cochlear implantation in subjects with unilateral sensorineural deafness and tinnitus. Audiol Neurootol. 2009;14(3):163–71.
8. Deep NL, Gordon SA, Shapiro WH, Waltzman SB, Roland JT Jr, Friedmann DR. Cochlear implantation in children with single-sided deafness. Laryngoscope. 2021;131(1):E271–e7.
9. Friedmann DR, Ahmed OH, McMenomey SO, Shapiro WH, Waltzman SB, Roland JT Jr. Single-sided deafness cochlear implantation: candidacy, evaluation, and outcomes in children and adults. Otol Neurotol. 2016;37(2):e154–60.
10. Golub JS, Lin FR, Lustig LR, Lalwani AK. Prevalence of adult unilateral hearing loss and hearing aid use in the United States. Laryngoscope. 2018;128(7):1681–6.
11. Bess FH, Dodd-Murphy J, Parker RA. Children with minimal sensorineural hearing loss: prevalence, educational performance, and functional status. Ear Hear. 1998;19(5):339–54.

12. Ross DS, Visser SN, Holstrum WJ, Qin T, Kenneson A. Highly variable population-based prevalence rates of unilateral hearing loss after the application of common case definitions. Ear Hear. 2010;31(1):126–33.
13. Usami SI, Kitoh R, Moteki H, Nishio SY, Kitano T, Kobayashi M, et al. Etiology of single-sided deafness and asymmetrical hearing loss. Acta Otolaryngol. 2017;137(Suppl 565):S2–s7.
14. Pollaers K, Thompson A, Kuthubutheen J. Cochlear nerve anomalies in paediatric single-sided deafness – prevalence and implications for cochlear implantation strategies. J Laryngol Otol. 2020:1–4.
15. Ghogomu N, Umansky A, Lieu JE. Epidemiology of unilateral sensorineural hearing loss with universal newborn hearing screening. Laryngoscope. 2014;124(1):295–300.
16. Flint PW, Haughey BH, Robbins KT, Thomas JR, Niparko JK, Lund VJ, et al. Cummings otolaryngology-head and neck surgery e-book. Elsevier Health Sciences; 2014.
17. Perkins E, Rooth M, Dillon M, Brown K. Simultaneous labyrinthectomy and cochlear implantation in unilateral Meniere's disease. Laryngoscope Investig Otolaryngol. 2018;3(3):225–30.
18. Sykopetrites V, Giannuzzi AL, Lauda L, Di Rubbo V, Bassi M, Sanna M. Surgical labyrinthectomy and cochlear implantation in Menière's disease. Otol Neurotol. 2020;41(6):775–81.
19. Zeitler DM, Dorman MF, Natale SJ, Loiselle L, Yost WA, Gifford RH. Sound source localization and speech understanding in complex listening environments by single-sided deaf listeners after cochlear implantation. Otol Neurotol. 2015;36(9):1467–71.
20. Arndt S, Aschendorff A, Laszig R, Beck R, Schild C, Kroeger S, et al. Comparison of pseudo-binaural hearing to real binaural hearing rehabilitation after cochlear implantation in patients with unilateral deafness and tinnitus. Otol Neurotol. 2011;32(1):39–47.
21. Dorman MF, Zeitler D, Cook SJ, Loiselle L, Yost WA, Wanna GB, et al. Interaural level difference cues determine sound source localization by single-sided deaf patients fit with a cochlear implant. Audiol Neurootol. 2015;20(3):183–8.
22. Dillon MT, Buss E, Anderson ML, King ER, Deres EJ, Buchman CA, et al. Cochlear implantation in cases of unilateral hearing loss: initial localization abilities. Ear Hear. 2017;38(5):611–9.
23. Van de Heyning P, Vermeire K, Diebl M, Nopp P, Anderson I, De Ridder D. Incapacitating unilateral tinnitus in single-sided deafness treated by cochlear implantation. Ann Otol Rhinol Laryngol. 2008;117(9):645–52.
24. Ito J, Sakakihara J. Tinnitus suppression by electrical stimulation of the cochlear wall and by cochlear implantation. Laryngoscope. 1994;104(6 Pt 1):752–4.
25. Mertens G, De Bodt M, Van de Heyning P. Cochlear implantation as a long-term treatment for ipsilateral incapacitating tinnitus in subjects with unilateral hearing loss up to 10 years. Hear Res. 2016;331:1–6.
26. Bess FH, Tharpe AM, Gibler AM. Auditory performance of children with unilateral sensorineural hearing loss. Ear Hear. 1986;7(1):20–6.
27. Griffin AM, Poissant SF, Freyman RL. Speech-in-noise and quality-of-life measures in school-aged children with normal hearing and with unilateral hearing loss. Ear Hear. 2019;40(4):887–904.
28. Reeder RM, Cadieux J, Firszt JB. Quantification of speech-in-noise and sound localisation abilities in children with unilateral hearing loss and comparison to normal hearing peers. Audiol Neurootol. 2015;20 Suppl 1(01):31–7.
29. Hornsby BW, Werfel K, Camarata S, Bess FH. Subjective fatigue in children with hearing loss: some preliminary findings. Am J Audiol. 2014;23(1):129–34.
30. Bess FH. The unilaterally hearing-impaired child: a final comment. Ear Hear. 1986;7(1):52–4.
31. Lieu JE, Tye-Murray N, Karzon RK, Piccirillo JF. Unilateral hearing loss is associated with worse speech-language scores in children. Pediatrics. 2010;125(6):e1348–55.
32. Purcell PL, Shinn JR, Davis GE, Sie KC. Children with unilateral hearing loss may have lower intelligence quotient scores: a meta-analysis. Laryngoscope. 2016;126(3):746–54.
33. Arndt S, Prosse S, Laszig R, Wesarg T, Aschendorff A, Hassepass F. Cochlear implantation in children with single-sided deafness: does aetiology and duration of deafness matter? Audiol Neurotol. 2015;20(Suppl 1):21–30.

34. Benchetrit L, Ronner EA, Anne S, Cohen MS. Cochlear implantation in children with single-sided deafness: a systematic review and meta-analysis. JAMA Otolaryngol Head Neck Surg. 2021;147(1):58–69.
35. Zeitler DM, Sladen DP, DeJong MD, Torres JH, Dorman MF, Carlson ML. Cochlear implantation for single-sided deafness in children and adolescents. Int J Pediatr Otorhinolaryngol. 2019;118:128–33.

# Hearing Preservation and Electro-acoustic Stimulation in Cochlear Implants

15

Emily Kay-Rivest, J. Thomas Roland Jr, and Daniel Jethanamest

## 15.1 Introduction

The indications for cochlear implantation (CI) have changed significantly over the past three decades. Initially, a CI was reserved for bilateral, profound deafness. More recently, indications have expanded and include single-sided deafness (SSD), as well as patients with significant low-frequency hearing with a steeply sloping high-frequency (HF) hearing loss. Previously, this last group, sometimes referred to as having a *ski-slope pattern* of hearing loss, may have been considered to be hearing too well to benefit from a cochlear implant. It was believed that the insertion of a CI electrode would completely eliminate all residual hearing. That idea has since been disproven, and hearing preservation has become a realistic and common goal. In 1989, Boggess et al. reported conserving hearing in approximately one-third of their patients [1]. In 2006, a hearing preservation rate of 89% in a cohort of 28 patients was reported, when specific surgical techniques were employed [2].

Electro-acoustic stimulation (EAS) is defined as the delivery of both acoustic and electric information to the cochlea. In theory, the advantages of preserved acoustic hearing include better spectral information and improved fine temporal structure that may not be delivered with electric stimulation [3]. Preservation of low-frequency

**Supplementary Information** The online version contains supplementary material available at [https://doi.org/10.1007/978-981-19-0452-3_15].

E. Kay-Rivest · J. T. Roland Jr
Department of Otolaryngology—Head and Neck Surgery, Division of Otology and Neurotology, New York University, New York, NY, USA

D. Jethanamest (✉)
Division of Otology and Neurotology, New York University, New York, NY, USA
e-mail: daniel.jethanamest@nyulangone.org


S. DeSaSouza (ed.), *Cochlear Implants*,
https://doi.org/10.1007/978-981-19-0452-3_15

acoustic hearing is thought to improve the recognition of speech in noise in cochlear implant recipients [4] and may also contribute to music enjoyment [5].

The ability to preserve residual hearing has now become an important topic of discussion and research. Residual hearing may be lost through several mechanisms and often occurs at the time of surgery or immediately postoperatively. However, there are also instances in which hearing is preserved initially but may be lost in the months following implantation. This can happen both gradually or suddenly, and the mechanism of this occurrence remains unknown. Theories for hearing loss at the time of surgery include trauma to the basilar membrane, osseous spiral lamina, spiral ligament, Reissner's membrane and spiral ganglion cells, all of which have been described in cadaveric models [6, 7]. When occurring in delayed fashion, proposed theories for hearing loss include fibrosis within the cochlea, inflammation and endolymphatic hydrops [8]. Another possible mechanism of injury is damage to the blood vessels within the lateral wall of the scala tympani [9].

## 15.2 Techniques for Hearing Preservation

It has become clear that hearing preservation is an achievable goal, and a great amount of research has been performed to explore various techniques that can result in the maximal amount of hearing preservation. These include modifications of insertion techniques, different routes of insertion (round window, peri-round window or traditional cochleostomy), use of different electrodes and administration of peri-operative steroids. Despite the various techniques which are described in detail below, patient factors also come into play and may determine the ability to preserve residual hearing. Duration of deafness, stability of SNHL, sex and noise exposure are important considerations when planning for hearing preservation surgery. In a review of 85 patients, Kopelovich et al. evaluated factors related to low-frequency hearing preservation. They found that the loss of residual hearing at 1-year post-activation was related to older age, male gender and an etiology of noise-induced hearing loss (NIHL) [10]. They also identified a trend in which patients with more co-morbidities lost residual hearing more frequently, although their sample size was limited, and statistical significance was not achieved.

Wanna et al. reviewed short- and long-term rates of hearing preservation in their cohort of 196 patients [11]. They noted a 38% rate of hearing preservation in the short term, which dropped to a rate of 18% long-term. They found that better preoperative hearing predicted hearing preservation on the long term, which has been demonstrated in other studies [12–14]. Lateral wall and mid-scala electrodes had 3.4 and 5.6 times higher odds of hearing preservation compared to perimodiolar electrodes in the short-term only. Follow-up studies from the same institution using a newer, thinner perimodiolar electrode reported 60% of patients preserved residual hearing (<80 dB HL LF PTA) at 6 months. In a matched cohort comparison of slim perimodiolar to slim lateral wall electrodes, the perimodiolar group showed better preservation of low-frequency hearing [15, 16]. A review from the United Kingdom looked at their population of hearing preservation candidates [17]. Their overall rate of hearing preservation was 52.9%. Sex, age at implantation, depth of insertion, lateral wall versus perimodiolar and pre-operative hearing levels did not affect the rates of hearing preservation in their cohort. It is clear that determining the factors most affecting hearing preservation remains elusive and will require further investigation.

### 15.2.1 Insertion Technique

Limiting intracochlear trauma is an important but controversial topic. The term *soft surgery* has been used increasingly when referring to an attempt at limiting trauma to the cochlear. Whether through a round window insertion or a cochleostomy, principles of *soft surgery* include minimizing drilling if a cochleostomy is performed, avoiding suctioning of perilymph, as well as properly sealing the cochleostomy.

Several techniques are employed to maximize hearing preservation. We perform a traditional mastoidectomy and facial recess for a majority of uncomplicated cases. The facial recess is opened widely, and care is taken not to disrupt or drill on the ossicles. Regardless of the planned insertion point, the round window must be fully visualized, so the bony overhang of the round window niche is carefully removed with a 1 mm diamond burr. Being able to see the entire round window is important for a precise scala tympani insertion. The surgical cavity is well-irrigated to remove and bone dust and blood from the field. When a cochleostomy is created, it is drilled anterior and inferior to the round window membrane, in order to avoid potentially violating the scala media. While drilling the promontory cochleostomy, the endosteum of the scala tympani is identified and kept intact until drilling is completed. A lubricant such as glycerin or hyaluronic acid gel may be used as a lubricant and deterrent to blood. Prior to electrode insertion, we always ensure that the electrode itself is free of bone dust and the electrode is inserted with careful attention to any form of resistance. Suctioning of any perilymph is avoided from around the round window or cochleostomy, and the opening is sealed with small pieces of fascia. Intra-operative telemetry and X-ray are performed for every case. Care is taken to avoid displacement of the electrode during this monitoring and during closure.

Two examples of EAS systems in use can be found in Fig. 15.1. A sample of audiologic criteria for EAS candidacy can be found in Fig. 15.2. An example of an

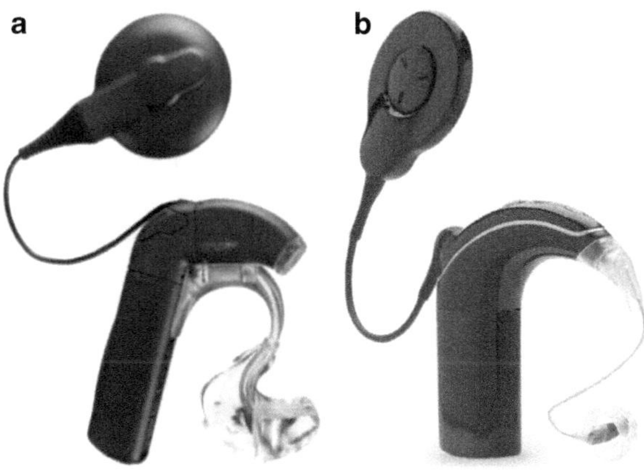


**Fig. 15.1** (**a**) DUET 2 processor. Courtesy of MED-EL Corp. (**b**) Nucleus Hybrid processor (can be used with all electrodes). Courtesy of Cochlear Corp

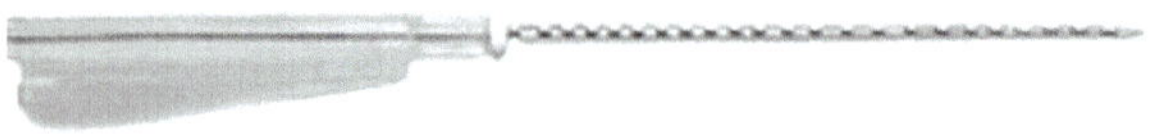

**Fig. 15.2** Hybrid L24 electrode, intended for patients with stable hearing loss with residual hearing in the low frequencies. Courtesy of Cochlear Corp

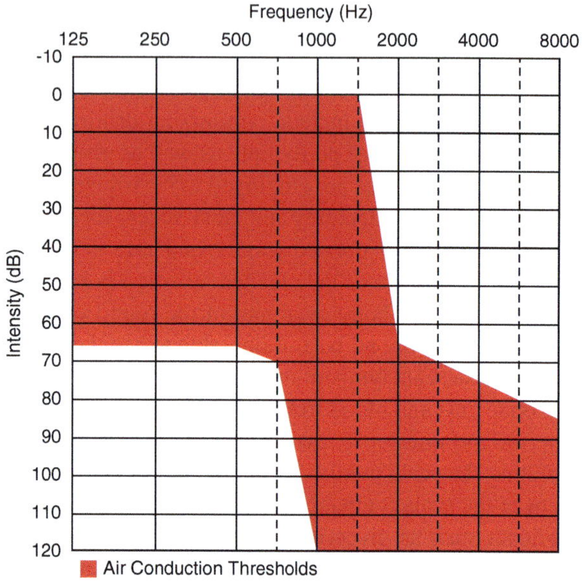


**Fig. 15.3** Red area: unaided air conduction thresholds for candidacy for the SYNCHRONY EAS Cochlear Implant System. With permission from MED-EL

electrode intended for EAS, the Hybrid L24 by Cochlear Corp can be found in Fig. 15.3. A video can be found of a cochleostomy and insertion of a Hybrid electrode performed at our center.

### 15.2.2 Route of Electrode Insertion and Speed of Insertion

Two major atraumatic techniques have been proposed: the round window insertion and the *soft* cochleostomy technique. Previously, the round window insertion carried concerns of injury and trauma to the spiral osseous lamina. This however was in the context of the prior generation electrodes, which tended to be larger and more rigid. Currently, with the advent of softer and thinner electrodes, the round window insertion technique has regained interest. Some advocate that avoiding a cochleostomy will allow for less noise-induced trauma from drilling, and less risk of bone dust accumulation within cochlea.

Berrettini et al. compared three surgical techniques head to head in 30 patients with residual hearing [18]. The first group underwent a classic round window approach (with insertion of a Nucleus 24 M-K standard electrode array). The second group underwent a *soft* surgical technique (with insertion of a Nucleus 24

Contour electrode array). They described their *soft* technique as a 1–1.2 mm cochleostomy performed 2 mm anterior to the round window niche and opening the endosteum only after completing the drilling. The third group underwent a modified antero-inferior cochleostomy near the round window (with a Nucleus 24 Contour Advance electrode array, using the Advance Off Stylet technique). In this third group, the bony overhang of the round window niche was drilled completely. For groups 1, 2 and 3, the percentages of completely preserved hearing were 12.5%, 27.3% and 54.5%, respectively. Overall, the best results were found in the group that underwent a modified anterior inferior cochleostomy and insertion of a full-length electrode. With this technique, hearing preservation occurred at least partially in 81.8% of patients.

As electrode arrays have evolved over time, the ideal approach is still unclear. Havenith et al. attempted to compare round window insertion to cochleostomy in a systematic review [19]. They found no clear benefit to one approach compared to the other, although they emphasized the lack of randomized controlled studies. The studies that they included also had a wide range of electrodes used, as well as follow-up times, ranging from 1 to 30 months. In another review, Snels et al. evaluated differences in hearing preservation between the cochleostomy and round window approaches at 1, 6 and 12 months after surgery [20]. The differences were 13.1%, 18.6% and 1.7%, respectively, favoring round window insertion. However, only the difference noted at 6 months was statistically significant.

Speed of electrode insertion was also evaluated by Snels et al. [20]. They compared articles that explicitly stated slow insertion and compared them to those that did not. Among this group of patients, there were no statistically significant differences in hearing preservation ($p = 0.722$). Unfortunately, a large number of articles did not report their speed of insertion. The research regarding speed of insertion is still in its early phases. Mittmann et al. measured cochlear pressures in an artificial cochlear model using a pressure sensor within the apex and noted that perimodiolar electrodes induced higher peak pressures compared to straight electrodes [21]. Another study aimed at investigating peak hydraulic pressure and peak forces on the cochlear wall during electrode insertion, using a variety of insertion techniques [22]. Interestingly, the results were slightly contradictory. Slower insertion resulted in higher peak hydraulic pressures, but also in lower forces on the cochlear wall. The clinical significance of these findings still needs to be clarified.

### 15.2.3 Electrode Design

The type of electrode that results in increased hearing preservation has also been an important subject of research. One consideration is the hypothesis that a shorter electrode is less likely to traumatize the apical hair cells, resulting in better low-frequency hearing preservation [11, 23]. Another option is to utilize a longer electrode, but only inserting it partially. Finally, some may argue that a thin, soft and full-length electrode may be preferable and will still allow for hearing preservation [24]. One must also consider the long-term outcomes of residual hearing, and the use of full-length contemporary electrodes, which can often be used and preserve low frequency hearing while providing greater coverage. If residual hearing is lost in the short or long term, having a full-length electrode in place may be favorable and avoid the potential need for revision. If a shorter electrode is chosen, however, it is important to confirm the stability of the hearing loss in the ear to be implanted [25, 26].

Roland et al. published the long-term outcomes of a trial with the Nucleus Hybrid L24 (Cochlear Ltd., Sydney, Australia) implant [27]. A total of 32 out of their 50 enrolled patients had 5-year follow-up data available. Their criteria for the use of the Hybrid L24 electrode was a severe HF SNHL (≥75 dB HL over 2 kHz, 3 kHz, and 4 kHz) with a residual LF hearing level ≤60 dB HL at 500 Hz and below. They defined *functional residual hearing* as a five-frequency LF PTA ≤90 dB HL. With these criteria, 72% of their cohort had a functional residual hearing at 5 years post-operatively. Furthermore, they evaluated the use of the acoustic component in this group. At 12 months, 84% used their acoustic component. This number dropped to 72% at 5 years post-activation. In a series of patients published by Gantz et al. who were implanted with short electrodes, they noted that low-frequency thresholds remained stable over several years (even up to 15 years), with an average loss of 0.75 dB per year [28].

A more recent update from Gantz et al. looked at three groups of patients: group 1 was implanted with the Nucleus Hybrid S8 electrode (10 mm long), group 2 with the Nucleus Hybrid L24 electrode (16 mm long) and group 3 with the Nucleus Hybrid S12 electrode (10 mm long). Respectively, 83%, 92% and 86% of subjects maintained functional hearing [29]. In their cohort, they noted that the most important shifts in hearing occurred between the surgery and the initial activation, despite using hearing preservation techniques. The second decline in hearing occurred most commonly between 0.25 and 0.5 years after initial activation, and this is usually followed by long-term stability. The hypothesis for this second shift was fibrotic changes within the cochlea, as they were able to evaluate the temporal bone of a deceased patient who had lost low-frequency hearing between months one and four after activation. His temporal bone showed extensive fibrotic changes and bone debris and surprisingly revealed normal hair cell, and ganglion cell counts.

Helbig et al. examined the outcomes with another electrode intended for hearing preservation and possible EAS use: the MED-EL PULSAR cochlear implant with the FLEX24 electrode [30]. This 24 mm electrode was used in 18 patients. Hearing was preserved in all subjects and remained stable over a 1-year follow-up time. All patients experienced a slight decrease in hearing after insertion, and there were no differences between the patients who underwent a cochleostomy compared to a round window insertion. They demonstrated improved performance in the EAS condition compared to the CI-only condition on word and sentence testing, which persisted over the year of follow-up.

In 2018, a multicenter study conducted in the United States evaluated 73 subjects who were implanted with PULSAR or SONATA cochlear implant systems with FLEX24 electrode arrays [31]. They demonstrated that the MED-EL EAS system is safe and effective in patients with normal to moderate SNHL in the low frequencies.

Patients had significant improvements on sentence testing in noise in the EAS condition compared to preoperative aided conditions. Furthermore, compared to the CI-only condition, most patients in their cohort performed better in the EAS condition (1 patient out of 67 performed better with electric stimulation alone on City University of New York (CUNY) sentences in noise, and four subjects performed better with electric stimulation alone on consonant-nucleus-consonant (CNC) words in quiet).

Snels et al. attempted to clarify whether hearing preservation occurred more frequently with straight vs. perimodiolar electrode array at 1 and 6 months postoperatively [20]. There was a slight trend in favor of the straight electrode, although the differences in hearing preservation were only significant at the 1-month postoperative mark. They could not draw any conclusions at 12 months after insertion due to the small number of cases. Furthermore, the length of the inserted electrode (they defined short as ≤17 mm and long as >17 mm) showed no statistically significant differences in terms of hearing preservation.

Woodson et al. examine 121 patients who received either a slim perimodiolar electrode or a slim lateral wall array in the context of hearing preservation [32]. Their study groups were comparable in terms of age, gender, preoperative degree of hearing loss and duration of deafness. They found comparable results between both electrodes in terms of hearing preservation at all frequencies. Similar results were reported by others [33]. Despite this promising outlook for many electrode designs, more research is still needed to clarify the ideal properties for hearing preservation.

### 15.2.4 Corticosteroid Use

Corticosteroid use in cochlear implantation has the goal of decreasing the inflammation that is thought to occur within cochlea at the time of and after insertion. Glucocorticoid receptors can be found on the cochlear hair cells, the spiral ligament as well as the spiral ganglion neurons [34]. A systematic review and meta-analysis of animal studies by Shaul et al. evaluated the impact of corticosteroid use on hearing preservation [35]. They examined various methods of administration. For local application of glucocorticoids over the round window, they noted a possible benefit, although interestingly more so at high frequencies. Systemic glucocorticoids were noted to be beneficial across most frequencies at 1 month after implantation. Unfortunately, there was a lack of long-term data, making it difficult to conclude the presence of significant benefit. They were not able to draw any conclusions about drug-eluting electrodes due to small numbers of experiments.

Snels et al. divided corticosteroid use into four categories: not used, systemic administration, local application and both systemic and local administration [20]. At 1, 6 and 12 months postoperatively, no significant differences in hearing preservation were noted between groups, although there was a trend favoring corticosteroid administration of all kinds, they were not able to illicit a clear advantage. Sweeney et al. evaluated the efficacy of an oral steroid course [36]. They compared

20 patients who had received an oral corticosteroid taper to 7 who had not. They found that the degree of hearing preservation in patients treated with steroids was significantly higher. Although among a small number of patients, their findings do suggest that oral steroids may be a useful adjunct for hearing preservation. At our center, in both children and adults, a short course of high-dose prednisone (weight-based, 3 days before and 3 days after), is prescribed for hearing preservation. Different methods of administration of steroids are still being evaluated, including administration via catheter inserted into the cochlea directly [37].

## 15.3 Outcomes of Hearing Preservation and EAS

There are several potential benefits to hearing preservation in cochlear implant users. These included better speech perception in quiet [38], better speech perception in noise [4] and an increased appreciation of music [5]. Furthermore, maintaining low-frequency hearing may result in an overall improved sound quality, where sounds are described as more "natural" and less "raspy" [28].

**Hearing in Noise**

The most commonly discussed benefit of EAS is a significant advantage in noisy environments, likely due to the preservation of residual low-frequency hearing. Skarzynski et al. studied 10 patients with residual low-frequency hearing [39]. They reported that patients in the EAS condition had better performance outcomes in background noise and music appreciation. James et al. reported a 20% improved speech in quiet in their EAS patients, as well as high rates of satisfaction with EAS usage [40]. They also noted slightly better speech reception thresholds in noise compared to CI users alone, although it was among a very small number of patients. Adunka and colleagues compared EAS to electric stimulation alone, within the same subject group [41]. They noted that adding acoustic hearing allowed for better speech understanding compared to electric stimulation alone. This body of information suggests that low-frequency hearing preservation provides an advantage in discriminating speech and in music appreciation.

**Music Appreciation**

Certain cochlear implant users struggle with music identification and enjoyment. Elements such as differentiating pitch and recognizing melodies can be difficult. A significant amount of research emanates from the University of Iowa, putting forth the idea that preservation of low-frequency hearing may aid in music appreciation. Gantz et al. reviewed their patients with residual hearing in whom a short, 10 mm electrode was inserted [28]. Patients were tested in an electro-acoustic setting. They evaluated the ability to detect pitch changes as well as the ability to recognize the direction of pitch change. This last marker in particular is thought to be an important element needed for melody recognition. Within the group studied, they noted that 10 mm hybrid recipients performed closer to normal-hearing adults than patients with full length electrodes in all pitch identification tasks. Brockmeier et al. also noted significantly better frequency discrimination scores in the EAS condition [42]. On the other hand, rhythm perception, chord discrimination, dissonance rating and emotion rating subtest performance was no different between EAS groups and controls.

**Controversies**

This potential benefit is not agreed upon universally, however. A number of studies have shown minimal to no benefit for EAS [42, 43]. Incerti et al. performed a systematic review of electric-acoustic stimulation, with a focus on obtaining answers to several questions including who may not derive benefit from EAS [44]. They compiled 27 articles and concluded that three groups of patients may elect not to utilize their EAS: those with too little hearing, those with too much hearing, as well as those who thought supplementary hearing instruments were cumbersome and unpleasant. For example, a patient with chronic otitis externa may not elect to continue wearing their hearing aid. The above-mentioned factors can all lead to a patient rejecting their use of EAS.

A recent article focused on examining the benefit for speech perception and acceptance of EAS fitting [12]. In their cohort, patients with postoperative thresholds ≤75 dB HL for 125 and 250 Hz were eligible for EAS fitting. With this criterion, 55.7% of patients in their group were eligible for EAS at 3 months postoperatively. However, only approximately half of the patients eligible to use EAS chose to do so. The lack of perceived benefit, as well as fluctuations of low-frequency hearing, were among the reasons for rejecting EAS. Other reasons outlined in their study were difficulty with equipment, physical discomfort and preference of an off-ear processor. Overall, many questions still remain to understand the full range of benefits of EAS. Furthermore, there is an important need to delineate which patients will derive the most benefit from it.

## 15.4 Hearing Preservation in Children and in the Elderly

Hearing preservation in children is also a growing field of research and has gained acceptance over the past 15 years. The approach to hearing preservation in children at our center is very similar to that in adults, including our use of perioperative corticosteroids and our surgical technique.

Selleck et al. reviewed factors associated with low-frequency hearing preservation in children with cochlear implants [45]. They evaluated a group of 105 children and found that preoperative low-frequency PTA and method of implant insertion were the main factors influencing rates of hearing preservation, with lateral wall electrodes showing higher rates of hearing preservation. Interestingly, they found that electrodes that were inserted more deeply had higher hearing preservation rates. Finally, their group did not find a correlation between the presence of an enlarged vestibular aqueduct and the ability to preserve residual hearing. Gantz et al. also found that hearing preservation was an achievable goal in the adolescent population and that these patients received significant benefits compared to hearing aids alone [46]. Carlson et al. reviewed their pediatric population and found that 82% of patients maintained detectable thresholds, with 65% having functional low-frequency hearing [47]. Overall, current evidence would suggest that residual hearing may be maintained in children, similarly to adults.

Below in Fig. 15.4 is an example of a child with residual hearing who received a cochlear implant.

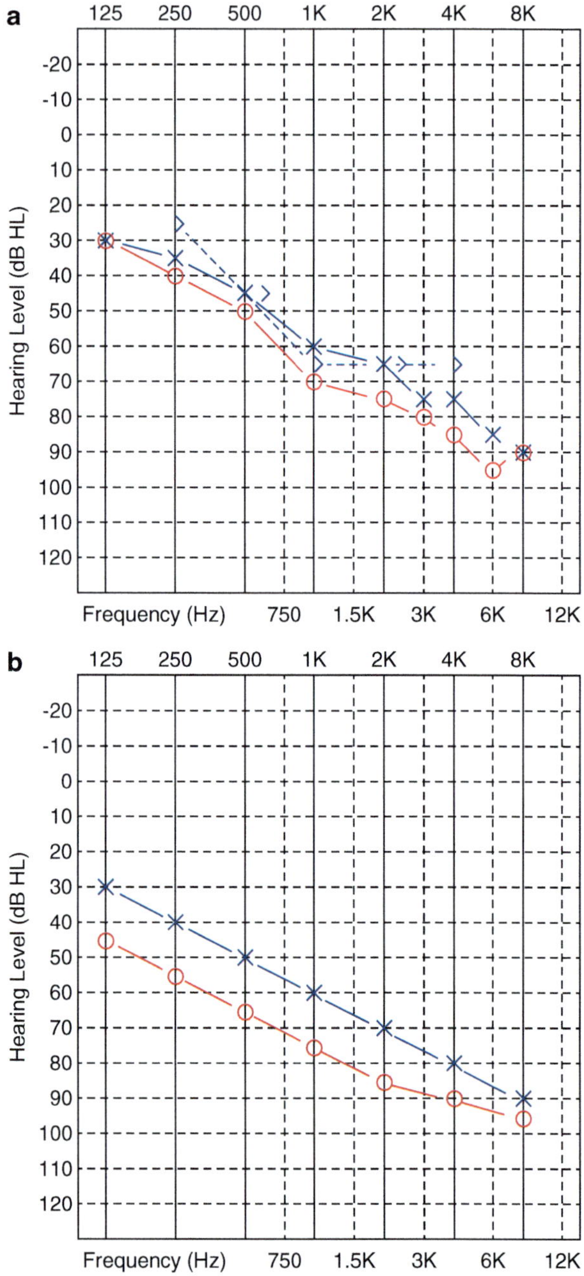


**Fig. 15.4** (**a**) Preoperative audiogram of a 10-year-old female with progressive hearing loss of unknown etiology. Speech discrimination on the right was 62% at 95 dB HL and on the left was 66% at 90 dB HL using CNC word scores. Her Right ear was implanted because subjectively she felt her left ear was more useful. A *soft* surgical technique was employed and a slim perimodiolar electrode was inserted through a cochleostomy. She received steroids 3 days before surgery and 3 days after (prednisone 1 mg/kg/day). (**b**) On most recent follow-up (6 months postoperatively) hearing is preserved (15 dB threshold decline). Currently prefers EAS to electric-only stimulation

The elderly population is another group in whom cochlear implantation is gaining attention. Patients are living longer and healthier lives and desire the best auditory function. One review looked at the rates of hearing preservation in the elderly and found that 60% of CI recipients had a least one postoperative threshold ≤85 dB HL [48]. Their findings suggest that measures to preserve low-frequency hearing, such soft techniques and even corticosteroid administration should not be overlooked in the elderly population.

## 15.5 Future Directions

**Real-Time Electrocochleography**

Electrocochleography (ECoG) is a method of recording hair cell and auditory nerve responses within the cochlea and can also be referred to as acoustically evoked inner ear potentials. The responses elicited by an acoustic stimulus include cochlear microphonics (CM), summating potentials (SP) as well as the compound action potential (CAP). The CM and SP are thought to reflect hair cell contribution, whereas the CAP reflects the potential of the entire auditory nerve. The CM reflect both the potentials of the inner and outer hair cells, although it is likely dominated by the outer hair cell responses. A drop in the amplitude of the ECoG signal without recovery may indicate poor hearing preservation, although the use of ECoG remains incompletely understood [49]. A systematic review of 21 articles evaluating intraoperative ECoG demonstrated that this clinical tool can provide important information allowing for a less traumatic CI insertion, and may eventually play a role in hearing preservation [50]. Another systematic review highlights the need for future research in this domain [51], noting that intraoperative ECoG recording were successfully obtained in 90% of patients, but their ability to predict postoperative residual hearing conservation was limited.

**Robotic-Assisted Insertion**

Robotically-assisted surgical insertion of the cochlear implant is one proposed mechanism for decreased insertion-related trauma. Kaufmann et al. compared the insertion of electrodes by hand ($n = 12$) versus robotic-assisted insertion ($n-12$) in a cadaveric study [52]. The insertions that were performed by robotically assisted mechanisms showed lower insertion forces and variability. Their group hypothesizes that the constant pressure spikes that occur when inserting the electrode by hand could have deleterious effects. Overall, the concept holds promise in terms of allowing for the most atraumatic insertion possible.

## 15.6 Conclusion

Several advantages to preserving residual hearing in cochlear implant patients have been reported in the large breadth of literature surrounding this topic. These patients, who were previously underserviced due to their remnant hearing, are now receiving a great deal of attention and for the most part, are thriving post-implantation. Hearing preservation is an achievable goal in children, adults and the elderly. Further research is still required to better understand the natural history of residual hearing, the ideal electrode for preserving hearing, as well as factors that will predict hearing preservation as well as benefit from it.

## References


1. Boggess WJ, Baker JE, Balkany TJ. Loss of residual hearing after cochlear implantation. Laryngoscope. 1989;99(10 Pt 1):1002–5.
2. Balkany TJ, Connell SS, Hodges AV, Payne SL, Telischi FF, Eshraghi AA, et al. Conservation of residual acoustic hearing after cochlear implantation. Otol Neurotol. 2006;27(8):1083–8.
3. Gifford RH, Dorman MF, Spahr AJ, Bacon SP. Auditory function and speech understanding in listeners who qualify for EAS surgery. Ear Hear. 2007;28(2 Suppl):114s–8s.
4. Turner CW, Gantz BJ, Vidal C, Behrens A, Henry BA. Speech recognition in noise for cochlear implant listeners: benefits of residual acoustic hearing. J Acoust Soc Am. 2004;115(4):1729–35.
5. Gfeller KE, Olszewski C, Turner C, Gantz B, Oleson J. Music perception with cochlear implants and residual hearing. Audiol Neurootol. 2006;11(Suppl 1):12–5.
6. Kennedy DW. Multichannel intracochlear electrodes: mechanism of insertion trauma. Laryngoscope. 1987;97(1):42–9.
7. Nadol JB Jr, Ketten DR, Burgess BJ. Otopathology in a case of multichannel cochlear implantation. Laryngoscope. 1994;104(3 Pt 1):299–303.
8. Nadol JB, Eddington DK. Histopathology of the inner ear relevant to cochlear implantation. Adv Otorhinolaryngol. 2006;64:31–49.
9. Wright CG, Roland PS. Vascular trauma during cochlear implantation: a contributor to residual hearing loss? Otol Neurotol. 2013;34(3):402–7.
10. Kopelovich JC, Reiss LA, Oleson JJ, Lundt ES, Gantz BJ, Hansen MR. Risk factors for loss of ipsilateral residual hearing after hybrid cochlear implantation. Otol Neurotol. 2014;35(8):1403–8.
11. Wanna GB, O'Connell BP, Francis DO, Gifford RH, Hunter JB, Holder JT, et al. Predictive factors for short- and long-term hearing preservation in cochlear implantation with conventional-length electrodes. Laryngoscope. 2018;128(2):482–9.
12. Spitzer ER, Waltzman SB, Landsberger DM, Friedmann DR. Acceptance and benefits of electro-acoustic stimulation for conventional-length electrode arrays. Audiol Neurootol. 2021;26(1):17–26.
13. Carlson ML, Driscoll CL, Gifford RH, Service GJ, Tombers NM, Hughes-Borst BJ, et al. Implications of minimizing trauma during conventional cochlear implantation. Otol Neurotol. 2011;32(6):962–8.
14. Moran M, Dowell RC, Iseli C, Briggs RJS. Hearing preservation outcomes for 139 cochlear implant recipients using a thin straight electrode array. Otol Neurotol. 2017;38(5):678–84.
15. Nassiri AM, Yawn RJ, Holder JT, Dwyer RT, O'Malley MR, Bennett ML, et al. Hearing preservation outcomes using a precurved electrode array inserted with an external sheath. Otol Neurotol. 2020;41(1):33–8.
16. Holder JT, Yawn RJ, Nassiri AM, Dwyer RT, Rivas A, Labadie RF, et al. Matched cohort comparison indicates superiority of precurved electrode arrays. Otol Neurotol. 2019;40(9):1160–6.

17. Harrison L, Manjaly JG, Ellis W, Lavy JA, Shaida A, Khalil SS, et al. Hearing preservation outcomes with standard length electrodes in adult cochlear implantation and the uptake of electroacoustic stimulation. Otol Neurotol. 2020;41(8):1060–5.
18. Berrettini S, Forli F, Passetti S. Preservation of residual hearing following cochlear implantation: comparison between three surgical techniques. J Laryngol Otol. 2008;122(3):246–52.
19. Havenith S, Lammers MJ, Tange RA, Trabalzini F, della Volpe A, van der Heijden GJ, et al. Hearing preservation surgery: cochleostomy or round window approach? A systematic review. Otol Neurotol. 2013;34(4):667–74.
20. Snels C, IntHout J, Mylanus E, Huinck W, Dhooge I. Hearing preservation in cochlear implant surgery: a meta-analysis. Otol Neurotol. 2019;40(2):145–53.
21. Mittmann P, Mittmann M, Ernst A, Todt I. Intracochlear pressure changes due to 2 electrode types: an artificial model experiment. Otolaryngol Head Neck Surg. 2017;156(4):712–6.
22. Snels C, Roland JT Jr, Treaba C, Jethanamest D, Huinck W, Friedmann DR, et al. Force and pressure measurements in temporal bones. Am J Otolaryngol. 2020;42(2):102859.
23. Gantz BJ, Turner C, Gfeller KE. Acoustic plus electric speech processing: preliminary results of a multicenter clinical trial of the Iowa/Nucleus Hybrid implant. Audiol Neurootol. 2006;11(Suppl 1):63–8.
24. Brant JA, Ruckenstein MJ. Electrode selection for hearing preservation in cochlear implantation: a review of the evidence. World J Otorhinolaryngol Head Neck Surg. 2016;2(3):157–60.
25. Mahmoud AF, Massa ST, Douberly SL, Montes ML, Ruckenstein MJ. Safety, efficacy, and hearing preservation using an integrated electro-acoustic stimulation hearing system. Otol Neurotol. 2014;35(8):1421–5.
26. Novak MA, Black JM, Koch DB. Standard cochlear implantation of adults with residual low-frequency hearing: implications for combined electro-acoustic stimulation. Otol Neurotol. 2007;28(5):609–14.
27. Roland JT Jr, Gantz BJ, Waltzman SB, Parkinson AJ. Long-term outcomes of cochlear implantation in patients with high-frequency hearing loss. Laryngoscope. 2018;128(8):1939–45.
28. Gantz BJ, Turner C, Gfeller KE, Lowder MW. Preservation of hearing in cochlear implant surgery: advantages of combined electrical and acoustical speech processing. Laryngoscope. 2005;115(5):796–802.
29. Gantz BJ, Dunn CC, Oleson J, Hansen MR. Acoustic plus electric speech processing: Long-term results. Laryngoscope. 2018;128(2):473–81.
30. Helbig S, Baumann U, Hey C, Helbig M. Hearing preservation after complete cochlear coverage in cochlear implantation with the free-fitting FLEXSOFT electrode carrier. Otol Neurotol. 2011;32(6):973–9.
31. Pillsbury HC III, Dillon MT, Buchman CA, Staecker H, Prentiss SM, Ruckenstein MJ, et al. Multicenter US clinical trial with an electric-acoustic stimulation (EAS) system in adults: final outcomes. Otol Neurotol. 2018;39(3):299–305.
32. Woodson E, Smeal M, Nelson RC, Haberkamp T, Sydlowski S. Slim perimodiolar arrays are as effective as slim lateral wall arrays for functional hearing preservation after cochlear implantation. Otol Neurotol. 2020;41(6):e674–e9.
33. Friedmann DR, Kamen E, Choudhury B, Roland JT Jr. Surgical experience and early outcomes with a slim perimodiolar electrode. Otol Neurotol. 2019;40(3):e304–e10.
34. Meltser I, Canlon B. Protecting the auditory system with glucocorticoids. Hear Res. 2011;281(1–2):47–55.
35. Shaul C, Venkatagiri PK, Lo J, Eastwood HT, Bester CW, Briggs RJS, et al. Glucocorticoid for hearing preservation after cochlear implantation: a systemic review and meta-analysis of animal studies. Otol Neurotol. 2019;40(9):1178–85.
36. Sweeney AD, Carlson ML, Zuniga MG, Bennett ML, Wanna GB, Haynes DS, et al. Impact of perioperative oral steroid use on low-frequency hearing preservation after cochlear implantation. Otol Neurotol. 2015;36(9):1480–5.
37. Prenzler NK, Salcher R, Lenarz T, Gaertner L, Warnecke A. Dose-dependent transient decrease of impedances by deep intracochlear injection of triamcinolone with a cochlear catheter prior to cochlear implantation-1 year data. Front Neurol. 2020;11:258.

38. Büchner A, Illg A, Majdani O, Lenarz T. Investigation of the effect of cochlear implant electrode length on speech comprehension in quiet and noise compared with the results with users of electro-acoustic-stimulation, a retrospective analysis. PLoS One. 2017;12(5):e0174900.
39. Skarzynski H, Lorens A, Piotrowska A, Anderson I. Partial deafness cochlear implantation provides benefit to a new population of individuals with hearing loss. Acta Otolaryngol. 2006;126(9):934–40.
40. James C, Albegger K, Battmer R, Burdo S, Deggouj N, Deguine O, et al. Preservation of residual hearing with cochlear implantation: how and why. Acta Otolaryngol. 2005;125(5):481–91.
41. Adunka OF, Dillon MT, Adunka MC, King ER, Pillsbury HC, Buchman CA. Hearing preservation and speech perception outcomes with electric-acoustic stimulation after 12 months of listening experience. Laryngoscope. 2013;123(10):2509–15.
42. Brockmeier SJ, Peterreins M, Lorens A, Vermeire K, Helbig S, Anderson I, et al. Music perception in electric acoustic stimulation users as assessed by the Mu.S.I.C. test. Adv Otorhinolaryngol. 2010;67:70–80.
43. Mamelle E, Granger B, Sterkers O, Lahlou G, Ferrary E, Nguyen Y, et al. Long-term residual hearing in cochlear implanted adult patients who were candidates for electro-acoustic stimulation. Eur Arch Otorhinolaryngol. 2020;277(3):705–13.
44. Incerti PV, Ching TY, Cowan R. A systematic review of electric-acoustic stimulation: device fitting ranges, outcomes, and clinical fitting practices. Trends Amplif. 2013;17(1):3–26.
45. Selleck AM, Park LR, Choudhury B, Teagle HFB, Woodard JS, Gagnon EB, et al. Hearing preservation in pediatric recipients of cochlear implants. Otol Neurotol. 2019;40(3):e277–e82.
46. Gantz BJ, Dunn C, Walker E, Van Voorst T, Gogel S, Hansen M. Outcomes of adolescents with a short electrode cochlear implant with preserved residual hearing. Otol Neurotol. 2016;37(2):e118–25.
47. Carlson ML, Patel NS, Tombers NM, DeJong MD, Breneman AI, Neff BA, et al. Hearing preservation in pediatric cochlear implantation. Otol Neurotol. 2017;38(6):e128–e33.
48. Bourn S, Goldstein MR, Jacob A. Hearing preservation in elderly cochlear implant recipients. Otol Neurotol. 2020;41(5):618–24.
49. Campbell L, Kaicer A, Sly D, Iseli C, Wei B, Briggs R, et al. Intraoperative real-time cochlear response telemetry predicts hearing preservation in cochlear implantation. Otol Neurotol. 2016;37(4):332–8.
50. Kim JS. Electrocochleography in cochlear implant users with residual acoustic hearing: a systematic review. Int J Environ Res Public Health. 2020;17(19).
51. Yin LX, Barnes JH, Saoji AA, Carlson ML. Clinical utility of intraoperative electrocochleography (ECochG) during cochlear implantation: a systematic review and quantitative analysis. Otol Neurotol. 2020;Publish Ahead of Print.
52. Kaufmann CR, Henslee AM, Claussen A, Hansen MR. Evaluation of insertion forces and cochlea trauma following robotics-assisted cochlear implant electrode array insertion. Otol Neurotol. 2020;41(5):631–8.

# Endoscopic-Assisted Cochlear Implantation

# 16

Davide Soloperto, Daniele Marchioni, Nicola Bisi, and Alessia Rubini

## 16.1 History of Endoscopic Ear Surgery

Middle ear surgery was revolutionized in the 1950s through the introduction of the binocular oto-microscope. Since the microscope had a direct view of the surgical field, blind spaces in the middle ear, like the retro tympanum and epitympanum, were investigated during surgery through micro-mirrors.

In 1966, Harrold Hopkins invented the Hopkins rod endoscope with Karl Storz's group for the exploration of the tympanic membrane. The endoscope was first employed for the observation of the tympanic membrane and for the investigation of the tympanic cavity, looking through a tympanic perforation, providing a more detailed view of the retrotympanic regions [1].

Wullstein popularized the use of angled endoscopes in 1984. Otosurgeons started using the 2.7 mm optical system with a 70° angle, Wullstein's scope, to monitor the posterior recesses of the tympanic cavity.

In 1988, a video-monitored endoscopic guided surgery was developed for the retro tympanum and the anterior epitympanum with special instruments, by matching the endoscope with a micro-camera.

In 1990, Thomassin first chronicled the endoscopic use to detect residual cholesteatoma during microscopic surgery [2].

The use of the endoscope for myringoplasty [3], for support during second look cholesteatoma surgery [4], to transtympanically recognize perilymphatic fistulae [5], to discover other middle ear lesions during the follow-up period and for the

**Supplementary Information** The online version contains supplementary material available at [https://doi.org/10.1007/978-981-19-0452-3_16].

D. Soloperto · D. Marchioni (✉) · N. Bisi · A. Rubini
Department of Otolaryngology Head and Neck Surgery, University of Verona, Verona, Italy


S. DeSaSouza (ed.), *Cochlear Implants*,
https://doi.org/10.1007/978-981-19-0452-3_16

handling of previously canal wall up approach treated cholesteatomas [6], dates back to the 1990s.

Tarabichi first examined the results of endoscopic ear surgery (EES) for cholesteatomas in 1997, describing the transcanal endoscopic tympanotomy and the extended atticotomy techniques for cholesteatoma sac removal [7].

During the "8th International Conference on Cholesteatoma and Ear Surgery" in Antalia (Turkey) Dr. Stephane Ayache proposed to create an otosurgeon group from all over the world, who was beginning to use the endoscope for otologic procedures. This international working group on Endoscopic Ear Surgery (IWGEES) was initially formed by Dr. Mohamed Badr-El-Dine (Egypt), Muaaz Tarabichi (Dubai), Livio Presutti (Italy), Daniele Marchioni (Italy), Stephan Ayache (France) David Pothier (Canada), and Seiji Kakehata (Japan).

The possibility of using the endoscope as an assisting or operative tool for cholesteatoma surgery started spreading worldwide at the beginning of the twenty-first century.

Thanks to the experience of the IWGEES, many courses and congresses were organized worldwide, in order to teach and spread the new endoscopic technique of middle ear surgery. In particular, the teachings were based on new anatomical concepts regarding the tympanic cavity and new physiopathological principles.

In fact, the use of endoscopy during cholesteatoma surgery has allowed surgeons to analyze and redefine the anatomical knowledge of the tympanic cavity. Many studies, from our school Marchioni/Presutti, have been crucial to systematically organize the anatomical and physiological principles. This is nowadays the basis of endoscopic ear surgery, such as the pathways of ventilation in the middle ear, the anatomical classification of the retrotympanic spaces and structures, the selective attical dysventilation syndrome which is the rationale of the transcanal endoscopic approach to attical cholesteatoma.

The advantages of EES are many, including the chance of preserving the mastoid cavity and thus its functions, the conservation of the ossicular chain and the non-pathological mucosa. Moreover, the endoscope allows for the magnification of the middle ear blind recesses and for surgical work in these areas, preventing residual disease, and it allows for the restoration of the pathways of ventilation in the middle ear, thus preventing recurrence [8, 9].

The first experiences of the application of the endoscope in cholesteatoma surgery have shown a clear advantage over microscopic exclusive surgery, especially regarding residual rate.

In 2017, Panetti et al. compared the endoscopic-assisted surgical procedure to the microscopic procedure for the treatment of cholesteatoma and a lower residual cholesteatoma rate was observed when the endoscope was employed during surgery [10].

Badr-El-Dine deemed the sinus tympani to be the most frequent site of intraoperative residuals in both canal wall up (CWU) and canal wall down (CWD) groups by the following ones being the facial recess and the undersurface of the scutum in the CWU patients. The overall incidence of intraoperative residuals identified using the endoscope, in primary surgery after thorough microscopic cleaning was 22.8% [11].

Further advances in the endoscopic technique were introduced by our Italian school (Marchioni/Presutti), who codified the endoscopic transcanal approach to the inner ear, in particular, the transcanal transpromontorial route that allows for intralabyrinthine and intracanalicular vestibular schwannoma removal in patients with sensorineural hearing loss. This is a minimally invasive approach to the inner ear and internal auditory canal, avoiding extended transtemporal approaches and manipulation of the posterior and medial cranial fossa dura.

However, the endoscope also has some disadvantages including the one-handed nature of the technique, the two-dimensional vision of the surgical field, the difficult control of intraoperative bleeding.

Nowadays, the endoscopic technique is performed in many clinics worldwide for tympanic neoplasm, otosclerosis, chronic otitis media, and especially for cholesteatoma, as it has proved to be very advantageous for the treatment of the tympanic cavity, in association with the microscope if the pathology to be treated also extends to the mastoid.

### 16.1.1 Endoscopy in Cochlear Implantation

All the anatomical features of the round window district and inferior retrotympanum have been endoscopically inspected and outlined, being a crucial area of the middle ear [12, 13].

The present authors' studies on the endoscopic anatomy of the round window were the first to focus on the anatomy of the *fustis* and its implications on CI surgery.

The round window niche, an anatomical bony structure shaping the entry of the cochlear membrane, posteriorly merges into the inferior retrotympanum and is located between the *finiculus* (anteriorly and inferiorly) and the *subiculum* (posteriorly and superiorly). It has a trilateral shape, with the posterior pillar, the tegmen, and the anterior pillar as its boundaries and the RW membrane at its apex. The *subiculum* (from Latin, "support") expands from the posterior pillar to the styloid prominence, inferiorly limiting the sinus tympani. The *finiculus* (from Latin, "border") stretches from the anterior pillar to the jugular dome, dividing the retrotympanum from the hypotympanum. Proctor initially defined it as *sustentaculum promontori*, as it was believed to always encompass the inferior tympanic artery [14].

The *fustis* is a smooth bony element making up the floor of the round window chamber (a three-dimensional area lying between the round window niche and round window membrane). It runs from the styloid complex to the round window niche, and it represents an important landmark for the identification of the RW membrane and the scala tympani beyond it [15].

Two different types of *fustis* were defined, according to their orientation with the scala tympani: in type A it points to the *scala tympani*, while in type B the antero-superior limit of the *fustis* lies immediately below the *scala tympani* and it represents its floor.

Between the *fustis* and the *finiculus*, a wide tunnel is often noticeable which deeply extends below the cochlea, linking the tympanic cavity to the petrous apex cells stretching under the promontory. Different types of *subcochlear canaliculus* were defined by the current authors according to their grade of pneumatization and extension: Type A, the most pneumatized, was described as a deep and wide tunnel medially originating from the round window niche and extending under the cochlea and the internal auditory canal until the petrous apex, type B as a limited pneumatization under the cochlea, without a detectable relationship to the petrous apex. In Type C the *subcochlear canaliculus is absent,* without a pneumatized area under the cochlea and the petrous apex. These different conformations are age related, in fact, from 3 to 19 years pneumatization constantly increases, with a peak in adolescence. Then it progressively reduces; in fact, type C is more present from 19 years onward, and the lowest percentage of pneumatization is reached in elderly patients [16] (Fig. 16.1).

Clinical applications of the endoscopic study of the retrotympanum and the round window chamber anatomy are important for cholesteatoma and cochlear implantation surgery. In these surgeries, the knowledge of the round window anatomy is relevant, in particular, the morphology of the *fustis* and its different inclinations that indicate the round window membrane and the *subcochlear canaliculus*, to understand the position of the round window membrane and guide array insertion in difficult cases, or for removal of residual disease in pediatric cholesteatoma [12, 16].

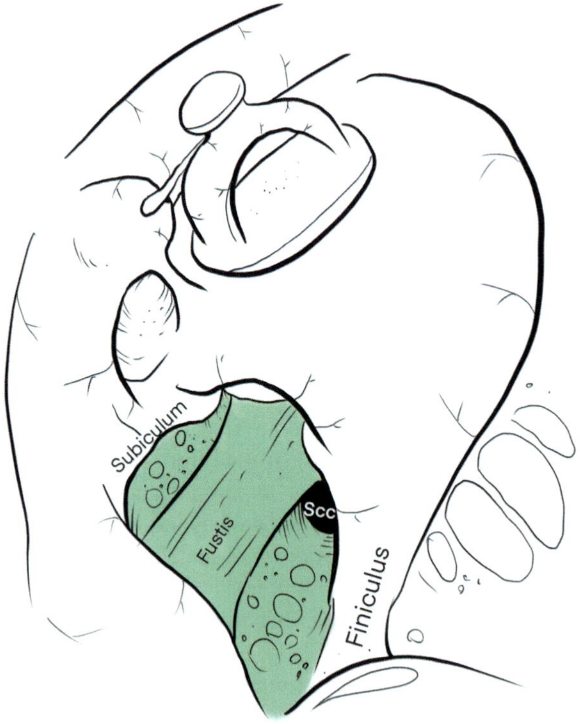


**Fig. 16.1** Drawing showing the round window niche with its anatomical boundaries, the *subiculum* and the *finiculus*. The round window chamber floor is made up of the *fustis* that points to the *scala tympani*. The *subcochlear canaliculus* (Scc) can be identified between the *fustis* and the *finiculus*

Therefore, we believe the endoscope can be particularly helpful especially in case of malformed anatomy, since the tympanic cavity can be magnified thanks to this valuable tool.

Middle and inner ear malformations prove technically challenging for CI surgery, when the facial nerve has an anomalous course or in case of cerebrospinal fluid gusher.

Endoscopy associated with CI placement is described in literature as a microscopic-endoscopic assisted or transcanal exclusive endoscopic procedure.

The first endoscopic assisted surgical approaches described in our articles introduced two different types of microscopic endoscopic-assisted cochlear implantation: an endoscopic approach with a small transmastoid tunnel for array placement to avoid array extrusions and a trans-attical approach in case of malformations (codified by Marchioni/Presutti) that requires a regular mastoidectomy and an array insertion through a trans-attical route.

A third approach described in literature requires an exclusively transcanal endoscopic technique.

### 16.1.2 Endoscopic-Assisted CI Placement

The first application of the endoscope in cochlear implantation was associated to a microscopic retroauricular procedure. It required endoscopic steps in which a transcanal endoscopic approach to tympanic cavity was performed to check the anatomical features and to obtain a clear view of the round window to carry out an endoscopic cochleostomy through the round window membrane or, in case of inaccessible round window, a promontorial cochleostomy. After that the microscopic steps included a retro auricular incision and a mastoidectomy with an anterior atticotomy, thus opening an ample connection between the posterior epitympanum and the mesotympanic spaces. The array was gently pushed from the epitympanum into the mesotympanum, through the passage which had been created, then the array was carefully introduced into the cochleostomy, working through the external auditory canal. Indications for this trans-attical endoscopic-assisted CI placement approach are an atypical course of the facial nerve and anomalies of the inner ear (i.e., CHARGE syndrome), a high jugular bulb that forbids an explorative tympanotomy and a sclerotic mastoid.

As stated above, patients suffering from CHARGE syndrome or other ear malformations which discourage traditional transmastoid facial recess access surgery, need an endoscopic transcanal approach to the round window niche that enables the surgeon to better identify the promontorial structures [17].

Along with anatomical malformations, the assistance of the endoscope is also useful in case of cochlear implantation in ossified cochlea (meningitis, autoimmune inner ear diseases, advanced otosclerosis, temporal bone traumas, other pathological conditions). It avoids a blind dissection thanks to the magnification of the anatomical features of the round window and the subsequent identification of the surrounding anatomical structures of the niche [18].

This technique enables the surgeon to increase the number of cases in which cochlear implantation is feasible, and, we believe, it will also lower the morbidity rate linked to this surgical technique.

Further development in the use of the endoscope for CI surgery is the transcanal endoscopic-assisted procedure, which allows for CI placement without a mastoidectomy. This technique provides a viable option which allows for an optimal view of the RW niche for a secure identification of the scala tympani [19].

Using micro-loupes or a microscope, the skin of the posterior portion of the EAC is carefully detached from the bony section of the canal, lifting the tympanic membrane to enter the tympanic cavity. Under endoscopic magnification of the round window, its membrane is identified and a cochleostomy is performed. A 4-mm wide bony groove is then fashioned in the facial recess in the posterior-superior portion of the EAC, employing a diamond burr to identify the facial nerve course. Behind Henle's spine, another corridor is then opened in the mastoid section, so the array is inserted in this tunnel and then, under endoscopic magnification, it is gradually pushed into the previously identified RW membrane.

### 16.1.3 Totally Endoscopic CI Placement

Abdulrahman Dia et al. analyzed 25 transcanal exclusively endoscopic cochlear implantations carried out in 24 ears [20].

In this procedure, the external auditory canal skin is endoscopically lifted from the bony wall of the canal and by drilling, a groove is created to place the proximal segment of the array. Then the electrode array is inserted via the canal into the RW or into a cochleostomy.

All implants were fully introduced into the scala tympani, and 24 of them showed a regular function with appropriate thresholds. No relevant complications were observed, the implant array was visible through the external auditory canal skin, while not exposed, in 6 out of 24 ears. Sixteen months was the mean follow-up time [20].

This approach was largely discussed, due to the possible complications connected to the array extrusion, since the array is placed underneath the skin of the external auditory canal. Among the possible problems, skin infections and the formation of iatrogenic cholesteatoma are worthy of note.

Some authors state that the endoscopic approach does not provide a useful contribution to cochlear implant surgery. Tarabichi et al., for instance, maintain that the transcanal approach provides access to the basal turn of the cochlea at a significant angle to the axis of the scala tympani, in comparison to the traditional microscopic approach through a posterior tympanotomy, therefore a deflection of the electrode off the wall of the cochlea would be called for to follow the trajectory of the basal turn [21].

Moreover, using the external auditory canal as a path for the electrodes might lead to extrusion, epithelial ingrowth, and chronic infection. The above-mentioned authors found a consistent number of electrode extrusion cases in the canal and an

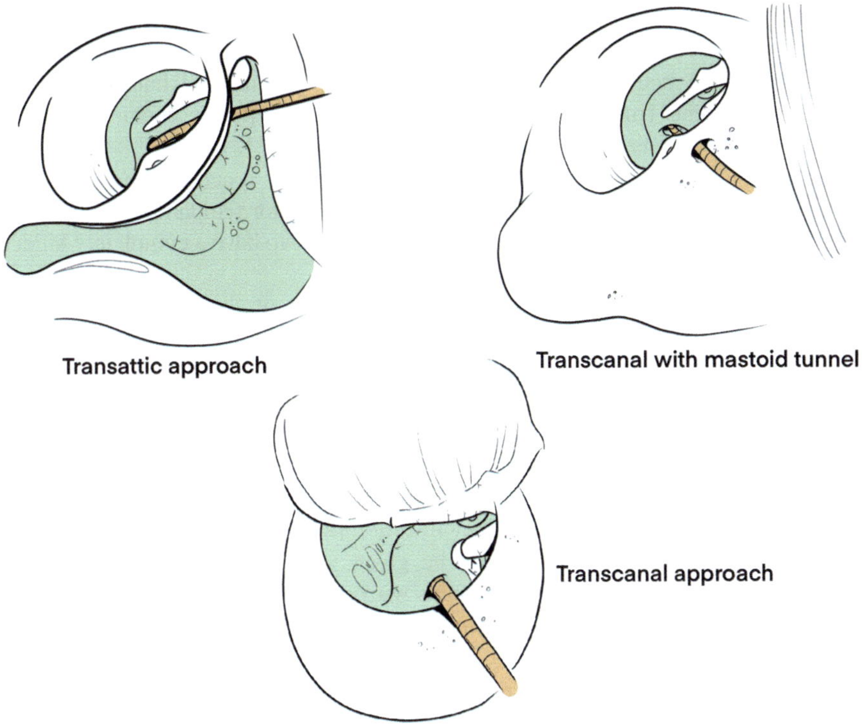


**Fig. 16.2** Drawing showing the array positioning during the endoscopic assisted transattic approach, the endoscopic assisted transcanal approach with mastoid tunnel and during the totally endoscopic transcanal cochlear implantation approach

amount of acquired cholesteatomas, probably due to transcanal wiring. They reached the conclusion that cochlear implantation through a posterior tympanotomy is a low morbidity and highly effective surgical operation so, in their opinion, the endoscopic technique is not that useful in regular CI surgery.

The trans-attical endoscopic-assisted CI placement procedure and the transcanal endoscopic-assisted one through a small tunnel posterior to Henle's spine, avoid the above-mentioned complications by placing the array through the mastoid and the attic or through the facial recess, so the electrode is stored in a considerable bone chuck, far from the ear canal (Fig. 16.2).

## 16.2 Surgical Considerations

Nowadays, indications for cochlear implantation (CI) are expanding and difficult cases require a prompt preoperative radiological assessment of middle ear, cochlea, and mastoid anatomy.

Bone malformations of the labyrinth have been found in 20% of all cases of congenital profound hearing loss [22] and the incidence has recently increased to 30% due to the betterment in high-resolution CT scanning techniques and the improved awareness of cochlear malformations, as a consequence, cochlear implants are increasingly being inserted in malformed cochleae [23].

When middle and inner ear abnormalities are present, it can be difficult to gain access to the promontory and RW via a standard posterior tympanotomy. In literature, 4%–14% of patients with ear anomalies are found to have a completely hidden or absent RW, during CI surgery [24, 25].

In these circumstances, the microscopic insertion of the electrodes into the cochlea might endanger the facial nerve (FN) and the presence of a partially or totally concealed RW niche and membrane might make it unfeasible to approach the cochlea [26].

Therefore, it is of paramount importance for a safe and successful surgery to correctly expose the anatomical landmarks and to be aware of the relation among the atypical middle ear structures to prevent facial nerve damage and to produce the correct cochleostomy position for array insertion [27].

Furthermore, consideration should be given whether to the present practice might lead to gusher in syndromic patients with ear anomalies and the condition of the cochlear nerve in the internal auditory canal (IAC) must be taken into account before surgery [28].

Even in cases without complex malformations, a sclerotic mastoid with no air cells and a high jugular bulb could represent difficult conditions for the surgeon.

The endoscopic assisted CI approach devised in the last few years, as previously stated, might therefore represent a good solution for the management of these difficult cases.

### 16.2.1 Surgical Endoscopes

Different types of rigid endoscopes are normally used for ear surgery. They are either 2.7, 3, or 4 mm in diameter. The working lengths are 18, 15, 14, 11, and 6 cm.

The 0° and 30° angled endoscopes are the most widespread, followed by the 45° endoscope. An endoscope with a greater angle (70°) is only employed for the inspection and management of limited spaces like the sinus tympani. The current authors recommend the use of endoscopes with 3 mm diameter and 15 cm length, with angles of 0° and 45°; a 4-mm endoscope should be considered only in case of a wide external auditory canal (Fig. 16.3).

### 16.2.2 Surgical Steps

#### 16.2.2.1 Endoscopic Steps

A 0° endoscope, 15 cm in length, is introduced into the external auditory canal and employed to fashion a tympano-meatal flap (Fig. 16.4a). This is commonly elevated

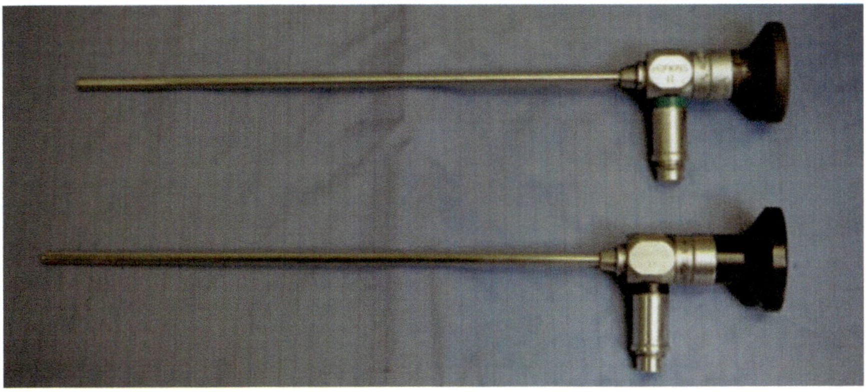

**Fig. 16.3** Karl Storz Hopkins endoscopes of 15 cm length, 4 mm diameter, with different angles (0° and 45°)

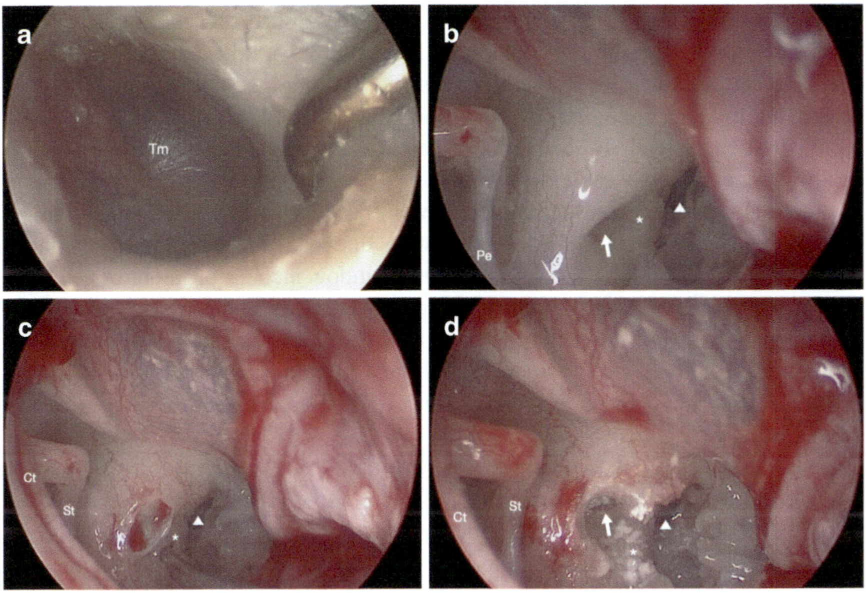


**Fig. 16.4** (**a–d**) Transcanal endoscopic approach to the RW. The tympano-meatal flap is harvested, gaining access to the promontory region. The RW region is visualized, with the tegmen procidence, obscuring the RW membrane. Fustis type B helps in the visualization of the RW position. After drilling the tegmen area, the RW membrane is finally shown. Ct, Chorda tympani; St, stapes; Pe, pyramidal eminence; Tm, tympanic membrane; *, fustis; white arrow, RW membrane; white triangle, subcochlear canaliculus

under endoscopic view, gaining access to the tympanic cavity. The flap is then anteriorly pulled, until the posterior border of the malleus is detectable. After lifting the timpano-meatal flap, an endoscopic check of the tympanic cavity anatomical structures is carried out (Fig. 16.4b). When the facial nerve is discovered to have an

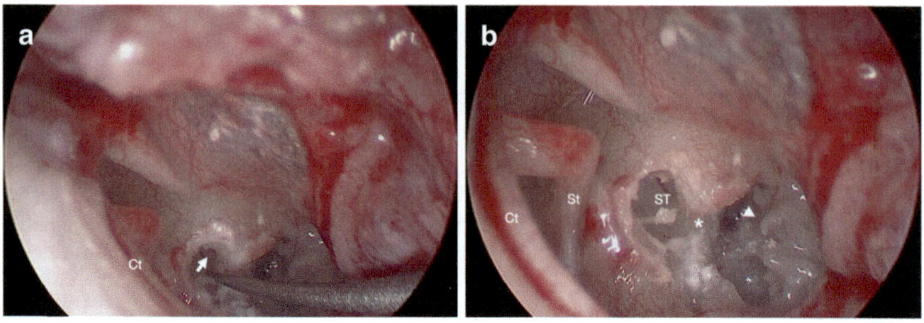


**Fig. 16.5** (**a**, **b**) Transcanal endoscopic approach to the RW. The RW is well identified and opened with a micro-hook, exposing the scala tympani. Notice the parallel orientation of the fustis in relation to the scala tympani. Ct, chorda timpani; St, stapes; ST, scala tympani; *, fustis; white arrow, direction of the scala tympani; white triangle, subcochlear canaliculus

atypical course, an inspection of the correlation between the nerve and the ossicular structures, RW niche and promontory, is due. Once the surgeon defines the anatomical connection among the surrounding structures of the middle ear, the RW niche is distinctly detected and its accessibility assessed. A diamond burr can be employed to drill out the tegmen, to improve the exposure of the RW (Fig. 16.4c, d).

When such exposure is obtained, the membrane is opened through a micro-hook, crafting access to the scala tympani (Fig. 16.5a, b). Afterward, a fragment of Gelfoam is positioned on the opened RW. In case a disadvantageous anatomy is discovered and when the RW is not accessible, due to an altered course of the facial nerve or a huge jugular bulb hiding the round window niche, a promontorial cochleostomy can be carried out. In such instances, during promontorial cochleostomy endoscopic control of the facial nerve and the RW niche is paramount to preserve the nerve itself. The scala tympani can be gently opened, performing a cochleostomy just anteriorly and inferiorly to the RW. Eventually, Gelfoam is set on the cochleostomy aperture.

#### 16.2.2.2 Microscopic Steps

A retroauricolar skin incision is produced, detecting the plane of the temporal muscle fascia; a posterior periosteal flap is fashioned and lifted, revealing the mastoid bone (Fig. 16.6a–c). When the mastoid cells are there and no ossicle or facial nerve imperfection is found, the surgical steps are the ones of a suprameatal approach. An antrotomy, with an anterior atticotomy, is carried out, following the conventional landmarks, and preserving the posterior wall of the external auditory canal (Fig. 16.6d). The anterior atticotomy continues through the suprameatal route to expose the incudo-malleolar joint and the anterior attic.

When the mastoid air cells are missing and there is not enough space through the suprameatal route, the incus is taken away, thus producing an ample link between the posterior epitympanum and the mesotympanic spaces (Fig. 16.7a–d). When the mastoid air cells are abundant, a limited posterior tympanotomy is carried out, to widen the surgical area for array introduction, keeping the ossicles intact.

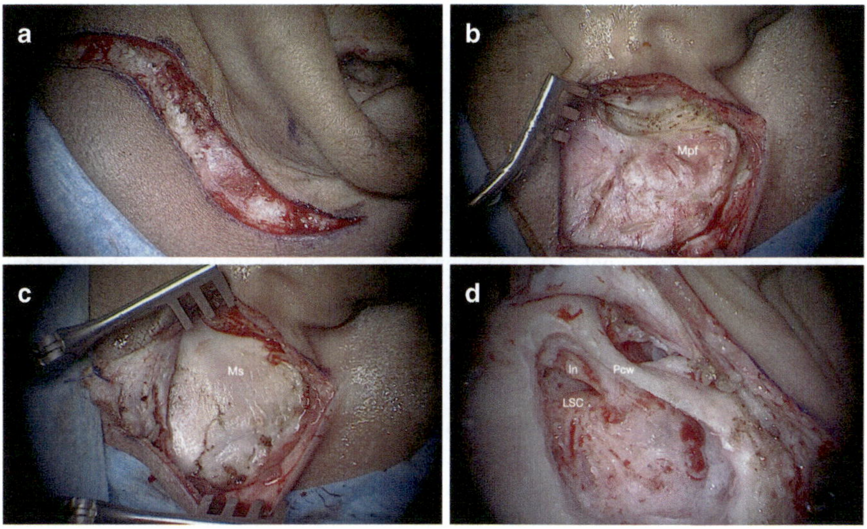


**Fig. 16.6** (**a–d**) Microscopic steps. A postero-superiorly extending retroauricolar incision is performed. The plane of the temporalis fascia is found, then the muscolar-subperiostal flap is elevated and fixed with a stitch. The mastoid bone is uncovered. After cortical mastoidectomy, the traditional landmarks are exposed. In, incus; LSC, lateral semicircular canal; Mpf, mastoid periostal flap; Ms, mastoid bone; Pcw, posterior canal wall

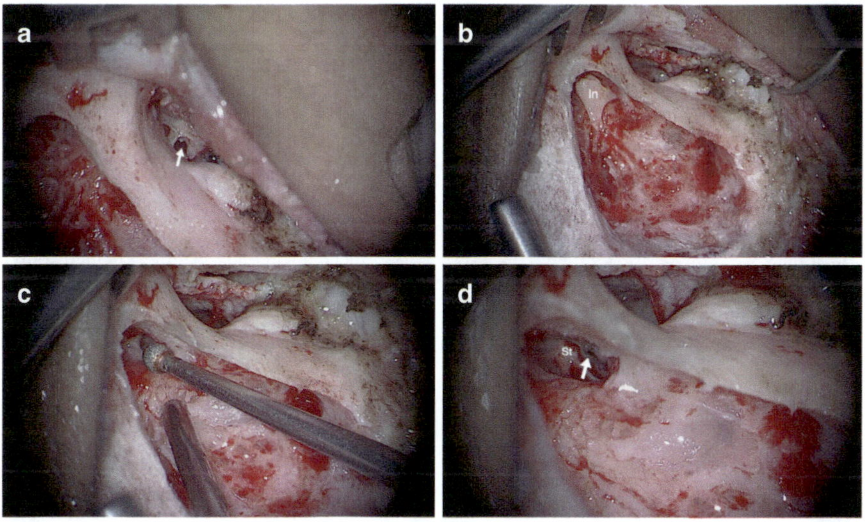


**Fig. 16.7** (**a–d**) Microscopic steps. The previously endoscopically opened RW is visualized under microscopic view (white arrow). The incus is removed (**b**), the attic is well opened to better expose the trans mastoid route for the insertion of the array (**c**, **d**). In, incus; St, stapes

The receiver–stimulator of the implant is introduced and encased under the temporalis muscle. The array is smoothly driven through the corridor which has been crafted, from the epitympanum into the mesotympanum; the array is then covered and carefully introduced into the cochleostomy, through the external auditory canal (Fig. 16.8a–d). Intraoperative X-rays are carried out to validate the correct position of the array.

The cochleostomy is sealed with a small piece of temporalis fascia along with fibrin glue. The timpano-meatal flap is repositioned, and Gelfoam is used to pack the external auditory canal. The receiver body is covered under the subperiosteal flap and the retroauricolar skin incision is closed (Video 16.1).

Several surgical approaches are reported in literature to treat difficult cases in CI surgery. Some authors recommend a transcanal or osteoplastic technique through the posterior canal [29] or a suprameatal approach (SMA), in which a full mastoidectomy is avoided but a suprameatal tunnel is carried out. Vascular anomalies may hinder the realization of this tunnel [30].

Singh et al. favored a canal wall down (CWD) tympanomastoidectomy in case of ear malformations [31]. However, this approach has many drawbacks including electrode extrusion, mastoid cavity maintenance, and the risk of infection.

Sennaroglu et al. proposed access to the middle ear through an endaural incision with a timpano-meatal flap as a replacement of the CWD technique [32]. They decided to cover the electrode creating a groove in the posterior ear canal while

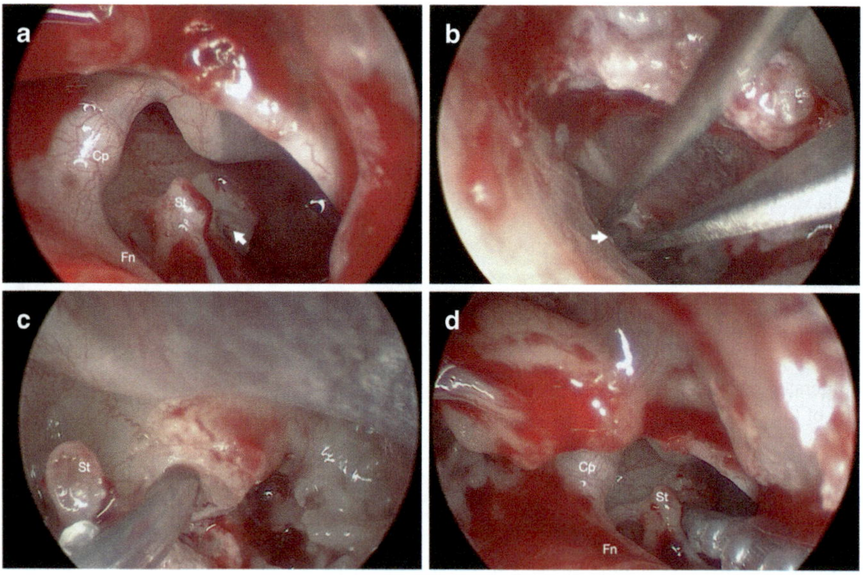


**Fig. 16.8** (**a**–**d**) Endoscopic view through the transmastoid transattic route before array insertion (**a** white arrow). The array is gently pushed inside the cochlea (**b** white arrow). Endoscopic transcanal check of the correct array insertion (**c**, **d**). Cp, cochleariform process; Fn, facial nerve; St, stapes

moving the electrode into the mastoid cavity. However, a mastoidectomy was still required, thus making these approaches potentially more challenging for syndromic people, like CHARGE suffering patients. The Modified Rambo transcanal approach is another viable option. A laterally based tragal skin flap is fashioned and the skin covering the concha cartilage is lifted back, then a blind sac closure after the circumferential dissection of the soft tissue around the cartilaginous canal is performed and the skin is everted outside the meatus [33].

Eventually, some authors recommend a subtotal petrosectomy to secure a better field of vision and better gusher control [34]. This approach grants a better management of the CSF leakage, through the obliteration of the Eustachian tube orifice and cavity, but this surgical procedure poses some risks, namely the chance of fat infection, which can spread through the cochleostomy, leading to meningitis, and the occurrence of entrapped cholesteatoma in the cavity.

From our experience, we strongly recommend an endoscopic-assisted cochlear implant in all patients, both adults and children, with possible unfavorable anatomical exposure of the RW, because of the advantages offered by this approach. First, the transcanal corridor should be preferred since it produces the clearest frontal direct view of the RW area [24, 35].

This feature, along with structure magnification, with a full HD view and the opportunity to work really close to the anatomical landmarks, represents the major benefit of this kind of approach. Moreover, angled endoscopes allow for a visualization around the corner, granting a panoramic view of the anatomical structures, which would be impossible through the direct line of vision of the microscope. This turns out to be of paramount importance to gain access to the RW area and for a correct introduction of the electrodes into the ST [36].

The morphology of the RW membrane, the fustis, the area concamerata, and the subcochlear canaliculi are well visible in all conditions [15, 17].

The use of the endoscope also enables the surgeon to clearly detect the orientation of the ST of the basal turn, producing valuable details about the orientation of the modiolus and guaranteeing a correct positioning and progress of the array into the cochlea.

Another relevant aspect to be considered concerns a possible iatrogenic damage to the facial nerve which still represents a major surgical complication after cochlear implant placement, especially in malformed ears [25]. During the endoscopic step of a cochleostomy, the facial nerve is always under direct and magnified observation, even in case of an atypical course, therefore the use of the endoscope allows for a much safer transmastoid/suprameatal microscopic step, by pointing out the precise course of the facial nerve in the middle ear. In addition, through this technique the chorda tympani is preserved, since it gets mobilized during the endoscopic step and it is not drilled during the microscopic trans-attic step.

Eventually, the endoscopic use protects the integrity of the posterior canal wall and avoids a subtotal petrosectomy or any other of the previously described open approaches [17].

Downsides mainly concern the long learning curve, enhancing the risk of damage to the tympano-meatal flap, such as tympanic membrane perforation with a consequent possible infection through the defect, because of inexperienced hands. Also, the bleeding management affects the choice of the physician's surgical technique. Despite the possibility of avoiding it, at times, an endoscopic assisted CI requires also the incus removal, limiting the use of the stapedial reflex for the evaluation of the C-level (i.e., comfort or maximal stimulation level). For syndromic young children, with a developmental delay this can be regarded as a drawback [35].

Other reported disadvantages are a higher electrode extrusion risk, chronic infections and acquired cholesteatoma. Finally, a transcanal approach would grant access to the basal turn of the cochlea at a substantial angle to the axis of the cochlear basal turn [21].

In conclusion, we recommend endoscopic assistance, in particular when complex anatomy is foreseen, in subjects requiring cochlear implantation. Unlike the traditional microscopic approach, it grants a better observation of the promontorial structures, even in malformed ears, where conventional approaches and also neuroradiological investigation do not always lead to suitable solutions to the patients' and the otosurgeon's necessities.

## References


1. Marquet J, Boedts D. Otology. Acta Otorhinolaryngol Belg. 1975;29(2):299–316.
2. Thomassin JM, Inedjian JM, Rud C, Conciatori J, Vilcoq P. Otoendoscopy: application in the middle ear surgery. Rev Laryngol Otol Rhinol. 1990;111(5):475–7.
3. El-Guindy A. Endoscopic transcanal myringoplasty. J Laryngol Otol. 1992;106(6):493–5.
4. McKennan KX. Endoscopic "second look" mastoidoscopy to rule out residual epitympanic/mastoid cholesteatoma. Laryngoscope. 1993;103(7):810–4.
5. Poe DS, Rebeiz EE, Pankratov MM. Evaluation of perilymphatic fistulas by middle ear endoscopy. Am J Otol. 1992;13(6):529–33.
6. Thomassin JM, Braccini F. Role of imaging and endoscopy in the follow up and management of cholesteatomas operated by closed technique. Rev Laryngol Otol Rhinol. 1999;120(2):75–81.
7. Tarabichi M. Endoscopic management of acquired cholesteatoma. Am J Otol. 1997;18(5):544–9.
8. Alicandri-Ciufelli M, Marchioni D, Kakehata S, Presutti L, Villari D. Endoscopic management of attic cholesteatoma. Otolaryngol Clin N Am. 2016;49(5):1265–70.
9. Presutti L, Anschuetz L, Rubini A, Ruberto M, Alicandri-Ciufelli M, Dematte M, et al. The impact of the transcanal endoscopic approach and mastoid preservation on recurrence of primary acquired attic cholesteatoma. Otol Neurotol. 2018;39(4):445–50.
10. Panetti G, Cavaliere M, Panetti M, Marino A, Iemma M. Endoscopic tympanoplasty in the treatment of chronic otitis media: our experience. Acta Otolaryngol (Stockh). 2017;137(3):225–8.
11. Badr-el-Dine M. Value of ear endoscopy in cholesteatoma surgery. Otol Neurotol. 2002;23(5):631–5.
12. Marchioni D, Alicandri-Ciufelli M, Pothier DD, Rubini A, Presutti L. The round window region and contiguous areas: endoscopic anatomy and surgical implications. Eur Arch Otorhinolaryngol. 2015;272(5):1103–12.
13. Marchioni D, Alicandri-Ciufelli M, Piccinini A, Genovese E, Presutti L. Inferior retrotympanum revisited: an endoscopic anatomic study: inferior retrotympanum revisited. Laryngoscope. 2010;120(9):1880–6.
14. Proctor B, Bollobas B, Niparko JK. Anatomy of the round window niche. Ann Otol Rhinol Laryngol. 1986;95(5):444–6.

15. Marchioni D, Soloperto D, Colleselli E, Tatti MF, Patel N, Jufas N. Round window chamber and fustis: endoscopic anatomy and surgical implications. Surg Radiol Anat. 2016;38(9):1013–9.
16. Marchioni D, Gazzini L, Bisi N, Barillari M, Rubini A. Subcochlear canaliculus patterns in the pediatric and adult population: radiological findings and surgical implications. Surg Radiol Anat [Internet]. 2021 Feb 20 [cited 2021 May 9].
17. Marchioni D, Soloperto D, Guarnaccia MC, Genovese E, Alicandri-Ciufelli M, Presutti L. Endoscopic assisted cochlear implants in ear malformations. Eur Arch Otorhinolaryngol. 2015;272(10):2643–52.
18. Marchioni D, Soloperto D, Bianconi L, Guarnaccia MC, Genovese E, Presutti L. Endoscopic approach for cochlear implantation in advanced otosclerosis: a case report. Auris Nasus Larynx. 2016;43(5):584–90.
19. Marchioni D, Grammatica A, Alicandri-Ciufelli M, Genovese E, Presutti L. Endoscopic cochlear implant procedure. Eur Arch Otorhinolaryngol. 2014;271(5):959–66.
20. Dia A, Nogueira JF, O'Grady KM, Redleaf M. Report of endoscopic Cochlear implantation. Otol Neurotol. 2014;35(10):1755–8.
21. Tarabichi M, Nazhat O, Kassouma J, Najmi M. Endoscopic cochlear implantation: call for caution: endoscopic Cochlear implantation. Laryngoscope. 2016;126(3):689–92.
22. Jackler RK, Luxfor WM, House WF. Congenital malformations of the inner ear: a classification based on embryogenesis. Laryngoscope. 2009;97(S40):2–14.
23. McClay JE, Tandy R, Grundfast K, Choi S, Vezina G, Zalzal G, et al. Major and minor temporal bone abnormalities in children with and without congenital sensorineural hearing loss. Arch Otolaryngol Neck Surg. 2002;128(6):664.
24. Chen YH, Liu TC, Yang TH, Lin KN, Wu CC, Hsu CJ. Using endoscopy to locate the round window membrane during cochlear implantation: our experience with 25 patients. Clin Otolaryngol. 2018;43(1):357–62.
25. Vesseur AC, Verbist BM, Westerlaan HE, Kloostra FJJ, Admiraal RJC, van Ravenswaaij-Arts CMA, et al. CT findings of the temporal bone in CHARGE syndrome: aspects of importance in cochlear implant surgery. Eur Arch Otorhinolaryngol. 2016;273(12):4225–40.
26. Leong AC, Jiang D, Agger A, Fitzgerald-O'Connor A. Evaluation of round window accessibility to cochlear implant insertion. Eur Arch Otorhinolaryngol. 2013;270(4):1237–42.
27. Marchioni D, Carner M, Soloperto D, Sacchetto A, Genovese E, Presutti L. Endoscopic-assisted cochlear implant procedure in CHARGE syndrome: preliminary report. Acta Oto-Laryngol Case Rep. 2017;2(1):52–8.
28. Mylanus EAM, Rotteveel LJC, Leeuw RL. Congenital malformation of the inner ear and pediatric Cochlear implantation. Otol Neurotol. 2004;25(3):308–17.
29. Jang JH, Song J-J, Yoo JC, Lee JH, Oh SH, Chang SO. An alternative procedure for cochlear implantation: transcanal approach. Acta Otolaryngol (Stockh). 2012 Jun;5:1–5.
30. Kronenberg J, Baumgartner W, Migirov L, Dagan T, Hildesheimer M. The suprameatal approach: an alternative surgical approach to cochlear implantation. Otol Neurotol. 2004;25(1):41–5.
31. Singh RS. Modification of the standard surgical approach for cochlear implants. Ann Otol Rhinol Laryngol Suppl. 1995 Sep;166:432–4.
32. Sennaroglu L, Aydin E. Anteroposterior approach with split ear canal for Cochlear implantation in severe malformations. Otol Neurotol. 2002 Jan;23(1):39–43.
33. Wick CC, Moore AM, Killeen DE, Isaacson B. The modified Rambo Transcanal approach for Cochlear implantation in CHARGE syndrome. Otol Neurotol. 2017 Oct;38(9):1268–72.
34. Free RH, Falcioni M, Di Trapani G, Giannuzzi AL, Russo A, Sanna M. The role of subtotal Petrosectomy in Cochlear implant surgery: a report of 32 cases and review on indications. Otol Neurotol. 2013;34(6):1033–40.
35. Carner M, Sacchetto A, Bianconi L, Soloperto D, Sacchetto L, Presutti L, et al. Endoscopic-assisted Cochlear implantation in children with malformed ears. Otolaryngol Neck Surg. 2019 Oct;161(4):688–93.
36. Güneri EA, Olgun Y. Endoscope-assisted Cochlear implantation. Clin Exp Otorhinolaryngol. 2018;11(2):89–95.

# Robot-Assisted Cochlear Implantation 17

Daniele De Seta, Yann Nguyen, Renato Torres,
Isabelle Mosnier, and Olivier Sterkers

## 17.1 Introduction

Robotic surgery in the last few years has gained popularity in ear surgery as an effective tool to improve the accuracy of surgical gesture by reducing involuntary movements of the surgeon such as tremor, drift, undershoot and overshoot, and the

**Supplementary Information** The online version contains supplementary material available at [https://doi.org/10.1007/978-981-19-0452-3_17].

D. De Seta
Inserm/Institut Pasteur, Institut de l'Audition, Technologie et thérapie génique de la surdité, Paris, France

Unit of Otolaryngology, San Giovanni-Addolorata Hospital, Rome, Italy

Y. Nguyen · O. Sterkers (✉)
Inserm/Institut Pasteur, Institut de l'Audition, Technologie et thérapie génique de la surdité, Paris, France

GHU Pitié-Salpêtrière, DMU ChIR, Service ORL, GRC Robotique et Innovation Chirurgicale, AP-HP/Sorbonne Université, Paris, France

R. Torres
Inserm/Institut Pasteur, Institut de l'Audition, Technologie et thérapie génique de la surdité, Paris, France

Facultad de Medicina, Departamento de Ciencias Fisiologicas, Universidad Nacional de San Agustin de Arequipa, Arequipa, Peru

I. Mosnier
Inserm/Institut Pasteur, Institut de l'Audition, Technologie et thérapie génique de la surdité, Paris, France

GHU Pitié-Salpêtrière, DMU ChIR, Service ORL, GRC Robotique et Innovation Chirurgicale, AP-HP/Sorbonne Université, Paris, France

GHU Pitié-Salpêtrière, Unité Fonctionnelles Implants cochléaires, AP-HP/Sorbonne Université, Paris, France



S. DeSaSouza (ed.), *Cochlear Implants*,
https://doi.org/10.1007/978-981-19-0452-3_17

jerk, a sudden reflex or spasmodic muscular movement related to lack of experience or to tiredness. Other advantage reported by the use of robotic devices is the improvement of the force control feedback. Recent studies report that cochlear implantation may take advantage from robotic assistance in all the steps of the surgery: (i) the approach to the middle ear by automated mastoidectomy and posterior tympanotomy through a tunnel also known as direct cochlea access (DCA); (ii) a minimally invasive cochleostomy by means of robot-assisted drilling tool; (iii) the alignment of the correct insertion axis on the cochlear basal turn; and (iv) the insertion of the electrode array via motorized insertion tools [1].

The reduction of the intracochlear trauma during cochlear implant (CI) insertion is currently the standard care in cochlear implantation surgery with the objective of maintaining the integrity of inner ear structures for all cochlear implant recipients, even for those candidates with severe-to-profound hearing loss where there is no residual hearing to preserve. The reduction of the trauma during implantation offers several advantages indeed. The preservation of the residual low-frequency hearing is necessary for the electro-acoustic stimulation, but has also been demonstrated to contribute to better speech perception scores in patients with only classic electric stimulation [2]. Moreover, limiting the scalar translocation and thus the intracochlear damage has been proved to be a positive prognostic factor of hearing performances also for those patients without preoperative residual hearing [3, 4]. In addition, the reduced trauma limits the intracochlear fibrosis and/or ossification facilitating the possible revision surgery, especially for children who will probably require one or more reimplantation during their lifetime. Other advantages of limiting intracochlear injury include the potential application of future technologies, such as cellular regeneration or other novel cochlear nerve stimulation modalities [5]. In fact, providing a reversible atraumatic gesture may leave the possibility to remove the intracochlear device and eventually perform a reimplantation without compromising the inner ear structures.

The use of robotic devices in CI surgery has been demonstrated to be reliable in experimental models, to improve structure and hearing preservation in animals [6] or temporal bone cadaveric model [7], and more recently to have excellent postoperative results in implanted patients [8]. Different groups have studied and developed CI robotic devices, during the last two decades. In this chapter, a review of the different robots and automated devices capable of improving the surgeon gesture in the different steps of the cochlear implant surgery, from the inner ear access to the electrode array insertion, is presented.

## 17.2 Direct Access to the Cochlea

The standard and mostly used access to the cochlea for CI surgery requires a mastoidectomy and the passage of the electrode array through the posterior tympanotomy, although alternative and less invasive approaches have been described (trans-canal or supra-meatal) [9, 10]. The conventional approach needs significant drilling of the mastoid cells to identify the anatomical landmarks and to obtain a sufficient field of vision before opening the facial recess in safe conditions. A direct percutaneous tunnel from the retro-auricular mastoid region to the cochlear basal turn would reduce the invasiveness of the surgical procedure and, probably, the surgical time. During the last few decades, the improvement of imaging resolution and the development of surgical navigation systems, also known as image-guided systems, provided a solution to compensate the loss of visual control over the tunnel to be drilled to reach the inner ear. In fact, the development and the recent improvements of this technology allowed the landmark recognition and real-time positioning of the surgical instruments in the temporal bone.

Several laboratory experimental studies have been performed in the past few years to test the different variables for obtaining a reliable and safe direct cochlear access (DCA) for CI insertion [11–15] (Fig. 17.1).

Currently, several systems are able to create a straight trajectory from the mastoid surface to the scala tympani at the ideal approach angle for entering the cochlea through the round window in temporal bone; two of them have been used in clinical practice (see section: clinical applications).

### 17.2.1 HEARO® System

The group from Bern, Switzerland, developed a robot, named HEARO®, which was designed for drilling a preoperatively planned tunnel based on CT images, passing through the facial recess with close proximity and sufficient margin to the facial nerve (>0.4 mm) [16]. The device is controlled by either a computer or manually

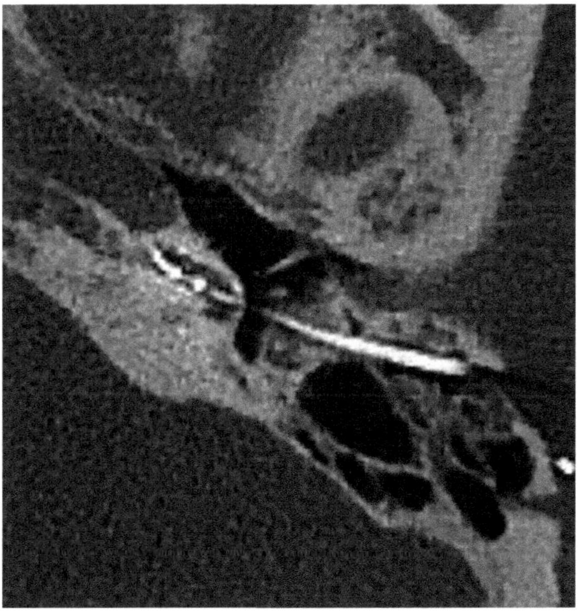

**Fig. 17.1** Direct cochlear access. Postoperative CT scan. Note the intact mastoid compartment and the direct linear access to the inner ear. The tunnel drilled by the Hearo® system allowed the implantation of a MED-EL electrode array in the scala tympani. Modified from Caversaccio, et al. (2019) Robotic middle ear access for cochlear implantation: First in man. PLoS One 14(8): e0220543. https://doi.org/10.1371/journal.pone.0220543

using a 3D mouse. The robotic arm attaches directly to the operating table and controls the position of the surgical tool using active optical tool tracking relative to the patient via a bone-anchored active dynamic reference base (DRB) marker. All robot movements remain under the control of the user via an activation hand switch [17].

In the preoperative phase, four surgical screws are positioned into the mastoid under local anesthesia. A CT scan of the temporal bone is then performed and the images are transferred to a custom-developed planning software system to create a drilling plan based on the individual patient's anatomy. The software enables automatic location of the implanted fiducial screws and the segmentation of anatomical structures to define a safe drilling trajectory from the mastoid surface to a target selected on the cochlea (round window or cochleostomy). Distances to surrounding anatomy are automatically calculated and displayed by the software, to assist in optimizing the trajectory for a scala tympani placement of the electrode array.

In the operating room, the patient's head is secured in a head-holder and the robot is fixed onto the surgical table (Fig. 17.2). The surgical plan is subsequently transferred to the robotic system. The process starts with recording the fiducial screw positions by an optically tracked system. Once all fiducial screws locations have been digitized by the camera, the tracked tool is displayed in the surgical plan on the graphical user interface for navigation. The DRB is then attached to the temporal bone, and a second patient-to-image registration is performed relative to the DRB. The DRB allows the robot system to compensate for small changes in patient position during drilling. Robotic drilling of the tunnel is controlled by the surgeon using a hand-held switch and is performed using a custom heat-reducing drill to reduce the thermal damage to the facial nerve. Electromyographic facial nerve monitoring performed at preoperatively planned positions controls the facial functioning during the procedure. When the last portion of the tunnel is completed and the middle ear is reached, a tympano-meatal flap is performed to allow microscopic supervision of electrode array insertion in the cochlea.

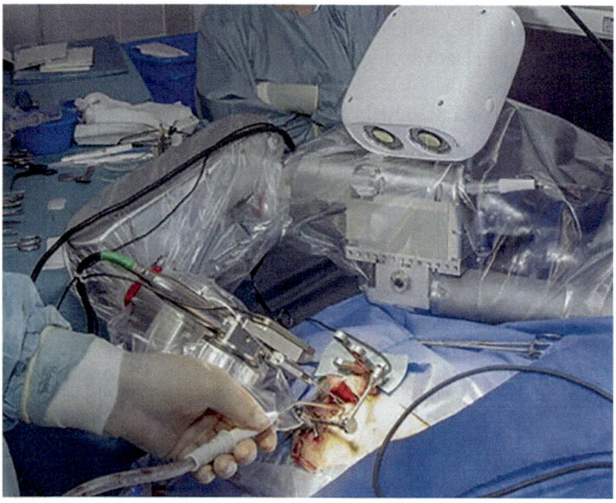

**Fig. 17.2** The Hearo® robotic system during a cochlear implantation procedure. Modified from Caversaccio, et al. (2019) Robotic middle ear access for cochlear implantation: First in man. PLoS One 14(8): e0220543. https://doi.org/10.1371/journal.pone.0220543

### 17.2.2 Vanderbilt Robotic System

Bone-attached parallel robot requires neither head fixation nor intraoperative registration. The systems are based on a patient's customized stereotaxic frame directly fixed on the head during both imaging and surgical intervention [18]. The group of Labadie and colleagues from Vanderbilt University (Nashville, USA) designed and developed a robotic system for DCA by using a micro-stereotactic frame attached to the patient skull via three rigid bone anchors [18]. In the preoperative CT scan, the anatomy of interest is automatically segmented and a safe linear trajectory avoiding vital anatomical structures and targeting the scala tympani is defined. Segmentation is accomplished via atlas-based segmentation for the external ear canal and ossicles and active shape modeling for the labyrinth and its subcomponents for facial nerve and chorda tympani. Trajectory generation specifies avoidance of the facial nerve and external ear canal but does allow violation of the chorda tympani if no other solutions are possible. In the operating room, three titanium self-tapping anchors attached to extenders with spherical tip are screwed into the skull. The spherical tips act both as fiducials for registering the patient's anatomy to the CT scan and as attachment points for a miniature stereotactic frame. An intraoperative cone-beam CT scan is performed, and the segmented anatomy and drill trajectory from the preoperative CT scan are mapped to the intraoperative CT scan. A miniature tabletop that mounts onto the spherical fiducial markers via legs of specified lengths is then fabricated "on-the-fly" using a computer-numeric-control machine [19]; a specifically designed drill is attached to the micro-stereotactic frame, and then mounted on the fiducial markers. A cutaneous incision is made and the temporal bone is exposed. The tunnel is wider when lateral to the facial nerve (3.797 mm diameter) and then smaller at the level of the facial recess (1.59 mm diameter). A second intraoperative CT scan is obtained for additional safety to confirm the correct position of the drill and then confirmed under endoscopic vision. A tympano-meatal flap is lastly raised to allow access to the middle ear and perform the cochleostomy. Finally, the electrode array is passed into the drilled tunnel, and inserted in the cochlea under direct visualization. Confirmation of correct insertion and assessment of intracochlear positioning is made with a final intraoperative CT scan.

### 17.2.3 Hannover Robotic Systems

The group from Hannover, Germany, developed during the last decade different robot-based systems with the principal aim of reaching the inner ear via a minimally invasive approach, which can be divided into three technologies:

(i) System based on an industrial robot adapted to the cochlear implant surgery: The KR3 (KUKA GmbH, Augsburg, Germany) is a six-joint light robot, with 6 degrees of freedom, a maximum operating distance of 635 mm in *x*/*y*-axis, and maximum loading capacity of 3 kg [13].

(ii) Custom-made parallel kinematics with optimized structural elements [20, 21]: These devices have passive legs made of micrometer gauges and mounted via magnetic bearings directly on the skull. The more recent one is based on a spherical platform, using three non-rigid bone anchors letting the possibility to change the anchors location, adapting to each patient, so that the device provided a straight-line trajectory guidance. The device was tested on an artificial temporal and the target accuracy was 0.4 ± 0.12 mm, a result potentially suitable for minimally invasive cochlear implant surgery.
(iii) Customized targeting platforms, consisting of a reusable base frame and a disposable patient-specific instrument: The disposable template was customized in the operating room to set the correct drill position. The plates are positioned with a mechatronics system in the desired position for the correct drilling of the tunnel, and the fixation methods for the micro-stereotactic frame were based on bone cement-filled struts [22].

## 17.3 Robot-Based Cochleostomy

The access to the scala tympani can be achieved by either a cochleostomy or direct round window insertion. Several studies compared the two techniques with some advantages reported in favor of the round window membrane insertion. Wanna et al. [23] showed the cochleostomy to be more traumatic and prone to scalar translocation than pure round window insertion. Nevertheless, considering the trajectory of the electrode array during the insertion, the first point of contact of lateral wall arrays is the 180° region in case of cochleostomy insertion, while in pure round window membrane insertion the array tip would hit the modiolar region before continuing its trajectory in the basal turn [24]. The choice of the entry point in the cochlea should be done on the basis of the anatomical variation of the hook region of cochlea [25].

Cochleostomy is a delicate step in the cochlear implantation surgery and consists in drilling the promontory to access the scala tympani to insert the electrode array. When drilling through the bone tissue of the cochlea, the inadvertent protrusion of the drill through the endosteal membrane can lead to its perforation in more than 60% of cases and inner ear damages [26]. Recent studies showed that manual opening of the endosteal membrane was a predictive factor of residual hearing preservation. On the contrary, a perforation of such a thin membrane (0.1–0.2 mm thick) by a rotating drill can lead to (i) increase of pressure into the endolymphatic fluids; (ii) direct trauma to the basilar membrane; and (iii) contamination of the fluids with bone dust [27]. To facilitate such a gesture, a smart hand-guided robotic microdrill system, coupled to a force sensor, was developed by Brett and colleagues [26]. The device was able to sense the changes in force transients and to stop on the interface of bone and soft tissue, preserving the endosteal membrane. Set at 700 RPM at a progression speed of 0.1 mm/s [28], and compared to manual drilling, robotic drilling reduced to 1% of the velocity induced on the endosteal membrane [29] with a mean force level of 1°N (0.6°N–1.3°N).

Klenzer and colleagues developed a force-controlled robot system with a conventional industrial robot (RX90CR, Staeubli AG, PfäYkon, Switzerland) using articulated arm kinematic structures coupled to a registration software to program a semi-automated cochleostomy. Coupled to 2D images and virtual endoscopic vision, the ideal localization of the cochleostomy was chosen and the cochleostomy performed with a target error of 0.25 mm [0.13–0.37 mm] [12].

## 17.4 Motorized Electrode Array Insertion Tool

Standard insertion of the electrode array is in general manually performed with limited visual and tactile feedback with the use of forceps possibly aided with micro-forks. In order to further control this high accuracy step, several insertion tools have been designed and commercialized. Indeed, the insertion technique is influenced by many factors, and some of them such as tremor, fits and starts, and insertion speed can be controlled with the use of such devices.

The motorized insertion tools have been designed to assist robotic implantation. Motorization of the insertion procedure could minimize intracochlear trauma as it allows for (i) standardization of the insertion, independently by the electrode array characteristics or surgical expertise; (ii) smoothing the insertion forces profile, and elimination of human tremor; and (iii) a very low speed and continuous insertion beyond those which are manually feasible.

Experimental insertion tools were developed by several groups (Hannover, Nashville, New York, Paris) [30–36]. The different automated motorized insertion tools allowed the insertion of straight electrodes, pre-curved electrodes, or both, enabling even a controlled stylet removal.

JT Roland (NYU, New York) and colleagues designed and developed an insertion device for a robotic advance-off-stylet (AOS) pre-curved electrode insertion. The device was intended for the bench evaluation of cochlear implant electrode insertion dynamics by fluoroscopic analysis and intracochlear hydraulic and mechanical force and lastly to evaluate the histological intracochlear trauma, and not for clinical application [30].

The group from Hannover, Germany, developed a first automated insertion tool in 2008 for AOS insertion and was tested and validated in synthetic scala tympani and cadaveric temporal bone models [31, 32]. Successively in cooperation with the Department of Mechanical Engineering, Vanderbilt University, Nashville, USA, they developed a force sensing unit which can be attached to the automated insertion tool (force resolution: 1000 μN) [33]. The tool was secondarily developed with another integrated force sensor (force resolution: 30 μN) and was designed to insert a straight electrode array, but could also pull the stylet during AOS insertion [34]. Recently, the same group proposed a new concept of a simple tool designed to automate the intracochlear cochlear insertion of electrode array with an easy adaptation to electrode arrays from different manufacturers, and meeting all sterility needs and regulations for intraoperative use [35]. The prototype facilitates automated forward motion using a syringe connected to an infusion pump. The design of the device purposes a commercially available, sterile, disposable syringe as hydraulic cylinder that provides automated hydraulic actuation. The plunger of the syringe serves as a piston and transforms the pressure inside the barrel into a continuous and linear movement at constant speed that pushes the electrode array into the scala tympani. The prototype is then connected to a standard surgical retractor with a flexible arm for manually adjusting the correct positioning under the direct control of the surgeon. Insertion velocity can be controlled via the infusion pump by setting a corresponding flow rate according to the desired insertion speed.

The group from Paris, France (Sorbonne University/Inserm), developed their first version of a motorized insertion tool a decade ago [36]. The tool was composed of a rotary electrical motor mounted on a micromanipulator. A threaded screw on the micromanipulator converted the rotary movement into a linear actuation. Motor speed was controlled via the input voltage current using an analog-to-digital interface card. The linear movement of the micromanipulator pushed the array via a blunt pin inside an insertion tube in order to eject the array. With this device, smooth slow insertion could be obtained, to achieve a reproducible insertion quality, necessary to evaluate force profiles in artificial cochleae and trauma in temporal bones. In the experimental insertion model, a 6-axis force was placed under the temporal bone. Force profiles for normal insertions, complete fold-over, or incomplete insertion could be measured with this test bench [37]. The current version of the tool took into consideration the visual field impairment and the possibility to be connected to a robotic arm (RobOtol®, Collin, Bagneux, France). The actuator speed was controlled via laboratory power supply and set at 0.8 mm/s. This tool was validated on plastic scala tympani model, in temporal bones, and in an animal model [36, 37].

## 17.5 Robot-Assisted Electrode Array Insertion

The most important phase of cochlear implantation surgery is the insertion of the electrode array. The optimal array insertion includes both a full insertion into the scala tympani and a preservation of the inner ear structures. In addition to array specifications (size, shape, stiffness, etc.), different predictive factors have been correlated to an atraumatic insertion of the electrode array, mainly depending on the human hand accuracy and therefore on the surgeon's experience. The insertion axis, ideally aligned to the basal turn of the cochlea [38], a low speed of insertion (0.25 mm/s) [39], and low forces applied during insertion were correlated to a high number of electrodes correctly inserted in the scala tympani, and reduced intracochlear trauma [40].

### 17.5.1 RobOtol® System, Paris, France

A robot-based arm developed to be able to operate in restrained areas was first designed to be dedicated to middle ear procedures, for the assistance of precise gestures such as otosclerosis surgery [41]. The current version of the RobOtol® is a

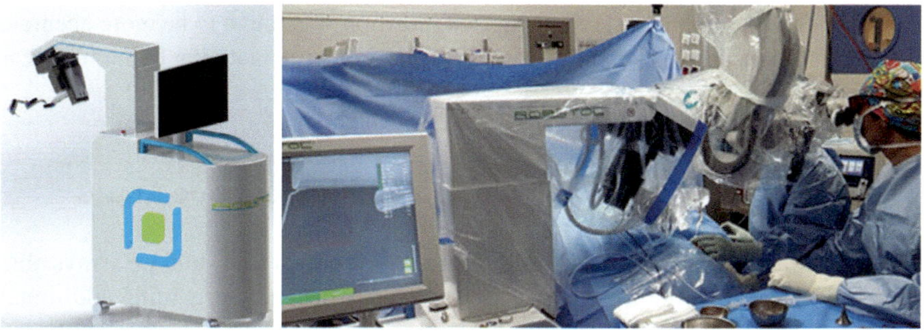

**Fig. 17.3** Left: Overall view of the RobOtol®. The system comprises a cart carrying a controller, a human–machine interface and a slave robot-based arm. Right: operating room setting where both the microscope and the robot with the instrument holder arm are present. Modified from Vittoria S., et al. Robot-based assistance in middle ear surgery and cochlear implantation: first clinical report. Eur Arch Otorhinolaryngol. 2021;278:77–85. https://doi.org/10.1007/s00405-020-06070-z

6 degrees-of-freedom (DOF) teleoperated robot arm [42–44] (Fig. 17.3). It is provided by two adjustable arms that can be used separately: one is a dedicated micro-instrument holder and the other is an endoscope holder. Three linear actuators were integrated into a XYZ cross-table. The table was built with 2 orthogonal (X–Y) precision linear stages with 70 mm travel, and a Z precision linear stage with 95 mm travel. Three DC micromotors with a magnetic incremental encoder were used for all rotary actuators. These were connected to a harmonic drive gearhead with a 100:1 reduction ratio. Two command modes are available to teleoperate the RobOtol® system: (i) The Phantom Omni® (SensAble Technologies, Inc., Woburn, MA) a pen-like interface with 6 DOF. It works with a position-to-position command from the master to the slave arms. The command is based on a registered correspondence between the local stylus frame and the robot tool frame. (ii) The Space-Mouse (3Dconnexion, Waltham, MA), with a position-to-velocity command. The registration mode allows master arm configuration to be uncoupled from the robot, and allows indirect visual feedback (e.g., angled endoscope). In the velocity command mode, stylus motion codes for robot speed (as with a joystick). In this mode, the user has to release the dead man's foot switch (DMFS) to stop the robot. In both modes, the DMFS allows the surgeon to confirm movement commands. In both command modes, a down-scale ratio between the master and slave arms can be implemented to enhance control for a more accurate movement. The use of RobOtol® system in cochlear implantation is with micro-instrument holder arm, the robot to align the motorized insertion tool, or the other dedicated electrode array's holder instrument for the insertion in the scala tympani. After the round window membrane opening, the array is pushed in the scala tympani by the motorized insertion tool or, in the clinical setting, directly by the forward movement of the robotic arm. In the latter scenario, all the axes of freedom of the robot are blocked (X-, Y-, and all rotation axes), with the exception of the Z-axis that allowed the robot arm to move only linearly along the chosen insertion trajectory toward the scala tympani. Using a constant speed insertion of 0.25 mm/s and compared to a manual

insertion on temporal bones, robot-assisted insertion was found to be more accurate if the optimal insertion axis was respected [7] and less traumatizing to the inner ear structures [45].

## 17.6 Curvature-Controlled and Steerable Electrode Arrays

Two different groups [46, 47] worked on the development of prototype arrays able to bend or curve in order to facilitate the surgical insertion by providing additional degrees of freedom to achieve more precise control of the array trajectory during insertion. The aim of these prototypes is to guide the trajectory of the insertion following the cochlear coiling and thus to minimize the contact with the lateral wall or modiolar region so that the occurrence of an insertion trauma would be limited.

Zhang and colleagues developed a robot capable of achieving a cochlear implantation with a controlled steerable electrode array. In their actively electrodes, a strand is embedded off the centerline of an elastomeric electrode array and attached internally to the tip of the electrode inside. The rest of the strand can move inside the electrode. When pulling the strand while holding the base of the electrode array, the electrode array bends to predetermined shapes. The last prototype developed by the researchers was a parallel robot with force sensing capability, 6 actuators that manipulate its moving platform through 6 independently controlled linear actuators (cylinders) [46]. The base of this robot is held stationary during surgery through a mechanical lock. The steerable electrode is held on the moving platform. The electrode steering includes 2 levels of motions. First, the electrode itself can be bent to a certain shape by the embedded strand. Different amounts of pull on the strand correspond to different bent shapes of the steerable electrode. Second, the bent electrode as a whole unit can be rotated by the robot, which further increases its steerability. The rotation from the robot can adjust the electrode approach angle toward the scala tympani. The robot was controlled through a haptic joystick that allows surgeons to move the robot, following the hand motions of surgeons. The computer shows and records the surgery information, such as insertion depth, insertion speed, and sensed force.

Unfortunately, steerable electrode array technology, despite their promising results, has not yet been developed by cochlear implant manufacturers.

## 17.7 Clinical Applications

At present, three robots are used for cochlear implantations in patients. Two of them (Vanderbilt system and HEARO®) were designed for the DCA, the subsequent electrode array insertion being manually performed; the last one (RobOtol®) is not intended for a mastoid tunnel drilling but for the robotic alignment of the electrode array through a mastoidectomy and its subsequent insertion in the scala tympani.

### 17.7.1 Vanderbilt System

The first preliminary report showed 9 patients who underwent a CI surgery. Eight of them had a successful intracochlear insertion of the array, although one procedure has to be converted to standard open technique. Mean surgical time was 182 ± 36 min. Styleted CI electrode arrays were used in 6 patients, and the other 3 patients received lateral wall electrode array. As major complication, one patient developed a mild postoperative permanent mild facial nerve palsy due to overheating [48]. No further clinical studies have been performed pending improvement of safety mechanisms to protect against possible mechanical or thermal damage [49].

### 17.7.2 HEARO® System

Nine patients were enrolled for the first cochlear implantation trial with the robotic system [17], the mean total surgical time was 4 h, and the drilling accuracy was very high (0.2 ± 0.10 mm). In 3 cases, the procedure was converted to standard open technique due to critical distance of the tunnel to vital structures.

### 17.7.3 RobOtol® System

The RobOtol® was available from February 2018 at Pitié-Salpetrière Hospital (Paris, France) where the first clinical trial took part [50] and successively was adopted in other centers in Europe and China (Video 17.1). Cochlear insertions were possible using specific tools available for different devices (straight electrode array of Advanced Bionics® (Valencia, CA, USA), Cochlear® (Sydney, Australia), MED-EL® (Innsbruck, Austria), Nurotron® (Hangzhou, China), and Oticon Medical® (Vallauris, France) [8, 50–52]. The AOS insertion of a pre-curved electrode array (Advanced Bionics, Mid-Scala®) was also possible, but was partially robot-assisted. The stylet was positioned and maintained by the robot arm, and then the electrode array was pushed manually into the cochlea [52]. At present, more than one-hundred CIs were implanted with the aid of RobOtol® system and the numbers are rapidly increasing. Published data reported that the robot-assisted insertion of straight electrode array is less traumatizing for the inner ear, compared to the manual one, with 7% versus 16% of translocated electrodes, respectively ($p < 0.001$) [52]. The average total time of surgery (including mastoidectomy and posterior tympanotomy) was 138 ± 7.1 min, an acceptable performance with approximately 30 min more than the manual technique (average of 109 ± 4.0 min). The group from Liege, Belgium, reported the preliminary results of their first five MED-EL® Flex 24 electrodes implanted with the robotic system. The insertion speed was 0.88 ± 0.12 mm/s, the mean postoperative PTA (500–4000 Hz) hearing loss was 13.60 ± 7.70 dB, and the postoperative radiological analysis did not show any electrodes translocation or damage to the inner ear structures [8].

## 17.8 Future Perspectives

The ideal robot for cochlear implantation should encompass all the best characteristics from the available devices, from both the direct cochlear access systems and the robotic arm and insertion tools.

To date, among the 3 robotic systems that have been used for cochlear implantation in patients, the RobOtol® is the more widespread used. Considering the intracochlear trauma, the RobOtol®, compared to standard manual cochlear implantation surgery, has been demonstrated to reduce the intracochlear forces in temporal bones and to correctly position the array in the scala tympani with both low translocation and high hearing preservation rates in patients; partial hearing preservation rate after the HEARO® system procedure was reported in 4 out of 9 patients, while the Vanderbilt robot mainly designed for a mini-invasive inner ear access does not have yet published data concerning hearing preservation results.

### 17.8.1 Robotic Arm Alignment for Insertion Axis Control

The optimal insertion axis of the electrode array is parallel to the basal turn of the cochlea. Torres et al. [38] showed that the mental representation of the basal-turn anatomy was experience-dependent but that even experts had non-optimal representation to some extent (<7 degrees error). In successive studies, the same authors reported that the robotic alignment of the insertion tool with the aid of a navigation system reduced the angle error with an optimal insertion vector below 2 degrees in temporal bone models [7]. Successive temporal bone studies indicate that the angle of approach to the scala tympani centerline is a critical factor in intracochlear trauma [45]. Unpublished data show that the automated insertion system (RobOtol® + navigation system) could accurately align the tip of the pre-curved Advanced Bionics Mid-scala® electrode array to the axis of the basal turn and then the subsequent coiling of the scala tympani, and dramatically reduce intracochlear trauma and translocation. Considering these results, we can assume that the application of the image guidance systems to the RobOtol® for cochlear implantation on patients should improve the hearing preservation rate and therefore ameliorate the postoperative auditory outcomes for these patients.

### 17.8.2 Insertion Force and Electrocochleography (EcochG) Feedback Control During CI Insertion

Preserving the amplitude of EcochG responses has shown to predict the extent of hearing preservation [53]. Moreover, the electrode insertion forces were demonstrated to be correlated with structural damage in human temporal bone [40] and by extension with the level of post-implantation hearing loss. In a guinea pig model study, by Lo and colleagues from Melbourne, Australia, modified cochlear implants were inserted while monitoring the ECochG responses and insertion forces. Results showed that intraoperative compound action potential (CAP) amplitude during implantation was predictive of an atraumatic insertion and reduced post-implantation hearing loss [54]. A rise in force usually preceded the reporting of resistance, although by less than 1 s. These results suggest that intraoperative CAPs may offer a robust feedback mechanism for improving hearing preservation rates than electrode insertion force recordings, especially considering the rapid changes in insertion force and relatively slow human reaction times. However, a recent systematic review concluded that ECochG recordings were achieved in over 90% of patients, but accuracy to predict postoperative hearing loss remained limited [55].

New robotic insertion tools should be provided with loop feedback systems capable of modifying the insertion parameters on the basis of both insertion forces and electrocochleographic responses.

### 17.8.3 Electrode Insertion Path Planning

In a recent study, Wang et al. [56] proposed a method to study the optimal insertion path into the scala tympani of a perimodiolar electrode array and plan a strategy for a robotic insertion following the designed path (centerline of scala tympani). The coordinate information of the optimal path was combined with the stylet extraction state to conduct the path planning for robotic cochlear implant, and the result was sent to the robot for kinematic inverse solution to obtain the robot motion trajectory. The results of the study showed a reduction of the insertion forces using the path planning insertion method. The path planning methodology seems to be a promising tool to reduce intracochlear trauma and could be in further studies modified for the application to other electrode array (e.g., steerable or straight electrodes).

## 17.9 Conclusion

First clinical trials in patients implanted with robotic devices began a few years ago, and since then, three different systems have been successfully used. Robotic cochlear implantation is currently used in few centers, but its application and the number of procedures is rapidly increasing. Moreover, a great acceptance of patients and parents toward task-autonomous robotic cochlear implantation was recently reported in a survey in patients scheduled for manual cochlear implantation [57]. Considering the promising results in terms of mini-invasiveness, reduced trauma, and better hearing preservation, further laboratory research and clinical studies should continue with the aim of improving the results of robotic cochlear implantation making the implant insertion an atraumatic and reversible gesture for a total preservation of the inner ear structure and physiology.

## References


1. Daniele, De Seta Hannah, Daoudi Renato, Torres Evelyne, Ferrary Olivier, Sterkers Yann, Nguyen. Robotics automation active electrode arrays and new devices for cochlear implantation: A contemporary review. Hear Res. 2022. 414108425-10.1016/j.heares.2021.108425.
2. Schaefer S, Sahwan M, Metryka A, et al. The benefits of preserving residual hearing following cochlear implantation: a systematic review. Int J Audiol. 2021;60:1–17. https://doi.org/10.1080/14992027.2020.1863484.
3. Aschendorff A, Kromeier J, Klenzner T, et al. Quality control after insertion of the nucleus contour and contour advance electrode in adults. Ear Hear. 2007;28:75S–9S. https://doi.org/10.1097/AUD.0b013e318031542e.
4. Finley CC, Skinner MW. Role of electrode placement as a contributor to variability in cochlear implant outcomes. Otol Neurotol. 2008;29:920–8. https://doi.org/10.1097/MAO.0b013e318184f492.
5. Devare J, Gubbels S, Raphael Y. Outlook and future of inner ear therapy. Hear Res. 2018;368:127–35. https://doi.org/10.1016/j.heares.2018.05.009.
6. Mamelle E, Kechai NE, Granger B, et al. Effect of a liposomal hyaluronic acid gel loaded with dexamethasone in a Guinea pig model after manual or motorized cochlear implantation. Eur Arch Otorhinolaryngol. 2017;274:729–36. https://doi.org/10.1007/s00405-016-4331-8.
7. Torres R, Kazmitcheff G, De Seta D, et al. Improvement of the insertion axis for cochlear implantation with a robot-based system. Eur Arch Otorhinolaryngol. 2017;274:715–21. https://doi.org/10.1007/s00405-016-4329-2.
8. Barriat S, Peigneux N, Duran U, et al. The use of a robot to insert an electrode array of Cochlear implants in the cochlea: a feasibility study and preliminary results. Audiol Neurotol. 2021;26(5):361–7.
9. Kiratzidis T. "Veria operation": cochlear implantation without a mastoidectomy and a posterior tympanotomy. A new surgical technique. Adv Otorhinolaryngol. 2000;57:127–30. https://doi.org/10.1159/000059218.
10. Kronenberg J, Migirov L, Dagan T. Suprameatal approach: new surgical approach for cochlear implantation. J Laryngol Otol. 2001;115:283–5. https://doi.org/10.1258/0022215011907451.
11. Caversaccio M, Stieger C, Weber S, et al. Navigation and robotics of the lateral skull base. HNO. 2009;57:975–82. https://doi.org/10.1007/s00106-009-1985-1.
12. Klenzner T, Ngan CC, Knapp FB, et al. New strategies for high precision surgery of the temporal bone using a robotic approach for cochlear implantation. Eur Arch Otorhinolaryngol. 2009;266:955–60. https://doi.org/10.1007/s00405-008-0825-3.
13. Majdani O, Rau TS, Baron S, et al. A robot-guided minimally invasive approach for cochlear implant surgery: preliminary results of a temporal bone study. Int J Comput Assist Radiol Surg. 2009;4:475–86. https://doi.org/10.1007/s11548-009-0360-8.
14. Stieger C, Caversaccio M, Arnold A, et al. Development of an auditory implant manipulator for minimally invasive surgical insertion of implantable hearing devices. J Laryngol Otol. 2011;125:262–70. https://doi.org/10.1017/S0022215110002185.
15. Nguyen Y, Miroir M, Vellin J-F, et al. Minimally invasive computer-assisted approach for Cochlear implantation: a human temporal bone study. Surg Innov. 2011;18:259–67. https://doi.org/10.1177/1553350611405220.
16. Anso J, Balmer TW, Jegge Y, et al. Electrical impedance to assess facial nerve proximity during robotic Cochlear implantation. IEEE Trans Biomed Eng. 2019;66:237–45. https://doi.org/10.1109/TBME.2018.2830303.
17. Caversaccio M, Gavaghan K, Wimmer W, et al. Robotic cochlear implantation: surgical procedure and first clinical experience. Acta Otolaryngol (Stockh). 2017;137:447–54. https://doi.org/10.1080/00016489.2017.1278573.
18. Kratchman LB, Blachon GS, Withrow TJ, et al. Design of a bone-attached parallel robot for percutaneous cochlear implantation. IEEE Trans Biomed Eng. 2011;58:2904–10. https://doi.org/10.1109/TBME.2011.2162512.

19. Labadie RF, Mitchell J, Balachandran R, et al. Customized, rapid-production microstereotactic table for surgical targeting: description of concept and in vitro validation. Int J Comput Assist Radiol Surg. 2009;4:273–80. https://doi.org/10.1007/s11548-009-0292-3.
20. Kobler J-P, Kotlarski J, Oltjen J, et al. Design and analysis of a head-mounted parallel kinematic device for skull surgery. Int J Comput Assist Radiol Surg. 2012;7:137–49. https://doi.org/10.1007/s11548-011-0619-8.
21. Kobler J-P, Nuelle K, Lexow GJ, et al. Configuration optimization and experimental accuracy evaluation of a bone-attached, parallel robot for skull surgery. Int J Comput Assist Radiol Surg. 2016;11:421–36. https://doi.org/10.1007/s11548-015-1300-4.
22. Vollmann B, Müller S, Kundrat D, et al. Methods for intraoperative, sterile pose-setting of patient-specific microstereotactic frames. Proc SPIE. 2015;9415(2015):94150M.
23. Wanna GB, Noble JH, Carlson ML, et al. Impact of electrode design and surgical approach on scalar location and cochlear implant outcomes. Laryngoscope. 2014;124(Suppl 6):S1–7. https://doi.org/10.1002/lary.24728.
24. Zhou L, Friedmann DR, Treaba C, et al. Does cochleostomy location influence electrode trajectory and intracochlear trauma? Laryngoscope. 2015;125:966–71. https://doi.org/10.1002/lary.24986.
25. Atturo F, Barbara M, Rask-Andersen H. On the anatomy of the "hook" region of the human cochlea and how it relates to cochlear implantation. Audiol Neurootol. 2014;19:378–85. https://doi.org/10.1159/000365585.
26. Brett PN, Taylor RP, Proops D, et al. A surgical robot for cochleostomy. Annu Int Conf IEEE Eng Med Biol Soc. 2007;2007:1229–32. https://doi.org/10.1109/IEMBS.2007.4352519.
27. Coulson CJ, Reid AP, Proops DW. Robotics can lead to a reproducibly high-quality operative result for ear, nose, and throat patients. Proc Inst Mech Eng. 2010;[H] 224:735–42. https://doi.org/10.1243/09544119JEIM714.
28. Coulson CJ, Assadi MZ, Taylor RP, et al. A smart micro-drill for cochleostomy formation: a comparison of cochlear disturbances with manual drilling and a human trial. Cochlear Implants Int. 2013;14:98–106. https://doi.org/10.1179/1754762811Y.0000000018.
29. Assadi MZ, Du X, Dalton J, et al. Comparison on intracochlear disturbances between drilling a manual and robotic cochleostomy. Proc Inst Mech Eng. 2013;227:1002–8. https://doi.org/10.1177/0954411913488507.
30. Roland JT. A model for Cochlear implant electrode insertion and force evaluation: results with a new electrode design and insertion technique. Laryngoscope. 2005;115:1325–39. https://doi.org/10.1097/01.mlg.0000167993.05007.35.
31. Hussong A, Rau T, Eilers H, et al. Conception and design of an automated insertion tool for cochlear implants. Annu Int Conf IEEE Eng Med Biol Soc. 2008;2008:5593–6. https://doi.org/10.1109/IEMBS.2008.4650482.
32. Hussong A, Rau TS, Ortmaier T, et al. An automated insertion tool for cochlear implants: another step towards atraumatic cochlear implant surgery. Int J Comput Assist Radiol Surg. 2010;5:163–71. https://doi.org/10.1007/s11548-009-0368-0.
33. Schurzig D, Webster RJ, Dietrich MS, et al. Force of cochlear implant electrode insertion performed by a robotic insertion tool: comparison of traditional versus advance off-stylet techniques. Otol Neurotol. 2010;31:1207–10. https://doi.org/10.1097/MAO.0b013e3181f2ebc3.
34. Majdani O, Schurzig D, Hussong A, et al. Force measurement of insertion of cochlear implant electrode arrays in-vitro: comparison of surgeon to automated insertion tool. Acta Otolaryngol (Stockh). 2010;130:31–6. https://doi.org/10.3109/00016480902998281.
35. Rau TS, Zuniga MG, Salcher R, et al. A simple tool to automate the insertion process in cochlear implant surgery. Int J Comput Assist Radiol Surg. 2020;15:1931–9. https://doi.org/10.1007/s11548-020-02243-7.
36. Miroir M, Nguyen Y, Kazmitcheff G, et al. Friction force measurement during cochlear implant insertion: application to a force-controlled insertion tool design. Otol Neurotol. 2012a;33:1092–100. https://doi.org/10.1097/MAO.0b013e31825f24de.

37. Nguyen Y, Miroir M, Kazmitcheff G, et al. Cochlear implant insertion forces in microdissected human cochlea to evaluate a prototype array. Audiol Neurootol. 2012;17:290–8. https://doi.org/10.1159/000338406.
38. Torres R, Kazmitcheff G, Bernardeschi D, et al. Variability of the mental representation of the cochlear anatomy during cochlear implantation. Eur Arch Otorhinolaryngol. 2016;273:2009–18. https://doi.org/10.1007/s00405-015-3763-x.
39. Rajan GP, Kontorinis G, Kuthubutheen J. The effects of insertion speed on inner ear function during cochlear implantation: a comparison study. Audiol Neurootol. 2013;18:17–22. https://doi.org/10.1159/000342821.
40. De Seta D, Torres R, Russo FY, et al. Damage to inner ear structure during cochlear implantation: correlation between insertion force and radio-histological findings in temporal bone specimens. Hear Res. 2017;344:90–7. https://doi.org/10.1016/j.heares.2016.11.002.
41. Nguyen Y, Bernardeschi D, Sterkers O. Potential of robot-based surgery for otosclerosis surgery. Otolaryngol Clin N Am. 2018;51:475–85. https://doi.org/10.1016/j.otc.2017.11.016.
42. Kazmitcheff G, Miroir M, Nguyen Y, et al. Evaluation of command modes of an assistance robot for middle ear surgery. In: Presented at the 2011 IEEE/RSJ International Conference on Intelligent Robots and System, International Conference on Intelligent Robots and Systems. San Francisco, CA, USA: IEEE; 2011. p. 2532–8. https://doi.org/10.1109/IROS.2011.6094634.
43. Miroir M, Nguyen Y, Szewczyk J, et al. Design, kinematic optimization, and evaluation of a teleoperated system for middle ear microsurgery. Sci World J. 2012;2012:e907372. https://doi.org/10.1100/2012/907372.
44. Miroir M, Nguyen Y, Szewczyk J, et al. RobOtol: from design to evaluation of a robot for middle ear surgery. In: Presented at the 2010 IEEE/RSJ International Conference on Intelligent Robots and Systems. San Francisco, CA, USA: IEEE; 2010. p. 850–6. https://doi.org/10.1109/IROS.2010.5650390.
45. Torres R, Jia H, Drouillard M, et al. An optimized robot-based technique for Cochlear implantation to reduce array insertion trauma. Otolaryngol Head Neck Surg. 2018;159:900–7. https://doi.org/10.1177/0194599818792232.
46. Zhang J, Wei W, Ding J, et al. Inroads toward robot-assisted cochlear implant surgery using steerable electrode arrays. Otol Neurotol. 2010;31:1199–206. https://doi.org/10.1097/MAO.0b013e3181e7117e.
47. Wu J, Yan L, Xu H, et al. A curvature-controlled 3D micro-electrode array for cochlear implants. In: The 13th International Conference on Solid-State Sensors, Actuators and Microsystems, 2005. Seoul, Korea: Digest of Technical Papers; 2005. p. 1636–9. https://doi.org/10.1109/SENSOR.2005.1497402.
48. Labadie RF, Balachandran R, Noble JH, et al. Minimally-invasive, image-guided Cochlear implantation surgery: first report of clinical implementation. Laryngoscope. 2014;124:1915–22. https://doi.org/10.1002/lary.24520.
49. Robert F, Labadie Katherine, Riojas Kathleen, Von Wahlde Jason, Mitchell Trevor, Bruns Robert, Webster Benoit, Dawant J. Michael, Fitzpatrick Jack, Noble. Clinical Implementation of Second-generation Minimally Invasive Image-guided Cochlear Implantation Surgery. Otol Neurotol. 2021. Publish Ahead of Print https://doi.org/10.1097/MAO.0000000000003025
50. Sykopetrites V, Lahlou G, Torres R, et al. Robot-based assistance in middle ear surgery and cochlear implantation: first clinical report. Eur Arch Otorhinolaryngol. 2020;278(1):77–85. https://doi.org/10.1007/s00405-020-06070-z.
51. Jia H, Pan JX, Li Y, et al. Preliminary application of robot-assisted electrode insertion in cochlear implantation. Zhonghua Er Bi Yan Hou Tou Jing Wai Ke Za Zhi. 2020;55:952–6. https://doi.org/10.3760/cma.j.cn115330-20200228-00141.
52. Daoudi H, Lahlou G, Torres R, et al. Robot-assisted Cochlear implant electrode array insertion in adults: A comparative study with manual insertion. Otol Neurotol. 2021;42(4):e438–44. https://doi.org/10.1097/MAO.0000000000003002.
53. O'Connell BP, Holder JT, Dwyer RT, et al. Intra- and postoperative electrocochleography may be predictive of final electrode position and postoperative hearing preservation. Front Neurosci. 2017;11:291. https://doi.org/10.3389/fnins.2017.00291.

54. Lo J, Bester C, Collins A, et al. Intraoperative force and electrocochleography measurements in an animal model of cochlear implantation. Hear Res. 2018;358:50–8. https://doi.org/10.1016/j.heares.2017.11.001.
55. Yin LX, Barnes JH, Saoji AA, Carlson ML. Clinical utility of electrocochleography (ECochG) during cochlear implantation: a systematic review and quantitative analysis. Otol Neurotol. 2021;42:363–71. https://doi.org/10.1097/MAO.0000000000002996.
56. Labadie RF, Riojas K, Von Wahlde K, Mitchell J, Bruns T, Webster III R, Dawant B, Fitzpatrick JM, Noble J. Clinical implementation of second-generation minimally invasive image-guided cochlear implantation surgery. Otol Neurotol. 2021;42(5):702–5. https://doi.org/10.1097/MAO.0000000000003025.
57. De Seta D, Daoudi H, Torres R, Ferrary E, Sterkers O, Nguyen Y. Robotics automation active electrode arrays and new devices for cochlear implantation: A contemporary review. Hear Res. 2021;414:108425. https://doi.org/10.1016/j.heares.2021.108425

# Structure Preservation of the Inner Ear in Cochlear Implantation

# 18

William Crohan and Gunesh P. Rajan

## 18.1 Introduction

It has long been appreciated that the act of inserting an electrode into the cochlea has the potential to damage delicate inner ear structures [1]. However, the priorities, techniques, and technologies since cochlear implantation was first performed have changed over time. Initially, it was arguably agreed upon that the potential for loss of residual hearing was considered to be an acceptable casualty in those who were severe to profoundly deaf, with the loss of vestibular function not prioritised [2].

As the clinical observations of hearing preservation after cochlear implantation emerged in the late 1980s, surgeons heralded the advent of a new field of research looking into the vulnerability of inner ear structures to trauma due to cochlear implantation. This has subsequently resulted in a broader understanding of the nature of the trauma to the cochlea and highlighted the vulnerability of the basilar membrane and organ of Corti, as well as the secondary involution of spiral ganglion cells due to inflammation, fibrosis, and a lack of auditory stimuli [3–7] (Fig. 18.1).

The term "soft surgery" as a means of preserving inner ear structures was first used in 1993 [8], before the benefits of structure preservation became properly appreciated. As the research has now progressed further, several explanations have emerged extolling the importance of structure preservation in cochlear

W. Crohan (✉)
Otolaryngology, Head & Neck Surgery, Division of Surgery, Medical School, University of Western Australia, Perth, WA, Australia

G. P. Rajan
Otolaryngology, Head & Neck Surgery, Division of Surgery, Medical School, University of Western Australia, Perth, WA, Australia

Department of Otorhinolaryngology, Head & Neck Surgery, LUKS, Lucerne, Switzerland


S. DeSaSouza (ed.), *Cochlear Implants*,
https://doi.org/10.1007/978-981-19-0452-3_18

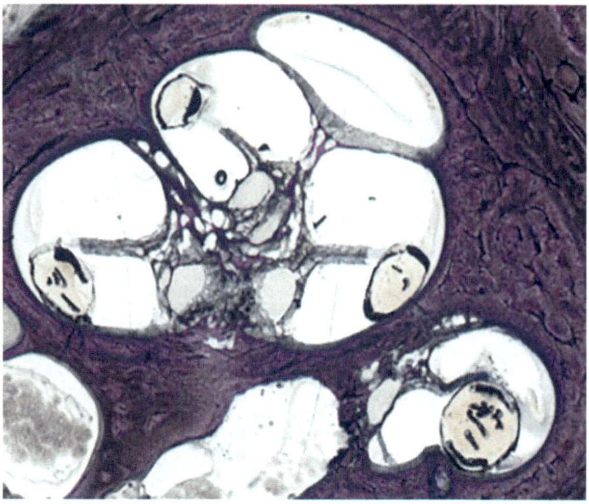

**Fig. 18.1** Cochleostomy with associated basilar translocation and inflammation in the basal turn (lower right). It is expected with time that spiral ganglion cells would begin to involute [80]

implantation, including functional hearing benefits, vestibular preservation, and futureproofing for potential therapies.

## 18.2 Functional Hearing Benefits

The benefits of *bimodal hearing*, where residual hearing or aided hearing is supplemented with a cochlear implant, began to gain appreciation in the late 1990s [9–12].

The deficiencies of hearing aids and the understanding that there was a "gap" that could be addressed through cochlear implants became better understood, from research that demonstrated that hearing aids resulted in only partial hearing improvement for individuals with hearing thresholds beyond 55–60 dB hearing loss and individuals with ski-slope hearing loss [13–15].

With respect to the cochlea, it was postulated by Adunka in his 2010 paper [16] that the preservation of residual hearing is necessitated by the inherent deficiencies in cochlear implants. Adunka surmised that acoustic input from a cochlear implant must undergo signal processing prior to presentation of a signal to the inner ear, which alters the volume and depth of information delivered to the auditory system. Furthermore, the signal received in the cochlear implant is split into tonotopic spectral segments, rather than presenting the smooth frequency continuum to the inner ear, such as a hearing aid would function, further compromising signal quality. [16] Lastly, the direct electric stimulation of the spiral ganglion by the cochlear implant has a compressed dynamic range of only 10 dB, compared to over 100 dB in a healthy ear [16].

The combination of the shortcomings of cochlear implants identified manifest in a clear argument for advocating hearing preservation, in order to achieve better patient outcomes. Clinically, it has been established that preserving residual hearing during cochlear implantation leads to better speech recognition, speech perception in noisy environments, sound localisation [9, 11, 14, 15, 17–22], and music perception [23].

Further, with respect to *bimodal hearing*, it has been established that the two methods of hearing are complementary rather than competitive following rehabilitation. In his 2014 paper [13], Skarzynski explored the impact of aiding preserved low-frequency residual hearing with hearing bestowed by a cochlear implant. Skarzynski resolved that speech recognition scores improved significantly in both quiet (76% vs 36%) and in background noise of 10 dB (68% vs 9%). Skarzynski also found that subjects with stronger preoperative low-frequency hearing experienced equal or greater improvements in speech perception, therein suggesting cochlear implantation had an additive and synergistic effect on hearing.

## 18.3 Preservation of the Vestibular System

Vestibular loss has a tragic effect on an individual's quality of life and is regarded as a significant disability. Short-term vestibular insult from implantation, including vertigo, nystagmus, and disequilibrium, has an incidence of 15–20% [24], whilst permanent debilitating injury is as high as 2% [25, 26]. With increasing knowledge about the vestibular system and the impact of vestibular malfunction, it is now accepted that the concept of hearing preservation needs to be expanded and include the vestibular system. This has marked the beginning of structure preservation in cochlear implantation, which aims at preserving the entire inner ear function after cochlear implantation.

It is unlikely that direct histological trauma to the vestibular apparatus during surgery is the cause of vestibular dysfunction [24]. Rather it is likely significantly transmitted intracochlear pressure variations which are discussed further below. Vestibular preservation has recently emerged as an important objective of cochlear implantation given the close association between trauma to the cochlea and vestibular loss relating to pressure variations being better appreciated in recent years [24]. With hearing preservation and vestibular preservation closely associated in implanted individuals [27], structure preservation strategies have been held as a means for both vestibular and residual hearing preservation.

Preservation of vestibular function is crucial in modern cochlear implantation when considering the increasing number of children and adults receiving bilateral cochlear implants. A bilateral loss of vestibular function in these patients after cochlear implantation can result in a severe permanent disability which can be avoided using the principles of structure preservation surgery.

## 18.4 Futureproofing for Emerging Therapies of Hearing Loss

New treatments enabled by biotechnological developments, such as hair cell regeneration or stem cell therapies could be implemented for hearing loss, however, it is indicated that these treatments will require a viable substrate in the inner ear [28]. Accordingly, it has been postulated that surgeons should seek to preserve inner ear structures in preparation for the possible availability of future technologies designed to restore hearing, such as stem cell therapy.

## 18.5 Key Considerations for Structure Preservation

### 18.5.1 Anatomic and Physiologic Considerations

#### 18.5.1.1 Anatomical Factors

The cochlea is a spiral-shaped structure divided into three compartments: the Scala Tympani Scala Media, and Scala Vestibuli. The chemical composition of the Scala Tympani and Scala Vestibuli imitates that of an extracellular environment, with high levels of sodium and low levels of potassium. In contrast, the Scala Media may be likened to an intracellular environment with comparatively high potassium and low sodium concentrations. Whilst the electrochemical gradient created by this disparity is essential to the perception of sound, a breach of these chemically distinct areas through a traumatic insertion is associated with a loss of hearing [2, 29].

The first 180 degrees of insertion beyond the basal turn (corresponding to between 90 degrees and 270 degrees) is a significant region of the cochlea for the preservation of residual hearing (Fig. 18.2). It contains a larger number of spiral

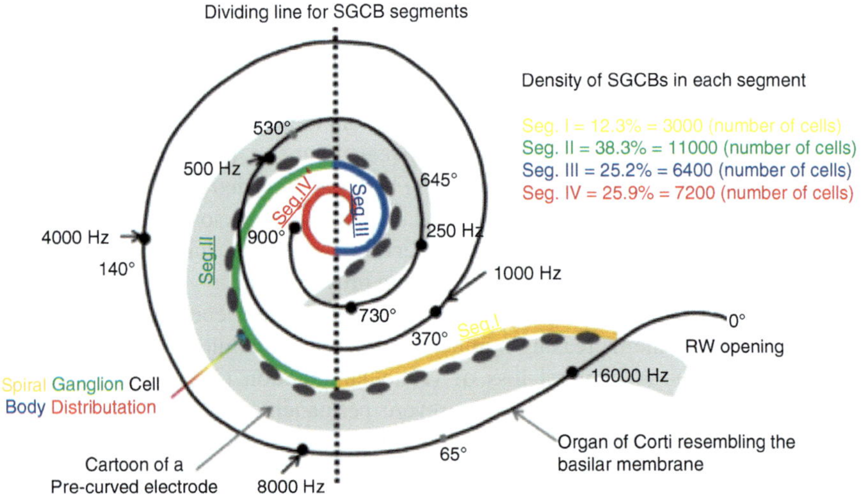


**Fig. 18.2** Relative distribution of spiral ganglion cell bodies. The organ of Corti (black line) with Greenwood Frequency distribution along the angular depth, measured from the round window. The spiral ganglion cell body distribution is shown by a prominent coloured spline line with the dotted grey line differentiating between four segments [30]

ganglion cells than any other segment of the cochlea, the successful stimulation of which is essential for optimal implantation outcomes [30]. This turn has also frequently presented as a particularly vulnerable region during cochlear implantation [31–35]. In a histological study, Biedron [36] demonstrated that the cochlear duct diameter does not decrease in diameter in a linear fashion, but rather varies in rate at which the diameter decreases. The combined ducts are significantly narrowed at the ascending portion of the first basal turn, which is a significant finding considering the amount of trauma that is found to occur at this location. It is theorised that the regional narrowing may be attributable to the close proximity of the carotid artery during development [36]. Whilst the narrowing of this portion of the cochlea may leave it vulnerable to electrode insertion trauma, it has also been demonstrated that a straight trajectory of insertion to the basal turn may produce higher insertion forces, and consequently more focal trauma at the basal turn. This effect may be particularly pronounced with the use of a cochleostomy [31, 33].

#### 18.5.1.2 Physiological Considerations

It is important to understand the transference of acoustic sound into intracochlear pressure variations, when considering the association between intracochlear pressure variations and trauma to the inner ear. Greene [37] makes an important contribution to explaining intracochlear pressure variations by demonstrating the two pressure levels (of the external auditory canal and intracochlear pressure levels) to be roughly comparable during implantation. This is due to the frequency of transient intracochlear pressure variation. In Vitro models frequently find these transients to last 0.1–0.2 s [37, 38], equivalent to 5–10 Hz. At these low frequencies, the sound transfer function of the middle ear is 1, or unamplified when travelling through the middle ear and accordingly, the consequences of intracochlear pressure variation are clear. A particularly good insertion may see a transient rise in pressure of ~100 Pa inside the cochlea, and a poor insertion possibly ~2.0 kPa [39, 40], (this translates to ~133–160 dB). Of comparable sound frequencies, the effect of this is most similar to a gunshot adjacent to the ear or blast trauma [41].

Initial studies investigating the causes of residual hearing loss identified key histopathological events outlined above, such as basilar translocation, as critical events during structure preservation implantation. Even with major advances in soft surgery techniques, however, 100% hearing preservation remains elusive [42]. With speed [43], CSF Gusher [44], and electrode stabilisation [45] all demonstrating a significant effect on hearing preservation, it is highly likely that minimising intracochlear pressure variation has a significant yet underappreciated role in structure preservation.

In addition to sensible attempts to reduce histological trauma to the ear, future methodology for hearing preservation during cochlear implantation should hold the reduction of intracochlear pressure variation as an important goal for surgery.

### 18.5.2 Patient Factors

With the emergence of electric-acoustic stimulation and partial deafness, the indications for cochlear implantation have expanded dramatically, as has the number of patients who can benefit from the extended applications of cochlear implantation. There are several crucial patient factors that influence the indication and subsequent decision-making for structure preservation during cochlear implantation.

#### 18.5.2.1 Assessing the Impact of Residual Hearing

Dorman and Gifford demonstrated the significant range of the overall hearing benefit achieved from bimodal treatment for hearing loss amongst patients with a similar amount of residual hearing [46] (Fig. 18.3). Whilst at one end of the spectrum the patients obtain an incredible amount of sound information from their residual hearing, there are other patients with the same hearing levels who appear to be profoundly deaf.

This leads to two questions. Firstly, why is that so? Secondly, how can we identify the benefit of the patients' residual hearing and predict the impact of preserving residual hearing? Answering the first question will merit a book dedicated solely to this question as the answers are found in the many dimensions of hearing and thus

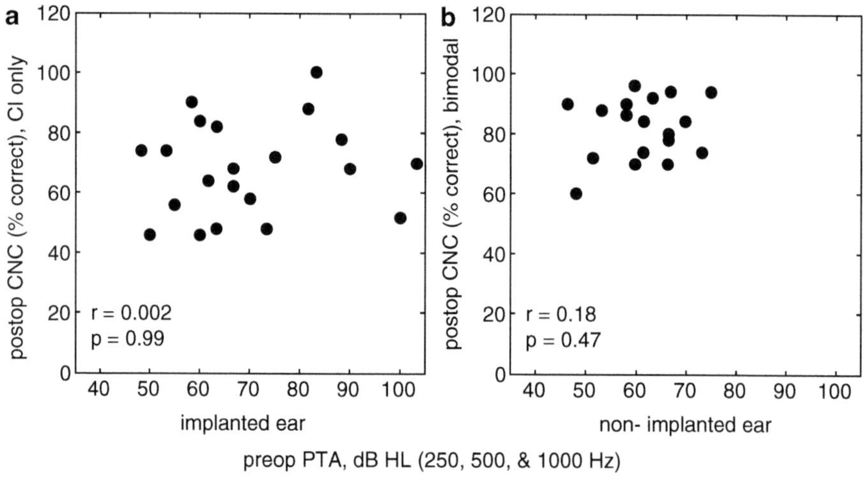


**Fig. 18.3** Panel (**a**) displays postoperative Consonant word scores (in percent correct) for the electric (E) only condition as a function of the preoperative, implant ear pure-tone average, in dB HL, for frequencies 250, 500 and 1000 Hz. Panel (**b**) displays postoperative Consonant word scores for the bimodal condition as a function of the preoperative, nonimplanted ear pure-tone average at 250, 500 and 1000 Hz. Gifford RH, Dorman MF, Shallop JK, Sydlowski SA. Evidence for the expansion of adult cochlear implant candidacy. Ear Hear. 2010 Apr;31(2):186–94. https://doi.org/10.1097/AUD.0b013e3181c6b831. PMID: 20071994; PMCID: PMC4092164

beyond the scope of this chapter. From the practical point addressing the second question is important for hearing health professionals and the processes that are in place to guide their decision-making.

Specific auditory testing such as sound localisation testing, measurements of the acoustic dynamic range and speech intelligibility provide important information in addition to the standard workup performed for cochlear implantation [47] which assist hearing professionals to determine the benefits of preserving the residual hearing in these patients. Emerging audiologic assessments such as measurement of spectral resolution and modulation [48, 49] and considering the quality of low-frequency acoustic hearing also provide objective tools to better predict the benefits of preserving the residual hearing.

#### 18.5.2.2 Age and Structure Preservation

Numerous studies have shown that the age of the patient is a variable that has a significant influence on structure preservation outcomes [45]. There are significant differences between children and adults, with children demonstrating far superior sustained hearing preservation after cochlear implantation [44, 45]. It has been postulated that the inner ear structures in children are likely to have different tissue properties, able to better attenuate the inner trauma occurring during and after cochlear implantation [45]. However, for the postoperative hearing outcomes there is little objective or experimental data that provide further insight into the mechanisms responsible for the different outcomes found between children and adults.

#### 18.5.2.3 Genetics and Structure Preservation

The ongoing research and increasing knowledge on the relationship between genetics and hearing loss have arguably reshaped the hearing professional's understanding of structure preservation, and decision-making with regard to managing cochlear implant patients. Mapping the genetic mutations for various kinds of hearing loss phenotypes together with an understanding on the natural course of these phenotypes, allows us to progressively personalise the hearing rehabilitation and implant strategy for the patients [50] (Fig. 18.4). Consequently, the body of data that shows structure preservation outcomes associated with the various genetic hearing loss mutations, in combination with knowledge on the nature of a hearing loss due to a specific mutation (i.e. whether the hearing loss is likely to remain stable over a lifetime such as GJB-24 or is likely to rapidly progress in childhood) has a significant impact on patient and family counselling regarding the prognosis and possible hearing rehabilitation strategies. Further, in considering the increasing availability and access to rapid genetic testing, it is very likely that genetic profiling of the patient's hearing loss pattern will soon be included as part of the standard workup of patients considered for cochlear implantation.

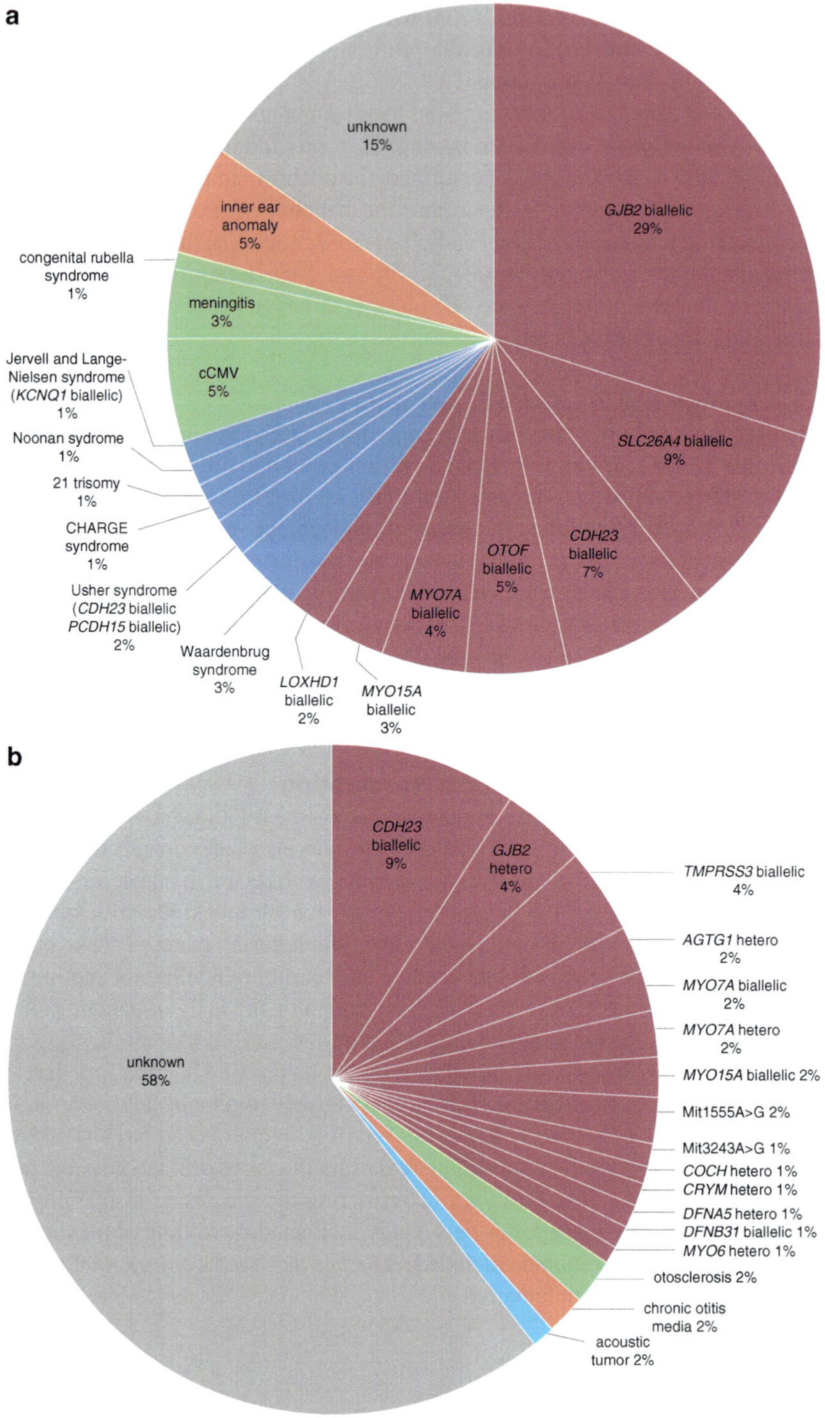


**Fig. 18.4** Genetic Background of cochlear implant patients. Genetic testing successfully identified causative mutations in deafness genes in (**a**) ~60% of prelingual hearing patients and (**b**) ~30% of post-lingual hearing loss patients [50]

## 18.6 Principles of Structure Preservation Surgery in Cochlear Implantation

### 18.6.1 Mechanisms of Inner Ear Injury During Cochlear Implantation: The 2-Hit Model

A concept that describes the processes responsible for the inner ear trauma during cochlear implantation is the "Two Hit Hypothesis". The *First Hit* occurs during the cochlear implantation surgery as a consequence of various mechanical forces. The *Second Hit* consists of the different responses of the inner ear after the electrode array insertion. In the following section, we discuss the *Two Hit Hypothesis* in greater detail to provide a better understanding into the mechanisms of inner ear trauma due to cochlear implantation.

#### 18.6.1.1 The *First Hit*

The inner ear is a delicate, complex structure. Certain structures within the inner ear are more susceptible to trauma than others, the consequences of which can be seen in the immediate loss of residual hearing experienced by some patients.

Certain complications during cochlear implantation surgery logically produce an immediate drop in all or a residual portion of a subject's hearing, for example (but not limited to):

- Tears of the basilar membrane, such as in electrode translocation, allowing intermixing of the perilymph and endolymph, exposing the organ of Corti and stria vascularis to a microenvironment lethal for hair cells [51].
- Damage or violation of the (endostium for example) during the drilling of a cochleostomy, resulting in an inflammatory response of the pancochlear endosteum, which in turn may lead to neoosteogenesis [52].
- Penetration of the spiral ligament compromising the blood flow through the stria vascularis, invoking an inflammatory response [53].
- Disruption of the osseous spiral lamina, likely disrupting the dendrites from spiral ganglion cells present within, causing immediate hearing loss and eventual spiral ganglion cell degeneration [54].

With respect to the vulnerable structures within the inner ear, it has been theorised that trauma to the stria vascularis, based laterally in the spiral, risks blood vessels that are susceptible to trauma, such as the posterior spiral vein and its tributaries. The lateral wall of the cochlear lumen also contains microchannels through the spiral ligament connecting the scala tympani to the scala vestibuli, as evidenced by the presence of identical micropores on the surface of the round ligament, above and below the basilar membrane [54, 55] (Fig. 18.5). Given the delicate structure of micropores, it can be theorised that these micropores when damaged may block off and prevent the balance of fluid between the scala vestibuli and scala tympani. This is supported experimentally by observations demonstrating the swelling of the scala tympani postoperatively, presumed to be a largely inflammatory reaction [54].

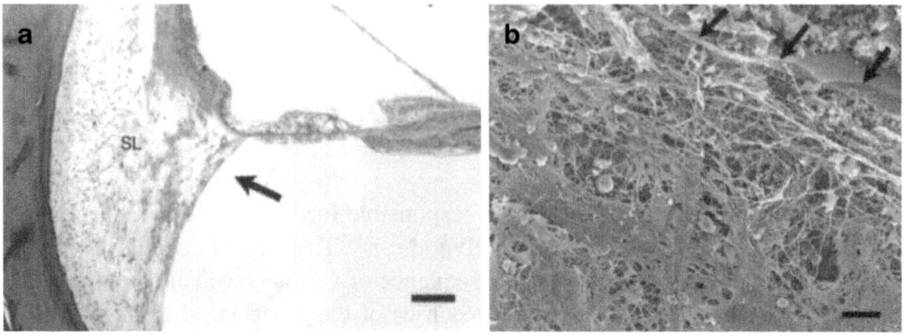


**Fig. 18.5** Micropores in the cochlear lumen. Illustrated is the spiral ligament (SL). The arrow inside the scala tympani indicates the angle of view for the electron micrograph in (**b**), in which the surface of the spiral ligament facing the scala tympani is shown. The arrows at the upper right indicate the area of attachment of the basilar membrane, which was cut away to prepare this specimen. Note the porous, irregular meshwork of connective tissue at the spiral ligament surface beneath the basilar membrane attachment. Scale bar = 100 μm (**a**), 20 μm (**b**) [54]

Within the medial aspect of the cochlea, it has been shown that the osseous matrix (such as that covering the spiral ganglion and modiolar vasculature) is more fragile and fractures more easily relative to other aspects of the cochlea [54]. Even without an osseous fracture, deviation of structures by electrode pressure may be enough to compromise blood flow, tear the basilar membrane, and accordingly induce an inflammatory response [54–57]. As such, as noted above, the medial aspect of the cochlea is more sensitive to electrode trauma, and especially meticulous care should be taken of medial structures intraoperatively [54].

Even without obvious evidence of histological trauma, there may be damage during implantation. This is particularly relevant for intracochlear pressure variation. As mentioned previously, blast trauma may be the most analogous comparison of intracochlear pressure during surgery due to the frequency and magnitude of pressure variation.

Despite the obvious trauma and damage by blast trauma, profoundly deaf cochleas post-blast trauma have often been found to have no histological evidence of trauma, aside from degeneration of outer hair cells and spiral ganglion nerve cells [58]. Importantly, they have not been found to have gross membranous rupture as is sometimes commonly believed [58]. Similarly, the exact mechanism of hearing loss due to variation in intracochlear pressure during implantation has not been determined either. It is possible that direct insult to outer hair cells is the cause of profound hearing loss during pressure variation.

#### 18.6.1.2 The *Second Hit*

The combination of direct tissue trauma during electrode insertion and the introduction of a foreign body into the inner ear leads to reactive processes whereby residual hearing is reduced through inflammatory responses, which are then followed by fibrosis, apoptosis of critical neural and cellular structures, ossification, and potentially focal necrosis of the inner ear [59].

These changes exhibit themselves in a manner commencing at the basal turn 12 h post-traumatic insertion, with a progressive increase in radicals and products associated with necrosis [60]. Reactive cytokines and inflammatory products including TNF-a, IL-1B, iNOS, COX-2, Caspase C [61], and JNK [60, 62, 63] are critical to the inflammatory cascade and have been demonstrated as potential pharmacological targets.

Fibrosis and ossification are natural scar responses following inflammation, but have been demonstrated to be counterproductive to the preservation of residual hearing [64]. Products such as TGF-B1, TGF-B3, CTGF are known to proliferation of the scar response [59, 61, 65], and have been shown to be particularly responsive to topical corticosteroids. As well as proliferation, inflammatory signals have also been demonstrated to be critical to the initial apoptotic signal via the classical pathway that disproportionately effects neural tissue [16, 59]. The outer hair cells and spiral ganglion neuron fibres have shown to be particularly vulnerable to apoptosis [66]. This appears mediated by p-c-Jun, Caspase3 amongst other factors, and is supported by the presence of reactive oxygen species and antihydroxynonenal, a highly reactive membrane peroxidation product, in apoptotic environments [67].

### 18.6.2 Tackling the *First Hit*

#### 18.6.2.1 Cochleostomy Versus Round Window Access

The merits accessing the cochlea through a cochleostomy or via the round window have been fiercely debated like few other areas within cochlear implant research. Compelling arguments have been historically made for both cases, with a consensus regarding the round window as the superior access point emerging in recent years.

Briggs et al. [68] in 2005 argued that *soft surgery* necessitates the use of a cochleostomy to guarantee insertion into the scala tympani because of the complexity of the hook region of the cochlea at the opening of the round window. Specifically, it was argued that cochleostomy should be placed inferior rather than anterior to the round window niche due to the risk of insertion into the scala vestibuli, and the risk of exposing the attachment of the basilar membrane and spiral ligament. Additionally, sub-optimal insertion trajectory associated with round window insertion could result in a loss of hearing preservation. Whilst an acute angle of trajectory when inserting the electrode has been correlated with increased insertion forces [33], and histological trauma [69, 70], no study has clinically demonstrated a link between poor trajectory in round window implantations and residual hearing loss thus far.

Studies that have found cochleostomy to be inferior to round window insertion have typically had small round window cohorts [21, 71], though the possibility of achieving hearing preservation through cochleostomy has been clearly demonstrated [68, 72, 73].

Evidence from large cochlear implantation institutions suggests that round window insertions are superior to cochleostomy for hearing preservation [42, 74, 75]. Although results vary between different academic institutions, it has been suggested that hearing preservation in over 90% of patients is routinely possible through round window insertion [42, 76, 77], whereas even experienced cochlear implant surgeons will not be able to achieve hearing preservation in more than 80% of patients using a cochleostomy [78, 79]. The reason for the reduced outcome abovementioned has been attributed to the significant histological trauma and subsequent inflammatory response potentially initiated by a cochleostomy [6, 75, 80–82]. Histological trauma is not always guaranteed, occurring in 40–50% of cochleostomies, and appears most pronounced in the first 90 degrees of insertion [31, 75, 80].

An important criticism of round window insertions is the anatomic variation of the round window and the resulting electrode trajectory. A medial trajectory has the potential to cause significant histological trauma, as demonstrated in several cadaver studies [33, 70]. To prevent such trauma, it is critical to drill the bony overhang of the round window and increase exposure. Particularly in those patients with a posterior-facing round window, drilling of the bony overhang therein improving surgical access can prevent significant histological trauma in almost 90% of patients [69]. It is important to acknowledge however that far more fibrosis and ossification is produced as a product of drilling a cochleostomy, than is seen with round window insertion [75].

Accepting that a round window insertion is optimal for hearing preservation, there are numerous methods for opening the round window such as a $CO_2$ laser, diode laser, scalpels, or microhooks. In Vitro studies by Todt and Mittman have demonstrated that a large, central round window opening opened using a scalpel or microhook under moist or "underwater" conditions is optimal for hearing preservation [40, 83–85]. In addition, good visualisation of the round window is essential [86].

#### 18.6.2.2 Further Consideration of Surgical Factors

It is essential to stabilise the electrode both during the insertion (such as through a two hand technique or insertion tool), and after when fixing the electrode in the middle ear [39, 45, 87]. Not fixing the electrode post insertion can cause significant pressure changes in the cochlea, thereby compromising hearing preservation [45].

Opening the cochlea and performing the insertion underwater has been studied extensively within the last decade. Whilst In Vitro experimentation is inconclusive [83], In Vivo clinical trials have more importantly found hearing preservation to be optimised during underwater insertion where the middle ear is filled with perilymph fluid immediately prior to surgery [88, 89]. We believe that the difference seen between In Vivo and In Vitro trials seen here is attributable to the large amounts of water used in In Vitro studies, producing large fluid shifts.

A slow electrode insertion speed has been conclusively demonstrated to be essential to hearing preservation. Clinically, it has been associated with improved hearing preservation when an electrode is inserted over 2 min [43]. In Vitro studies have attributed this to a reduction in intracochlear pressure variation during insertion [39, 90]. The relationship between hearing preservation and the speed of insertion has been shown to extend to "ultra-slow insertions", with insertions of up to 30 min having a statistically discernible impact on insertion forces [91, 92].

Following a successful insertion, the round window may be sealed. The optimal method for this is open to conjecture, but packing the opening has been shown to cause significant intracochlear pressure variation and should be avoided [87]. Likewise, a drop in residual hearing has been associated with artificial grafts, possibly due to a foreign body/inflammatory response [75].

#### 18.6.2.3 Perimodiolar Versus Lateral Wall Electrodes

The choice between a perimodiolar electrode and lateral wall electrode is again a debate only settled in recent years, and both electrodes may still be associated with significant intracochlear trauma in certain circumstances. Whilst preserved residual hearing is technically possible for either technique [42, 93], scientific advances in understanding over the last decade have made a clear case for a lateral wall electrode more compelling.

Aside from the obvious advantage of not needing to perform a cochleostomy, it is worth acknowledging that a perimodiolar design necessitates a stiffer electrode [54, 94]. Whilst hearing preservation may be achieved, the cochlea is an asymmetric structure with an inconsistently narrowing lumen diameter [33] that varies between individuals [33, 95]. Given the inconsistent anatomy of the cochlea, a stiff, uniformly shaped electrode is at risk of applying excessive traumatic force to surrounding inner ear structures. It has also been argued that the loss of residual hearing seen in perimodiolar implantation can be attributed to surgical error [93], and whilst this may sometimes be true, it does not allow the surgeon to be flexible in their approach and further any error in technique or inherent deficiencies may have significant traumatic impact.

Lastly, as discussed above, it is known that the medial structures within the cochlea are more susceptible to clinically significant trauma than the lateral wall [54]. Whilst meaningful trauma may be inflicted through trauma to the stria vascularis, the modiolus is a more delicate structure, and should be preferentially protected [45, 54].

#### 18.6.2.4 Further Consideration of Electrode Characteristics

Certain electrode characteristics have been shown to have a significant impact on residual hearing preservation. Larger volume electrodes correlate with larger intracochlear pressure variation in keeping with Poisson's equation of fluid dynamics [94, 96–98], whilst stiffer electrodes have been experimentally shown to lead to greater insertion forces, intracochlear fluid changes, and histological trauma [80, 94, 99].

Shorter electrodes, whilst innervating a smaller proportion of the cochlea, have classically been associated with preservation of residual hearing, particularly at lower frequencies [38, 94, 97, 100]. This is likely explained by the drastic increase in insertion forces seen at greater angles of insertion. Beyond 180 degrees of insertion, the insertion force has been shown to significantly rise [33], potentially causing greater histological trauma. However, recent findings with experimental ultra-slow insertions demonstrated how the insertion forces can further be significantly reduced, even with the use of longer electrode arrays and deeper insertions. It is crucial to further improve and augment current surgical techniques and tools so that structure preservation can be consistently and reliably achieved [101].

### 18.6.3 Minimising the Second Hit: The Impact of Pharmacology

#### 18.6.3.1 Corticosteroids

Even with a perfect insertion, it has been suggested that the sheer presence of an electrode as a foreign body produces an inflammatory response, evidenced by the histological obliteration of the scala tympani by fibrosis as a response to an inert foreign body [102]. The perioperative administration of corticosteroids has been shown to be integral to the preservation of residual hearing, with a strongly significant association between high dose dexamethasone applied topically, and a reduction in inflammatory products and apoptosis [59, 61]. Further, there is convincing evidence to support the administration of topical steroids, which have been shown to provide relief from an inflammatory response in a dose-dependent fashion [66, 103–105]. The effect of the topical steroids is strongest at the basal turn and opening of the round window, however, and comparatively weaker at the apex of the cochlea. In turn, there has been evidence to support the adjunctive and synergistic use of intravenous corticosteroids which likely have better distribution to the apex of the cochlea [103, 106]. Several studies have also shown that the glucocorticoids and certain anti-inflammatory medications can also offer protection of the vestibular hair cells and neural elements [107] (Fig. 18.6).

The authors therefore suggest a combination of intravenous and high-dose topical glucocorticosteroids such as dexamethasone or methylprednisolone, operating in a synergistic fashion, to best optimise structure preservation. Regarding future developments, preliminary studies have demonstrated that drug-eluting electrode arrays have significant potential to mitigate and block the inflammatory processes causing the second hit [56].

#### 18.6.3.2 Other Therapies

Products that may reduce inflammation have been investigated as potential pharmacological targets in residual hearing preservation. Although no products are yet commercially available, JNK Inhibitors, IGF1, HGF, and Etanercept have all shown significant promise within animal studies [67, 108, 109]. Importantly, different pharmacological agents have been shown to work with corticosteroid application in a synergistic fashion, heralding a promising role for future therapies [110].

A study by Ihler in 2014 demonstrated that the ultra-slow infusion of immune modulator etanercept via an intracochlear pump was able to preserve residual hearing. Surprisingly, however, the study also found a significant improvement within the control group, with continuous infusion of perilymph bestowing a statistically significant improvement in hearing preservation. This was attributed to the flushing of intracochlear cytokines which had been released in response to an initial inflammatory insult [111].

A further potential option for hearing preservation may be the use of topical hypothermia to ameliorate the inflammatory response. Not dissimilar to principles of clinical hypothermia already used in cardiothoracic surgery and neurosurgery, in a 2016 animal study Tamames demonstrated a significant improvement in hearing preservation with the use of intraoperative localised hypothermia [112]. In his study,

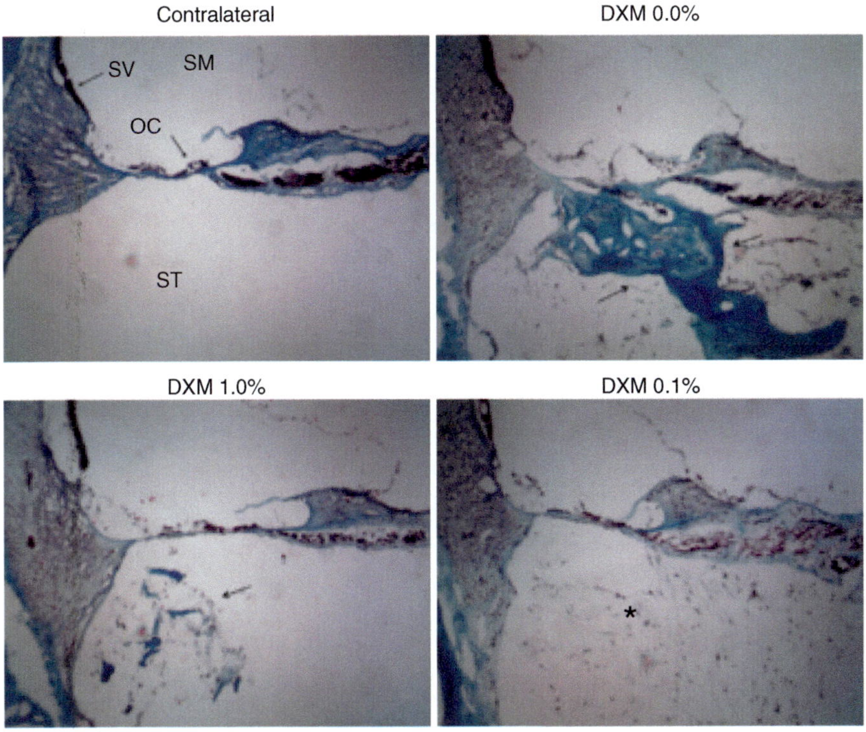


**Fig. 18.6** Masson's trichrome staining for the presence of fibrotic tissue. Representative micrographs of the midmodiolar cross-sections of control and implanted cochleae. Upper left panel shows an unimplanted cochlea, upper right panel shows an implanted cochlea with an electrode with dexamethasone, lower right shows an image of a cochlea with an electrode infused with 0.1% Dexamethasone, and lower left panel shows an image of a specimen with 1.0% Dexamethasone electrode [56]

the cochlea was cooled with a copper middle ear probe for 20 min prior to surgery and 20 min post-operatively. From Tamames study, it was found that hearing thresholds were significantly lower immediately post-operatively in the hypothermic group across all frequencies and improved across all frequencies to become comparable to control groups after a month. Finally, models illustrating focal control of temperature have demonstrated theoretical feasibility in humans [113] (Fig. 18.7).

## 18.7 Future Directions

The expanding indications for cochlear implantation over the last decade now encompass patients with varying levels of residual hearing and/or single sided deafness. The realisation that future hearing restoration treatments rely on viable tissue in the inner ear and that the paediatric patients implanted today are likely to need future reimplantation underpins the importance of preserving the inner ear structure

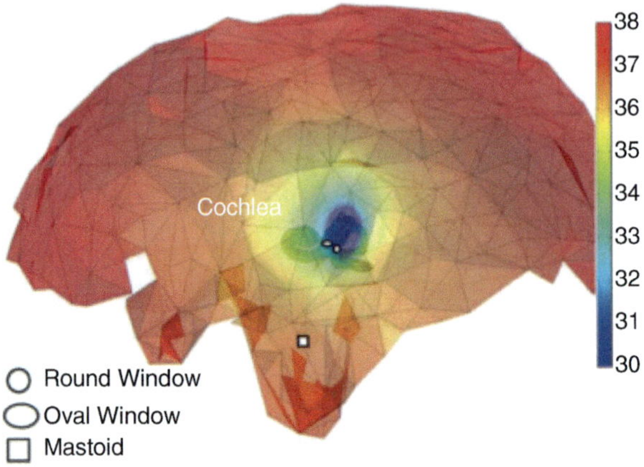


**Fig. 18.7** Localised hypothermia. Numerical 3D model of the temporal bone with the temperature distribution achieved from localized mild hypothermia. Locations of the round window, oval window, and mastoid thermistors are represented. Temperature contour was obtained at 18 min into the hypothermia protocol. The representative colour scale was fixed between 30 and 38 °C [113]

and function. Ongoing research is promising, and the growing knowledge gained from understanding the genetic landscape of hearing loss, and more sophisticated assessment will allow us to recognise different kinds of hearing loss patterns and provide unprecedented anatomical detail, thus redefining patient selection and personalised hearing restoration.

Automated insertion tools and robotic insertion devices [114] may overcome the current limitations of manual insertions, and together with ongoing improvements of electrode design could lead to a further improvement of insertion mechanics, reducing the effects of the *First Hit*. Furthermore, new and more selective pharmacological agents should improve hair cell and spiral ganglion protection during the *Second Hit* resulting in enhanced inner ear protection in cochlear implantation.

A new developing field is the use of robots to carry out implant insertions. Perhaps most critically to the development of structure preservation, more clinical trials are needed to test and validate findings seen in In Vitro Models, animal studies, and smaller pre-existing studies. Through the establishment and greater acceptance of principles of structure preservation during cochlear implantation, the future is likely to hold even broader indications for cochlear implantation, e.g. for disabling tinnitus in near-normal hearing ear.

## 18.8 Conclusion

Complete preservation of cochleovestibular function during cochlear implantation is the aspirational intent of current research efforts. The importance of an atraumatic insertion has been discussed extensively in the pursuit of hearing preservation and optimisation of surgical outcomes. Unfortunately, traditional cochlear implantation surgery is inherently limited.

Trauma to the delicate structures of the inner ear appears defined by discrete periods of damage, caused either by the initial mechanical trauma of surgery or by the inflammatory and proliferative response thereafter.

Intensive research has demonstrated nuanced patterns of hearing loss and residual hearing preservation, defined by age, genetics, and the medical decisions made perioperatively. What has followed has been efforts to optimise outcomes through changes to surgical technique, and pharmacological agents designed to further improve hearing preservation.

Currently, optimal structure preservation appears to be facilitated by:

1. Liberal use of both topical and intravenous glucocorticoids throughout surgery. Other synergistic anti-inflammatory agents are likely to soon become clinically available.
2. Minimisation of both insertional forces and intracochlear pressure variation.
3. Round window approach with good visualisation and a wide opening using a microinstrument such as microhook or needle, performed underneath a small pool of fluid within the middle ear.
4. Slow insertion of a soft lateral wall electrode using a very steady support system.
5. Extreme care to be taken if a decision is made to seal the round window.
6. Fixation of the electrode lead following insertion to prevent post-operative movement.

The future holds great promise for structure preservation during implantation. With optimisation of surgical outcomes comes a likely expansion of indications for implant surgery, the possibility of helping more individuals, and an exciting future for the specialty.

## References


1. Schindler RA, Bjorkroth B. Traumatic intracochlear electrode implantation. Laryngoscope. 1979;89(5 Pt 1):752–8.
2. Boggess WJ, Baker JE, Balkany TJ. Loss of residual hearing after cochlear implantation. Laryngoscope. 1989;99(10 Pt 1):1002–5.
3. O'Leary MJ, Fayad J, House WF, Linthicum FH Jr. Electrode insertion trauma in cochlear implantation. Ann Otol Rhinol Laryngol. 1991;100(9 Pt 1):695–9.
4. Fayad J, Linthicum FH Jr, Otto SR, Galey FR, House WF. Cochlear implants: histopathologic findings related to performance in 16 human temporal bones. Ann Otol Rhinol Laryngol. 1991;100(10):807–11.
5. Welling DB, Hinojosa R, Gantz BJ, Lee JT. Insertional trauma of multichannel cochlear implants. Laryngoscope. 1993;103(9):995–1001.
6. Shepherd RK, Clark GM, Xu SA, Pyman BC. Cochlear pathology following reimplantation of a multichannel scala tympani electrode array in the macaque. Am J Otol. 1995;16(2):186–99.
7. Nadol JB Jr. Patterns of neural degeneration in the human cochlea and auditory nerve: implications for cochlear implantation. Otolaryngol Head Neck Surg. 1997;117(3 Pt 1):220–8.

8. Lehnhardt E. Intracochlear placement of cochlear implant electrodes in soft surgery technique. HNO. 1993;41(7):356–9.
9. von Ilberg C, Kiefer J, Tillein J, Pfenningdorff T, Hartmann R, Sturzebecher E, et al. Electric-acoustic stimulation of the auditory system. New technology for severe hearing loss. ORL J Otorhinolaryngol Relat Spec. 1999;61(6):334–40.
10. Rossi G, Bisetti MS. Cochlear implant and traumatic lesions secondary to electrode insertion. Rev Laryngol Otol Rhinol (Bord). 1998;119(5):317–22.
11. Gstoettner W, Kiefer J, Baumgartner WD, Pok S, Peters S, Adunka O. Hearing preservation in cochlear implantation for electric acoustic stimulation. Acta Otolaryngol. 2004;124(4):348–52.
12. Gstoettner W, Plenk H Jr, Franz P, Hamzavi J, Baumgartner W, Czerny C, et al. Cochlear implant deep electrode insertion: extent of insertional trauma. Acta Otolaryngol. 1997;117(2):274–7.
13. Skarzynski H, Lorens A, Matusiak M, Porowski M, Skarzynski PH, James CJ. Cochlear implantation with the nucleus slim straight electrode in subjects with residual low-frequency hearing. Ear Hear. 2014;35(2):e33–43.
14. Hogan CA, Turner CW. High-frequency audibility: benefits for hearing-impaired listeners. J Acoust Soc Am. 1998;104(1):432–41.
15. Ching TY, Dillon H, Byrne D. Speech recognition of hearing-impaired listeners: predictions from audibility and the limited role of high-frequency amplification. J Acoust Soc Am. 1998;103(2):1128–40.
16. Adunka OF, Pillsbury HC, Buchman CA. Minimizing intracochlear trauma during cochlear implantation. Adv Otorhinolaryngol. 2010;67:96–107.
17. Nguyen S, Cloutier F, Philippon D, Cote M, Bussieres R, Backous DD. Outcomes review of modern hearing preservation technique in cochlear implant. Auris Nasus Larynx. 2016;43(5):485–8.
18. Huarte RM, Roland JT Jr. Toward hearing preservation in cochlear implant surgery. Curr Opin Otolaryngol Head Neck Surg. 2014;22(5):349–52.
19. Gstoettner WK, Van de Heyning P, O'Connor AF, Kiefer J, Morera C, Sainz M, et al. Assessment of the subjective benefit of electric acoustic stimulation with the abbreviated profile of hearing aid benefit. ORL J Otorhinolaryngol Relat Spec. 2011;73(6):321–9.
20. von Ilberg CA, Baumann U, Kiefer J, Tillein J, Adunka OF. Electric-acoustic stimulation of the auditory system: a review of the first decade. Audiol Neurootol. 2011;16(Suppl 2):1–30.
21. James C, Albegger K, Battmer R, Burdo S, Deggouj N, Deguine O, et al. Preservation of residual hearing with cochlear implantation: how and why. Acta Otolaryngol. 2005;125(5):481–91.
22. Hochmair ES. Surgical implications of perimodiolar cochlear implant electrode design: avoiding intracochlear damage and scala vestibuli insertion. Cochlear Implants Int. 2001;2(2):135–49.
23. Brockmeier SJ, Peterreins M, Lorens A, Vermeire K, Helbig S, Anderson I, et al. Music perception in electric acoustic stimulation users as assessed by the Mu.S.I.C. test. Adv Otorhinolaryngol. 2010;67:70–80.
24. Sosna M, Tacikowska G, Pietrasik K, Skarzynski H, Lorens A, Skarzynski PH. Effect on vestibular function of cochlear implantation by partial deafness treatment-electro acoustic stimulation (PDT-EAS). Eur Arch Otorhinolaryngol. 2019;276(7):1951–9.
25. Enticott JC, Tari S, Koh SM, Dowell RC, O'Leary SJ. Cochlear implant and vestibular function. Otol Neurotol. 2006;27(6):824–30.
26. Vibert D, Hausler R, Kompis M, Vischer M. Vestibular function in patients with cochlear implantation. Acta Otolaryngol Suppl. 2001;545:29–34.
27. Handzel O, Burgess BJ, Nadol JB Jr. Histopathology of the peripheral vestibular system after cochlear implantation in the human. Otol Neurotol. 2006;27(1):57–64.
28. Okano T, Kelley MW. Stem cell therapy for the inner ear: recent advances and future directions. Trends Amplif. 2012;16(1):4–18.
29. Adunka O, Kiefer J, Unkelbach MH, Radeloff A, Gstoettner W. Evaluating cochlear implant trauma to the scala vestibuli. Clin Otolaryngol. 2005;30(2):121–7.

30. Dhanasingh A, C NJ, Rajan G, van de Heyning P. Literature review on the distribution of spiral ganglion cell bodies inside the human Cochlear central Modiolar trunk. J Int Adv Otol. 2020;16(1):104–10.
31. Adunka O, Gstoettner W, Hambek M, Unkelbach MH, Radeloff A, Kiefer J. Preservation of basal inner ear structures in cochlear implantation. ORL J Otorhinolaryngol Relat Spec. 2004;66(6):306–12.
32. Kennedy DW. Multichannel intracochlear electrodes: mechanism of insertion trauma. Laryngoscope. 1987;97(1):42–9.
33. Avci E, Nauwelaers T, Hamacher V, Kral A. Three-dimensional force profile during Cochlear implantation depends on individual geometry and insertion trauma. Ear Hear. 2017;38(3):e168–e79.
34. Tykocinski M, Cowan RSC. Poly-vinyl-alcohol (PVA) coating of cochlear implant electrode arrays: an in-vivo biosafety study. Cochlear Implants Int. 2005;6(1):16–30.
35. Wardrop P, Whinney D, Rebscher SJ, Luxford W, Leake P. A temporal bone study of insertion trauma and intracochlear position of cochlear implant electrodes. II: comparison of spiral clarion and HiFocus II electrodes. Hear Res. 2005;203(1–2):68–79.
36. Biedron S, Westhofen M, Prescher A. Evaluation of the cochlear micro-morphology and the internal dimensions of the cochlear scalae with special reference to insertional trauma during cochlear implantation. Cochlear Implants Int. 2010;11(Suppl 1):153–7.
37. Greene NT, Mattingly JK, Banakis Hartl RM, Tollin DJ, Cass SP. Intracochlear pressure transients during Cochlear implant electrode insertion. Otol Neurotol. 2016;37(10):1541–8.
38. Mittmann M, Ernst A, Mittmann P, Todt I. Insertional depth-dependent intracochlear pressure changes in a model of cochlear implantation. Acta Otolaryngol. 2017;137(2):113–8.
39. Todt I, Mittmann P, Ernst A. Intracochlear fluid pressure changes related to the insertional speed of a CI electrode. Biomed Res Int. 2014;2014:507241.
40. Todt I, Ernst A, Mittmann P. Effects of round window opening size and moisturized electrodes on intracochlear pressure related to the insertion of a Cochlear implant electrode. Audiol Neurotol Extra. 2016;6(1):1–8.
41. Reed JW. Atmospheric attenuation of explosion waves. J Acoust Soc Am. 1977;61(1):39–47.
42. Skarzynski H, Lorens A, Zgoda M, Piotrowska A, Skarzynski PH, Szkielkowska A. Atraumatic round window deep insertion of cochlear electrodes. Acta Otolaryngol. 2011;131(7):740–9.
43. Rajan GP, Kontorinis G, Kuthubutheen J. The effects of insertion speed on inner ear function during cochlear implantation: a comparison study. Audiol Neurootol. 2013;18(1):17–22.
44. Crohan W, Krishnaswamy J, Rajan G. The effects of gusher-related Intracochlear pressure changes on hearing preservation in Cochlear implantation: a comparative series. Audiol Neurootol. 2018;23(3):181–6.
45. Bruce IA, Todt I. Hearing preservation Cochlear implant surgery. Adv Otorhinolaryngol. 2018;81:66–73.
46. Gifford RH, Dorman MF. Bimodal hearing or bilateral Cochlear implants? Ask Patient Ear Hear. 2019;40(3):501–16.
47. Group H. Quality standards for cochlear implantation in adults and older adults. 2017.
48. Gifford RH, Noble JH, Camarata SM, Sunderhaus LW, Dwyer RT, Dawant BM, et al. The relationship between spectral modulation detection and speech recognition: adult versus pediatric Cochlear implant recipients. Trends Hear. 2018;22:2331216518771176.
49. Landsberger DM, Padilla M, Martinez AS, Eisenberg LS. Spectral-temporal modulated ripple discrimination by children with Cochlear implants. Ear Hear. 2018;39(1):60–8.
50. Usami SI, Nishio SY, Moteki H, Miyagawa M, Yoshimura H. Cochlear implantation from the perspective of genetic background. Anat Rec (Hoboken). 2020;303(3):563–93.
51. Duvall AJ 3rd, Rhodes VT. Ultrastructure of the organ of Corti following intermixing of cochlear fluids. Ann Otol Rhinol Laryngol. 1967;76(3):688–708.
52. Ishiyama A, Doherty J, Ishiyama G, Quesnel AM, Lopez I, Linthicum FH. Post hybrid Cochlear implant hearing loss and endolymphatic hydrops. Otol Neurotol. 2016;37(10):1516–21.
53. Nadol JB Jr, Shiao JY, Burgess BJ, Ketten DR, Eddington DK, Gantz BJ, et al. Histopathology of cochlear implants in humans. Ann Otol Rhinol Laryngol. 2001;110(9):883–91.

54. Roland PS, Wright CG. Surgical aspects of cochlear implantation: mechanisms of insertional trauma. Adv Otorhinolaryngol. 2006;64:11–30.
55. Wardrop P, Whinney D, Rebscher SJ, Roland JT Jr, Luxford W, Leake PA. A temporal bone study of insertion trauma and intracochlear position of cochlear implant electrodes. I: comparison of nucleus banded and nucleus contour electrodes. Hear Res. 2005;203(1–2):54–67.
56. Bas E, Bohorquez J, Goncalves S, Perez E, Dinh CT, Garnham C, et al. Electrode array-eluted dexamethasone protects against electrode insertion trauma induced hearing and hair cell losses, damage to neural elements, increases in impedance and fibrosis: a dose response study. Hear Res. 2016;337:12–24.
57. Wright CG, Roland PS. Vascular trauma during cochlear implantation: a contributor to residual hearing loss? Otol Neurotol. 2013;34(3):402–7.
58. Cho SI, Gao SS, Xia A, Wang R, Salles FT, Raphael PD, et al. Mechanisms of hearing loss after blast injury to the ear. PLoS One. 2013;8(7):e67618.
59. Bas E, Dinh CT, Garnham C, Polak M, Van de Water TR. Conservation of hearing and protection of hair cells in cochlear implant patients' with residual hearing. Anat Rec. 2012;295(11):1909–27.
60. Eshraghi AA, Lang DM, Roell J, Van De Water TR, Garnham C, Rodrigues H, et al. Mechanisms of programmed cell death signaling in hair cells and support cells post-electrode insertion trauma. Acta Otolaryngol. 2015;135(4):328–34.
61. Bas E, Gupta C, Van De Water TR. A novel organ of corti explant model for the study of cochlear implantation trauma. Anat Rec (Hoboken). 2012;295(11):1944–56.
62. Eshraghi AA. Prevention of cochlear implant electrode damage. Curr Opin Otolaryngol Head Neck Surg. 2006;14(5):323–8.
63. Eshraghi AA, He J, Mou CH, Polak M, Zine A, Bonny C, et al. D-JNKI-1 treatment prevents the progression of hearing loss in a model of cochlear implantation trauma. Otol Neurotol. 2006;27(4):504–11.
64. Jia H, Wang J, Francois F, Uziel A, Puel JL, Venail F. Molecular and cellular mechanisms of loss of residual hearing after cochlear implantation. Ann Otol Rhinol Laryngol. 2013;122(1):33–9.
65. Ordonez F, Riemann C, Mueller S, Sudhoff H, Todt I. Dynamic intracochlear pressure measurement during cochlear implant electrode insertion. Acta Otolaryngol. 2019;2019:1–6.
66. Ye Q, Tillein J, Hartmann R, Gstoettner W, Kiefer J. Application of a corticosteroid (Triamcinolon) protects inner ear function after surgical intervention. Ear Hear. 2007;28(3):361–9.
67. Eshraghi AA, Gupta C, Van De Water TR, Bohorquez JE, Garnham C, Bas E, et al. Molecular mechanisms involved in cochlear implantation trauma and the protection of hearing and auditory sensory cells by inhibition of c-Jun-N-terminal kinase signaling. Laryngoscope. 2013;123(Suppl 1):S1–S14.
68. Briggs RJ, Tykocinski M, Stidham K, Roberson JB. Cochleostomy site: implications for electrode placement and hearing preservation. Acta Otolaryngol. 2005;125(8):870–6.
69. Shapira Y, Eshraghi AA, Balkany TJ. The perceived angle of the round window affects electrode insertion trauma in round window insertion - an anatomical study. Acta Otolaryngol. 2011;131(3):284–9.
70. Zhou L, Friedmann DR, Treaba C, Peng R, Roland JT Jr. Does cochleostomy location influence electrode trajectory and intracochlear trauma? Laryngoscope. 2015;125(4):966–71.
71. Rowe D, Chambers S, Hampson A, Eastwood H, Campbell L, O'Leary S. Delayed low frequency hearing loss caused by cochlear implantation interventions via the round window but not cochleostomy. Hear Res. 2016;333:49–57.
72. Tykocinski M, Saunders E, Cohen LT, Treaba C, Briggs RJS, Gibson P, et al. The contour electrode array: safety study and initial patient trials of a new perimodiolar design. Otol Neurotol. 2001;22(1):33–41.
73. Punke C, Zehlicke T, Sievert U, Pau HW. Acoustic-mechanical trauma during cochleostomy: animal experimental studies. HNO. 2011;59(6):570–4.

74. Rau TS, Suzaly N, Pawsey N, Hugl S, Lenarz T, Majdani O. Histological evaluation of a cochlear implant electrode array with electrically activated shape change for perimodiolar positioning [conference abstract]. Biomed Tech. 2018;63(Suppl 1):S135.
75. Burghard A, Lenarz T, Kral A, Paasche G. Insertion site and sealing technique affect residual hearing and tissue formation after cochlear implantation. Hear Res. 2014;312:21–7.
76. Skarzynski H, Lorens A, Piotrowska A, Zgoda M, Skarzynski PH. Hearing preservation after atraumatic round window deep insertion in partial deafness treatment (PDT) [conference abstract]. Int J Pediatr Otorhinolaryngol. 2011;75(Suppl 1):27.
77. Skarzynski H, Lorens A, Piotrowska A, Podskarbi-Fayette R. Results of partial deafness cochlear implantation using various electrode designs. Audiol Neurootol. 2009;14(Suppl 1):39–45.
78. Skarzynski H, Lorens A, D'Haese P, Walkowiak A, Piotrowska A, Sliwa L, et al. Preservation of residual hearing in children and post-lingually deafened adults after cochlear implantation: an initial study. ORL J Otorhinolaryngol Relat Spec. 2002;64(4):247–53.
79. Baumgartner WD, Jappel A, Morera C, Gstottner W, Muller J, Kiefer J, et al. Outcomes in adults implanted with the FLEXsoft electrode. Acta Otolaryngol. 2007;127(6):579–86.
80. Adunka O, Kiefer J. Impact of electrode insertion depth on intracochlear trauma. Otolaryngol Head Neck Surg. 2006;135(3):374–82.
81. Adunka OF, Pillsbury HC, Kiefer J. Combining perimodiolar electrode placement and atraumatic insertion properties in cochlear implantation - fact or fantasy? Acta Otolaryngol. 2006;126(5):475–82.
82. Hoskison E, Mitchell S, Harterink E, Coulson C. Systematic review: the radiological and histological evidence of cochlear trauma following implant insertion [conference abstract]. J Laryngol Otol. 2016;130(Suppl 3):S178–S9.
83. Mittmann P, Ernst A, Todt I. Intracochlear pressure changes due to round window opening: a model experiment. Sci World J. 2014;2014:341075.
84. Mittmann P, Ernst A, Mittmann M, Todt I. Optimisation of the round window opening in cochlear implant surgery in wet and dry conditions: impact on intracochlear pressure changes. Eur Arch Otorhinolaryngol. 2016;273(11):3609–13.
85. Martins Gde S, Brito Neto RV, Tsuji RK, Gebrim EM, Bento RF. Evaluation of intracochlear trauma caused by insertion of Cochlear implant electrode arrays through different quadrants of the round window. Biomed Res Int. 2015;2015:236364.
86. Mirsalehi M, Mohebbi S, Ghajarzadeh M, Lenarz T, Majdani O. Impact of the round window membrane accessibility on hearing preservation in adult cochlear implantation. Eur Arch Otorhinolaryngol. 2017;274(8):3049–56.
87. Todt I, Utca J, Karimi D, Ernst A, Mittmann P. Cochlear implant electrode sealing techniques and related intracochlear pressure changes. J Otolaryngol Head Neck Surg. 2017;46(1):40.
88. Anagiotos A, Beutner D, Gostian AO, Schwarz D, Luers JC, Huttenbrink KB. Insertion of Cochlear implant electrode Array using the underwater technique for preserving residual hearing. Otol Neurotol. 2016;37(4):339–44.
89. Stuermer KJ, Schwarz D, Anagiotos A, Lang-Roth R, Huttenbrink KB, Luers JC. Cochlear implantation using the underwater technique: long-term results. Eur Arch Otorhinolaryngol. 2018;275(4):875–81.
90. Kontorinis G, Lenarz T, Stover T, Paasche G. Impact of the insertion speed of cochlear implant electrodes on the insertion forces. Otol Neurotol. 2011;32(4):565–70.
91. Hugl S, Rulander K, Lenarz T, Majdani O, Rau TS. Investigation of ultra-low insertion speeds in an inelastic artificial cochlear model using custom-made cochlear implant electrodes. Eur Arch Otorhinolaryngol. 2018;275(12):2947–56.
92. Rau TS, Hugl S, Lenarz T, Majdani O. On the benefit of ultra-slow insertion speed: reduced insertion forces in cochlear implantation surgery [conference abstract]. Laryngorhinootologie. 2018;97(Suppl 2):S163.
93. Risi F. Considerations and rationale for Cochlear implant electrode design - past, present and future. J Int Adv Otol. 2018;14(3):382–91.

94. Jolly C, Garnham C, Mirzadeh H, Truy E, Martini A, Kiefer J, et al. Electrode features for hearing preservation and drug delivery strategies. Adv Otorhinolaryngol. 2010;67:28–42.
95. De Seta D, Torres R, Russo FY, Ferrary E, Kazmitcheff G, Heymann D, et al. Damage to inner ear structure during cochlear implantation: correlation between insertion force and radio-histological findings in temporal bone specimens. Hear Res. 2017;344:90–7.
96. Todt I, Mittmann M, Ernst A, Mittmann P. Comparison of the effects of four different cochlear implant electrodes on intra-cochlear pressure in a model. Acta Otolaryngol. 2017;137(3):235–41.
97. Lenarz T, Stover T, Buechner A, Paasche G, Briggs R, Risi F, et al. Temporal bone results and hearing preservation with a new straight electrode. Audiol Neurotol. 2006;11(Suppl 1):34–41.
98. Lauer G, Ucta J, Decker L, Ernst A, Mittmann P. Intracochlear pressure changes after cochlea implant electrode pullback-reduction of Intracochlear trauma. Laryngoscope Investig Otolaryngol. 2019;4(4):441–5.
99. Lo J, Bester C, Collins A, Newbold C, Hampson A, Chambers S, et al. Intraoperative force and electrocochleography measurements in an animal model of cochlear implantation. Hear Res. 2017;09:09.
100. Adunka O, Kiefer J, Unkelbach MH, Lehnert T, Gstoettner W. Development and evaluation of an improved cochlear implant electrode design for electric acoustic stimulation. Laryngoscope. 2004;114(7):1237–41.
101. Skarzynski H, Matusiak M, Furmanek M, Skarzynski PH. Deep insertion - round window approach by using SRA electrode. Cochlear Implants Int. 2014;15(Suppl 1):S4–7.
102. Braun S, Ye Q, Radeloff A, Kiefer J, Gstoettner W, Tillein J. Protection of inner ear function after cochlear implantation: compound action potential measurements after local application of glucocorticoids in the Guinea pig cochlea. ORL J Otorhinolaryngol Relat Spec. 2011;73(4):219–28.
103. Wang Y, Han L, Diao T, Jing Y, Wang L, Zheng H, et al. A comparison of systemic and local dexamethasone administration: from perilymph/cochlea concentration to cochlear distribution. Hear Res. 2018;370:1–10.
104. Eastwood H, Chang A, Kel G, Sly D, Richardson R, O'Leary SJ. Round window delivery of dexamethasone ameliorates local and remote hearing loss produced by cochlear implantation into the second turn of the Guinea pig cochlea. Hear Res. 2010;265(1–2):25–9.
105. Malkoc G, Dalgic A, Koc M, Kandogan T, Korkmaz S, Ceylan ME, et al. Histopathological and audiological effects of mechanical trauma associated with the placement of an intracochlear electrode, and the benefit of corticosteroid infusion: prospective animal study. J Laryngol Otol. 2014;128(8):702–8.
106. Acharya AN, Tavora-Vieira D, Rajan GP. Using the implant electrode Array to conduct real-time intraoperative hearing monitoring during pediatric Cochlear implantation: preliminary experiences. Otol Neurotol. 2016;37(2):e148–53.
107. Matsui JI, Haque A, Huss D, Messana EP, Alosi JA, Roberson DW, et al. Caspase inhibitors promote vestibular hair cell survival and function after aminoglycoside treatment in vivo. J Neurosci. 2003;23(14):6111.
108. Yamahara K, Nishimura K, Ogita H, Ito J, Nakagawa T, Furuta I, et al. Hearing preservation at low frequencies by insulin-like growth factor 1 in a Guinea pig model of cochlear implantation. Hear Res. 2018;368:92–108.
109. Gur H, Alimoglu Y, Duzenli U, Korkmaz S, Inan S, Olgun L. The effect of local application of insulin-like growth factor for prevention of inner-ear damage caused by electrode trauma. J Laryngol Otol. 2017;131(3):245–52.
110. Eshraghi AA, Roell J, Shaikh N, Telischi FF, Bauer B, Guardiola M, et al. A novel combination of drug therapy to protect residual hearing post cochlear implant surgery. Acta Otolaryngol. 2016;136(4):420–4.
111. Ihler F, Pelz S, Coors M, Matthias C, Canis M. Application of a TNF-alpha-inhibitor into the scala tympany after cochlear electrode insertion trauma in Guinea pigs: preliminary audiologic results. Int J Audiol. 2014;53(11):810–6.

112. Tamames I, King C, Bas E, Dietrich WD, Telischi F, Rajguru SM. A cool approach to reducing electrode-induced trauma: localized therapeutic hypothermia conserves residual hearing in cochlear implantation. Hear Res. 2016;339:32–9.
113. Tamames I, King C, Huang CY, Telischi FF, Hoffer ME, Rajguru SM. Theoretical evaluation and experimental validation of localized therapeutic hypothermia application to preserve residual hearing after Cochlear implantation. Ear Hear. 2018;39(4):712–9.
114. Crohan W. Mechanical factors affecting intracochlear pressure variation during in-vitro electrode implantation, 2021.

# Candidacy Considerations and Other Medical and Surgical Issues for Cochlear Implantation in Children

19

William P. R. Gibson and Catherine S. Birman

## 19.1 Candidacy

The cochlear implant candidacy is becoming wider as children with more and more residual hearing are now considered. The children considered for a cochlear implant can be classified into a pre-lingual category when the hearing loss has occurred before the child has been able to hear and learn to copy speech; a peri-lingual category, when the child has been deafened during the initial acquisition of speech; and a post-lingual category when the hearing loss has occurred after the child has acquired speech. Sadly, the peri-lingual category will lose their ability to speak if no intervention occurs. Recent studies [1] suggest that cochlear implant surgery for pre-lingually hearing impaired children should be undertaken under the age of 1 year to achieve the optimal speech and language outcome.

**Supplementary Information** The online version contains supplementary material available at [https://doi.org/10.1007/978-981-19-0452-3_19].

W. P. R. Gibson (✉)
Nextsense Cochlear Implant Centres (formerly Sydney Cochlear Implant Centres), The University of Sydney, Sydney, NSW, Australia
e-mail: Bill.Gibson@nextsense.org.au

C. S. Birman
Nextsense Cochlear Implant Centres (formerly Sydney Cochlear Implant Centres), The University of Sydney, Sydney, NSW, Australia

Nextsense Cochlear Implant Centres, Macquarie University, Macquarie Park, NSW, Australia
e-mail: Catherine.Birman@nextsense.org.au


S. DeSaSouza (ed.), *Cochlear Implants*,
https://doi.org/10.1007/978-981-19-0452-3_19

### 19.1.1 Medical Considerations: Discovering the Cause of the Hearing Loss

The cause of the hearing loss should be determined where possible, as this may influence the surgical technique and the cochlear implant outcome. Knowing the cause of the hearing loss is essential for counselling the parents and deciding on the appropriate post-implant training.

#### 19.1.1.1 Intrauterine Causes: Intrauterine Infection, Ototoxic Medications and Genetics

Genetic hearing loss can be subdivided into syndromic and non-syndromic causes. The syndromic causes may be linked to other disabilities such as loss of vision, kidney failure, developmental delay or heart disease that need evaluation prior to any surgical intervention. Often there are facial clues such as the white forelock, different coloured eyes and a wide space between the eyes seen in Waardenburg syndrome [2]. Jervill Lange Nielson syndrome is a profound hearing loss associated with a prolonged QT interval on the electrocardiogram that results in faints and loss of consciousness and causes sudden death in half the sufferers before the age of 15 years [3].

The commonest non-syndromic cause is due to Connexin 26 [4]. A genetic defect that affects the intracellular gaps and causes loss of electrical ionic charges within the cochlea. There are many other genetic causes of hearing loss. One example is 'large (or enlarged) vestibular aqueduct syndrome' (LVAS), which is often associated with Pendred syndrome [5] (Fig. 19.1a, b). The hearing loss may deteriorate during childhood. These children usually experience transient dizziness during the recovery after cochlear implant surgery.

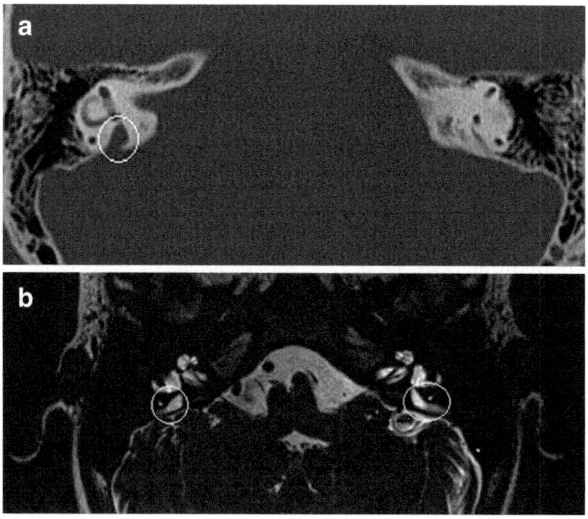


**Fig. 19.1** (LVAS CT (**a**) and LVAS MRI (**b**)) where I have put a white circle around the relevant areas

Viral illnesses during the first trimester of pregnancy can cause hearing loss, such as rubella [6] and CMV [7]. Rubella may be associated with eye and cardiac problems. Fortunately, rubella deafness is rare now in developed countries where vaccination occurs. Intra-uterine CMV may give no hearing loss or varying levels of hearing loss up to profound hearing loss, which can be unilateral or bilateral. It may be associated with other conditions such as developmental delay. If CMV can be detected by neonatal (PCR) screening and, if the appropriate treatment (Valganciclovir) can be given within the first 21 days a profound sensorineural hearing loss may be prevented [8].

Ototoxic drugs, especially during the first trimester may also cause hearing loss as the mother may have been unaware she was pregnant. In some countries, antibiotics such as gentamicin are frequently prescribed.

#### 19.1.1.2 Birth Events: Prematurity, Hypoxia and Jaundice

Prematurity (below 32 weeks gestational age) can be associated with hypoxia at birth and this is a major cause of perinatal hearing loss. Hypoxia is common in premature infants.

Hypoxia can cause a form of auditory neuropathy spectrum disorder (ANSD), which causes a loss of inner hair cells with survival of outer hair cells [9]. Using otoacoustic emissions as a screening tool to detect congenital hearing loss can lead to false reassurance and, later, the children may have difficulty perceiving speech using conventional hearing aids [10]. In the past, this was attributed to 'central auditory dysfunction (CAD)' and it was initially believed that a cochlear implant would be unhelpful. Fortunately, ANSD associated with birth hypoxia offers a favourable outcome using a cochlear implant. Unfortunately, other forms of ANSD may not be so amenable. Genetic forms of ANSD can be divided into pre- and post-synaptic causes [11]. Post-synaptic causes are often associated with abnormalities of the cochlear nerve and other disabilities such as visual loss.

Perinatal jaundice is common and usually settles within a few days. Kernicterus occurs with excessive bilirubin levels. A common cause is a mismatch of the Rhesus factor between the mother's blood and the neonate's blood [12]. Deafness due to kernicterus occurs because the cochlea fills with bile pigments causing loss of hair cells. Neurological problems, such as cerebral palsy, can also arise because the bile pigments damage nuclei within the brainstem.

#### 19.1.1.3 Post-natal Causes: Meningitis, Trauma and Ototoxic Medications

Severe or profound hearing loss can occur during infancy and childhood. Meningitis causes cochlear damage when the organism passes up the cochlear aqueduct to reach the inner ear. The inflammatory debris (pus) may become ossified and block the scala tympani. The cochlear aqueduct closes in most humans later in life and the threat of cochlear damage is lessened. Ossification within the cochlea prevents

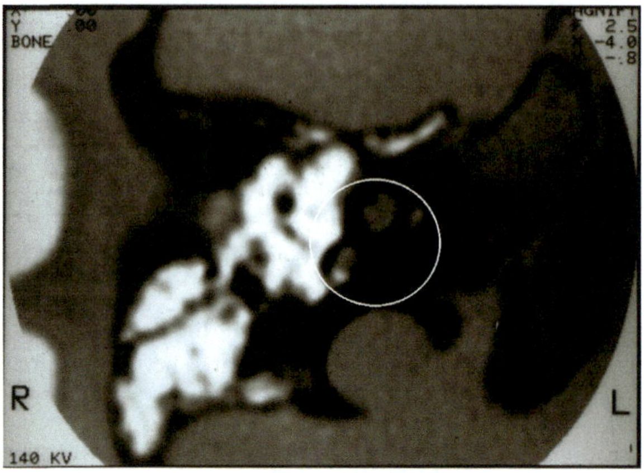


**Fig. 19.2** Obliteration of the basal cochlear turn due to osteogenesis as shown by CT. (The CT is reversed to show bone as a black image)

electrode insertion (Fig. 19.2). So meningitis in infants is treated as an emergency and cochlear implantation should not be delayed once the hearing loss has been verified [13]. Other viral illnesses causing encephalitis such as measles, mumps and rubella can have a similar effect.

Other causes of post-natal hearing loss include trauma, ototoxic agents, severe middle ear infections and cholesteatoma. Large vestibular aqueduct syndrome (LVAS) may only become evident during childhood with stepwise drops in hearing, particularly after head injuries.

### 19.1.2 Medical Considerations: Laboratory Investigations

Some investigations should always be undertaken prior to surgery. Some conditions may require special investigation. If the investigations show there would be an adverse outcome, the parents or guardians need to be informed and counselled.

**Electrocardiogram (ECG)** This test is done routinely for children with severe or profound congenital hearing loss, especially if there is any history of falls or blackouts to exclude Jervill Lange Nielson syndrome.

*Blood tests* may have been performed as part of the investigation for the initial hearing loss. For cochlear implant surgery routine blood tests are not normally required, unless there is a family history of excessive bleeding or bruising, tests to check platelet and coagulation factors may be required.

Genetic testing can be undertaken. Tests for connexin 26 and 30 are now easily available in Australia but tests for other genes such as the Pendred gene are more complex to obtain. It is anticipated that broader genetic testing will become more readily available for hearing loss.

#### 19.1.2.1 Radiology: CT Scan and MRI

Computerised tomography (CT) is often avoided because of radiation concerns as most abnormalities can be detected on magnetic resonance imaging (MRI).

MRI has a definite role and is always required. The MRI scan shows the fluid space of the cochlea, vestibule and semi-circular canals, allowing identification of any abnormal anatomy. After meningitis, the patency of the cochlear turns can be determined (Fig. 19.1a, b). LVAS can be detected (Fig. 19.2). Mondini and Michel abnormalities are evident on MRI. The vestibular labyrinth is abnormal in some ears affected, for example after intra-uterine rubella, and this can make identifying the entrance to the basal coil difficult to locate. Inner ear abnormalities may be associated with an abnormality in the course of the facial nerve; in these cases, a CT scan can be helpful.

Most importantly, the contents of the internal acoustic meatus (IAM) can be seen on a transcanal view. Normally four separate nerves can be seen (Fig. 19.3a). In Fig. 19.3b, only the facial nerve is present and the cochlear nerve is not visualised. Even, if only three or two nerves are counted, it is possible that cochlear nerve elements are absent or hypoplastic and may have fused with another nerve or are too small to see on the MRI scan resolution.

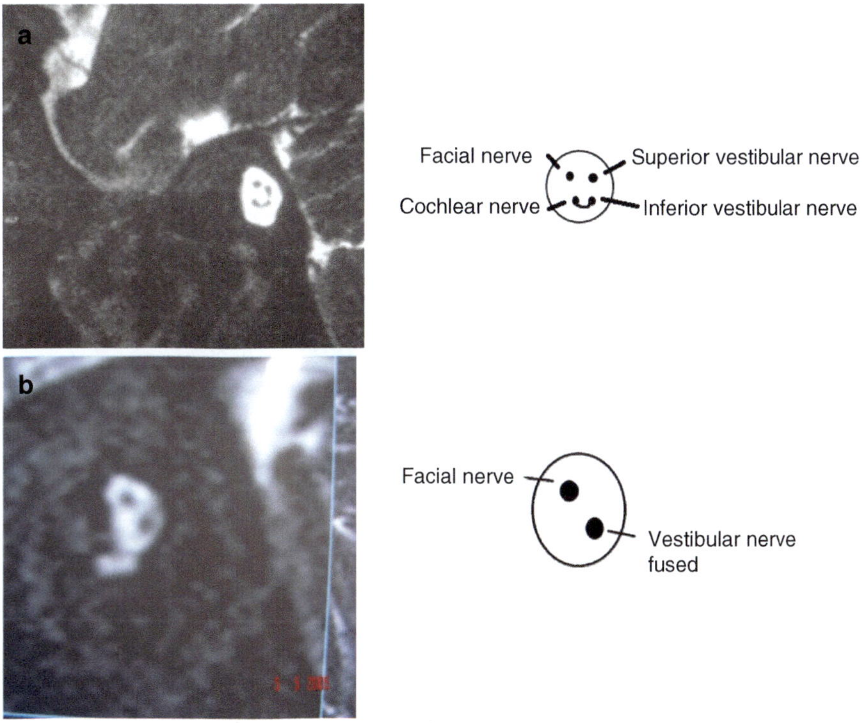


**Fig. 19.3** (a) A MRI transcanal view of the contents of the internal acoustic meatus showing the presence of all four nerves (cochlear nerve, facial nerve, superior vestibular nerve and inferior vestibular nerve). (b) A MRI transcanal view showing absence of the cochlear nerve in its normal position

#### 19.1.2.2 Electrophysiology: Electrocochleography and Electric Auditory Brainstem Potentials

The introduction of neonatal hearing screening and follow-up diagnostic auditory brainstem responses (ABR) enables children to be identified early and accurately within a few months of their birth.

In some cases, further electrophysiological testing is used to determine candidacy for cochlear implant surgery and can be performed with an audiologist or biomedical engineer. A surgeon inserts the electrode through the tympanic membrane to perform transtympanic electrocochleography (TTECochG) and transtympanic electric auditory brainstem potentials (TTEABR).

Transtympanic electrocochleography has become virtually redundant for the majority of paediatric candidates, as it can be replaced by auditory brainstem responses (ABR). It still has a role for cochlear nerve dysplasia, for older children who cannot be tested except under general anaesthetic, and those who have otitis media with effusion as well as significant hearing loss. The ECochG is quick to obtain and does not need any masking of the contralateral ear. The author utilises a 'golf club' electrode, which is inserted through a posteriorly placed myringotomy incision under direct vision [14]. Although it is very rare for a needle electrode to perforate an abnormal round window, the 'golf club' has a rounded surface making any round window damage unlikely (Fig. 19.4). The input impedance of a 'golf club' electrode is far less than a needle and allows larger recordings, which are not vulnerable to electrical interference within operating suites.

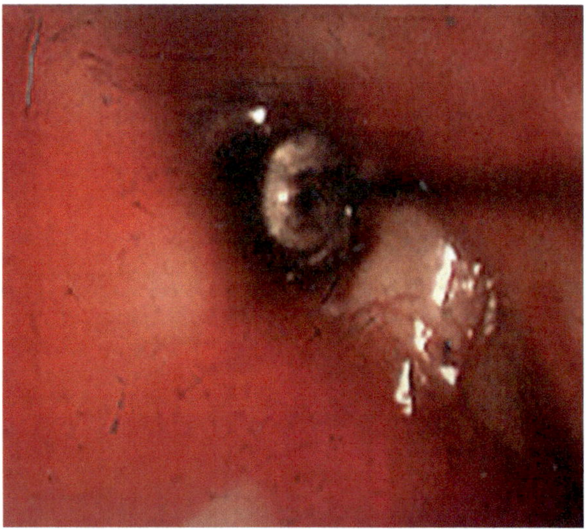

**Fig. 19.4** The golf club electrode positioned in the round window niche

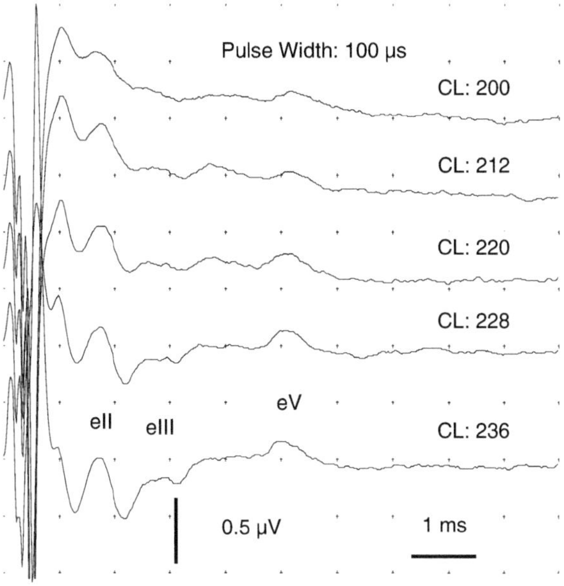


**Fig. 19.5** Electric auditory brainstem responses (EABR). Note the wave V has a latency of about 4 ms as there is no time lag due to sound conduction into the cochlea

Transtympanic electric auditory brainstem response (TTEABR) testing can indicate if there are any useable cochlear nerve fibres (Fig. 19.5). TTEABRs are difficult to obtain and require a 'golf club' electrode or a silver ball electrode placed accurately in the round window niche [14] (Fig. 19.4). The output of a cochlear implant is used to stimulate the cochlea via the cochlear implant software, which is synchronised to the recording equipment. The stimulating electrical charge must be delivered directly into the basal coil of the cochlea without diffusion into the middle ear tissues. The presence of otitis media with effusion makes TTEABR recording difficult.

TTEABR is undertaken when the cochlear nerve cannot be identified using transcanal MRI. In these cases, it is not known if the dysplastic cochlear nerve is entirely absent, or whether the nerve is hypoplastic or fused with an adjacent nerve. A recent consensus stated that a conventional cochlear implant should be offered first when a cochlea is present, and the auditory brainstem implant be offered only if the cochlear implant fails to provide adequate stimulation. A positive or negative TTEABR provides extra information when counselling the carers.

#### 19.1.2.3 Vaccinations: Rubella and Meningitis

**Rubella** Intrauterine rubella was one of the commonest causes of congenital deafness until the measles, mumps and rubella (MMR) vaccine was introduced in the 1980s [6]. Rubella; caused eye and heart problems in addition to hearing loss. The hearing loss was often associated with abnormal development of the otic capsule.

**Meningitis** Three types of meningitis occur: bacterial meningitis, viral meningitis and aseptic meningitis [15]. There is no vaccine for viral meningitis. Bacterial meningitis is the most serious illness and it is most often due to pneumococcus. There are several different strains of pneumococcal meningitis. Prevenar® vaccine is given in two doses initially. Pneumovax® vaccine is usually given after the age of 2 years and should not be given with Prevenar® vaccine but several weeks later.

### 19.1.3 Age Considerations: Auditory Plasticity

**Age** It has now been shown convincingly that the optimal speech and language outcome occurs when a child receives a cochlear implant when under 2 years of age [1, 16–18]. Profoundly deaf children who receive a cochlear implant after the age of 8 years have a far less favourable outcome, with little language understanding. This is due to the process of auditory plasticity.

Neural plasticity is the ability of the brain to develop certain neural pathways whilst the brain has the ability to change. The more essential the task, the more critical the time period for the development. For example, a foal should stand next to its mother within a few hours of birth. If the foal cannot stand within a day, the foal will never develop the ability to walk as the brain no longer has the ability to learn the task (loss of plasticity). In humans, both audition and vision have a critical time period for development after birth. Auditory plasticity is the ability to learn to hear, understand speech and this leads to the ability to produce speech. A baby listens and learns to babble using the sounds of speech soon after birth. By the age of 2 years, most children have developed some meaningful speech.

Auditory plasticity declines as the child ages. For a profoundly deaf child, if there has been no audition even using hearing aids, only limited benefit from a cochlear implant can be expected if the child receives a cochlear implant after the age of 6 years. Various studies have shown the benefit of early cochlear implantation and an ongoing study in Australia is suggesting that the optimal time for implant surgery is below 1 year of age [1].

Similarly, auditory plasticity affects the ability to utilise bilateral cochlear implants and to develop directional hearing and the benefits of binaural hearing. A teenager who has successfully received a cochlear implant in early childhood and then receives the contralateral cochlear implant when older, may have less speech discrimination from the second implant than from their first implant and is unlikely to develop directional hearing.

### 19.1.4 Surgical Considerations: Age, Blood Volume, Incision, Mastoid, Skull and Skull Abnormalities and Osteogenesis

Surgery for infants, especially if under the age of 1 year, requires careful evaluation and surgical expertise. Blood loss is to be avoided, especially if bilateral simultaneous surgery is performed. The average blood volume of a 7 kg infant is 560 ml (approximately weight in kg multiplied by 80). Underweight or frail infants may need to defer surgery until they are sufficiently robust.

Large incisions are more likely to become infected and to suffer keloid formation. A small postaural incision is better because the skin is elastic in young children [18, 19]. A pocket can be made, posteriorly, to hold the receiver snugly. The modern cochlear implant packages are thin, but the parents should be informed that the packages of the implants can be prominent in infants for several months after the surgery. Antibiotics are given prophylactically after induction and continued for 5 days after the surgery.

The development of the cochlea, middle ear and mastoid affect the surgery in infants. Fortunately, the cochlea is fully developed during the first trimester of pregnancy. The middle ear, ossicles and the antrum are at adult proportions but the mastoid bone develops considerably during the first few years of life [20]. The mastoid bone expansion is about 0.6–0.9 cm/year in length and width and 0.4 cm/year in depth in the first year, followed by half that rate until the age of 607 years. At puberty, there was a slower growth to reach adult size.

At surgery, there is limited access through the mastoid and this contain haematopoietic marrow that can bleed and needs special attention. Once the limited mastoid space is secured, the posterior tympanotomy and middle ear structures are viewed as in adult surgeries (Video 19.1), however, in infants, the petrous bone is slightly superiorly rotated, and the round window will be found slightly higher. The horizontal facial nerve is often seen from the antrum and even the stapes superstructure may be seen through the aditus in young children (Fig. 19.6).

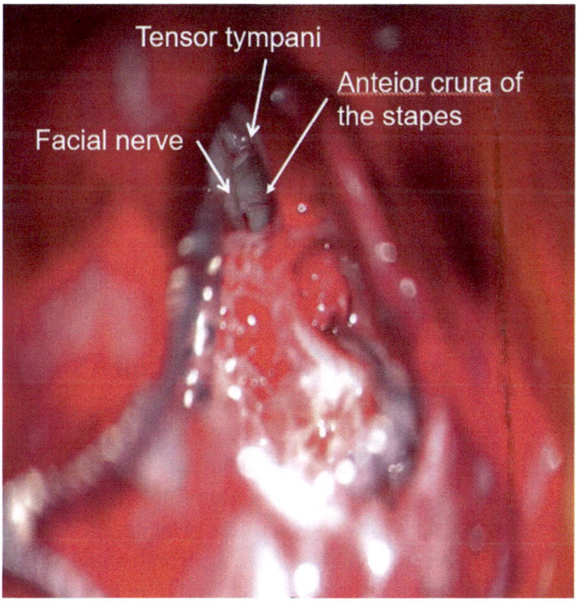


**Fig. 19.6** A view of the middle ear through the aditus in a 7-month-old child, note you can see through the aditus—the anterior crura of the stapes and the horizontal facial nerve to the region of the cochleariform process along with tensor tympani. Cochlear implant is in place in the mastoid and passing through the posterior tympanostomy

The thickness of the temporal bone may be only a few millimetres in infants under 1 year of age. A bony well is drilled to anchor the receiver-stimulator, but this is often shallower in a small infant compared with an adult. There is significant posterior growth of the temporal bone during early childhood [21]. The electrode lead wire can be subject to 2 cm of growth. All current cochlear implants have an expandable electrode lead which can lengthen to accommodate this growth. The bony bridge remaining above the tympanotomy does not alter significantly and can be utilised to fixate the medial end of the array.

## 19.2 Osteogenesis

The formation of bone within the cochlea occurs after meningitis in young children, but can also occur in adults, particularly with pneumococcal meningitis. The cochlear aqueduct is patent in the first few years of human life and infection from the cerebrospinal fluid can pass into the basal turn of the cochlea. The exudate can ossify within a few months. Initially, the soft new bone can be scooped out but after time it hardens and it may not be possible to insert a cochlear implant array. It may be possible to insert the array through the scala vestibule, in front of the oval window. There are also some special arrays provided by the manufacturers that are inserted through channels superior to the promontory and inferior to the promontory.

Urgent referral to a cochlear implant programme is essential if a child has severe or profound hearing loss following meningitis, as early surgery may ensure a cochlear implant can be placed.

## 19.3 Soft Surgery

Ears that have some low-frequency residual hearing can be implanted in the hope that the low-frequency hearing can be retained, and a 'hybrid device' can be utilised.

The hair cells are in the scala media and the implant array is inserted into the scala tympani so inserting the fine array slowly and gently can prevent displacing the basilar membrane and causing trauma to the hair cells. If the array is inserted too quickly, it can send the perilymph surging down the cochlea like a tsunami causing possible trauma. Often steroids are given to limit any inflammatory response.

## 19.4 Surgery in Presence of Skull Abnormalities: CHARGE and Other Dysplasias

The letters in CHARGE syndrome stand for: Coloboma of the eye, Heart defects, Atresia of the choanae, Retardation of growth and development, Genital hypoplasia and Ear abnormalities and deafness. The diagnosis is via major and minor features, and the majority of children have a chromosomal abnormality. In these children, the cochlea may be malformed (small and hypoplastic) with absent lateral semicircular canals causing the cochlea to rotate posteriorly [22]. Atresia or hypoplasia of the oval and round windows may occur. It can be difficult to locate the round window and the basal cochlear coil. CT-guided image surgery may be necessary to insert the array.

The cochlear nerve may be hypoplastic or absent. A trans-canal MRI view is essential and TTEABR may be helpful in reaching a decision to use a conventional cochlear implant or to consider a brainstem cochlear implant. Sometimes a favourable outcome occurs despite a seemingly compromised cochlear nerve. [23] Initially, the brainstem cochlear implants were used only for neurofibromatosis type two (NF2) patients and the results were often disappointing. Ten years ago, Collettti began using brainstem implants in non-NF2 cases including children with often encouraging results [24]. The surgical team must include an electrical neurophysiologist to help correctly place the electrodes in the brainstem and to avoid any unwanted stimulation of adjacent nuclei.

## 19.5 Further Surgical Considerations and Risks

Both the surgeon and the anaesthetist usually undertake the normal immediate preoperative checks. The surgeon sees the child and the parents prior to the surgery date. The surgeon should enquire about previous anaesthetics and if there were any complications. Any previous anaesthetic difficulties, any allergies and any recent or present infection should be noted.

The surgeon and the anaesthetist have to inform the parents of any potential risks.

## 19.6 Immediate Possible Complications of Surgery: Facial Nerve Palsy and Misplaced Electrode Array

The risk of damaging the facial nerve when undertaking the posterior tympanotomy is no greater than in adult surgeries. The mastoid cavity can be smaller, but the risk is very minimal with a well-trained surgeon. The risk of a delayed facial palsy in children is less than in older people as avascular changes are uncommon.

The electrode array can be misplaced, particularly in children with abnormal anatomy. Misplacements into a hypotympanic cell, the vestibule, semicircular canals or the internal auditory meatus are possible. These problems can be detected using intraoperative electrophysiological tests. [25] Neural Response Telemetry (Cochlear®) or the equivalent tests using other manufacturer's devices, show the neural responses and that the electrodes are correctly placed. If there is no response then intraoperative radiology should be requested.

Intraoperative cochlear implant evoked EABR testing does require a dedicated electrical neurophysiologist or audiologist and provides a robust means of testing the function of each electrode. This is most helpful in children with cochlear nerve dysplasia, as the mapping parameters can be adjusted to obtain an optimal cochlear implant evoked ABR response.

## 19.7 MRI After Cochlear Implantation

The cochlear implant receiver-stimulator package contains a magnet, which can be dragged or even displaced during a MRI examination. Furthermore, the MRI can heat long electrode leads causing tissue damage. Initially, the solution was to explant the magnet, perform the 1.5-Tesla MRI and then reimplant the magnet after the examination. An incision in the scalp is made behind the stimulator package and the magnet is removed and then replaced after the MRI has been performed. As this requires surgery, there is always a risk of damaging the device or infection. The next solution was for 1.5 Tesla MRI compatible cochlear implant devices, when a very tight bandage was wrapped around the head to prevent the magnet from moving. This can be painful and unfortunately, there are case reports of the magnet being displaced from the package and even tearing the retaining sialastic [26].

Most manufacturers now offer a 3.0-Tesla MRI compatible device. At time of writing, the limit seems to be 3.0 Teslas and the head shadow effect is still evident. MedEl was the first to provide a magnet that could align itself to the MRI. The other manufacturers are now offering similar solutions.

## 19.8 Delayed Complications of Surgery [27]: Infection, Cholesteatoma, Displacement of the Receiver-Stimulator Package, Extrusion of Electrodes, Device Extrusion, Electrode Malfunction and Failure of the Magnet to Keep Contact

Post-operative infection can occur some months or even a year after the surgery. If an infection occurs around the receiver-stimulator package, antibiotics may not be able to control the infection if a biofilm is present. A broad-spectrum antibiotic should be prescribed, and often given intravenously and continued orally for several weeks. If the infection appears to have settled but when the antibiotics are ceased, if the infection recurs a few weeks later, there is no option but to remove the package and wait for resolution of the infection in the wound before inserting another cochlear implant. The electrode array can be left in the cochlea by cutting the array close to the round window/cochleostomy but the package and leads must be removed. Leaving the array in the cochlea helps to identify the position of insertion and also lessens the risk of fibrosis closing the cochlea or infection entering the cochlea and causing osteogenesis.

Cholesteatoma formation within the implanted ear is uncommon. If this occurs, surgery is needed. Depending on the size of the cholesteatoma, it may be necessary to remove the cochlear implant, and a blind sac closure of the external meatus is performed. Most surgeons stage the procedure and wait for 3 months before re-exploring the ear to ensure the cholesteatoma is completely eradicated. Occasionally, when the cholesteatoma is caught early, only local surgery is required and it is possible to preserve the cochlear implant.

Displacement of the stimulator receiver package is rare. If the device was placed in a tight periosteal pocket, then it can only displace towards the external meatus. This can be prevented by drilling a socket in the skull bone or by placing a tie around where the electrode array leaves the package. If the head coil can still be placed, then there is no need for surgery to reposition the package unless it is too close to the pinna. If surgery is undertaken, then care should be taken not to pull the array out from the cochlea.

Extrusion of electrodes can occur if the implant was performed at an early age and there has been considerable skull growth during childhood or following infection or a significant knock to the head. The problem can be detected on device programming (mapping) and on radiology. Often the array can be reinserted if picked up early. Sometimes the existing cochlear implant array cannot be reinserted, or shows evidence of damage after reinsertion so it may be necessary to reinsert another device. The new array can usually be reinserted into the scala tympani, but if there is considerable fibrosis it may still be possible to insert it through the scala vestibuli.

Electrode malfunction is not uncommon. All the leading brands have had to recall devices when a manufacturing fault occurs. The companies have been exemplary in admitting the fault and offering assistance to replace the faulty devices.

Malfunction of a few of the electrodes occurs in some of the devices, especially after several years. In Cochlear® devices, up to 5 of the 22 electrodes can be faulty without significant impact on the recipient's hearing, depending on the location of the faulty electrodes. The ultimate decision to replace the device is not dependent on the number of faulty electrodes but on whether or not the hearing has been compromised.

Failure of the magnet to keep contact occurs due to thickening of the scalp or very strong sturdy hair. For obese children, it is better to place the receiver/stimulator package upright above the ear where the scalp remains thinner. In some children of African descent, the hair is very strong and a small circle of hair has to be shaved away to allow the head coil to stay in contact.

## 19.9 Pain After Cochlear Implantation

Cochlear implant surgery is not very painful, on average children use paracetamol for 2 days following surgery [28]. Long-term pain around the site of the stimulator-receiver package following surgery is rare. It is necessary to exclude an infection. The area should be palpated to see if there is any swelling and the tympanic membrane is checked for any sign of otitis media. An ultrasound examination can show if there is fluid (haematoma or seroma) around the package. If the magnet is too strong, it may cause reddening of the skin but rarely causes any significant pain.

Skin erosion due to the magnet is rare in children but can be a problem in elderly patients.

Sadly, some congenitally deaf recipients may have received the implant at an older age and have not been able to distinguish useable sounds and wish to be disassociated with a cochlear implant. Similarly, we have seen a few older teenagers, develop a sensation of pain associated with a previously fine, functioning device. Investigations may show no cause, however, sometimes there is co-existing anxiety or depression. Some have had the device removed due to their symptoms of pain and have felt that their pain was relieved.

## 19.10 Loss of Residual Hearing

If residual low frequency has been retained after surgery, a 'hybrid device' can be used which combines a cochlear implant and a hearing aid. Sadly, often the residual hearing slowly declines over time and the hearing aid component may is no longer be viable. In some ears, the residual hearing is lost suddenly about 2–3 months after the surgery. Various explanations have been offered. One possibility is that the vein of the modiolus, which drains venous blood from the hair cells becomes obstructed as fibrosis occurs around the electrode array. Even after successfully retaining some low-frequency hearing, some patients may elect to just use the cochlear implant, rather than a hybrid device, as they find the sound provided by the cochlear implant is clearer. For this reason, a full-length electrode array is preferable to a shortened array.

## 19.11 Removal of a Malfunctioning Cochlear Implant: Indications and Outcome

### 19.11.1 Indications for Removal of the Cochlear Implant, Outcome After Reinsertion

*Indications for removal*, commonest reasons are device malfunction or infection (especially if cholesteatoma has occurred). Less common reasons are device or electrode extrusion, pain, or just the wish of the recipient. Details of these complications have previously been discussed.

*Outcome after reinsertion*, it appears that there is little change in the performance of the cochlear implant after reinsertion [29]. On removing the array, the exact site of reinsertion should be noted, as there have been cases when the array is inserted into a false tract. The insertion can be checked by electrically using neural responses such as NRT or ART. It may be difficult to remove the array if there is osteogenesis and the array can be snapped if excess traction is applied. In such cases, it is often possible to reinsert into the scala vestibuli.

## 19.12 Conclusions

Paediatric cochlear implants are a modern success story, allowing children with severe or profound hearing loss to learn to listen, hear and speak. For the majority of children, timely provision of a cochlear implant allows the child to have sufficient hearing and language to go to a regular school. This chapter covers aspects that the surgeon in the cochlear implant team may encounter. The surgeon is not only involved in the surgery, but also in the pre-operative candidacy evaluation and in the long-term follow-up of the recipients.

## References


1. Ching TYC, Dillon H, Leigh G, Cupples L. Learning from the longitudinal outcomes of children with hearing impairment (LOCHI) study: summary of 5-year findings and implications. Int J Audiol. 2018;57(suppl 2):S105–11. https://doi.org/10.1080/14992027.2017.1385865.
2. Ahmed Jan N, Mui RK, Masood S. Waardenburg Syndrome. [Updated 2020 Sep 25]. In: StatPearls [Internet]. Treasure Island, FL: StatPearls Publishing; 2020 Jan. Available from https://www.ncbi.nlm.nih.gov/books/NBK560879/
3. Pabba K, Chakraborty RK. Jervell and Lange Nielsen Syndrome. [Updated 2021 Mar 1]. In: StatPearls [Internet]. Treasure Island, FL: StatPearls Publishing; 2021 Jan. Available from https://www.ncbi.nlm.nih.gov/books/NBK537300/
4. Kenna MA, Wu B, Cotanche DA, Korf BR, Rehm HL. Connexin 26 studies in patients with sensorineural hearing loss. Arch Otolaryngol Head Neck Surg. 2001;127(9):1037–42. https://doi.org/10.1001/archotol.127.9.1037.
5. Pryor SP, Madeo AC, Reynolds JC, Sarlis NJ, Arnos KS, Nance WE, Yang Y, Zalewski CK, Brewer CC, Butman JA, Griffith AJ. SLC26A4/PDS genotype-phenotype correlation in hearing loss with enlargement of the vestibular aqueduct (EVA): evidence that Pendred syndrome and non-syndromic EVA are distinct clinical and genetic entities. J Med Genet. 2005;42:159–65.
6. Brookhouser PE, Bordley JE. Congenital rubella deafness: pathology and pathogenesis. Arch Otolaryngol. 1973;98(4):252–7. https://doi.org/10.1001/archotol.1973.00780020262008.
7. American Academy of Pediatrics. Cytomegalovirus infection. In: Kimberlin DW, Brady MT, Jackson MA, Long SS, editors. Red Book. 2018 Report of the committee on infectious diseases. 31st ed. Itasca, IL: American Academy of Pediatrics; 2018. p. 310.
8. Nassetta L, Kimberlin D, Whitely R. Treatment of congenital cytomegalovirus infection: implications for future theurapeutic strategies. J Antimicrob Chem. 2009;63:862–7. https://doi.org/10.1093/jac.dkp/083.
9. Rea PA, Gibson WPR. Evidence for surviving outer hair cell function in deaf ears. Laryngoscope. 2003;113:2030–3. https://doi.org/10.1097/00005537-200311000-00033.
10. Gibson WP, Graham JM. Editorial: 'auditory neuropathy' and cochlear implantation - myths and facts. Cochlear Implants Int. 2008;9(1):1–7. https://doi.org/10.1179/cim.2008.9.1.1.
11. McMahon CM, Patuzzi RB, Gibson WP, Sanli H. Identification of different subtypes of auditory neuropathy using electrocochleography. In: Kaga K, Starr A, editors. Neuropathies of the auditory and vestibular eighth cranial nerves. Tokyo: Springer; 2009. https://doi.org/10.1007/978-4-431-09433-3_3.
12. Bhutani VK, Zipursky A, Blencowe H, Khanna R, Sgro M, Ebbesen F, Bell J, Mori R, Slusher TM, Fahmy N, Paul VK, Du L, Okolo AA, de Almeida MF, Olusanya BO, Kumar P, Cousens S, Lawn JE. Neonatal hyperbilirubinemia and Rhesus disease of the newborn: incidence and impairment estimates for 2010 at regional and global levels. Pediatr Res. 2013;74(Suppl 1):86–100. https://doi.org/10.1038/pr.2013.p208.

13. Dodds A, Tyszkiewicz E, Ramsden R. Cochlear implantation after bacterial meningitis: the dangers of delay. Arch Dis Child. 1997;76:139–40.
14. Wong SHW, Gibson WPR, Sanli H. Use of transtympanic round window electrocochleography for threshold estimations in children. Am J Otol. 1997;18:632–6.
15. Douglas SA, Sanli H. Gibson WPR meningitis resulting in hearing loss and labyrinthitis ossificans - does the organism matter? Cochlear Implants Int. 2008;9:90–6.
16. Kileny PR, Zwolan TA, Ashbaugh C. The influence of age at implantation on performance with a cochlear implant in children. Otol Neurotol. 2001;22(1):42–6.
17. Niparko JK, Tobey EA, Thal DJ, Eisenberg LS, Wang N-Y, Quittner AL, Fink NE. Spoken language development in children following cochlear implantation. JAMA. 2010;303(15):1498–506. https://doi.org/10.1001/jama.2010.451.
18. Gibson WPR, Harrison HC, Prowse C. A new incision for placement of the 'Cochlear' multichannel cochlear implant. J Laryngol Otol. 1995;109:821–5.
19. Ray JD, Gibson W, Sanli H. Surgical complications of 844 consecutive cochlear implantations and observations on large versus small incisions. Cochlear Implants Int. 2004;5:87–95.
20. Cinamon U. The growth rate and size of the mastoid air cell system and mastoid bone: a review and reference. Eur Arch Otorhinolaryngol. 2009;266:781–6.
21. Dahm MC, Shepherd RK, Clark GM. The postnatal growth of the temporal bone and implications for cochlear implantation in children. Acta Otolaryngol Suppl. 1993;505:1–39.
22. Birman CS, Brew JA, Gibson WPR, Elliott EJ. CHARGE syndrome and Cochlear implantation: difficulties and outcomes in the paediatric population. Int J Pediatr Otorhinolaryngol. 2015;79(4):487–92.
23. Birman CS, Powell RF, Gibson WPR, Elliott EJ. Cochlear implant outcomes in cochlear nerve aplasia and hypoplasia. Otol Neurotol. 2016;37:438–45.
24. Colletti V, Carner M, Miorelli V, Guida M, Colletti L, Fiorino F. Auditory brainstem implant (ABI): new Frontiers in adults and children. Otolaryngol Head Neck Surg. 2005;133(1):126–38. https://doi.org/10.1016/j.otohns.2005.03.022.
25. Pau H, Parker A, Sanli H, Gibson WP. Displacement of electrodes of a cochlear implant into the vestibular system: intraoperative and postoperative electrophysiological analyses. Acta Otolaryngol. 2005;125:1116–9.
26. Broomfield SJ, Da Cruz M, Gibson WP. Cochlear implants and magnetic resonance scans: a case report and review. Cochlear Implants Int. 2013 Jan;14(1):51–5. https://doi.org/10.1179/1754762811Y.0000000027.
27. Kempf HG, Johann K, Lenarz T. Complications in pediatric cochlear implant surgery. Eur Arch Otol. 1999;256:128–32. https://doi.org/10.1007/s004050050124.
28. Birman C, Gibson W, Elliott EJ. Pediatric cochlear implantation associated with minimal postoperative pain and dizziness. Otol Neurotol. 2015;36(2):220–2. https://doi.org/10.1097/AO.0000000000000569.
29. Toner F, Sanli A, Hall A, Birman C. Intraoperative Cochlear implant reinsertion effects evaluated by electrode impedance. Otol Neurotol. 2020;41(6):e695–9. https://doi.org/10.1097/MAO.0000000000002650.

# Explantation and Reimplantation of Cochlear Implants

# 20

Clarós Pedro and Koniewska Anna

## 20.1 Introduction

Cochlear implant (CI) is an excellent auditory rehabilitation for selected deaf adults and children who receive little or no benefit from hearing aids. It is the treatment of choice for patients with severe-to-profound sensorineural hearing loss. The first cochlear implantation was described by Drs. House and Doyle in 1961 [1]. Cochlear implant seems to be one of the great advances in modern medicine. Since a few decades ago, there is a constant improvement in medical and surgical care as well as technology associated with cochlear implants. Despite of that, it is still impossible to avoid some complications associated with implantation of CI, which can even lead to the necessity of CI explantation. Complications rates associated with CI are ranging from 7% to 19.9%, and are more frequent in cases with cochlear malformations. The rate of complications is much lower in cases of reimplantation than in the initial implantation [2].

Explantation is defined as the removal of an existing implant, with no subsequent replacement [3]. On the other hand, reimplantation is explantation of an existing device followed by the replacement of a new implant [3]. It is important to distinguish another possible surgical management performed in cases in which

**Supplementary Information** The online version contains supplementary material available at [https://doi.org/10.1007/978-981-19-0452-3_20].

C. Pedro (✉)
Clarós Clinic, Cochlear Implant Centre, Barcelona, Spain
e-mail: clinica@clinicaclaros.com

K. Anna
Department of Otorhinolaryngology and Oncological Laryngology, Medical University of Silesia, Zabrze, Poland


S. DeSaSouza (ed.), *Cochlear Implants*,
https://doi.org/10.1007/978-981-19-0452-3_20

explantation is not mandatory [3]. Proposed a third category in cochlear implant revision surgery, which is “minor revision surgery.” Minor revision surgeries are performed on the wound or the existing implant, and include receiver-stimulator reposition, skin flap revision, change of magnet, magnet reinsertion, and aeroseal operation.

## 20.2 Experience of the First Author

In Clarós Clinic Cochlear Implant Centre, Barcelona, Spain, the first cochlear implantation was performed in 1992 on an adult patient, and in 1993 on a child. Since then, we have implanted 1556 CI, 311 (20%) in adults, and 1244 (80%) in children.

## 20.3 Complications of Cochlear Implantation

Complications associated with CI can be related to surgical technique, patient anatomy, foreign body placement, dysfunction of the implanted device. Complications can be divided into major and minor. Major complications are defined as those which require reoperation or hospitalization for medical treatment or have caused permanent disability and severe symptoms. Minor complications could be treated in outpatients medically or by minor surgical intervention. We can distinguish also complications that occur during surgery and postoperatively. Complications during surgery may include cerebrospinal fluid leakage (Fig. 20.1), autonomic disorders, major bleeding, and neurological complications. Postoperative complications can include facial paralysis, disabling tinnitus or vertigo, debilitating pain, skin problems, electrode displacement, infections, hematomas, processor failures, and tympanic perforations. Another, very useful classification of CI postoperative complications was proposed by Parent et al. [2]. They divided postoperative complications into four groups: (1) device-related (malfunctions, poor electrode placements, movements of part of the implant), (2) local (pain, infections, scar problems, hematomas), (3) cochleovestibular (tinnitus, vertigo), and (4) related to lesions of adjacent structures (leakage of cerebrospinal fluid, facial paralysis, tympanic perforations). The incidence of complications after cochlear implantation varies, depending on research and defined criteria from 5.7% to 19.9% [4]. Cerebrospinal fluid leaks are the most frequent intraoperative complication with 0.40% incidence in all patients. The risk of device-related complications is higher in pediatric patients [2].

There is no proof of age effect on the risk of complications, CI surgery seems to be safe at the extreme ends of life [2].

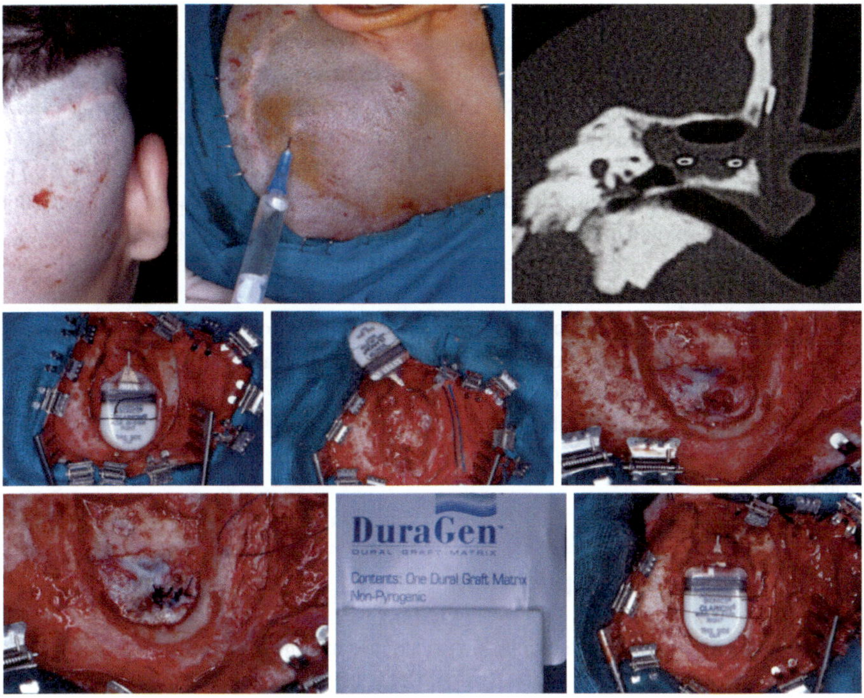


**Fig. 20.1** Cerebrospinal fluid leak as a result of having damaged the Dura during surgery. The difference between a hematoma, purulent collection, or CSF is in the aspiration of the liquid and screening its content

## 20.4 Epidemiology

Frequency of CI revision surgeries from recent studies varies from 5.0% to 8.3% [3, 5–8]. Children because of growing skull size which could lead to electrode or device migration, increased incidence of otitis media, and greater susceptibility to head injuries, more often require revision surgery [6].

## 20.5 Indications for CI Revision Surgery

Indications for revision surgery can be divided into: hard device failure, soft device failure, wound complications, magnet, or device migration [7]. Hard device failure is defined by lack of receiving useful auditory stimuli from their CI in patients associated with failed device integrity testing. Soft failures, according to soft failure consensus statement published in 2005 [9], are conditions in which suspicion of device malfunction could not be proven using currently available in vivo integrity testing. In case of soft failures, the patient could present auditory symptoms (buzzing, roaring, static, popping), nonauditory symptoms (dizziness, pain, shocking, burning, facial stimulation), or poor audiometric performance. Wound complications include: wound dehiscence, abscess formation, device extrusion (partial or complete), persistent foreign body reaction, or cutaneous fistula formation [7]. Another useful classification divides revision CI surgery into device- and patient-related. Device-related includes: hard device failure and soft device failure, allergies, persistent foreign body reaction, patient-related: wound infections and cholesteatoma [6].

CI revision surgeries can be divided into four categories: (1) reimplantation, (2) minor revision surgeries, (3) explantation without reimplantation, and (4) electrode array insertion. In the minor revision surgeries category we can include: procedures performed on the wound or the existing implant, including receiver-stimulator reposition, skin flap revision, change of magnet, magnet reinsertion, and aeroseal operation [3].

## 20.6 Infectious Complications

Infectious complications associated with cochlear implantation are followed by meningitis, petrositis, mastoiditis (Fig. 20.2), prosthetic inflammation/infection, labyrinthitis, post-auricular fistula, scalp cellulitis, or site-specific wound complications plus a *Staphylococcus* or general incision and drainage. The incidence rate of infections after cochlear implantation varies from 1.4% to 8.2%. Children aged 1 and 2 years are susceptible to infectious complications. Skin flap infection is the most common cause of device extrusion after CI surgery.

Prosthetic inflammation/infection is the most common infectious complication. The most common detected isolates, associated with flap infection, are *Staphylococcus aureus* and *Pseudomonas aeruginosa*. Infection of *Pseudomonas aeruginosa* with its ability for causing biofilm reaction, requires reimplantation because of colonization around the implant.

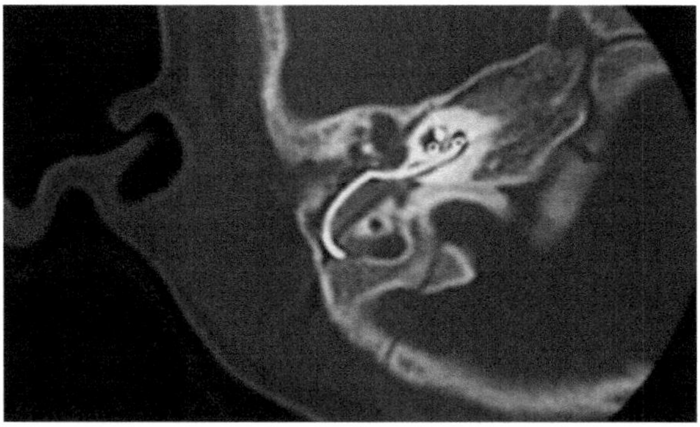

**Fig. 20.2** Acute mastoiditis in a case with CI. The existence of an infection in the middle ear can be complicated by acute meningitis

## 20.7 Flap Necrosis

Flap necrosis seems to be associated with size of skin incision. Lover incidence of flap necrosis was observed in cases of minimal retro auricular incision [10]. While performing the flap incision, it is also necessary to follow the course of the vascular pattern of the skin. An anteriorly based C-shaped flap for cochlear implantation can cut the blood supply from the occipital artery, causing flap-related complications. Therefore, an inferiorly based U-shaped flap is often recommended. Thinning of musculocutaneous flap should be avoided. Another cause of CI extrusion can be incision made parallel and too close to the implant edge.

Intravenous antibiotic therapy is strongly recommended in cases when the tissue surrounding the device becomes infected or the device is exposed. Flap necrosis can also occur due to foreign body reactions to the suture or excessive magnet pressure on the skin (Fig. 20.3).

Initial treatment of CI extrusion should include: antimicrobial and anti-inflammatory therapy, debridement of the wound, and elimination of the infected tissue. Failure of the initial treatment obliges performance reconstruction of the skin flap alone or with adjuvant hyperbaric oxygen therapy (HBOT). Introduction of HBOT in cases of wound infection/necrosis increases effectiveness of treatment [4]. HBOT with repeated pressure changes up to 6 atm abs is safe for implant components [11].

Surgical possibilities for treatment of CI extrusion are following: post-auricular pedicle skin flap, scalp rotational flaps, pericranial flaps, microvascular free flaps

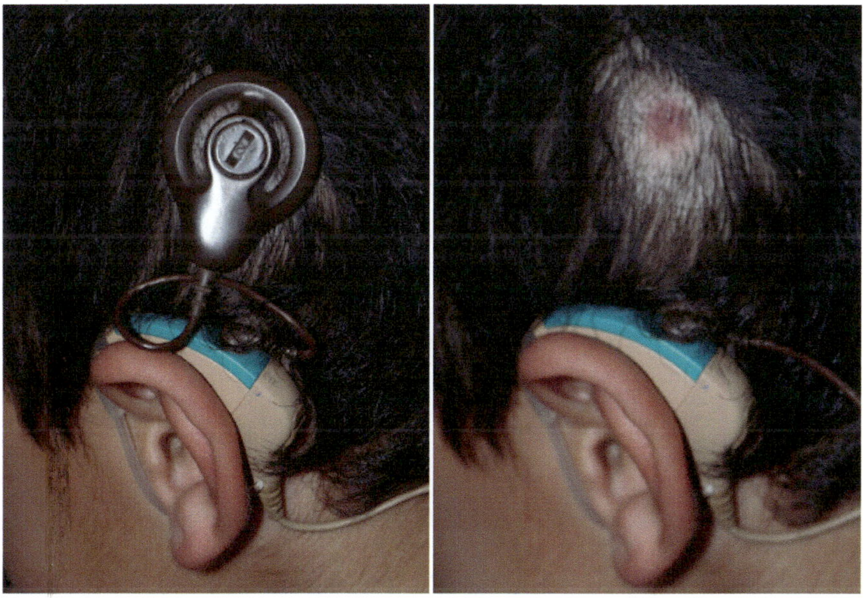

**Fig. 20.3** Skin flap lesion by a magnet

(e.g., Fasciocutaneous anterolateral thigh flap), and a pedicle temporalis muscle flap. Key to CI success is covered with healthy and vascularized tissue [4].

## 20.8 Flaps Technique

The Temporoparietal Fascia Flap (TPFF) technique is a simple procedure with limited morbidity. It consists of creating two well-vascularized pedicles that will join in the midline, once the damaged skin area has been removed.

The anterior flap is obtained through a preauricular incision that extends up the skull. Its vascularization is guaranteed by the superficial temporal artery. The posterior flap is obtained by anterior rotation until it joins in the midline. Its vascularization is guaranteed by the posterior occipital artery.

Both flaps include dermis, muscle, fascia, and subcutaneous fat. The results are satisfactory when the surgeon is experienced and knowledgeable about vascularization and reconstructive plastic surgery (Figs. 20.4, 20.5, 20.6, 20.7, and 20.8).

In Clarós Clinic, all patients were operated with a standardized procedure. CI skin incisions were inferiorly based inverted U-shaped. The skin flap with subcutaneous tissue covered the implant with margins of at least 1 cm. Thinning of the flap was avoided. Beneath the flap, the bone was exposed and drilled to create a 2–3 mm deep pocket in which the CI receiver/stimulator (R/S) was precisely placed [12]. To improve the device stability, two small bony canals were created for passage of nonresorbable tiedown sutures or titanium plates with screws (Fig. 20.9).

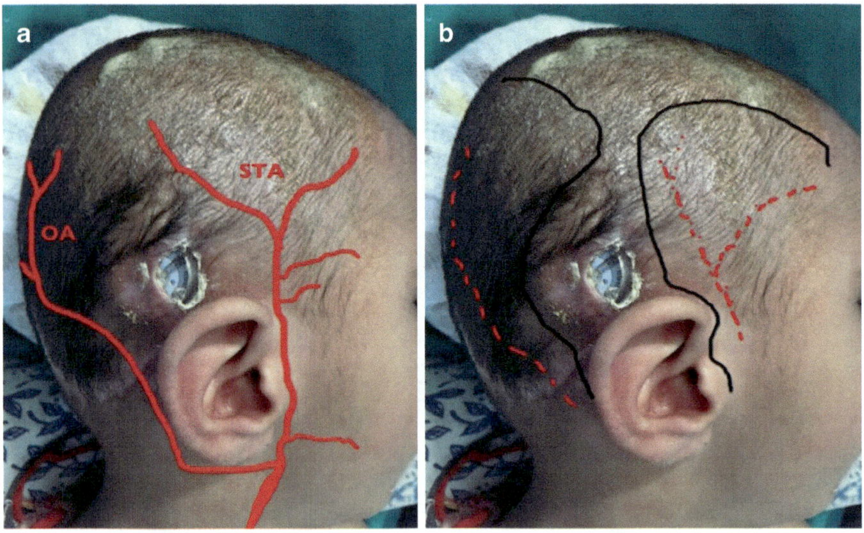


**Fig. 20.4** (**a**) In red, tracing of the facial arteries: Superficial temporal artery (STA) and posterior occipital artery (OA). (**b**) In black, tracing the skin incisions

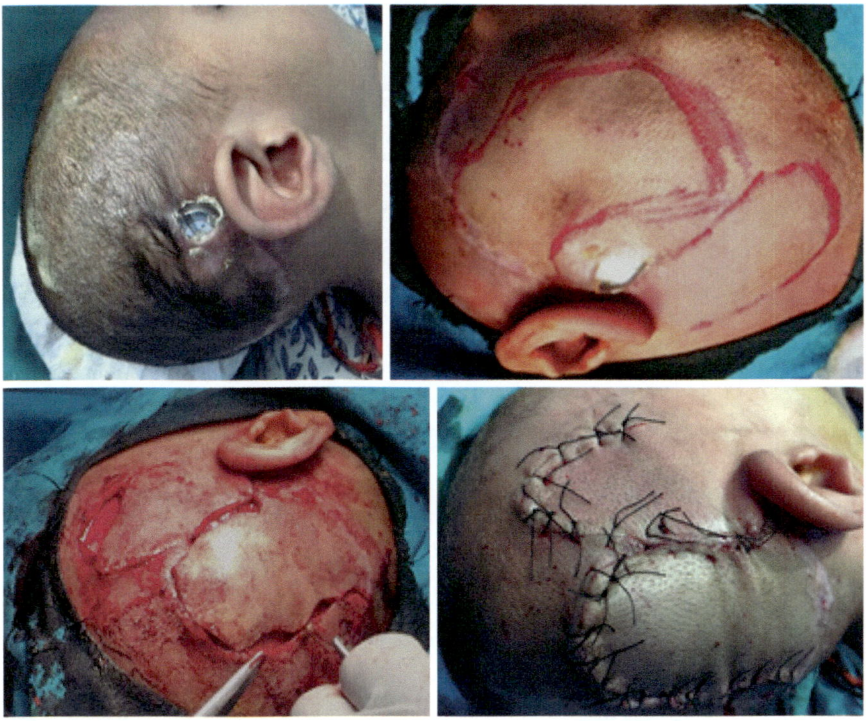

**Fig. 20.5** Double rotation skin flaps technique for wound closure

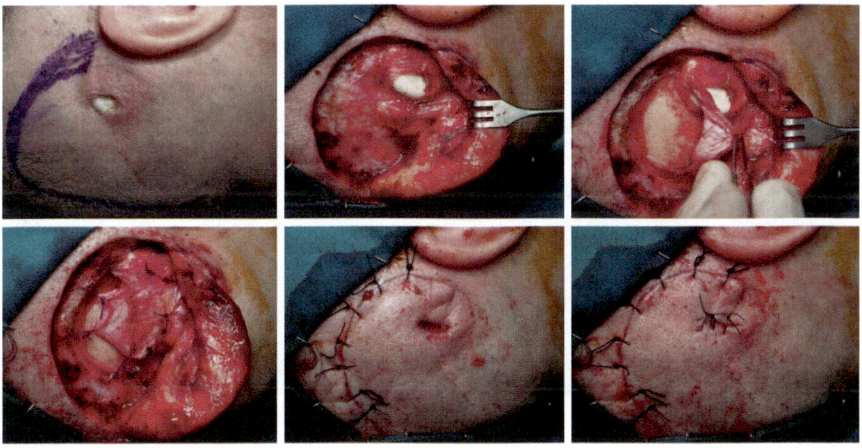

**Fig. 20.6** Advancing Rotating flap technique with temporoparietal subcutaneous periostium covering the stimulator/receiver

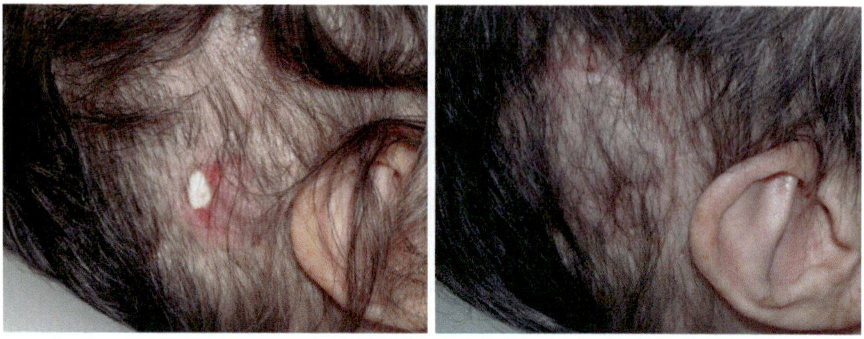

**Fig. 20.7** CI Extrusion preop and final results

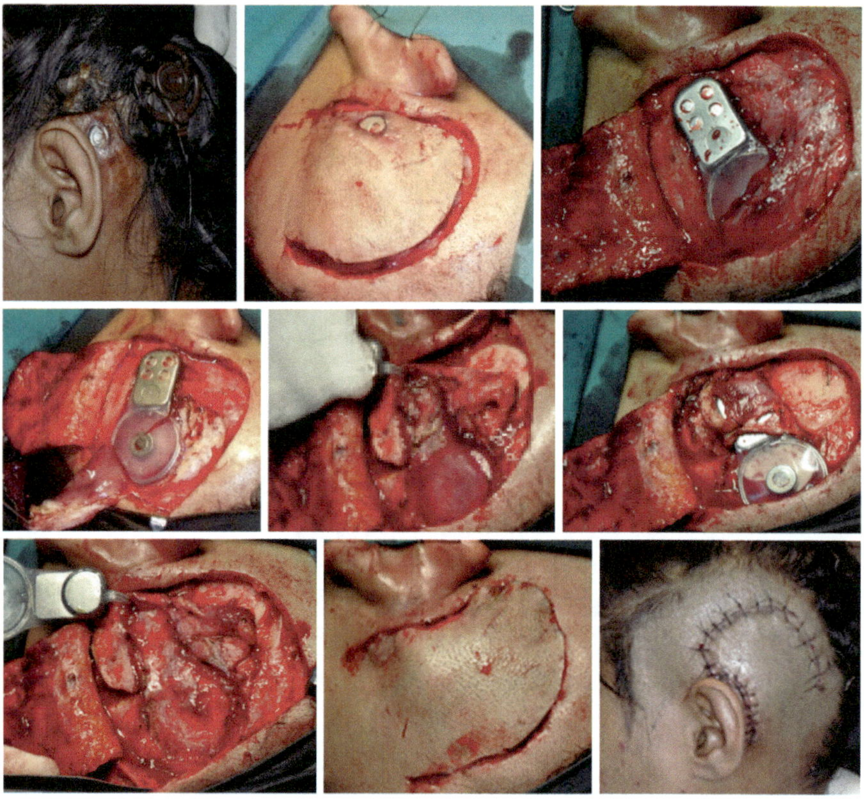

**Fig. 20.8** Extrusion of CI. Surgical Technique with *témporo-parietal* flap with removal of granulation tissue around, covering with fascia and advancing displacement of the skin, and preserving the same stimulator device

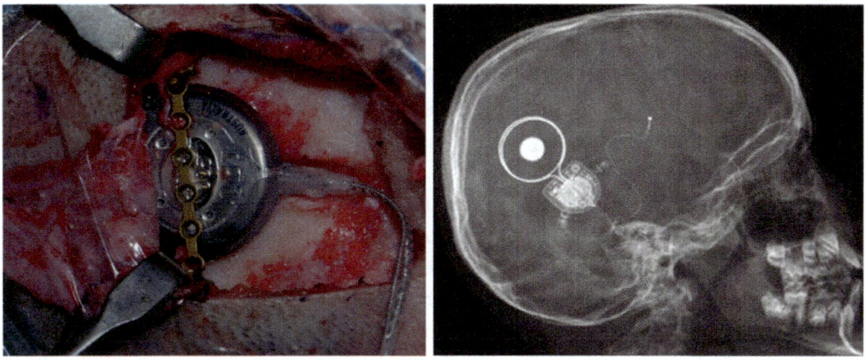

**Fig. 20.9** Titanium plates and screws to fix the CI receiver/stimulator. X-ray control

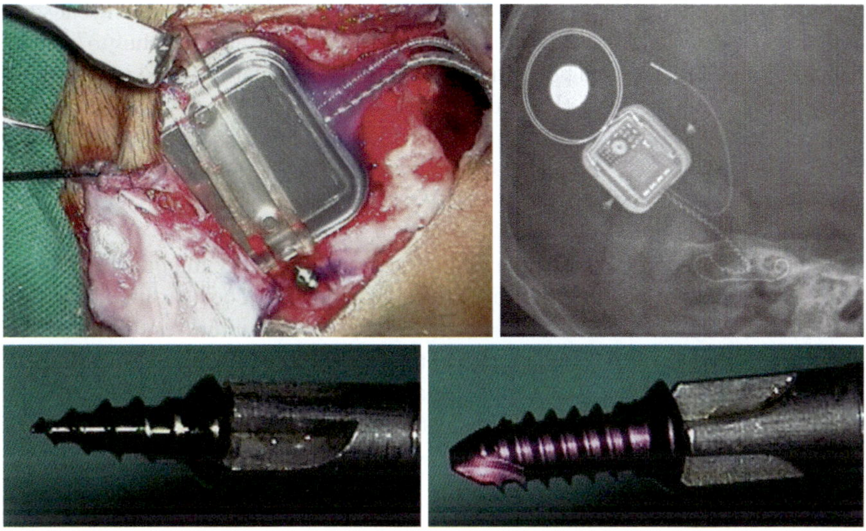

**Fig. 20.10** Lactosorb mini-plates fixation system and two 5 mm titanium screws. X-ray control does not find any devise displacement

Until October 2007, we used a fixation system with 1.2 mm pure titanium mini-plates and two titanium screws self-tapping and retaining. Since January 2009 we began using a new system, LactoSorb (82% poly-L-lactic acid-18% polyglycolic acid copolymer), the only clinically proven material that completely resorbs within 1 year. This technique is widely applicable, cost-effective, low time-consuming, and not associated with increased complications. This system allows a stable fixation with total resorption of the plate after 1 year. No complications have been observed. Secure fixation was successfully obtained in all cases (Fig. 20.10).

## 20.9 Pressure Injuries

National Pressure Ulcer Advisory Panel (NPAUP) proposed a pressure injury staging system (stage 1–4) for describing the severity of skin flaps reactions in the area of the external antenna.

Stage 1 is associated with erythema, slight irritation and requires stopping wearing the device for a brief period or to use a coil spacer. In stage 2, skin breakdown, redness and swelling are present, topical and oral antibiotics for at least 7–10 days should be recommended. Stage 4 with full-thickness skin loss requires topical and oral antibiotics for 7–10 days and stop wearing the external device for 2 weeks. In stage 4 we can observe exposed bone, muscle, or implant, and infection. In this stage, parenteral intravenous antibiotics for 7–10 days are required, as well as surgical intervention, or removal of the device. Most of those skin reactions are located at the central part of the antenna [13].

Significantly higher incidence of pressure injuries occurs in patients at age 7 years and younger (Fig. 20.11). According to Hsieh et al. [13] study, 7.0% of patients with CI suffer from pressure injuries. This complication could occur even a few years after surgery [13] (Fig. 20.12).

## 20.10 Allergy to Silicone

The silicone cover of CI can cause allergic reactions. Allergy to silicone is a rare cause of cochlear implant extrusion. Patients experiencing cochlear implant extrusion, particularly with a delayed onset and negative wound culture results, should be tested for silicone allergy. Comorbid infection cannot be excluded, so in each case, swab sampling from the wound should be taken. With a positive test result of allergy to silicone and negative culture, explantation of CI is necessary with subsequent reimplantation of custom-made cochlear implant without an allergenic silicone component.

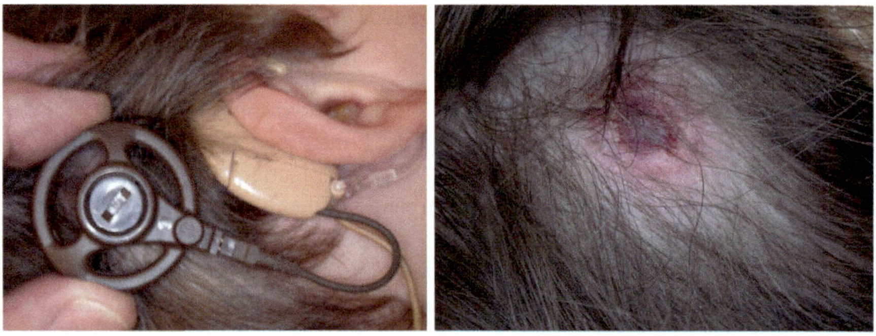

**Fig. 20.11** Pressure injuries are located at the central part of the antenna. It is a minor complication. With the non-use of the antenna, for 2 weeks it is usually resolved spontaneously

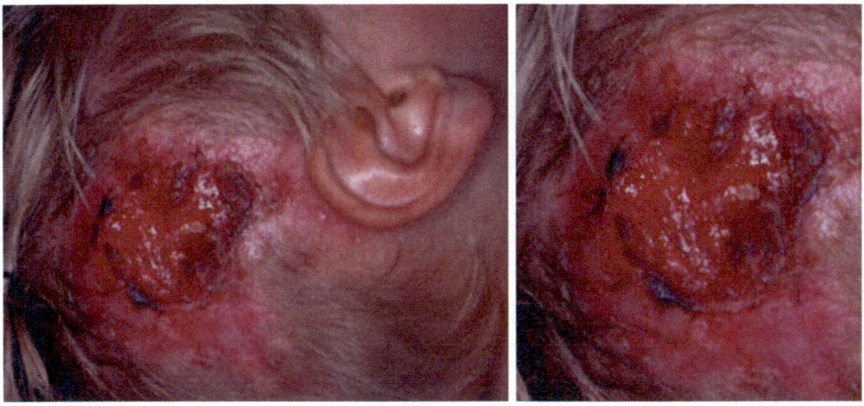

**Fig. 20.12** Magnet excessive pressure flap infection. It is a major complication few years after surgery because a flap will probably be needed to close it

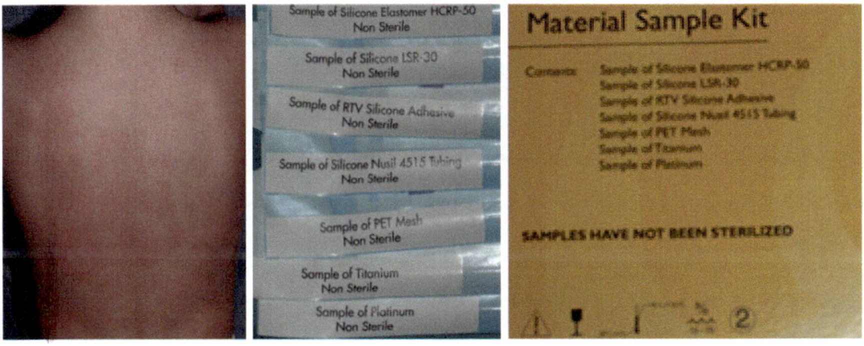


**Fig. 20.13** Kit to perform the silicone allergy test from the Cochlear Company

Diagnostic criteria of an allergy or a foreign body reaction can be reached when conditions such as chronic pain without fluctuation of the implant, negative laboratory culture, and positive test for allergy to silicone, are met (Fig. 20.13).

The only solution is to preserve the implant with a conservative technique where all the granulation tissue around the stimulator is removed and to make several injections with triamcinolone®. In case of failure, reimplantation with a new implant without silicone is mandatory (Figs. 20.14, 20.15, and 20.16). All CI-associated companies can provide a custom-made device. The intolerance of a cochlear implant can be caused by an allergic reaction or a reaction to a foreign body and with an appropriate technique; we can save the cochlear implant [14].

Uneventful wound healing and long-term extrusion-free follow-up, after the reimplantation with a custom-made cochlear implant, clinically prove the diagnosis.

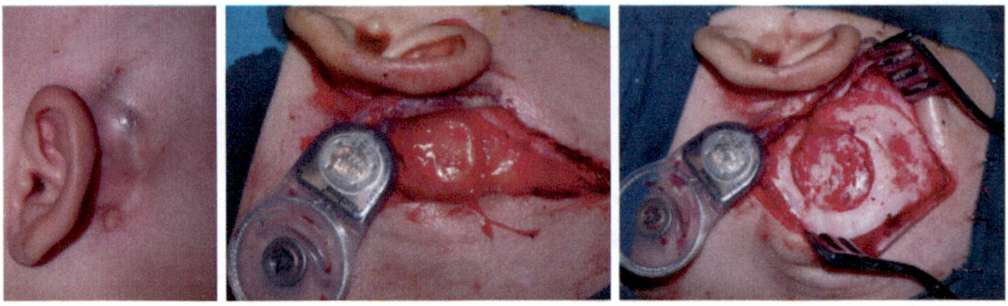

**Fig. 20.14** Case of reaction to CI. Surgical revision

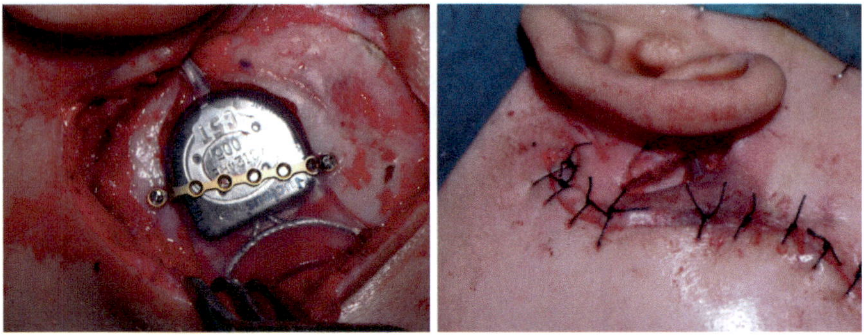

**Fig. 20.15** After all the inflammatory tissue is removed, triamcinolone is injected and the implant is fixed with a small titanium plate with two screws

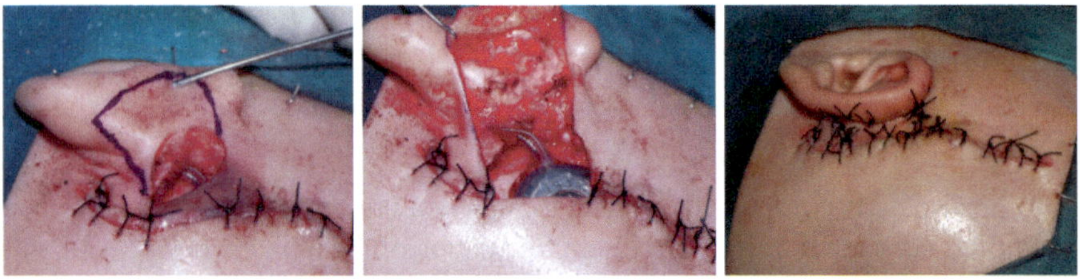

**Fig. 20.16** Cutaneous suture using a cutaneous flap of the external ear to be able to interpose the cartilage between the stimulator and the skin

## 20.11 Malposition of Electrode Array

Scala tympani is an appropriate place for electrode insertion during CI implantation. Malposition of electrode array is possible due to misplacement during surgery, migration (extrusion) out of the cochlea, or erosion through the rock-hard wall of the cochlea. The incidence of electrode misplacement during surgery is about 0.5% in cases of normal ear anatomy [15]. To avoid electrode migration, special attention should be paid to the reliable fixation of the electrode array during CI surgery.

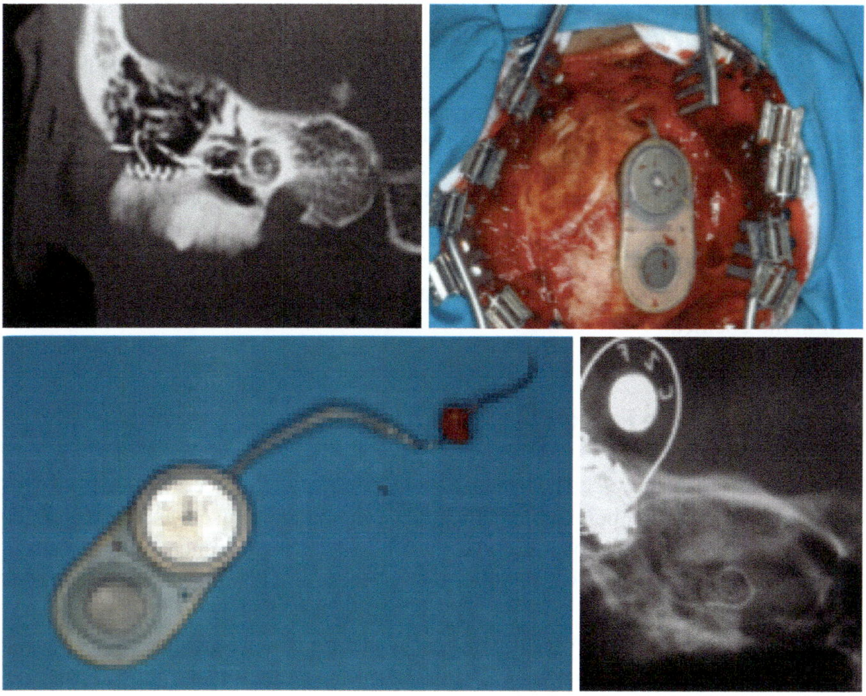

**Fig. 20.17** Electrode placed in the hypotympanum. X-ray of its repositioning in the cochlea

The possible locations of extra-cochlear electrode arrays are Eustachian tube, facial recess, vestibule, petrous apex, internal auditory canal, Hyrtl's fissure (i.e., incomplete ossification of the tympano-meningeal fissure), superior and horizontal semicircular canals, carotid canal, and hypotympanum (Fig. 20.17). Dietz et al. [16] proposed criteria for evidence of array migration: increase of the impedances and/or nonauditory percept in the basal channels. Migration of an electrode array can be caused by head injury or head growth in children. In case of total migration, reimplantation is necessary; partial migration could require only reprogramming of the device.

To avoid electrode migration, special attention should be paid to the reliable fixation of the electrode array during CI surgery. It is recommended to do an X-ray of the skull before the end of anesthesia after cochlear implantation. It can ensure the surgeon on the correct position of the CI. In some cases, CI extrusion can occur despite complete insertion of the entire electrode into cochlea, during the closing maneuvers of the incision.

Electrode migration does not always require revision surgery. If a decline of speech intelligibility is not present, only deactivation of some single channels is possible. In case of high impedance or nonauditory perception of the basal electrodes it would be enough to remove them from the stimulation map [16].

The most preferable radiological examination for imaging of the postoperative electrode placement is cone-beam computed tomography (CBCT). This procedure is extremely safe for the patients because it is possible to perform with low-dose radiation exposure. By using the CBCT technique, it is possible to achieve adequate image quality with minimal electrode artifact. Electrode position could be checked with respect to insertion depth and the insertion angle.

Another possible cause of incorrect electrode array placement is placing the electrode in an infra-cochlear air cell, mistaking it for the round window. It can occur even in experienced hands, if there is a fibrous or bony obliteration of the round window niche. In these cases, the only possibility is to reposition the implant within the cochlea.

## 20.12 Electrode Forced into Insertion

Sometimes, when the electrode matrix is inserted into the cochlea, an excess of force applied on it can be exerted, causing it to compact on itself and therefore the different electrodes come together producing electrical interferences. It can occur in cases where the cochlea is very narrow or with some ossification of the *Scala tympani* (Fig. 20.18).

In these cases, it is necessary to remove the electrode and reposition it again. The electrode should be checked; in case of damage, a new device should be used.

## 20.13 Tip Roll Over

The bent tip of the electrode can occur during insertion, especially in some brands of CIs with a soft matrix, causing the electrode to bend back on itself. This anomaly can be detected both radiographically and in the verification of intraoperative electrical measurements. It produces a dispersion of neuronal excitation around each electrode. The tip fold can be identified by an electrophysiological test that includes

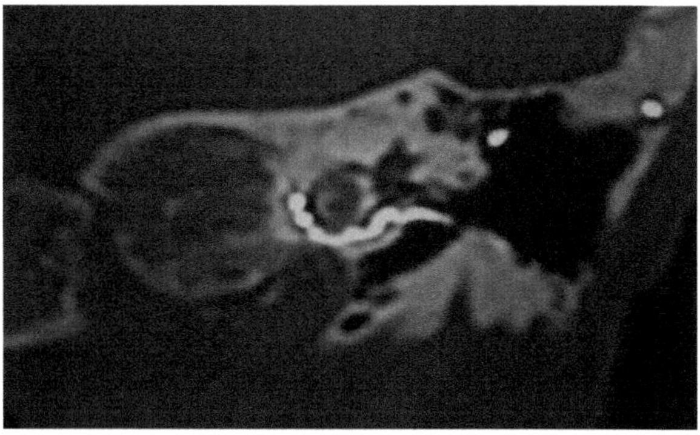

**Fig. 20.18** Electrode forced or compressed inside the cochlea. It occurs when the insertion force of the electrode is excessive. It causes interference in the process of the cochlea stimulation. Following, it is mandatory to remove it and if possible to reposition again or place a new one

excitation propagation, spread of excitation (SOE) or electric field imaging (EFI) (Fig. 20.19).

Once the malposition of the electrode is detected, it must be removed, straightened, and repositioned on the cochlea [17]. Deactivation of the involved electrodes can improve performance, possibly avoiding revision surgery.

## 20.14 Array Fibrosis

Fibrosis around the electrode holder is not frequent although possible. When this happens, there is a decrease in speech performance and perception, with the frequent need for reprogramming. Typical clinical signs are indicative of changes in device performance with increased electrode impedances.

CI explantation shows the existence of this fibrous tissue around the electrode and can be interpreted as a foreign body reaction or intolerance to CI materials. Before proceeding with reimplantation, we recommend administering local steroids into the cochlea as well as changing the implant brand (Fig. 20.20).

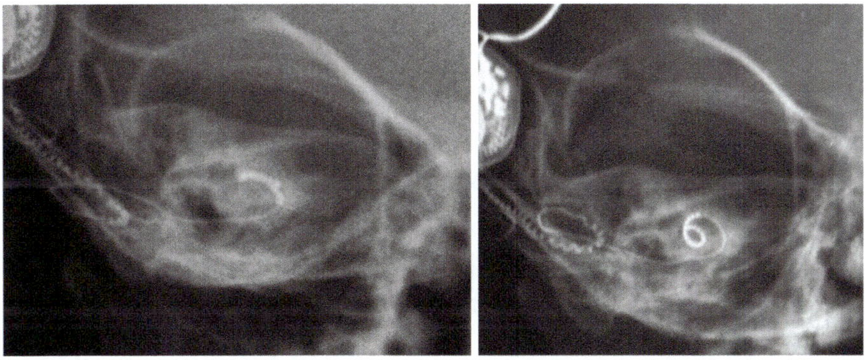

**Fig. 20.19** Electrode bent at its tip. Removal of the electrode and its repositioning in good condition

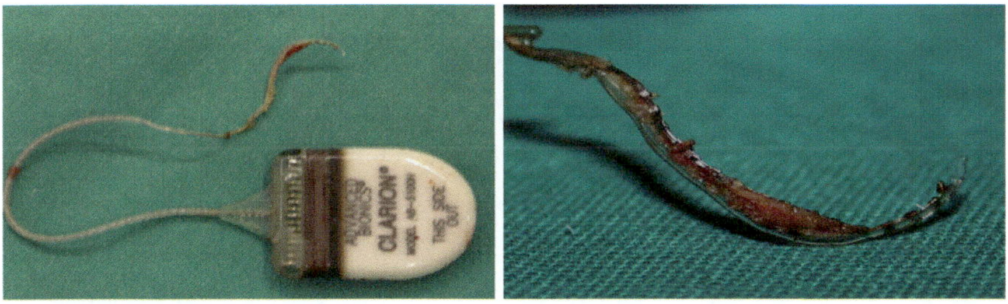


**Fig. 20.20** Clarion implant explanted with fibrous tissue in the electrode array that hinders the transmission of the electrical stimulus

## 20.15 Vestibular Insertion of the Electrode

It is possible that at the time of implantation the electrode can be inserted into the vestibular system, in either the superior or the lateral semicircular canal. In this position, vestibular symptoms, such as nystagmus and vertigo, are associated with nonauditory response, which will lead to suspect a wrong placement of the electrode array (Figs. 20.21 and 20.22) [18, 19].

## 20.16 Dislocation of Electrodes from Scala Tympani to Scala Vestibuli

The location of the electrode in the *Scala vestibuli* after a CI has low incidence, but we can estimate between 8% and 10% based on our experience. In these cases, the electrode array penetrates the basal membrane within 45° of the insertion of the electrode when inserted through the round window and dislocated in the first 45° segment when it was through a cochleostomy. The final placement of the electrode array can be evaluated using multiplanar reconstructed cone-beam CT images (Fig. 20.23).

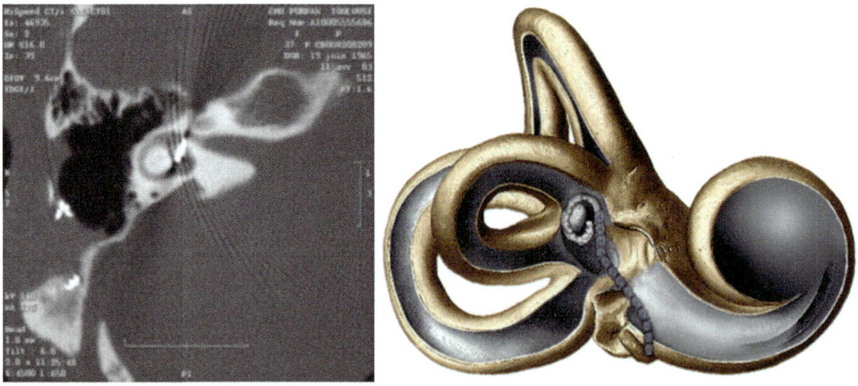

**Fig. 20.21** Electrode located in the vestibule and superior semicircular canal

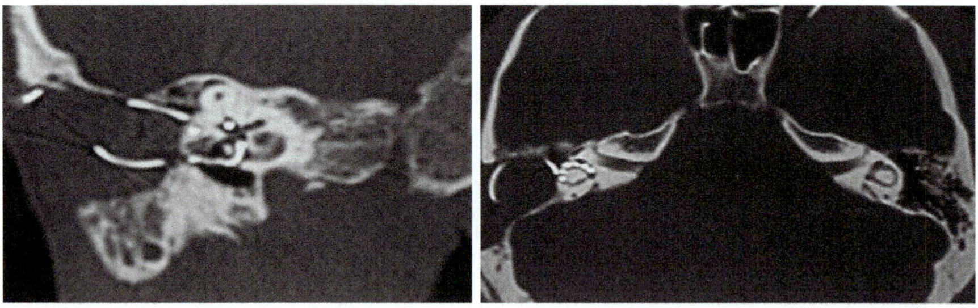

**Fig. 20.22** Electrode array located in the horizontal semicircular canal

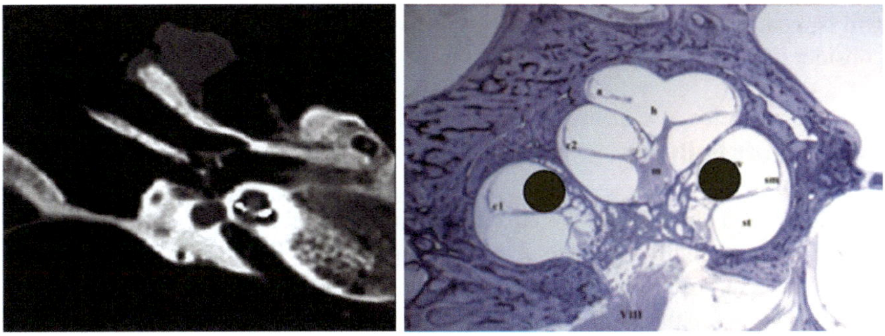

**Fig. 20.23** Insertion of the electrode in the *Scala Vestibuli*

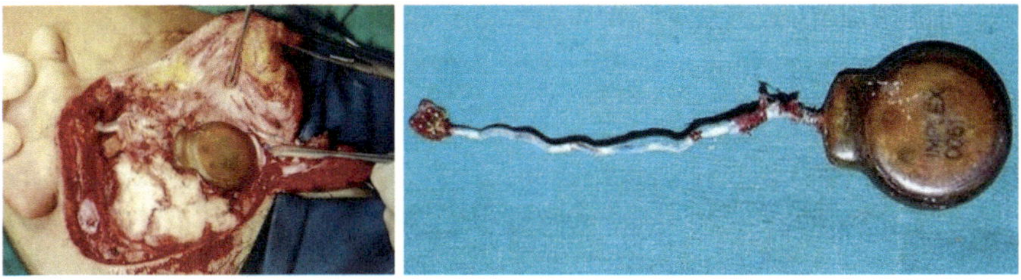


**Fig. 20.24** Hortmann Implex Cochlear Implant explantation. From Dr. DeDaSousa collection Mumbai, India

In these cases of Scala dislocation, although there are no hearing differences, it may require an increase in the necessary stimulus load and the load units of the maximum comfortable loudness level tend to increase with time [20].

This wrong anatomical position is explained in some cases by direct communication between the basal turn and the vestibule, as can occur in Mondini's malformation, in which there is an absence of ossification of the spiral lamina or opening of the vestibule during surgery.

## 20.17 Device Update

Another indication of explantation is to substitute the device for more modern equipment, option for those patients who are using some of the old technologies, such as Hortmann Implex (Fig. 20.24) or the House/3M mono-channel implants or some other brand with few hearing gains. The results in postlingual were superior with multi electrode implants and there was no significant difference between SPEAK, ACE, CIS, and SAS strategy users [21].

Although theoretically it represents a good change, it must be considered that a new replacement surgery may carry a risk of damaging the surviving auditory nerve [22]. It is a fact that we do not have the means to accurately predict the benefits that will be achieved in the postoperative period with the new technology, but we must consider it as a possibility of updating the system.

## 20.18 Soft Failures

Soft failure is a condition in which a device malfunction is suspected but cannot be proven using currently available in vivo testing methods [9]. In case of soft failures, the patient could present auditory symptoms (buzzing, roaring, static, popping), nonauditory symptoms (dizziness, pain, shocking, burning, facial stimulation), or poor audiometric performance. Soft failures are significantly more frequent in the population of adult CI patients [5].

According to the year 2005 consensus statement on soft failures, they are put in working diagnosis for cases with poor post-implant audiological performance or subjective adverse symptoms, like those mentioned before, with correct device integrity testing and normal radiographic studies. Approximately 30% or CI revision surgeries are due to soft failures [5].

Alleviation of symptoms after reimplantation with a new device supports the diagnosis of soft failure [9]. Soft failures can produce diagnostic difficulties in children, which is certainly easier to diagnose those in a cooperative, insightful adult.

## 20.19 Facial Nerve Stimulation

The facial nerve in patients with HF can be electrically stimulated with an incidence ranging from 1% to 15% [23]. The reason for this stimulation is possible electrical leakage from the electrode that can reach the proximity of the facial nerve, especially after extensive reaming of the mastoid bone and when high current intensities are applied to stimulate the auditory nerve.

Electrical discharges from the IC electrodes on the facial nerve cause facial spasms that can be mild to very extreme, preventing use of the implant. What should be first to change the stimulation strategies to effectively control the action on the facial nerve. With this procedure, it is possible to control this uncomfortable sequel of IC use (Fig. 20.25, Video 20.1).

## 20.20 Hard Failures

Hard device failure is defined by lack of receiving useful auditory stimuli from their CI in patients associated with failed device integrity testing. It is the most common indication for CI revision surgery. More than a half of CI revision surgeries are due to hard failure. Improvement could be achieved in more than 80% of reoperated patients [6].

Ceramic implants break more easily. The electronics can be damaged for other reasons, such as a failure of its components or the loss of tightness. Head injuries,

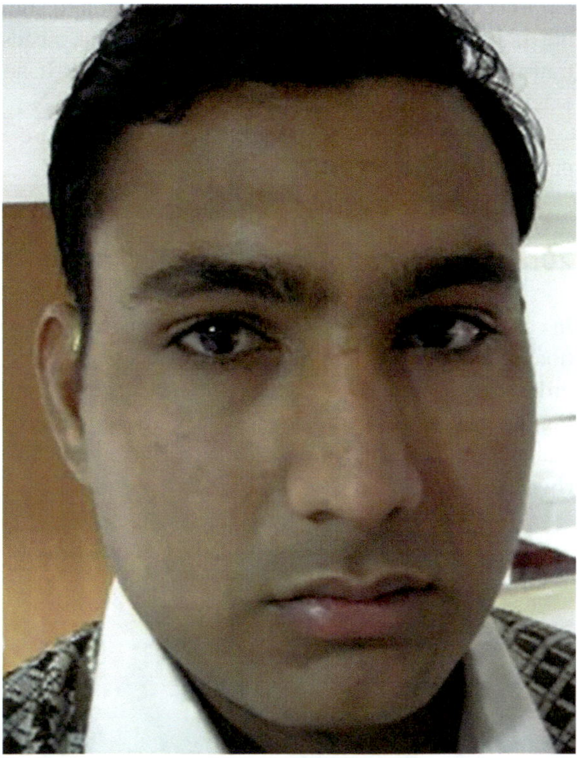

**Fig. 20.25** Facial nerve stimulation video. Click on the Video 20.1

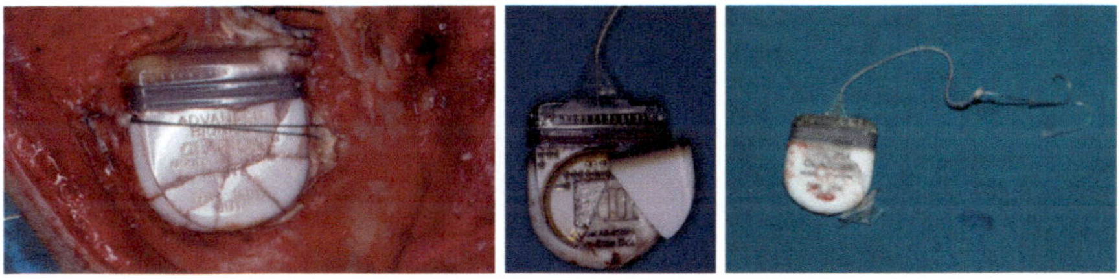

**Fig. 20.26** Explantation due to fracture of the ceramic capsule

whether due to traffic accidents or falls, cause damage to the stimulator/receiver, so the electronics inside can be damaged. In this case, a surgical exploration with or without explantation and/or reimplantation will be required (Fig. 20.26).

Once the interruption of electronics has been detected, the integrity tests must be carried out and proceed to the explantation and immediate reimplantation. The time it takes will be detrimental to the user of a CI.

The detection of failure is made by the following concepts: patient suddenly stopped responding to sound, showed some response to sound for a short period then stopped responding to sound, reports permanent or intermittent sound/speech quality deterioration, reports intermittent noise, reports noise only when switching on processor or patient shows aversive reaction to stimulation. To detect the possible failure, the speech processor, microphone, headset cable, transmitter cable, transmitter coil, and batteries must be checked. If necessary, all elements of the external equipment should be changed.

Next, we will proceed to verify that the software is correct and review all the parameters and strategies.

## 20.21 Explantation

In cases where the skin infection or the skin is completely destroyed, only one solution exists, explantation. Likewise, in cases where previous flaps have been done, in order to try to save the stimulator without success. In these cases, proceed by removing the body of the stimulator, but leaving the intracochlear part so that when reimplantation is necessary, the cochlea is permeable and this maneuver can be performed (Fig. 20.27).

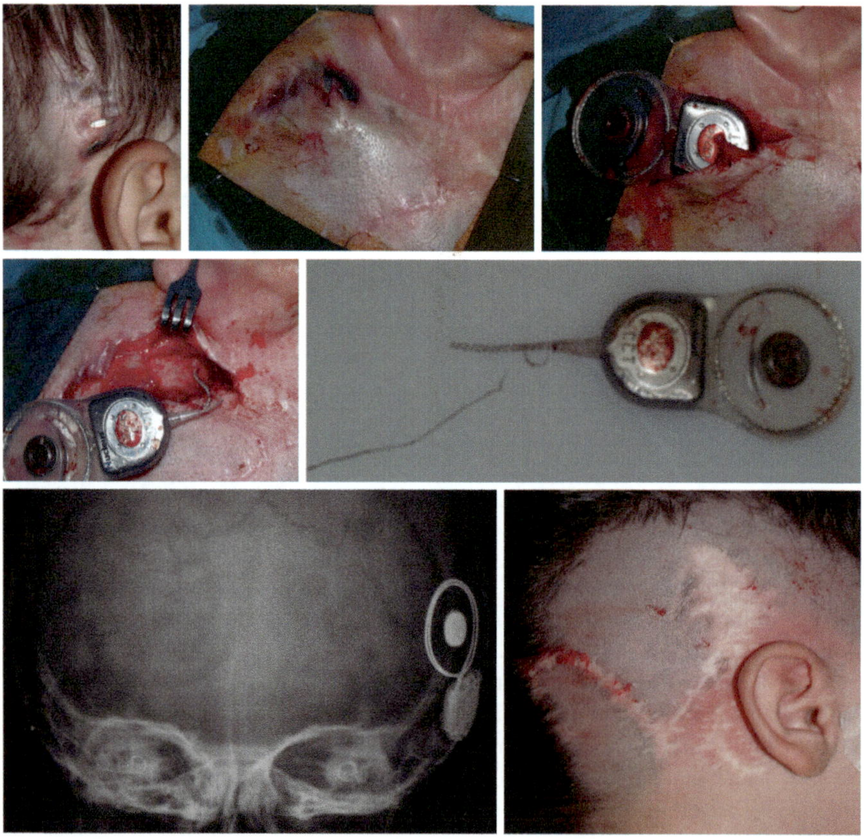

**Fig. 20.27** Explantation is the last measure to take into account. First, you have to try to save the implant, although in certain cases it is impossible and the only solution is to remove the stimulator

The need to do a CI explantation is evident when the implant is not working properly or when there are intermittent failures that affect the use of it, or there is a skin infection that has pierced the skin. Early recognition of complications from surgeries is critical. The effectiveness of CIs in deep deafness in both children and adults is demonstrated, but these devices are subject to breakdowns, damage, failures, and the need for upgrade. Another consideration we have to make is with regard to revision surgery in which, under different circumstances, it is necessary to have a direct view of the problem existing in the CI. Both in the first case and in the second case, the reimplantation should be performed by an experienced surgeon.

## 20.22 Conclusions

The number of reimplantation increases over time. We should remember that every patient with a cochlear implant is a potential candidate for cochlear reimplantation, especially in children. With development of new technologies more patients would decide to change their old CI for a modern one. There is no evidence that reimplantation leads to increasing number of medical complications or hearing impairment. The cochlear implant failure rates vary between children and adults as well as between different implant manufacturers. However, well-planned cochlear reimplantation is a safe procedure with excellent and predictable results in audiological performance.

The majority of reimplanted patients have comparable or better results than in their first implantation. Hard failures are most common indication for CI revision surgery and also tended to have the best outcomes following the reoperation. On the other hand, soft failure group has the lowest rate of performance improvement after revision surgery.

The functional results of a CI obtained after a reimplantation are usually the same as after the first CI. This means that the prosthetic performance is not lost in 90% of the cases, even in certain cases it is better.

Children because of growing skull size (which can lead to electrode or device migration), increase the incidence of otitis media and greater susceptibility to head injuries more often require revision surgery. It is also very important to make an early diagnosis, especially in children. Their auditory and speech performance would lag if reimplantation were delayed.

Careful analysis of HRCT temporal bone before CI implantation helps to better understand the patient's anatomy and allows limiting possible complications, which can lead to necessity of revision surgery [6].

The Cochlear Implant Manufacturers respond with improvements after analyzing each case. All involved companies are always supporting us in our failure cases. Reimplantation may be also an opportunity to update the patient's electronic system (Videos 20.2 and 20.3).

## References


1. Mudry A, Mills M. The early history of the cochlear implant: a retrospective. Otolaryngol Head Neck Surg. 2013;139(5):446–53. https://doi.org/10.1001/jamaoto.2013.293.
2. Parent V, Codet M, Aubry K, Bordure P, Bozorg-Grayeli A, Deguine A, et al. The French Cochlear Implant Registry (EPIIC): Cochlear implantation complications. Eur Ann Otorhinolaryngol Head Neck Dis. 2020;137(Suppl 1):S37–43. https://doi.org/10.1016/j.anorl.2020.07.007.
3. Wang JT, Wang AY, Psarros C, Da Cruz M. Rates of revision and device failure in cochlear implant surgery: a 30-year experience. Laryngoscope. 2014;124(10):2393–9. https://doi.org/10.1002/lary.24649.
4. Clarós P, Końska N, Clarós-Pujol A, Pujol C, Clarós A. Hyperbaric oxygen therapy as a therapeutic option in cochlear implants extrusion treatment in infected wounds. Acta Otolaryngol. 2020;140(7):544–7. https://doi.org/10.1080/00016489.2020.1744721.
5. Kimura KS, O'Connell BP, Nassiri AM, Dedmon MM, Haynes DS, Bennett ML. Outcomes of revision Cochlear implantation. Otol Neurotol. 2020;41(6):e705–11. https://doi.org/10.1097/MAO.0000000000002659.
6. Rayamajhi P, Kurkure R, Castellino A, Kumar S, Nandhan R, Kameswaran M. A clinical profile of revision cochlear implant surgery: MERF experience. Cochlear Implants Int. 2020;29:1–7. https://doi.org/10.1080/14670100.2020.1823128.
7. Stevens SM, Dougherty H, Wenstrup L, Hammer T, Cole T, Redmann A, Pensak ML, Samy RN. Is hard failure still a common indication for revision surgery in adult Cochlear implant recipients? Otol Neurotol. 2019;40(3):321–7. https://doi.org/10.1097/MAO.0000000000002118.
8. Wijaya C, Simões-Franklin C, Glynn F, Walshe P, Reilly R, Viani L. Revision cochlear implantation: the Irish experience. Cochlear Implants Int. 2019;20(6):281–7. https://doi.org/10.1080/14670100.2019.1647372.
9. Balkany TJ, Hodges AV, Buchman CA, Luxford WM, Pillsbury CH, Roland PS, Shallop JK, Backous DD, Franz D, Graham JM, Hirsch B, Luntz M, Niparko JK, Patrick J, Payne SL, Telischi FF, Tobey EA, Truy E, Staller S. Cochlear implant soft failures consensus development conference statement. Otol Neurotol. 2005;26(4):815–8. https://doi.org/10.1097/01.mao.0000178150.44505.52.
10. Dağkıran M, Tarkan Ö, Sürmelioğlu Ö, Özdemir S, Onan E, Tuncer Ü, Bayraktar S, Kıroğlu M. Management of Complications in 1452 pediatric and adult Cochlear implantations. Turk Arch Otorhinolaryngol. 2020;58(1):16–23. https://doi.org/10.5152/tao.2020.5025.
11. Backous D, Dunford RG, Segel P, Muhlocker MC, Carter P, Hampson NB. Effects of hyperbaric exposure on the integrity of the internal components of commercially available cochlear implant systems. Otol Neurotol. 2002;23(4):463–7.
12. Clarós P, Valor C. Two new systems in Cochlear implants: titanium and resorbable mini-plates. Cochlear Implants Int. 2010;11(1):176–80.
13. Hsieh HS, Lee CY, Wu HP, Zhuo MY, Hwang CF. Pressure ulcers and skin infections after cochlear implantation: a delayed yet serious issue. Int J Pediatr Otorhinolaryngol. 2020;138:110241.
14. Clarós P, Clavería MA, Pujol C, Suñol M, Cardesa A. Allergy or foreign body reaction in cochlear implant. How to save the implant. Int J Pediatr Otorhinolaryngol. 2011;75(S1):1–9.
15. Wendell Todd N, Fainberg JC, Kadom N. Into and out of the cochlea: a reimplantation saga. Cochlear Implants Int. 2020;18:1–5. https://doi.org/10.1080/14670100.2020.1780771.
16. Dietz A, Wennström M, Lehtimäki A, Löppönen H, Valtonen H. Electrode migration after cochlear implant surgery: more common than expected? Eur Arch Otorhinolaryngol. 2016;273(6):1411–8.
17. Zuniga MG, Rivas A, Hedley-Williams A, Gifford R, Dwyer R, Dawant BM, Sunderhaus L, Hovis KL, Wanna GB, Noble JH, Labadie RF. Tip fold-over in cochlear implantation: case series. Otol Neurotol. 2017;38(2):199–206. https://doi.org/10.1097/MAO.0000000000001283.

18. Jain R, Mukherji SK. Cochlear implant failure imaging evaluation of the electrode course. Clin Radiol. 2003;58(4):288–93. https://doi.org/10.1016/s0009-9260(02)00523-8.
19. Woolford TJ, Saeed SR, Boyd P, Hartley C, Ramsden RT. Cochlear re implantation. Ann Otol Rhinol Laryngol Suppl. 1995;166:449–53.
20. Fischer N, Pinggera L, Weichbold V, Dejaco D, Schmutzhard J, Widmann G. Radiologic and functional evaluation of electrode dislocation from the scala tympani to the scala vestibuli in patients with cochlear implants. AJNR Am J Neuroradiol. 2015;36(2):372–7. https://doi.org/10.3174/ajnr.A4189.
21. DeSaSouza S, D'Sousa N, D'Sousa DJF. Recent advances in cochlear implant devices and techniques in India. Int Congr Ser. 2003;1240:365–8. https://doi.org/10.1016/S0531-5131(03)00805-7.
22. Gantz BJ, Lowder MW, McCabe BF. Audiologic results following reimplantation of cochlear implants. Ann Otol Rhinol Laryngol. 1989;98:12–6.
23. Burmeister J, Rathgeb S, Herzog J. Cochlear implantation in patients with otosclerosis of the otic capsule. Am J Otolaryngol. 2017;38:556–9.

# Surgical Complications Following Cochlear Implantation

21

Ryan-William Grech and Iain A. Bruce

## 21.1 Introduction

Cochlear implantation (CI) is well established as a treatment modality in congenital and acquired severe-to-profound sensorineural hearing loss (SNHL), which cannot be adequately managed using conventional hearing aids. In common with other operative procedures involving the temporal bone, the proximity of the surgical field to a number of neurovascular structures, and the small size of the operative area mean that complications are inevitable. Fortunately, training in CI surgery is of a standard that limits the occurrence of serious or life-changing complications, and our understanding of techniques to reduce the risk and manage complications continues to evolve. For the purposes of this chapter, we will concentrate on complications directly related to the process of inserting a CI, and will not discuss device-related complications (hard and soft failures). Likewise, it is important to differentiate complications from post-operative events that have particular relevance or consequence

**Supplementary Information** The online version contains supplementary material available at [https://doi.org/10.1007/978-981-19-0452-3_21].

R.-W. Grech
Paediatric ENT Department, Royal Manchester Children's Hospital, Manchester University NHS Foundation Trust, Manchester Academic Health Science Centre, Manchester, UK

Department of ENT and Head and Neck Surgery, Mater Dei Hospital, Msida, Malta

I. A. Bruce (✉)
Paediatric ENT Department, Royal Manchester Children's Hospital, Manchester University NHS Foundation Trust, Manchester Academic Health Science Centre, Manchester, UK

Division of Infection, Immunity and Respiratory Medicine, Faculty of Biology, Medicine and Health, University of Manchester, Manchester, UK
e-mail: Iain.Bruce@manchester.ac.uk


S. DeSaSouza (ed.), *Cochlear Implants*,
https://doi.org/10.1007/978-981-19-0452-3_21

**Table 21.1** List of minor and major complications

| Minor complications | Major complications |
|---|---|
| Vertigo | Meningitis |
| Chorda tympani damage | Facial palsy |
| Headaches/pain | Cerebrospinal fluid (CSF) leak |
| Tinnitus | Cholesteatoma |
| Acute otitis media resolving with antibiotics | Extrusion of the receiver-stimulator package |
| Minor wound infection | Extrusion of the electrode array from the cochlea |
| Peri-auricular/hemifacial swelling | Dislocation of magnet |
| Transient facial palsy | Facial stimulation with implant requiring explantation |
| Perforated tympanic membrane | |

after implantation, without the existence of a direct causal relationship (acute otitis media with or without mastoiditis). 'Never events' (wrong side surgery and retained surgical instruments (e.g. templates)) are not included in this review.

The complications from cochlear implant surgery can be broadly divided into major and minor complications. Major complications are those that require explantation of the implant or surgical intervention, or permanent disability (e.g. facial paralysis), and complications causing continuous discomfort. Minor complications resolve with conservative management (medical or audiological) or resolve spontaneously. A list is provided in Table 21.1. To date, there is no standardized classification system for the complications of CI surgery, although a number of have been proposed [1–4].

The rate of complications after CI surgery has been reported as 3–60% [4–8], with the variability largely reflecting the lack of a standardized method for classification. Over time, the number of major complications has steadily decreased whilst the number of minor complications reported has remained fairly stable [4–8]. When considering the incidence of complications, one must keep in mind that the selection criteria for implantation continue to broaden; to include the extremes of age, those with inner ear malformations and cochlear nerve deficiency, and bilateral simultaneous implantation [9–11]. As such, it is perhaps inevitable that the technical challenge of CI surgery will continue to increase, as surgeons strive to better preserve cochlear fine structures and insert electrode arrays in the presence of significant cochlear dysplasia.

### 21.1.1 Peripheral Vestibular Dysfunction

The most common complication of CI surgery is vertigo [4–8]. This affects adults more often than children [5–8]. The postulated aetiologies for vertigo post-cochlear implantation are: (1) spread of electric impulses from the cochlea to the vestibular nerve [12] and the saccule [13], (2) persistent perilymphatic fistula through the round window membrane [1, 14], (3) trauma to the scala vestibuli during insertion, (4) mechanical disturbance of the membranous labyrinth [12, 15], and (5) benign positional paroxysmal vertigo (BPPV) [16, 17]. Peripheral vestibular lesions are more common in the adult population, with a prevalence that increases with age [18], compounded by deterioration in the function of organ and sensory systems that normally aid the vestibular system with balance control, namely, vision, oculomotor (via the vestibulo-ocular reflex), joint position sense (proprioception), peripheral sensation, and central input [19]. Consequently, any insult to the vestibular system may result in a lengthier recovery in older patients. In children, young people and younger adults imbalance is usually a transient problem that recovers within a few days or weeks.

Vestibular rehabilitation can be used to aid central compensation and return to normal daily activities in cases of persisting vestibular dysfunction. Some clinicians advocate pre-operative vestibular testing to identify unilateral or bilateral vestibular dysfunction, which can help with the decision-making process regarding laterality of implantation and counselling prior to the procedure [20]. Pre-habilitation (before CI) to improve existing vestibular function may be considered in those patients with significant pre-existing vestibular hypofunction.

In children, SNHL is often related to vestibular dysfunction [21, 22] due to the common embryological origin of the inner ear and vestibular structures. Due to this, combined with extrapolation from adult data, there have been concerns regarding the long-term vestibular effects of cochlear implantation in children, especially in bilateral CI surgery or surgery on the ear with the better vestibular function [23]. To date, this has not materialized in clinical practice, with no strong evidence to show clinically significant changes in vestibular function [24, 25]. Recent studies have suggested that CI in children with SNHL and associated balance disorders have improved balance function [26, 27]. The auditory cues received whilst moving are thought to contribute to this apparent improvement [28]. It has also been postulated that the electrical stimuli provided by the electrode array could be enhancing the processing pathways of the vestibular system [26].

Hearing preservation CI surgery appears to have a positive effect upon limiting vestibular complications [29], presumably as a consequence of attempts to limit the trauma and forces delivered to the inner ear, and possibly the anti-inflammatory properties of steroids used to protect the cochlea.

### 21.1.2 Tinnitus

Tinnitus is a recognized complication of cochlear implant surgery, with a variable proportion (1.5–20%) [30–33] of patients reporting a new tinnitus or worsening of a pre-existing tinnitus. The exact reason for this is not fully understood, but the creation of a cochleostomy rather than the use of the round window for insertion and disruption of the basilar membrane by the electrode array have been postulated [32, 34]. However, some adults are now undergoing CI primarily for intractable unilateral tinnitus associated with an ipsilateral hearing loss, and the authors' experience is that cochlear implantation is more likely to be associated with reduced perception of tinnitus when wearing the audioprocessor.

Although the exact aetiology remains contentious and is likely to be variable, damage to the auditory pathway as a result of inner and outer hair cell damage, cochlear hydrops, lesions of the vestibulocochlear nerve, and the cerebellopontine angle, is considered to be causal. As such, it is not surprising that around 65% [32, 34] of CI candidates suffer from tinnitus pre-operatively. It has long been proposed that electric impulses to the cochlea suppress tinnitus [35–37] with the exact mechanism of this suppression remaining elusive. It has been suggested that the enhancement of neural inputs to the auditory pathway could result in control of the tinnitus [38], as observed in hearing aid users. This improvement in tinnitus has also been observed post-cochlear implantation, with reduction or complete elimination of the tinnitus in 55–65% of recipients [31, 33, 34]. Patients with a higher burden of handicap from their tinnitus seem to benefit more from this intervention [39]. These favourable results make CI one of the treatment modalities in patients who suffer from intractable tinnitus and deafness [34, 39].

### 21.1.3 The Facial Nerve

The path of the facial nerve is aberrant in 10–15% of cases of inner ear malformations [40, 41]. This makes pre-operative imaging, surgical planning, and reliable facial nerve monitoring essential to avoid injury to the facial nerve. Likewise, in older children and adults with a history of chronic otitis media (COM) the fallopian canal may be eroded and the nerve dehiscent.

Dependent upon pre-existing or iatrogenic reduction in the bony covering of the facial nerve, further compounded by cochlear anomalies (common cavity and cochlear hypoplasia) [42], there is a risk of nonauditory stimulation (NAS) with stimulation of the facial nerve by the electrode array. Risk can be mitigated by surgical planning and choice of electrode array design (e.g. peri-modiolar), and symptom occurrence reduced by reprogramming (Fig. 21.1).

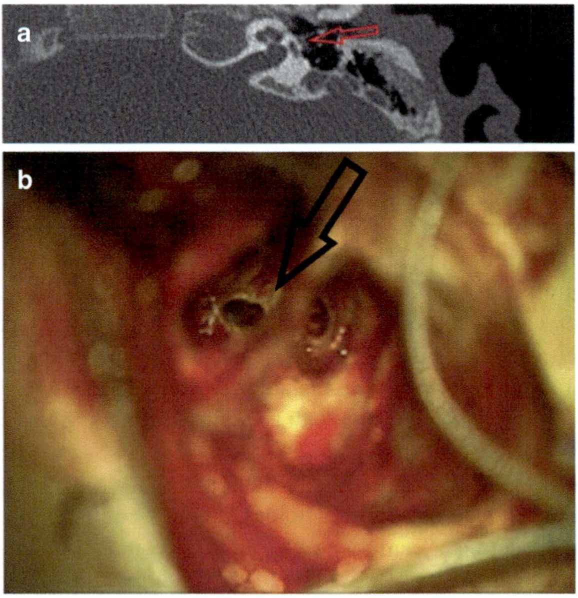


**Fig. 21.1** Anomalous facial nerve traversing the promontory in a child with CHARGE syndrome

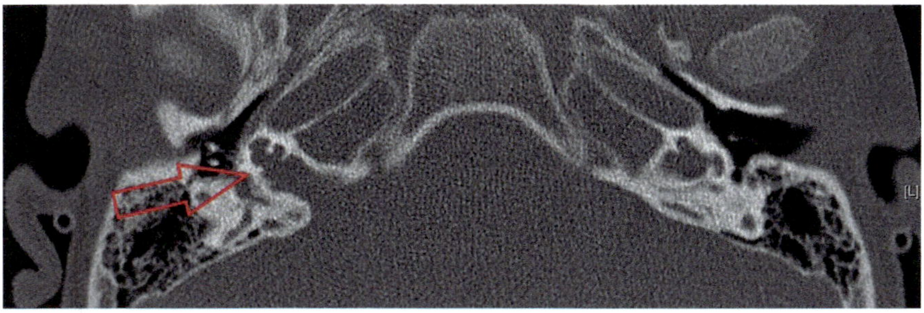


**Fig. 21.2** CT of an X-linked gusher (red arrow) showing the typical 'corkscrew appearance' in IP-III with the interscalar septa present, an absent modiolus, and an absent lamina cribrosa separating the basal turn of the cochlea from the internal auditory canal. A thin otic capsule is also a common feature

### 21.1.4 Perilymphatic Gusher

This is a problem mostly associated with X-linked deafness featuring an IP-III-type cochlear malformation [43, 44]. Apart from the intracochlear malformations associated with this anomaly there are other radiological features that predict the presence of this pathology: (1) thin otic capsule, (2) bulbous widening of the lateral aspect of the internal auditory canal, and (3) dysplastic vestibule, oval, and round window [45]. Intra-operatively, bulging of the stapes footplate has also been described [46].

The method used to manage a perilymphatic gusher is to lift the head of the operating table up and the use of a fascia/muscle graft and fibrin sealant to seal the cochleostomy (or round window) following insertion of the cochlear implant. It is important to anticipate such cases following review of the radiological images during the assessment phase before surgery. The senior author favours a cochleostomy approach in such cases as it aids packing of the entry point into the cochlea, and conversely a larger cochleostomy is preferable. Latterly, CI manufacturers have also developed silicone rings and electrodes with 'cork-like stoppers' to help seal perilymphatic leaks, which do not require a larger cochleostomy to be drilled (Fig. 21.2)

### 21.1.5 Extrusion of the Internal Component

Extrusion of the receiver-stimulator package (RSP) occurs at a rate of 0.5–1% and can happen up to several years after surgery [47, 48]. The pathogenesis of extrusion is thought to be *reduced skin viability* or *rejection*. Skin problems include necrosis and wound breakdown, which can happen post-operatively due to infection or poor vascularization of the flap. Thinning of the skin flap as a result of the pressure from the overlying magnet can also result in extrusion over the longer term. The RSP may be considered to have been 'rejected' when tissue cultures are negative, there is no bacterial biofilm over the RSP, and histology demonstrates evidence of giant cells and macrophages [49]. Allergy to silicone has been previously postulated as a cause for rejections [50, 51], but the literature regarding this is scant, possibly due to the very low incidence of this problem.

Viability of the overlying skin and soft tissue plays a major role in influencing the risk of extrusion, with repeat surgery, diabetes mellitus, smoking, and other conditions that affect microvascular circulation, being implicated. Pre-existing dermatological problems increase the risk of extrusion due to the recognized negative impact on skin healing. The choice of incision also should be taken into consideration, since it is preferable to avoid having an incision overlying the RSP. Closure of the wound in multiple layers, including periosteal and subcutaneous layers, is advised to limit the risk of exposure of the device in superficial wound infections with skin breakdown [52, 53]. The management of skin inflammation over the RSP is dependent upon the site of the irritation and the integrity of the skin. Whilst the rarity of the problem limits the availability of strong evidence, most clinicians will consider early systemic antibiotic treatment and 'resting' the skin and soft tissues by not wearing the audioprocessor and coil until the inflammation resolves. The length and type of antibiotic regime should be decided in conjunction with a Microbiologist, on the understanding that a prolonged course of treatment may be required. When the inflammation is localized solely to the area overlying the internal magnet in the RSP, reducing the strength of the external magnet may resolve the problem [54] (Fig. 21.3).

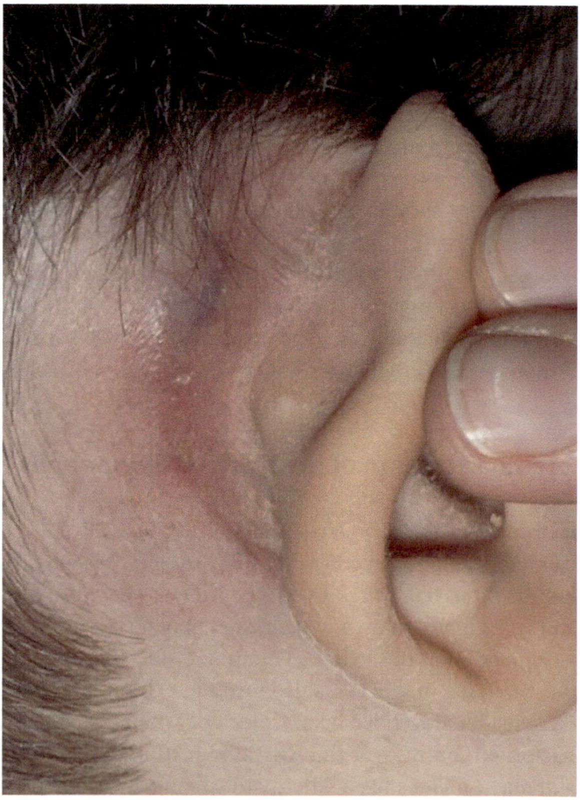

**Fig. 21.3** Developing stitch abscess in the post-auricular wound

Once the internal component of the cochlear implant becomes exposed there is a significant risk of 'losing' the implant. Several different methods have been suggested to attempt to salvage an exposed cochlear implant [55–62], including prolonged aggressive antibiotic management, 'washout' with chlorhexidine and erythromycin [59], optimization of physiological derangements (glycaemic control and thyroid levels) and the use of hyperbaric oxygen [57]. A number of techniques are described to cover the exposed RSP with a vascularized flap, including a temporo-parietal fascia flap [55, 60], rotational two-layered skin flaps [61], and temporalis myofascial flap [62]. Salvaging extruding receiver-stimulator packages remains a significant challenge, which often results in explantation (leaving the electrode array in the cochlea as a 'spacer') and reimplantation several months later when the inflammation has settled (Fig. 21.4a–d).

Extrusion of the electrode array from the cochlea is a rare finding, which may reflect initial over insertion of the electrode array, an obliterative process in the cochlea, or movement of the cable during, or after, coiling in the mastoid cavity. Damage to the posterior wall of the external auditory canal during the initial surgery carries the extremely uncommon risk of erosion by pressure of the electrode cable into the ear canal (Fig. 21.5).

### 21.1.6 Other Considerations

#### 21.1.6.1 Role of Intraoperative Imaging

There is a growing role for intraoperative imaging (X-ray, fluoroscopy, and CT scanning) in cases of cochlear malformation, difficult insertion or where the surgeon has doubts with regard to the placement of the electrode [63–66]. Intraoperative imaging has not been demonstrated to be advantageous for 'routine' cases.

#### 21.1.6.2 Inner Ear Malformations

As candidacy criteria for CI have evolved so has the technical challenge inherent in the surgical procedure of accessing and inserting an electrode array into the cochlea [9, 67, 68]. In the 1980s and early 1990s, all inner ear malformations were contraindications for cochlear implant surgery [69–71]. In the 1990s, small series of CIs in this patient cohort began to appear [72–74] prompting the realization that significant benefit could be expected, although it may not be readily measurable using existing outcome measurement instruments and may be influenced by the comorbidities (syndromic diagnosis and cognitive impairment) that can be associated with inner ear malformations. However, in some studies the improvement in speech perception [68] was comparable to that seen in patients with no apparent cochlear anomalies [75]. The only absolute anatomical contraindications to CI surgery are cochlear aplasia and absent cochlear nerve.

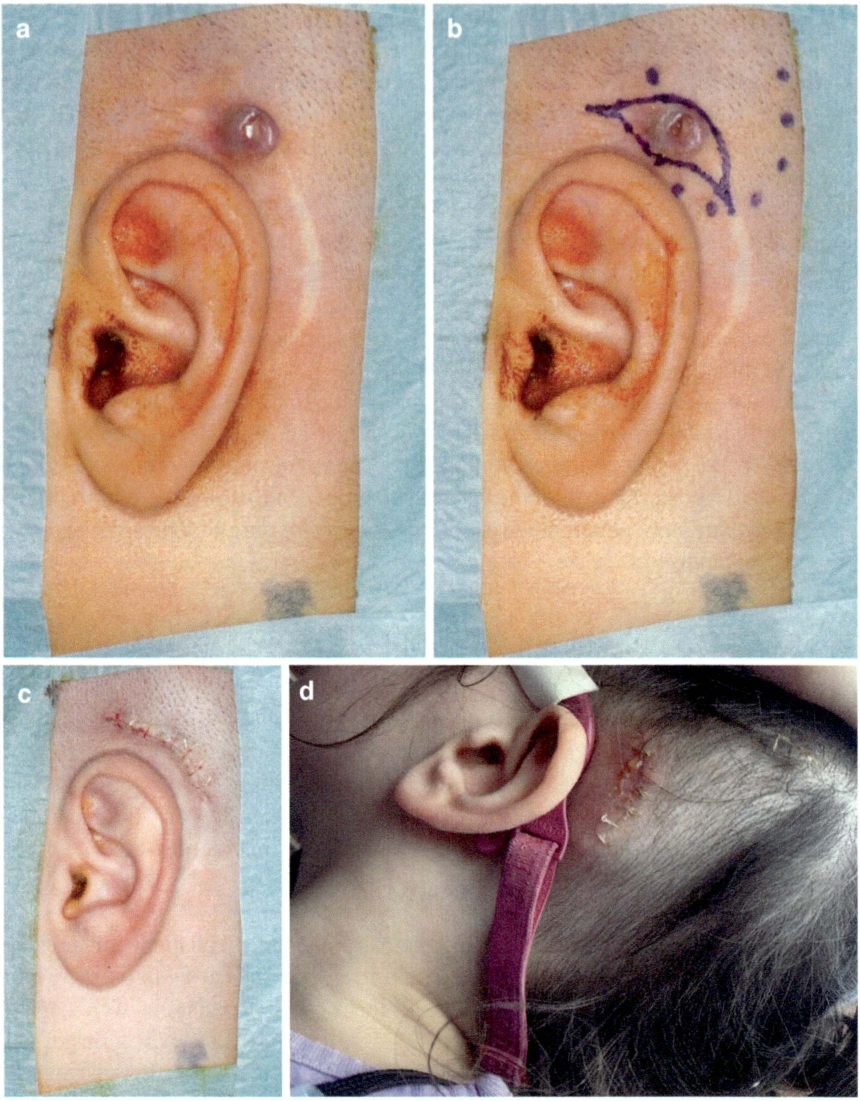


**Fig. 21.4** (**a**) Extrusion with exposure of the RSP. (**b**) Intraoperative image with the position of the underlying RSP marked. Note that the incision has healed such that it overlies the anterior edge of the RSP. (**c**) Initial closure following resection of the dehiscent skin. (**d**) Threatened extrusion in the child who subsequently needed an explant

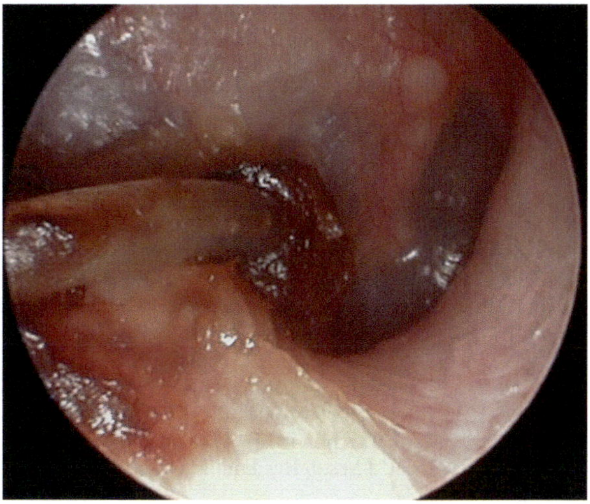

**Fig. 21.5** Erosion of the electrode array into the external ear canal

## References


1. Cohen NL, Hoffman RA, Stroschein M. Medical or surgical complications related to the nucleus multichannel Cochlear implant. Ann Otol Rhinol Laryngol. 1988;97(Suppl 2):8–13.
2. Hansen S, Anthonsen K, Stangerup S, Jensen JH, Thomsen J, Cayé-Thomasen P. Unexpected findings and surgical complications in 505 consecutive cochlear implantations: a proposal for reporting consensus. Acta Otolaryngol. 2010;130(5):540–9.
3. Theunisse HJ, Pennings RJE, Kunst HPM, Mulder JJ, Mylanus EAM. Risk factors for complications in cochlear implant surgery. Eur Arch Otorhinolaryngol. 2018;275(4):895–903.
4. Jeppesen J, Faber CE. Surgical complications following cochlear implantation in adults based on a proposed reporting consensus. Acta Otolaryngol. 2013;133(10):1012–21.
5. Venail F, Sicard M, Piron JP, Levi A, Artieres F, Uziel A, et al. Reliability and complications of 500 consecutive Cochlear implantations. Arch Otolaryngol Head Neck Surg. 2008 Dec 15;134(12):1276–81.
6. Farinetti A, Ben Gharbia D, Mancini J, Roman S, Nicollas R, Triglia J. Cochlear implant complications in 403 patients: comparative study of adults and children and review of the literature. Eur Ann Otorhinolaryngol Head Neck Dis. 2014;131(3):177–82.
7. Binnetoglu A, Demir B, Batman C. Surgical complications of cochlear implantation: a 25-year retrospective analysis of cases in a tertiary academic center. Eur Arch Otorhinolaryngol. 2020;277(7):1917–23.
8. Cohen NL, Hoffman RA. Complications of Cochlear implant surgery in adults and children. Ann Otol Rhinol Laryngol. 1991;100(9):708–11.
9. Varadarajan VV, Sydlowski SA, Li MM, Anne S, Adunka OF. Evolving criteria for adult and pediatric Cochlear implantation. Ear Nose Throat J. 2021;100(1):31–7.
10. Birman CS, Powell HRF, Gibson WPR, Elliott EJ. Cochlear implant outcomes in cochlea nerve aplasia and hypoplasia. Otol Neurotol. 2016;37(5):438–45.
11. Arnoldner C, Lin VYW. Expanded selection criteria in adult cochlear implantation. Cochlear Implants Int Interdiscip J. 2013;14:10.

12. Ito J. Influence of the multichannel cochlear implant on vestibular function. Otolaryngol Head Neck Surg. 1998;118:900–6.
13. Coordes A, Basta D, Götze R, Scholz S, Seidl RO, Ernst A, Todt I. Sound-induced vertigo after cochlear implantation. Otol Neurotol. 2012;33(3):335–42. https://doi.org/10.1097/MAO.0b013e318245cee3.
14. Kusuma S, Liou S, Haynes DS. Disequilibrium after cochlear implantation caused by a perilymph fistula. Laryngoscope. 2005;115(1):25–6. https://doi.org/10.1097/01.mlg.0000150680.68355.cc.
15. Huygen PL, Broek P, Spies TH. Does intracochlear implantation jeopardize vestibular function? Ann Otol Rhinol Laryngol. 1994;103:609–14.
16. Zanetti D, Campovecchi CB, Balzanelli C, Pasini S. Paroxysmal positional vertigo after cochlear implantation. Acta Otolaryngol. 2007;127(5):452–8. https://doi.org/10.1080/00016480600951442.
17. Limb CJ, Francis HF, Lustig LR, Niparko JK, Jammal H. Benign positional vertigo after cochlear implantation. Otolaryngol Head Neck Surg. 2005;132(5):741–5. https://doi.org/10.1016/j.otohns.2005.01.004.
18. Agrawal Y, Ward BK, Minor LB. Vestibular dysfunction: prevalence, impact and need for targeted treatment. J Vestib Res Equilib Orientat. 2013;23(3):113–7. https://doi.org/10.3233/VES-130498.
19. Lacour M, Bernard-Demanze L. Interaction between vestibular compensation mechanisms and vestibular rehabilitation therapy: 10 recommendations for optimal functional recovery. Front Neurol. 2015;5:285. https://doi.org/10.3389/fneur.2014.00285.
20. West N, Klokker M, Caye-Thomasen P. Vestibular screening before Cochlear implantation: clinical implications and challenges in 409 Cochlear implant recipients. Otol Neurotol. 2021;42(2):e137–44. https://doi.org/10.1097/MAO.0000000000002898.
21. Maes L, Kegel D, Alexandra, Waelvelde V, Hilde, Dhooge I. Rotatory and collic vestibular evoked myogenic potential testing in normal-hearing and hearing-impaired children. Ear Hear. 2014;35(2):e21–32. https://doi.org/10.1097/AUD.0b013e3182a6ca91.
22. Inoue A, Iwasaki S, Ushio M, Chihara Y, Fujimoto C, Egami N, Yamasoba T. Effect of vestibular dysfunction on the development of gross motor function in children with profound hearing loss. Audiol Neurootol. 2013;18(3):143–51. https://doi.org/10.1159/000346344.
23. Melvin TA, Della Santina CC, Carey JP, Migliaccio AA. The effects of cochlear implantation on vestibular function. Otol Neurotol. 2009;30(1):87–94. https://doi.org/10.1097/mao.0b013e31818d1cba.
24. Yong M, Young E, Lea J, et al. Subjective and objective vestibular changes that occur following paediatric cochlear implantation: systematic review and meta-analysis. J Otolaryngol Head Neck Surg. 2019;48(1):22. https://doi.org/10.1186/s40463-019-0341-z.
25. Eustaquio ME, Berryhill W, Wolfe JA, Saunders JE. Balance in children with bilateral cochlear implants. Otol Neurotol. 2010;32:424–7.
26. Gnanasegaram JJ, Parkes WJ, Cushing SL, McKnight CL, Papsin BC, Gordon KA. Stimulation from Cochlear implant electrodes assists with recovery from asymmetric perceptual tilt: evidence from the subjective visual vertical test. Front Integr Neurosci. 2016;13:32. https://doi.org/10.3389/fnint.2016.00032.
27. Wolter NE, Gordon KA, Campos J, Vilchez Madrigal LD, Papsin BC, Cushing SL. Impact of the sensory environment on balance in children with bilateral cochleovestibular loss. Hear Res. 2021;400:108134. https://doi.org/10.1016/j.heares.2020.108134.
28. Campos J, Ramkhalawansingh R, Pichora-Fuller MK. Hearing, self-motion perception, mobility, and aging. Hear Res. 2018;369:42–55. https://doi.org/10.1016/j.heares.2018.03.025.
29. Coordes A, Ernst A, Brademann G, Todt I. Round window membrane insertion with perimodiolar cochlear implant electrodes. Otol Neurotol. 2013;34(6):1027–32. https://doi.org/10.1097/MAO.0b013e318280da2a.
30. Hou JH, Zhao SP, Ning F, Rao SQ, Han DY. Postoperative complications in patients with cochlear implants and impacts of nursing intervention. Acta Otolaryngol. 2010;130(6):687–95. https://doi.org/10.3109/00016480903334445.

31. Kloostra FJ, Arnold R, Hofman R, Van Dijk P. Changes in tinnitus after cochlear implantation and its relation with psychological functioning. Audiol Neurootol. 2015;20(2):81–9. https://doi.org/10.1159/000365959.
32. Todt I, Rademacher G, Mutze S, Ramalingam R, Wolter S, Mittmann P, Wagner J, Ernst A. Relationship between intracochlear electrode position and tinnitus in cochlear implantees. Acta Otolaryngol. 2015;135(8):781–5. https://doi.org/10.3109/00016489.2015.1024332.
33. Di Nardo W, Cantore I, Cianfrone F, Melillo P, Scorpecci A, Paludetti G. Tinnitus modifications after cochlear implantation. Eur Arch Otorhinolaryngol. 2007;264(10):1145–9. https://doi.org/10.1007/s00405-007-0352-7.
34. Kloostra FJJ, Verbist J, Hofman R, Free RH, Arnold R, van Dijk P. A prospective study of the effect of Cochlear implantation on tinnitus. Audiol Neurootol. 2018;23(6):356–63. https://doi.org/10.1159/000495132.
35. Chouard CH, Meyer B, Maridat D. Transcutaneous electrotherapy for severe tinnitus. Acta Otolaryngol. 1981;91(5–6):415–22. https://doi.org/10.3109/00016488109138522.
36. Portmann M, Nègrevergne M, Aran JM, Cazals Y. Electrical stimulation of the ear: clinical applications. Ann Otol Rhinol Laryngol. 1983 Nov–Dec;92(6 Pt 1):621–2. https://doi.org/10.1177/000348948309200617.
37. Mielczarek M, Olszewski J. Direct current stimulation of the ear in tinnitus treatment: a double-blind placebo-controlled study. Eur Arch Otorhinolaryngol. 2014;271(6):1815–22. https://doi.org/10.1007/s00405-013-2849-6.
38. Surr RK, Montgomery AA, Mueller HG. Effect of amplification on tinnitus among new hearing aid users. Ear Hear. 1985;6(2):71–5. https://doi.org/10.1097/00003446-198503000-00002.
39. Dixon PR, Crowson M, Shipp D, Smilsky K, Lin VY, Le T, Chen JM. Predicting reduced tinnitus burden after Cochlear implantation in adults. Otol Neurotol. 2020;41(2):196–201. https://doi.org/10.1097/MAO.0000000000002481.
40. Sennaroğlu L, Tahir E. A novel classification: anomalous routes of the facial nerve in relation to inner ear malformations. Laryngoscope. 2020;130(11):E696–703. https://doi.org/10.1002/lary.28596.
41. Coudert A, Vigier S, Scalabre A, Hermann R, Ayari-Khalfallah S, Truy E. Analysis of inner ear malformations associated with a facial nerve anomaly in 653 children fitted with a cochlear implant. Clin Otolaryngol. 2019;44(1):96–101. https://doi.org/10.1111/coa.13246.
42. Berrettini S, Vito de A, Bruschini L, Passetti S, Forli F. Facial nerve stimulation after cochlear implantation: our experience. Acta Otorhinolaryngol Ital. 2011;31(1):11–6.
43. Talenti G, Manara R, Brotto D, D'Arco F. High-resolution 3 T magnetic resonance findings in cochlear hypoplasias and incomplete partition anomalies: a pictorial essay. Br J Radiol. 2018;91(1089):20180120. https://doi.org/10.1259/bjr.20180120.
44. Sennaroglu L, Sarac S, Ergin T. Surgical results of cochlear implantation in malformed cochlea. Otol Neurotol. 2006;27(5):615–23. https://doi.org/10.1097/01.mao.0000224090.94882.b4.
45. Hong R, Du Q, Pan Y. New imaging findings of incomplete partition type III inner ear malformation and literature review. AJNR Am J Neuroradiol. 2020;41(6):1076–80. https://doi.org/10.3174/ajnr.A6576.
46. Purcell DD, Fischbein N, Lalwani AK. Identification of previously "undetectable" abnormalities of the bony labyrinth with computed tomography measurement. Laryngoscope. 2003;113(11):1908–11. https://doi.org/10.1097/00005537-200311000-00009.
47. Petersen H, Walshe P, Glynn F, McMahon R, Fitzgerald C, Thapa J, Simoes-Franklin C, Viani L. Occurrence of major complications after cochlear implant surgery in Ireland. Cochlear Implants Int. 2018;19(6):297–306. https://doi.org/10.1080/14670100.2018.1513386.
48. Terry B, Kelt RE, Jeyakumar A. Delayed complications after Cochlear implantation. JAMA Otolaryngol Head Neck Surg. 2015;141(11):1012–7. https://doi.org/10.1001/jamaoto.2015.2154.
49. Xin Y, Yuan YS, Chi FL, Wang J, Yang JM. Foreign body reaction after Cochlear implantation: a case report. Chin Med J. 2015;128(15):2124–5. https://doi.org/10.4103/0366-6999.161402.

50. Kunda LD, Stidham KR, Inserra MM, Roland PS, Franklin D, Roberson JB Jr. Silicone allergy: a new cause for cochlear implant extrusion and its management. Otol Neurotol. 2006;27(8):1078–82. https://doi.org/10.1097/01.mao.0000235378.64654.4d.
51. Puri S, Dornhoffer JL, North PE. Contact dermatitis to silicone after cochlear implantation. Laryngoscope. 2005;115(10):1760–2. https://doi.org/10.1097/01.mlg.0000172202.58968.41.
52. Gluth MB, Singh R, Atlas MD. Prevention and management of cochlear implant infections. Cochlear Implants Int. 2011;12(4):223–7. https://doi.org/10.1179/146701011X12950038111576.
53. Almosnino G, Zeitler DM, Schwartz SR. Postoperative antibiotics following Cochlear implantation: are they necessary? Ann Otol Rhinol Laryngol. 2018;127(4):266–9. https://doi.org/10.1177/0003489418758101.
54. James AL, Daniel SJ, Richmond L, Papsin BC. Skin breakdown over cochlear implants: prevention of a magnet site complication. J Otolaryngol. 2004;33(3):151–4. https://doi.org/10.2310/7070.2004.02069.
55. Hariharan NC, Muthukumar R, Sridhar R, et al. Ideal flap cover for the salvage of exposed/infected Cochlear implants: a case series and literature review. Indian J Otolaryngol Head Neck Surg. 2020;72:292–6. https://doi.org/10.1007/s12070-019-01764-1.
56. Seo BF, Park SW, Han HH, Moon SH, Oh DY, Rhie JW. Salvaging the exposed cochlear implant. J Craniofac Surg. 2015;26(8):749–52.
57. Leach J, Kruger P, Roland P. Rescuing the imperiled cochlear implant: a report of four cases. Otol Neurotol. 2005;26(1):27–33.
58. Cunningham CD, Slattery WH, Luxford WM. Postoperative infection in cochlear implant patients. Otolaryngol Head Neck Surg. 2004;131(1):109–14.
59. Low WK, Rangabashyam M, Wang F. Management of major post-cochlear implant wound infections. Eur Arch Otorhinolaryngol. 2014;271:2409–13. https://doi.org/10.1007/s00405-013-2732-5.
60. Karimnejad K, Akhter AS, Walen SG, Mikulec AA. The temporoparietal fascia flap for coverage of cochlear reimplantation following extrusion. Int J Pediatr Otorhinolaryngol. 2017;94:64–7. https://doi.org/10.1016/j.ijporl.2017.01.020.
61. Gawęcki W, Karlik M, Borucki Ł, Szyfter-Harris J, Wróbel M. Skin flap complications after cochlear implantations. Eur Arch Otorhinolaryngol. 2016;273(12):4175–83. https://doi.org/10.1007/s00405-016-4107-1.
62. Bi Q, Chen Z, Lv Y, Luo J, Wang N, Li Y. Management of delayed-onset skin flap complications after pediatric cochlear implantation. Eur Arch Otorhinolaryngol. 2020;278(8):2753–61. https://doi.org/10.1007/s00405-020-06348-2.
63. Cosetti MK, Troob SH, Latzman JM, Shapiro WH, Roland JT Jr, Waltzman SB. An evidence-based algorithm for intraoperative monitoring during cochlear implantation. Otol Neurotol. 2012;33(2):169–76. https://doi.org/10.1097/MAO.0b013e3182423175.
64. Viccaro M, Covelli E, De Seta E, Balsamo G, Filipo R. The importance of intra-operative imaging during cochlear implant surgery. Cochlear Implants Int. 2009;10:198–202.
65. Molezini FD, Meira SG Jr, Neto DL, Filho OA. Cochlear implant radiography: technique adapted into a portable apparatus. Braz J Otorhinolaryngol. 2012;78(1):31–6. https://doi.org/10.1590/s1808-86942012000100005.
66. Yuan YY, Song YS, Chai CM, Shen WD, Han WJ, Liu J, Wang GJ, Dong TX, Han DY, Dai P. Intraoperative CT-guided cochlear implantation in congenital ear deformity. Acta Otolaryngol. 2012;132(9):951–8. https://doi.org/10.3109/00016489.2012.674214.
67. Hang AX, Kim GG, Zdanski CJ. Cochlear implantation in unique pediatric populations. Curr Opin Otolaryngol Head Neck Surg. 2012;20(6):507–17. https://doi.org/10.1097/MOO.0b013e328359eea4.
68. Pakdaman MN, Herrmann BS, Curtin HD, Van Beek-King J, Lee DJ. Cochlear implantation in children with anomalous cochleovestibular anatomy: a systematic review. Otolaryngol Head Neck Surg. 2012;146(2):180–90. https://doi.org/10.1177/0194599811429244.

69. Balkany T, Bird PA, Hodges AV, Luntz M, Telischi FF, Buchman C. Surgical technique for implantation of the totally ossified cochlea. Laryngoscope. 1998;108(7):988–92. https://doi.org/10.1097/00005537-199807000-00007.
70. Miyamoto RT, Robbins AJ, Myres WA, Pope ML. Cochlear implantation in the Mondini inner ear malformation. Am J Otol. 1986;7(4):258–61.
71. Sennaroglu L. Cochlear implantation in inner ear malformations: a review article. Cochlear Implants Int. 2010;11(1):4–41. https://doi.org/10.1002/cii.416.
72. Hoffman RA, Downey LL, Waltzman SB, Cohen NL. Cochlear implantation in children with cochlear malformation. Am J Otol. 1997;18:184–7.
73. Luntz M, Balkany T, Hodges AV, Telischi FF. Cochlear implants in children with congenital inner ear malformations. Arch Otolaryngol Head Neck Surg. 1997;123(9):974–7. https://doi.org/10.1001/archotol.1997.01900090090013.
74. Weber BP, Lenarz T, Hartrampf R, Dietrich B, Bertram B, Dahm MC. Cochlear implantation in children with malformation of the cochlea. Adv Otorhinolaryngol. 1995;50:59–65. https://doi.org/10.1159/000424436.
75. Papsin BC. Cochlear implantation in children with anomalous cochleovestibular anatomy. Laryngoscope. 2005;115:1–26.

# Recent Trends in Cochlear Implant Programming and (Re)habilitation

# 22

Colleen Psarros and Yetta Abrahams

## 22.1 The Starting Point

> "I know I felt great when I was switched on and I could hear a word. It is amazing technology. But when I left my switch on appointment, I broke down in tears, not that it was too much—but realising it hit me then this is something that isn't going to get much better than this—I'm going to have to wear the device all the time to hear and I'm going to have to work out how does the cochlear implant fit in with my life that I had before" … ML, 62 yrs

The ongoing cycle of lifelong cochlear implant care and management through mapping, ongoing (re)habilitation and evaluation is often shaped by the preoperative and surgical components which previous chapters have addressed. A typical cochlear implant journey irrespective of global and interclinic differences can be summarised by Fig. 22.1 [1] as shown.

The cochlear implant mapping and (re)habilitation process begins before surgery when goals and expectations are established. Clinical research on outcomes [2] and the recipient's own research can underpin goal setting and the steps taken toward optimal integration of device use in their everyday lives. Surgical decisions and outcomes will further determine the starting point of the cochlear implant mapping and rehabilitation. Mapping is setting a programme or code that can be sent to power and stimulate intra and extracochlear electrodes, which in turn stimulate nerve fibres, providing the auditory system access to sound that can be interpreted and refined through programming and rehabilitation.

**Supplementary Information** The online version contains supplementary material available at [https://doi.org/10.1007/978-981-19-0452-3_22].

C. Psarros · Y. Abrahams (✉)
Cochlear APAC, Macquarie Park, NSW, Australia
e-mail: cpsarros@cochlear.com; yabrahams@cochlear.com



S. DeSaSouza (ed.), *Cochlear Implants*,
https://doi.org/10.1007/978-981-19-0452-3_22

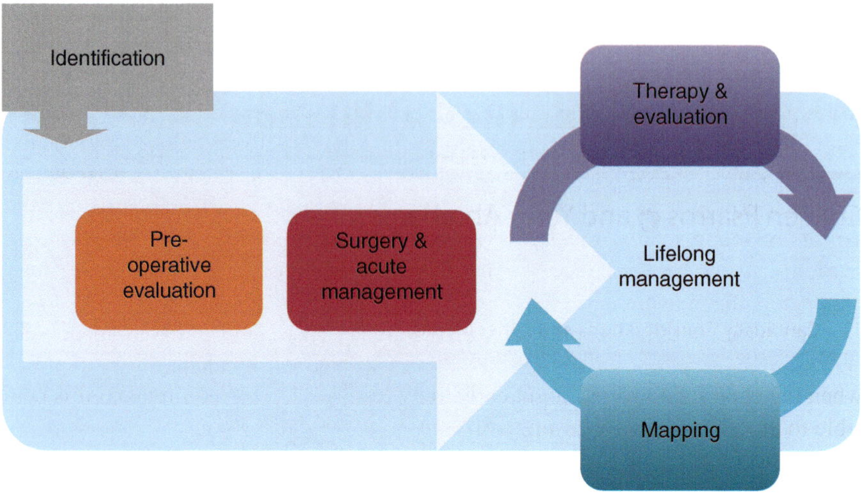


**Fig. 22.1** The cochlear implant journey [1]

## 22.2 Cochlear Implant Mapping: Why and How Is It Done

Changes in the recipient's "map" may occur due to changes in the biochemical and physiological composition of the cochlea [3]. Rance and Dowell [4] note there can also be some post-surgical changes that occur due to the healing mechanisms within the cochlea, such as fibrous sheath growing around the internal electrode array. This sheath can affect the current flow and result in changes in current requirements, which in some patients creates the need for regular adjustments of the CI "map" in the acute phase of CI management.

Traditionally mapping has relied on the behavioural feedback of the recipient to indicate the threshold and the maximum loudness level of sound percepts presented across individual electrodes. Behavioural methodology for gathering this information follows common practices used in audiometry which are adjusted according to age and cognitive abilities.

## 22.3 Map Verification

Verification that the map can comfortably provide access to the frequencies across the speech spectrum at levels of 25–30 dBA, has traditionally used any or a combination of sound field audiometry, speech perception assessment, functional questionnaires or clinical observation during (re)habilitation. The accuracy of such procedures can be impacted by the ability to reliably complete tasks considering developmental and cognitive limitations.

The use of free field cochlear implant-assisted audiograms in isolation to measure hearing sensitivity [5] is limited as the detection only information is not reflection of the auditory function that the access to sound is providing. The Ling [6] sound test is commonly used and is presented using an age or cognitively appropriate method.

Map verification with functional listening and speech identification tools such as The Speech Spatial Qualities [7] questionnaire can be used for children and adults. They provide a snapshot of cochlear implant use for participation and function in speech discrimination, localisation, spatial listening, listening effort and qualitative aspects of sound such as music. Review of functional listening prior to a mapping session can provide guidance for the clinician in counselling and targeting map parameters that may enhance hearing sensitivity and function.

The use of speech perception to verify the map must factor in the linguistic and neurocognitive factors which will be addressed later in this chapter. The trend to shift mapping to be less clinically bound and in real-world situations such as the café or in the home environment can provide a more realistic means of map verification [8].

## 22.4 What Constitutes a "Mapping" Session

Consensus on global good clinical practice (GCP) guidelines does not exist for cochlear implant programming of children or adults. Vaerenberg [9] surveyed 47 clinics from around the world who collectively used four manufacturers of cochlear implants: Advanced Bionics, Cochlear, Medel and Neurolec (now known as Oticon Medical). Recommendations for mapping were based on the responses of clinicians to interview questions that were reporting their individual clinical practices.

Considerable variability in approaches existed within and between clinics irrespective of the cochlear implant device manufacturer. Nonetheless, a checklist of recommended steps for cochlear implant programming was derived. It was recommended that there be four episodes of programming in the first year of cochlear implantation, with annual or six-monthly follow-ups thereafter.

Hour long mapping review sessions were recommended to include:

1. Perform pure tone audiometry and speech audiometry (in quiet)
2. Measure impedances and deactivate electrodes in case of short or open circuits.
3. Verify the levels on individual electrodes by loudness balancing.
4. Shift the profiles of the maximum and, if necessary, also of the minimum levels globally.
5. If deemed necessary, tilt the maximum levels globally.
6. Define own criteria to identify selected and exceptional cases in whom other MAP parameters are modified [9].

Deviation from these recommendations and more bespoke methods are becoming increasingly necessary with the expansion of candidacy criteria for cochlear implantation leading to more individual variability.

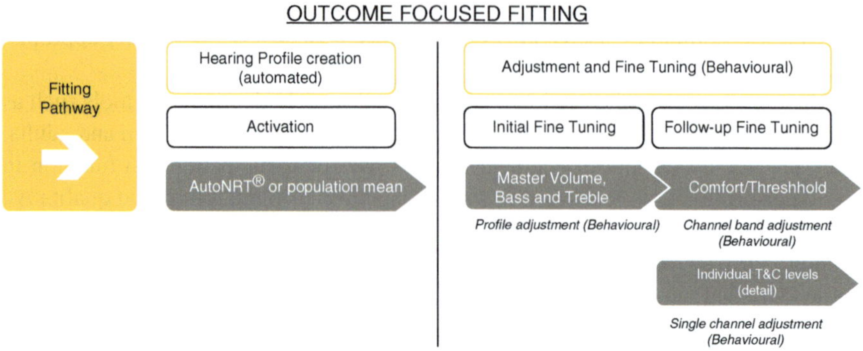


**Fig. 22.2** Outcome focussed fitting [8]

Botros [10] recommend Outcome Focused Fitting, a tiered clinical approach that can utilise information gathered from intraoperative testing into the initial fitting session and be used for subsequent sessions either directed by the clinician or by the recipient—or a combination of both [8].

The Outcome Focused Fitting (see Fig. 22.2) enables the clinician to verify the programme prior to implementing additional behavioural methods, which may actually be quite minimal such as single-channel adjustments.

This methodology, when used with children from the age of 7 months with an interdisciplinary team and caregivers, involves map verification in situ through functional assessment, including Ling [5] sounds [6]. The standard of care for infants with bilateral moderate-severe to profound hearing loss is increasingly becoming simultaneous bilateral cochlear implants [11]. The Outcome Focused Fitting session enables fitting of both ears whilst capitalising on the child's attention span, which may only last 10–15 min.

Programming software across manufacturers has evolved to reduce the amount of time that the recipient is "off the air". Previous versions of software have required adjustments which are conducted with the microphone deactivated and the recipient only having access to frequency-specific stimuli. Now adolescent and adult cochlear implant recipients who have challenges in certain listening situations such as a café or workplace are able to have their programming performed in these environments through the use of wireless programming devices and tablets or through the Nucleus Smart App rather than the traditional sound-treated room. When sound field audiogram or free field speech perception testing cannot be performed, use of functional questionnaires, and self-administered monitoring through the app-based Remote Check provides the recipient and or caregivers with the tools needed to ensure that their cochlear implant's sound processor has been programmed in a bespoke manner for their range of listening needs (Video 22.1).

The variability in the setting of children's maps within experienced cochlear implant centres in Australia was highlighted by Incerti [12]. They reviewed the map settings of 161 children at the age of 3 years and then at 5 years of age. Later implanted (>12 months) children had a significantly wider dynamic range at

6 months after device activation due to high comfort or loudness levels than those implanted at a younger age (<12 months of age). This was possibly due to older children being more involved and able to indicate when their comfort level had been reached, whereas clinicians may have been more conservative when working with the younger population. Narrower dynamic range and underestimated comfort levels could potentially contribute to restricted access to the speech range. Children who had neural or cochlear structural abnormalities had significantly higher threshold and comfort levels than those with normal neural and cochlear structures. It could be argued that an outcome fitting method could minimise the variability across these maps, especially if working with infants who are potentially unable to provide the behavioural information required for establishing level of comfort.

## 22.5 The First Mapping Session: Initial Activation

Device activation or switch on of the cochlear implant may deliver outcomes that do not match the expectations of the recipient and their family. Factors such as when the device is to be activated, the steps involved and maximising access to sound as early as possible can be pivotal in shaping outcomes. The objective for device activation is to ensure that the recipient has access to sound and is comfortable, it is unrealistic (although in some cases possible) to expect open set listening abilities at switch on.

## 22.6 Timing of the Initial Activation

Advances in surgical techniques include less invasive incisions leading to improvements in healing time. Initial activation of the cochlear implant is reliant on the healing of the post aural scar and reduction of resultant swelling. Historically the general timing of device activation ranged from 4 to 6 weeks following surgery [9] which has continued to be the standard of care for some clinics. A reduction to 2–4 weeks was observed in the early 2010s [13].

The timing of initial device activation continues to vary amongst and within clinics; however, evidence gathered over recent years has clearly demonstrated that device activation within 1 week [14] and as soon as 24 h after surgery is safe and feasible irrespective of the type of sound processor: behind the ear (BTE) or off the ear (OTE) [15, 16].

Electrode impedances were the only measurement that was found to be significantly different between early and later device activation, however, after 2 months of device use, impedances were not significantly different [14–16].

Some evidence exists suggesting that OTE sound processor fitting may need to be delayed due to the potential need for stronger magnets due to possible swelling around the implant site [15]. Individual variation exists in suitability for early device activation. Hence patient-centric care should consider factors such as healing rate, sound processor type (OTE fitting may be later due to post-surgical swelling and need to optimise magnet retention).

## 22.7 The Activation

Information used to set the first map on a recipient's sound processor will vary across clinics and manufacturers. The use of intraoperative measurements and surgical information can minimise the amount of behavioural information and potential variability that the recipient may experience.

In the early 2010s the suggested protocols and procedures for device activation were described as outlined in Table 22.1.

Technological differences cannot account for the disparity given these methodologies were advocated in 2013–2014. Neither framework is superior to the other,

**Table 22.1** Variations in the device activation process

| Steps/ Considerations | Vaerenberg [9] | Mueller and Reine [17] | Botros et al. [10] |
|---|---|---|---|
| 1 | Connect the processor 4 weeks after surgery | Device activation to be conducted by qualified personnel | Connect the processor any time from 1 day after surgery |
| 2 | Measure impedances and deactivate electrodes identified as short or open circuit | Equipment check | Impedances are automatically measured and faulty electrodes deactivated automatically |
| 3 | Measure maximum level behaviourally on a number of electrodes and interpolate others | Fitting according to manufacturer's specifications and directions | Use intraoperative eCAP measures or measure AutoNRT (eCAP) |
| 4 | Set the minimum level to 0 for Med-El, 10% for AB, and determine a minimum level and interpolate for Cochlear and Oticon Medical | Device orientation and explanation | Activate the microphone and increase the master volume |
| 5 | Perform loudness balancing by presenting a signal on all electrodes successively | Written materials are given | Check loudness and verify access to Ling sounds |
| 6 | Reduce the maximum level and then switch on the microphone | Open access to the clinic and ongoing support over time | Implement behavioural adjustment of threshold or comfort levels if indicated through verification |
| 7 | Let the CI recipient accommodate for a few minutes and then check loudness tolerance to voice and other sounds in the environment | | Two maps are automatically written |
| 8 | Put a number of progressive maps in the processor | | |
| 9 | The patient to accommodate to each programme for a couple of days and switch to the next one afterwards. | | |

however, the key criteria for considering which methodology to use will be based on the clinics understanding of the recipient and their needs, in particular for infants and children, or those with cognitive impairment that may be unable to perform the degree of behavioural testing required. Particularly at the time of device activation when such procedures are unfamiliar.

Methodologies that incorporate more objective measures that have the potential to minimise variability whilst optimising outcomes will be addressed below.

## 22.8 Binaural Integration and Maximising the Auditory Environment

It is essential to acknowledge the importance of the auditory system having good access to a symmetrical signal across the speech spectrum to minimise the disruption to binaural place level and timing cues [18].

Historically cochlear implants were only unilaterally implanted. Research and clinical outcomes have demonstrated the value of bilateral cochlear implantation, bimodal (hearing aid and cochlear implant) device use and with the preservation of residual hearing in the ear with the cochlear implant utilisation of an electroacoustic cochlear implant system. Simultaneous bilateral cochlear implant surgeries are recommended for children with symmetrical hearing losses and for adults who have vision impairment [11]. Unilateral cochlear implant recipients may benefit from a sequential cochlear implantation, with research indicating narrowing the gap between surgeries for both adults and children [19–21]. Implementation of these recommendations will differ according to the funding structures available within a country or region.

Maximising the binaural benefit requires programming of the both devices with verification to ensure a symmetrical signal irrespective of the device configuration. CI Manufacturer software has inbuilt mechanisms for the provision of bilateral balancing of loudness, and adjustments of acoustic components with devices. Bimodal programming for fitting a hearing aid and a cochlear implant within the one platform of software and hardware are quickly becoming an expected feature within manufacturer's software.

## 22.9 Standards of Care for Cochlear Implants

It is assumed clinics are aligned in achieving the best outcomes for their patients, yet explicit standards of care do not exist. The Delphi Consensus [22] is a landmark initiative to facilitate global well-being of adults with bilateral moderate-severe to profound hearing loss. The twenty statements of the consensus [22] stand to shape the clinical approach for adults who will benefit from cochlear implants and for those currently using them.

The Delphi consensus is aligned with trends over the past decade that place more emphasis on holistic models of service delivery [23] pre-empting the catalyst to question and revise approaches for the cochlear implant journey overall. Historically, procedures and protocols used for assessment and monitoring were focussed on gathering data originally needed to prove cochlear implant efficacy that is no longer required.

Consensus of CI care was initiated by a network of clinics that developed clinical standards, with adherence being voluntary [24]. The development of these standards highlighted the range of expertise and professionals who are delivering services. It was established cochlear implant programming was being conducted by audiologists, clinical scientists, physiologists, speech pathologists, engineers, clinical physiologists and medically trained doctors or otologists. The rehabilitation can be provided by all of the above mentioned in addition to specific roles of rehabilitation therapists, hearing therapists, and speech and language therapists [17]. Whilst each of these professionals has post-graduate training, the focus and interpretation of tasks may differ according to their areas of expertise. Due to rapid changes in the field, review of such standards are recommended every 5 years [25] to ensure they are reflective of current clinical practice.

In considering standard of cochlear implant care, The WHO International Classification of Function (ICF) [23] framework outlines a core set of classifications for hearing field and provides terms of reference in models of care. Facilitation of activity and participation through hearing health care is the imperative through addressing disability in body structure and function [26] (see Fig. 22.3).

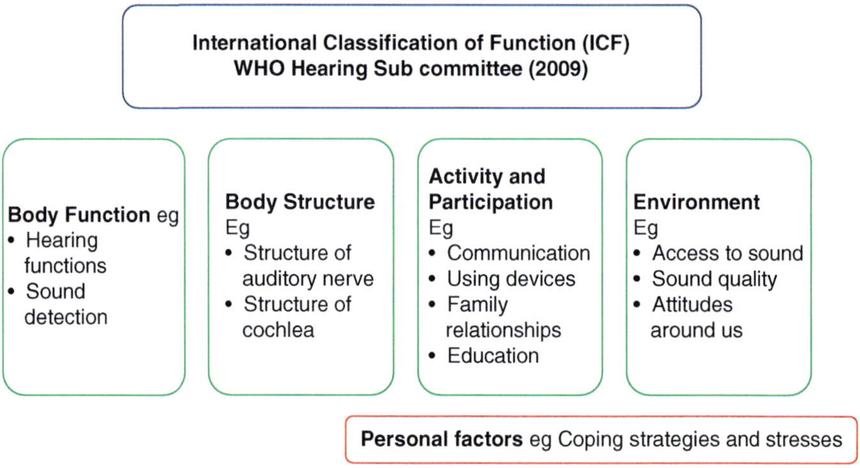


**Fig. 22.3** WHO-ICF [23] for hearing—whilst the fitting of cochlear implants addresses body function and structure consideration of how they can be used to facilitate activity and participation in various environments and individual characteristics underpins the recommendation for bespoke client centred care

## 22.10 Factors Impacting Variability in Cochlear Implant Programming

### 22.10.1 Self-Regulation of Clinical Training and Practice

With a range of commercially available cochlear implant systems, some clinics may specialise in one brand, either through choice or due to mandates from governing bodies. Other clinics may offer multiple brands to their patients. Training in cochlear implant programming is initially provided by cochlear implant manufacturers. There are very limited independently facilitated courses worldwide that will provide specific modules on cochlear implant programming, and certification is not available. Training usually occurs within the workplace by an internal subject matter expert.

This can lead to variability in approaches within clinics and between clinics in how cochlear implant recipients are managed. Research to reflect differences in approach is impacted by individual characteristics of recipients.

### 22.10.2 Increasing Installed Base of Cochlear Implant Recipient

Growth of cochlear implant recipients is exponential across the globe with activity increasing in emerging markets. Long established clinics have an increasing installed base that progressively increases over time. The level of care the clinic provides in the ongoing mapping and rehabilitation will be impacted by the capacity of the clinic to provide and afford to deliver such services. Modifications to protocols for scheduling recall appointments, reduction of appointment times, and increasing use of self-management are solutions that are being offered to facilitate more efficiencies within clinics, whilst shifting the loci of management to the recipient, thus endorsing patient-centred care practices.

Integration of cochlear implant services into mainstream clinical practices that are not specifically dedicated to cochlear implant programming has led to a shift in the genre of professions involved in mapping who may not have the length of experience or depth of knowledge that specialised clinics traditionally have held.

### 22.10.3 Reimbursement for Cochlear Implant Programming

Reimbursement for the provision of cochlear implant services differs across the globe from a total user pay to a total government-funded approach. The number of cochlear implant programming and or (re)habilitation sessions can often be determined by the cost implications for the clinic. The addition of self-management tools to recipients can potentially mitigate the number of sessions required in the future and make cochlear implant service delivery a more financially viable.

Psarros [27] performed a cost analysis of delivering 10 years of cochlear implant mapping and follow-up services to adult recipients. The financial impact of the frequency of appointments in the acute mapping phase led to a loss in revenue until the 5 years post-operative period. It is anticipated that self-management techniques, and more automated methods of programming over time, may reduce the time factors and number of episodes of service required.

## 22.11 Drivers of Methodological Changes in Cochlear Implant Mapping

### 22.11.1 Remote Programming

CI services are generally only available in larger cities [28] or via "outreach" services that require the audiologist/hearing health care provider to travel to different sites, potentially limiting access to programming and rehabilitation.

Difficulties with travel and the associated cost, possible time away from work or school, and the stress of travelling long distances to CI centres on a regular basis, raises many challenges for geographically remote patients and their families. Further, it is not always time- or cost-effective for the professionals providing the "outreach" services to travel to the patients. In other cases, the barrier may not always be distance. For example urban patients with social, economic, mobility, or transportation issues also may have difficulty accessing services.

The application of telepractice for CI management was first documented by Frank et al. [29] with their description of remote mapping and intraoperative monitoring. More recent research has demonstrated the use of remote intraoperative evaluation during CI surgery.

Telepractice has been well validated and is an efficient and effective method of delivering cochlear implant programming and rehabilitation [30]. The adoption of telepractice in cochlear implant service delivery was consolidated throughout the COVID-19 pandemic in 2020 and continues to be effectively used thereafter (Video 22.2).

As with device programming (re)habilitation can effectively be delivered within the clinic or using telepractice. Home-based interventions provide the natural environment specific to the child and family's needs [31]. The use of telepractice to provide habilitation for children with hearing loss has been well documented in the literature [2, 32]. Guiding principles for telepractice with children who have vision or hearing loss have been developed for this purpose [33]. This home-based model of service delivery has excellent application for consideration when extending telepractice to CI mapping.

## 22.12 Self-Management

Models of delivering remote programming are mostly still reliant on a clinician-led experience, and whilst the recipient plays and active role in the process, they do not have the autonomy to adjust their devices. Cullington [34] proposed that there be a shift toward removing the clinic-driven routine. Self-monitoring through a self-administered speech in noise test, self-adjustment of the device when indicated and online support was trialled. Outcomes measured found that functional listening performance was superior for the group who self-managed their cochlear implants compared to those who continued to use a traditional within clinic model. Feasibility and acceptance of a self-care model were determined with bilateral and unilateral cochlear implant recipients experiencing greater empowerment when accessing that model.

This project included users of devices from four cochlear implant manufacturers.

One manufacturer, Cochlear Ltd., had a commercially available tool, Remote Check, to deliver a self-care method of adjusting their device. Other components of the test battery such as the Triple Digit Test to check speech in noise required the use of a loan iPad and the functional listening questionnaire (the SSQ8) was administered at the end of the study. The online support group was accessed via the recipient's computer.

The Remote Check provides the same suite of tests that Cullington [35] used. Remote check runs through a series of assessments that can be tailored to the client's needs, and then reviewed by the clinician asynchronously. The recipient can perform some adjustments using their smartphone with the inclusion to review wound health through the use of the camera on the smartphone. Thus the steps in a typical clinic session can be self-managed by the recipient. This tool can be used for children by proxy through their parents or caregivers (Video 22.3).

## 22.13 Objective Measures from Surgery

Prior to the inclusion of a monopolar electrode on multichannel cochlear implants, objective measures relied on the use of additional equipment to perform intraoperative objective electrophysiological measurements. These measurements provide information intraoperatively to surgeons on device placement and integrity whilst providing the clinician information for device activation and potentially post-operative programming. Use of objective measures such as electrical auditory brainstem responses (EABR), electrical stapedius reflex thresholds (ESRT), electrical compound action potentials (eCAP), and cortical evoked potentials (CAEPs) have all been used to predict the mapping requirements of the initial and then ongoing cochlear implant mapping [36–38].

Experiments with eCAP [37] were the catalyst to the development of commercial platforms that are embedded in manufacturers programming software today. Wave [39] measurements can be obtained by clinicians and by surgical teams intraoperatively without the need for additional testing equipment. There is some conjecture about the validity of this information in predicting the setting of cochlear implant mapping [40, 41]. Botros [42] found that with machine learning principles and evidence from recipient performance that a profile scaling approach could be added to the cochlear implant programming software to provide a prediction of the initial mapping requirements of patients in device activation. In cases where the recipients' eCAP could not be measured intraoperatively a population mean could be used to estimate what was required [10].

Objective measures research stands to revolutionise device programming by utilising the internal electrode array for self-measurements with EEG recordings. Without the need for additional equipment, information can be transferred remotely to the clinician to facilitate changes required. It is proposed that instead of recipients needing to attend the clinic, the diagnostics of their device use in the real world will capture information and flag the need for changes that can enable remote adjustment of devices as required rather than scheduled appointments at the clinic [43, 44].

## 22.14 Imaging

Whilst there is agreement that the standard cochlea has 2.5 turns and is 30 mm in length, there is considerable variability in cochlear shape and size. The use of pre-operative imaging to determine the electrode type can forewarn the surgeon of any potential trauma during insertion enabling personalisation of implant selection and surgical planning [45].

Post-operative imaging has been used to guide the allocation of frequencies to individual electrodes. Characteristic frequency mapping studies [46] are based on the Greenwood function [47] of tonotopicity of the peripheral auditory system. Greenwoods function [47] calculated that the most apical electrode of a cochlear implant array and coding information for 80–120 Hz was typically placed at the temporal spatial point where spiral ganglion cells detect 513 Hz. This mismatch had implications for the rest of the array. Studies were performed on experienced users of cochlear implants, and outcomes did not demonstrate significant improvements. Tailoring and reallocating the frequency allocation, based on the insertion angle of the electrode array and using a logarithmic algorithm has shown some promise [48]. Continued improvements to imaging procedures and programming technologies could enable the ability to create frequency-tailored maps that could potentially enhance outcomes [49, 50].

Improved imaging techniques include the use of cone beam CT [51]. Imaging information from the preoperative scans and intra or immediately post-operative scans provide the basis for implementation of algorithms that can isolate parameters to individually tailor CI maps [52].

Emergence of manufacturer-specific tools to monitor electrode insertion during surgery and perform objective measures, will provide information to the clinician activating the device and for subsequent fittings.

## 22.15 The Role of "Big Data" and "Artificial Intelligence"

Big data is driving change across all fields of health care, influencing technology development and enabling patient-centric and user-driven approaches that have traditionally required direct clinical and clinician-driven intervention. Accordingly, manufacturers are utilising machine learning to automate routine processes in the cochlear implant recipients' journey as well as providing digital options for self-management in the form of apps.

Use of smartphones, smart watches and mobile devices has become integrated into the lifestyle of many for monitoring levels of exercise, heart rate, and more specifically, for management of chronic health conditions such as diabetes. Informatics and digital health ecosystem is in its infancy [53] with government regulators for health care developing guidelines for manufacturers and consumers to protect cyber security [54]. As cochlear implant recipients increasingly become technologically literate and technology is more capable of providing programming opportunities direct to the recipient, manufacturers are looking toward more automated processes for cochlear implant programming that can be driven by the recipient as well as the clinician.

Whilst there is some hesitancy amongst clinicians to enable recipients to manipulate their own devices [35], the algorithms used for these processes have been designed to minimise error that could result from non-familiarity or lack of experience with software or products.

By empowering recipients and carers to adjust their devices in their own sound environments, they are thus optimising their listening outside of the clinical setting; a setting that is not reflective of their regular listening needs.

Meeurs [55] developed a Fitting Outcomes eXpert (FOX), which has been developed further to a second-generation tool using artificial intelligence (machine learning). Through a series of psychoacoustic processes, a recipient can generate a map tailored to their specific needs. The battery of tests utilised in FOX provide a target driven and objective way to derive the cochlear implant mapping and reduces the variability that can occur across and within clinics due to the absence of standardised training and variability in experience each cochlear implant device and manufacturer.

It should be noted methods as such FOX may not be beneficial for infants and young children and a proportion of adult cochlear implant recipients because of the intensive behavioural component. Utilisation of a combination of behavioural, automated and objective measures procedures provides a safer and more viable alternative [10].

## 22.16 Lifelong Management of the Cochlear Implant

### 22.16.1 Troubleshooting

Irrespective of whether an optimal signal has been obtained in device programming sessions, ensuring the recipients can efficiently and effectively handle and care for the devices may circumvent additional appointments and episodes of care. Confidence and autonomy in device usage promote the empowerment of the recipient. Standard training of device handling, in line with other aspects of cochlear implant programming and rehabilitation does not exist. Tools such as the Cochlear Implant Management Skills survey [56], however, have been validated to have a good inter-user and intra-user reliability. Such tools enable a patient-centric approach to ensure individual recipient needs are addressed and circumvent potential shortcomings of device handling that would otherwise require additional or unscheduled appointment times, or potential time where the recipient is off air due to non-functioning equipment.

Device manufacturers provide access to written instructional material and guidelines for troubleshooting in both hard copy and online formats. Social media and websites also facilitate a collective sharing of ideas and support.

Diagnostic tools and apps such as the Nucleus Smart App are available to recipients to check the functionality of their sound processor.

### 22.16.2 Ongoing Appointments

Statement 14 of the Delphi consensus [22] "Adults who have undergone cochlear implantation should receive programming sessions as needed to optimise outcomes".

Existing guidelines generally indicate between 4 and 8 appointments for device programming in the first 12 months after surgery [17]. Ongoing follow-ups are suggested for 6 or 12 monthly intervals. Galvin [57] looked at the longitudinal mapping data of 680 recipients at the Royal Victoria Eye and Ear Hospital in Melbourne reviewing psychophysical changes in the first 2 years after device activation. Most changes occurred within the first 3 months of device activation with a plateau of psychophysical changes thereafter. A proposed scheduling of a cluster of appointments in the first 3 months with a follow up in the second-year post-surgery, then again at year 5 was felt to address the recipient need based on the psychophysical evidence.

As the install base of cochlear implant centres grow exponentially each year such regularity of appointments calls upon the need for alternative approaches to accommodate recipient need and clinical resourcing. The model of care proposed by Cullington et al. evokes empowerment and the autonomy of lifelong management of the cochlear implant with the recipient, and thus removing the clinic-driven schedule. The parallels of using such an approach in (re)habilitation are becoming more apparent.

> *"I thought I would be different..I expected too much too soon. I thought you would have this thing and bang I would hear everything ..even though I was told otherwise. Now I know by experience doing some listening practice earlier would have helped me on my hearing journey—GK after 12 month evaluation with her CI"*

### 22.16.3 Why (Re)habilitation?

Statement 12 of the Delphi consensus [22] confirms that even after 40 years of CI there is considerable variability in outcomes following CI: "Many factors impact cochlear implant outcomes; further research is needed to understand the magnitude of the effects". Hence predictions of the longitudinal CI journey are not possible. Traditionally, (re)habilitation for cochlear implant recipients has focussed on maximising the integration of the auditory signal provided through the device into communication contexts. Infants and children require regular intervention to utilise the signal to facilitate the development of speech and language (spoken, signed, or bilingual). Early generations of cochlear implant technology when signal processing was less sophisticated required a strong focus on auditory training. Recent trends have developed a more holistic approach to ensure generalisation and integration of the cochlear implant signal and a focus on psychosocial factors and function.

### 22.16.4 Differentiating Habilitation and Rehabilitation

For the purposes of this chapter, the focus will be on rehabilitation rather than habilitation. "Habilitation" is a process aimed at enabling the development of new skills and knowledge. Rehabilitation can arguably have more of a physiological focus and refers to regaining skills that may have been lost or compromised through an acquired disability or due to a change in one's circumstances. As can be seen in Fig. 22.4, habilitation is developmentally centred for children who have a disability from birth or early infancy [58].

As with device programming, the overarching approach underpinning (re)habilitation has alignment with the WHO ICF Hearing [59] (see Fig. 22.2).

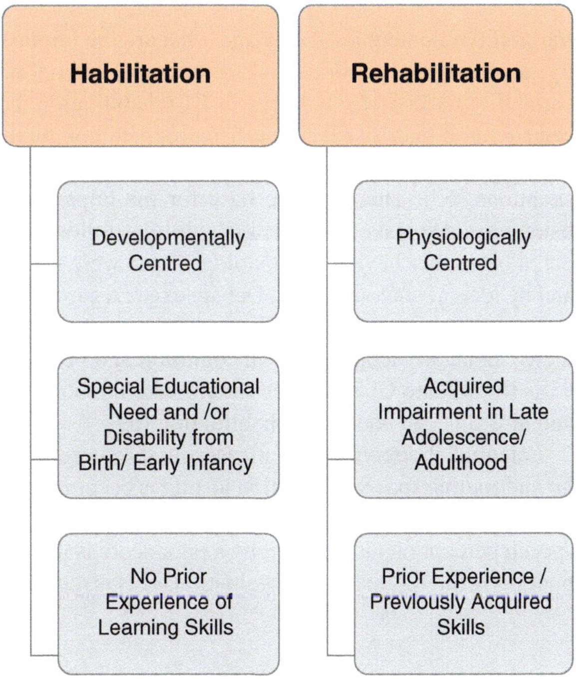


**Fig. 22.4** Key differences in habilitation and rehabilitation [58]

Traditionally cochlear implant rehabilitation has primarily focussed on the sensory management (Body Function and Body Structure) with minimal focus on activity and participation, environment and personal factors. Conversely, the focus on embedding habilitation within the achievement of developmental milestones provided a more holistic approach.

Following (ideally, early) identification of a moderate-severe to profound hearing loss, circumstances prevailing, infants and children begin the pathway to early cochlear implantation. This preoperative phase provides parents the opportunity to develop appropriate post-operative expectations that are pivotal in setting the foundation for optimal outcomes. Many studies have demonstrated the benefits of capitalising on the critical periods of neural development for amplification and cochlear implantation for bilateral and unilateral hearing loss [19, 60, 61]. Paediatric cochlear implant recipients are often enrolled in an early intervention, educational or a regular programme that integrates the use of listening into the child's environment using play and structure to develop communication (see Appendix). Early intervention programmes are recommended for children under the age of 6 years with the involvement of an interdisciplinary team to coach and support parents and caregivers in their child's habilitation [62, 63].

The benefits of family-focussed habilitation programmes for children have been published widely. Appendix provides links to a range of programmes across the globe that cater for paediatric habilitation.

### 22.16.5 Adult Rehabilitation

Variability in outcomes—why and what are the implications Considerable variability in outcomes for adults following cochlear implantation exists [39, 64]. Such variability necessitates tailoring of CI rehabilitation factoring in the recipients perceived and clinically identified listening and communication needs. These will be influenced by familiarity and experience with technology and their individual living situations [65]. The evidence base for the impact of rehabilitation on functional listening and social communication abilities following cochlear implantation is hindered by studies having methodologies that were not structured to identify absolute and incidental outcomes [66]. Debate exists regarding what skill adult rehabilitation is targeting. Listening is performed cognitively and perceived behaviourally, yet there can be an incongruence in cognition and behaviour [67, 68]. Development of tools to evaluate CI outcomes should take into consideration the role of cognition and how this can underpin rehabilitation [69].

Potential shortcomings of measuring the success of rehabilitation through regular and routine speech perception testing is becoming apparent [69]. Intrinsic factors such as verbal memory and neurocognitive function can influence performance on speech perception tasks, whereby a poor score is interpreted as the recipient being a poor performer. A battery of evaluation tools is required if measuring post-operative outcomes and the impact of rehabilitation. Studies to determine the efficacy of rehabilitation with adults need to focus on more than auditory training.

Setting, measuring, and achieving goals Aspects of auditory function as measured by reviewing client goals such as with the Client Oriented Scale of Improvement (COSI) [70] and functional performance questionnaires such as the SSQ and quality of life measures provide a much broader picture of client outcome as addressed in the WHO ICF model as shown in Lenarz [71]. Longitudinal improvements in quality of life and self-perceived benefits can provide closer assessment of real-world benefit for recipients [66].

The considerable variability in client outcomes [39] underpins the need for client-specific goals that are regularly tailored and adjusted at the individual's rate of progress. Realistic expectations and goals established well before device fitting pave the way to a smoother transition to acclimatisation to sound and the psychosocial implications of the access it provides [72]. Pichora-Fuller [73] highlights the cognitive energy needed to work on listening goals, particularly when adapting to a signal that is degraded for those who have previously had normal hearing. The degraded signal of the cochlear implant is even further highlighted for recipients who aspire for goals to appreciate music. The COSI [70] identifies up to five listening situations in which help with hearing is required. Attainable and measurable goals to reach in these listening situations are developed and reviewed at regular intervals with the recipient. The COSI [70] is a statistically valid measure that can be used routinely and has been integrated into the device programming software by Cochlear Ltd., Custom Sound Pro to facilitate the smooth link between device programming and rehabilitation. COSI goals can be updated and continue to be relevant throughout the recipient's entire cochlear implant journey as new listening experiences and challenges arise.

Evolution of rehabilitation and the emergence of holistic and patient-centred care Cochlear implant rehabilitation in the 1980s and early 1990s was structured around the principles used for working with severe to profoundly deaf adults who were gaining minimal benefits from hearing aids prior to the advent of cochlear implant technology. As described by Erber [74] "analytic auditory training takes a bottom-up approach, and is primarily focused on detection and discrimination of specific sounds, with the hope that the enhanced ability to detect and discriminate sounds will aid in identification and comprehension of a message".

Auditory training manuals that provided materials to move through the hierarchy (Fig. 22.5) were the focus of the "rehabilitation session". These manuals have been modified over the years [75] with a move toward more online materials. A key component of early auditory training included speech tracking [76] which more recently has been modified for a computer-based approach [77].

Auditory training was primarily conducted using the manuals, and as technology developed, more computer-based programmes. However, it was not until Martin [72] outlined the key principles for consideration in paediatric and adult (re)habilitation that a broadening of the key components required for effective rehabilitation

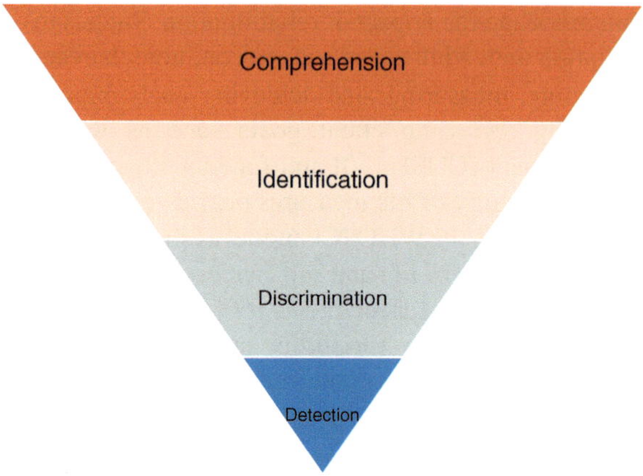


**Fig. 22.5** The auditory hierarchy

was outlined. Specifically, for adults, Martin [72] stressed prior to cochlear implant surgery, the need for clear post-operative systematic auditory and auditory visual training and communication skills training. Therapy was to include all or some the following

- Counselling.
- Auditory analytic and synthetic tasks.
- Speech reading.
- Communication skills training (conversation techniques, repair strategies, assertiveness training, interpersonal skills and coping mechanisms).
- Voice therapy (articulation, rhythm, and speech production).
- Guidance (information on the auditory system and hearing loss, effects of hearing loss on communication; impact of background noise and poor listening conditions; the importance of visual input, audio-visual integration and attending behaviour, the impact of speaker differences and social conditions; benefits and limitations of speech reading; benefits and limitations of the assistive devices; the use of community resources; self-help groups.
- Assistive listening devices.

Delivery of the rehabilitation could be individual and or within groups and could include significant others and should continue for the year after surgery and beyond.

Boothroyd [78] outlined that each recipient brings their own set of personal attributes (see Table 22.2). Clinical guidance and the provision of the relevant tools to derive measure and achieve goals must encompass intrinsic and extrinsic considerations.

Tang et al. [65] advocated for the consideration and inclusion of adjunct support and services, including the tailoring of CI rehabilitation sessions depending on the patient's familiarity with technology and living situation. Models of rehabilitation service delivery are not "one size fits all". The composition, intensity, and duration of rehabilitation will vary.

**Table 22.2** Boothroyd's [78] intrinsic and extrinsic factors impacting service delivery (2009)

| |
|---|
| Motivation |
| Readiness |
| Personality |
| Adaptability |
| Expectations |
| Perceived locus of control |
| Lifestyle |
| Function in other areas, e.g. cognition |
| Auditory ecology |
| Resources available to them |
| Support from significant others |

Holistic and patient-centred approaches such as informational counselling and self-management strategies as well as direct training approaches to listening have all been encouraged [78, 79]. At the core of these approaches is the bespoke approach that is taking the recipients intrinsic and extrinsic factors into account. Boothroyd [78] defines adult aural rehabilitation as a means of reducing hearing loss-induced deficits of function activity and participation and quality of life through a combination of sensory management, instructional, perceptual training and counselling in alignment with the WHO ICF Hearing outlined earlier in Fig. 22.2.

Boothroyd's [78] landmark paper outlines the key components of adult rehabilitation—managing the hearing loss (e.g. device fitting); instruction on how to use devices and expectations; specific perceptual training and counselling. All four components should be embedded and not approached in a linear fashion. By deeply embedding the goals and planning for cochlear implant rehabilitation in the preoperative process and within cochlear mapping sessions, the continuity of care for lifelong management of devices and maximising of outcomes can be achieved. The intrinsic and extrinsic considerations for rehabilitation for adults will inevitably change over time therefore rehabilitation and support needs to shift in accordance with the recipient needs over time. For example the lifestyle of a recipient when they are 21 will be quite different to when they are 50. Whilst they continue to use their devices, continuity of care can be adjusted to account for lifestyle changes (See Fig. 22.6).

Ferguson et al. [80] identified four cornerstones of rehabilitation. (1) Hearing and Listening devices. (2) Knowledge and skills. (3) Auditory and cognitive training. (4) Motivational engagement. Their research with models of rehabilitation using self-management and behaviour changes was found to be the core of patient-centred approaches to address the need to facilitate auditory function, activity, participation, and quality of life for adults with hearing loss [80].

More recently, in keeping with trends for programming to be less centre driven and more client driven, however, some of the barriers preventing these from being embraced are as follows:

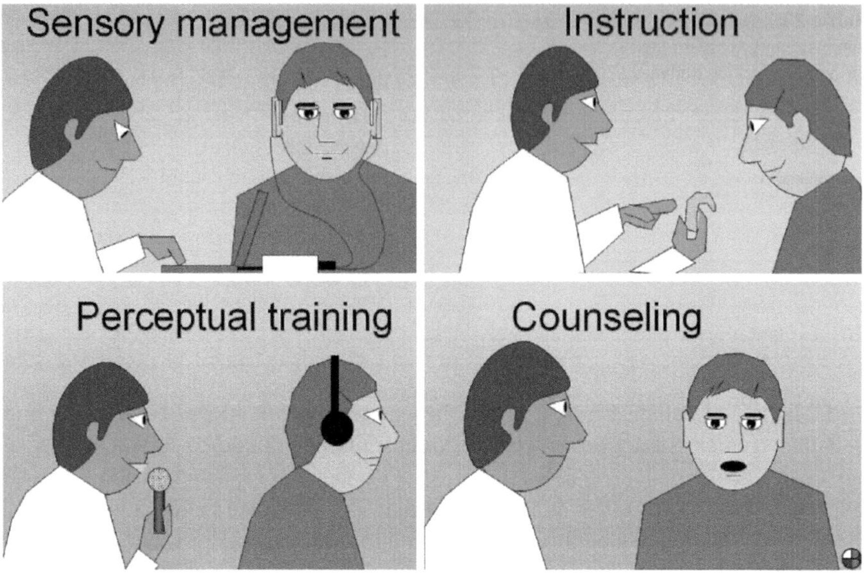


**Fig. 22.6** Key components of adult rehabilitation [78]

### 22.16.6 Barriers to Rehabilitation

1. Time and reimbursement

   Whilst it is clear that some form of rehabilitation including auditory training is recommended, 85.5% of 78 clinicians surveyed acknowledged the importance of auditory training following cochlear implantation [81]. However, the delivery of this was widely variable with the modality of service delivery either clinic-based, which was more costly to the clinician and the client, or home-based, which had lower costs. The provision of rehabilitation sessions in isolation to device programming sessions in some countries and clinics is not reimbursed and could be impacting on the delivery of essential standards of care. Dunn et al. [82] highlighted that the typical professional session with a cochlear implant recipient is bound by time constraints to focus more on the programming, testing, and troubleshooting with little time left for counselling let alone addressing some of the listening challenges experienced that could be addressed through rehabilitation.
2. Limitations of technology

   Whilst the focus of early cochlear implant rehabilitation was for auditory training the importance of inclusion of music perception in rehabilitation was the focus of research to address the issue that cochlear implant devices have limited capacity to process music to the same extent they can speech [83]. Cochlear implant recipients frequently reported a degraded appreciation of music through their cochlear implants than if they previously had normal hearing [84]. Music training programmes generally focus on melody, pitch, and timbre, however, those that have most real-world relevance are those requiring identification of sung lyrics with music that has close relevance to being able to process speech in background noise. Gfeller et al. [84] reported that 90% of her cohort of recipients were motivated to have rehabilitation specific to music, however preferred real-world "personally meaningful" tasks. Music training has however been found to have some overarching benefits for discrimination of speech in background noise [84].

3. Psychosocial factors

   The psychosocial implications of listening effort in real-world situations, in particular for music, has been observed to lead to withdrawal from social experiences that involve music (Dritsakis) [85] whilst other recipients can be motivated by the challenge to immerse themselves in tasks to improve performance [73]. Regardless, as Gfeller et al. [84] observed, the prevalence of CI users who exert effort in noisy listening situations can have long-term health implications. They found that therapy that targets culturally relevant and individualised music tastes may serve to circumvent some of the stresses. The psychosocial impact of struggling in adverse listening situations on social connection can be a significant barrier to optimising CI recipient outcomes. Hence, the development of problems solving strategies to mitigate this struggle will in turn help facilitate the integration of rehabilitation into real-world situations where recipients have experienced difficulty.

### 22.16.7 Facilitators for Rehabilitation

#### 22.16.7.1 m-Health (Mobile-Health)

With the emergence of m-health (mobile-health: using mobile devices and apps in health care), the use of App's for home-based monitoring and therapy has become more prevalent in health care. Figure 22.7 demonstrates the rate at which adults globally using m-health compared to other genre of Apps:

- https://www.statista.com/statistics/1180843/health-related-mobile-apps-worldwide-number-by-focus/

Olsen et al. [86] identified five out of 239 possible Apple's on App Stores that met the following criteria (1) available in English, (2) designed for adults, (3) included speech auditory training stimuli, (4) ability to download and use, (5) incorporation of evidence-based auditory learning principles (6) free and (7) potential for independent use by adult with hearing loss [86]. Olsen et al. [86] then submitted the Apps to the System Usability System to identify areas that would need to be trained specifically when supporting cochlear implant recipients of all ages when using these Apps. See Table 22.3.

In keeping with the patient centre holistic models advocated by Boothroyd [78] and Grenness [79], home-based auditory training apps can be included in a

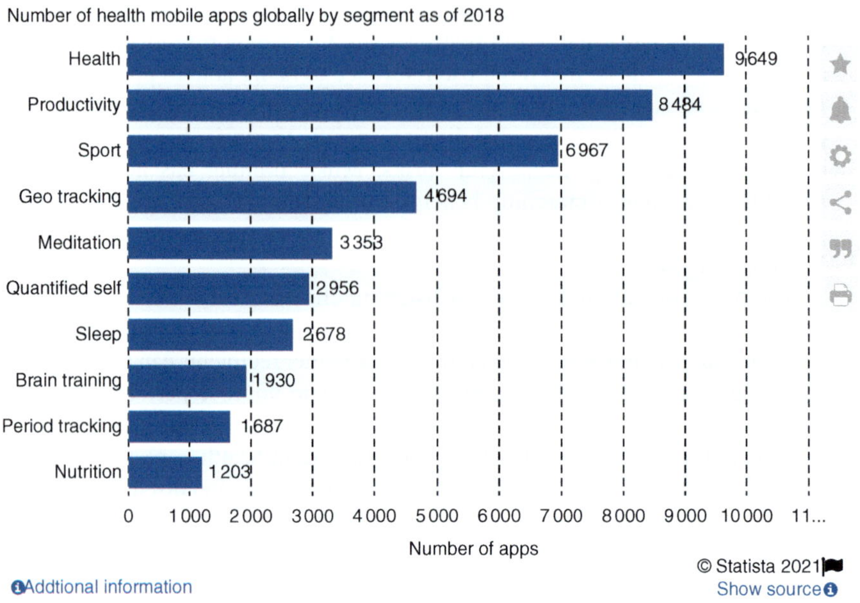


**Fig. 22.7** Number of health mobile apps by segment (Stata)

**Table 22.3** Auditory training App's for adults aged >65 years [86]

| Name | Clarity of visual layout | Instructions | Estimated need for training |
|---|---|---|---|
| | Relatively small font, good colour contrast | Instructions provided prior to each level of game, but no overall set of directions | Clients would need some training/guidance to determine which game to play |
| AB clix | Adequate font and colour contrast | Instructions appear when first opening app and for each level of activity selected | Clients would need some instruction on how to set up and use app |
| Games 4 Hearoes | Adequate font and clear icons used | Each game provides a set of instructions | Clients would need minimal instruction if any |
| Speech Banana | Clear icons, but relatively smaller font used | Minimal instruction provided | Clients would need some training to navigate different options when first using |
| iAngel sound | Relatively small font | Minimal instruction provided | Clients would need some training to navigate different options when first using |

recipient's rehabilitation programme. The clinician and the recipient can collaborate on relevance and content of Apps (collaborative decision making). The autonomy with the digital platforms can also serve to bridge the gap for the social connectivity that may emerge.

### 22.16.8 Self-Management in Adult Rehabilitation

Clinician support in rehabilitation can maximise the effectiveness of rehabilitation through the provision of clarity of direction, monitoring, establishment of support networks, feedback and encouragement, and ensuring that any self-driven training is at the level appropriate to optimise outcomes for the individual. Professionals and recipients can collaborate in lifelong cochlear implant support through the use of App's such as Cochlear CoPilot. Professionals work with the recipient to establish a personalised training and support path that can be implemented to build on knowledge of device use, develop, and refine auditory skills in a range of listening environments (see Fig. 22.8). The tasks are automatically updated as the APP tracks the recipient's usage and progress facilitating a specific tailoring of support.

Cochlear CoPilot focusses on the building of knowledge and the building of skills. The platform provides opportunities for recipient empowerment by keeping them well versed in latest trends, research, and advances to ensure the highest standard of care.

The evidence of the impact of rehabilitation is exacerbated when recipients have a plateau in their performance or the achievement's they make decline over time when rehabilitation is withdrawn and reduced [75]. Long-term users of cochlear implants have changing needs and requirements for their communication social demands and their cognitive ability to perform auditory processing. The Cochlear CoPilot addresses the need for "learning across the lifespan" (see Fig. 22.9a, b) by leveraging the principles of brain plasticity, perceptual learning and adult education. Further its health literacy focus ensures that the language and media used are relevant for the recipient. The empowerment principle of Cochlear CoPilot is through the focus and enrichment of what the client can do and places the control within their own means with the relevant support as required. The role of significant others

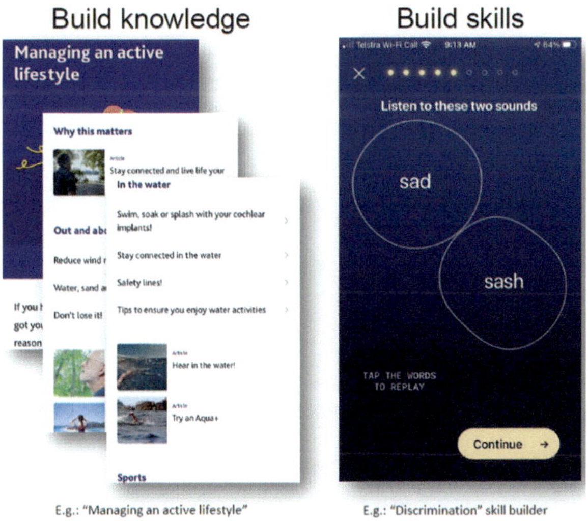


**Fig. 22.8** Cochlear CoPilot sample activities, e.g. Managing and active lifestyle and discrimination skill builder

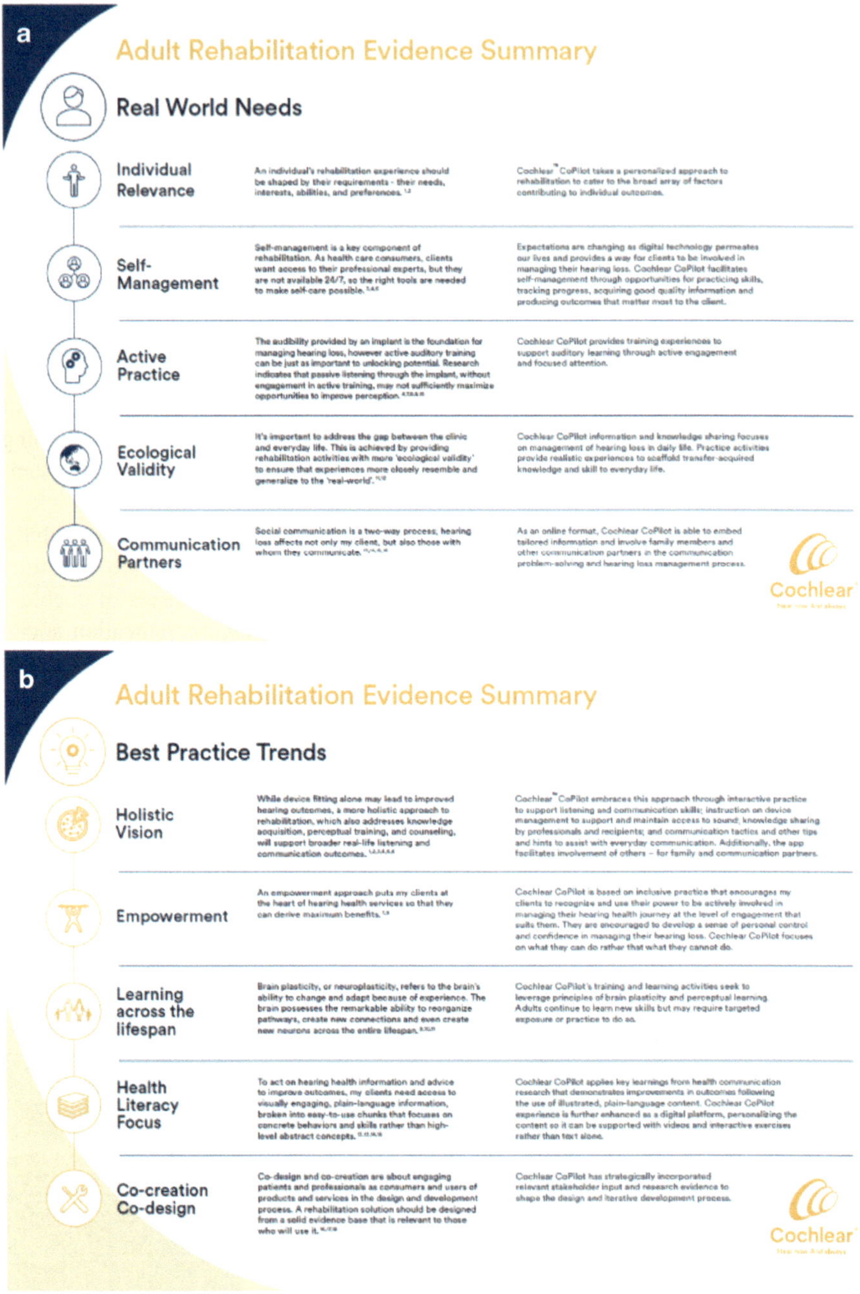


**Fig. 22.9** (**a**) Cochlear CoPilot best practice trends. (**b**) Cochlear CoPilot evidence summary

and communication partners is key to the success of the Cochlear CoPilot with tailored activities ensuring relevant stakeholders can engage in the recipient's rehabilitation process, which leads to more active engagement and more fluidity in the transition of the skills learnt into the recipients every day environment. This is further enhanced by the inclusion of active engagement in activities using artificial intelligence to emulate conversational exchange and the opportunity to practice "real life" situations.

Overcoming the issue of variability in outcomes Cochlear CoPilot provides individual relevance by accounting for the factors that have been identified to lead to variability in outcomes. Its holistic packaging of includes interactive practice of listening and communication skills, guideline's for device management and troubleshooting, collaborative support from other recipients and specific communication tactics and tips and hints.

Self-management of rehabilitation facilitates a longitudinal approach in which recipients continue to learn and refine auditory skills beyond passive assimilation of auditory input [87]. Drouin et al. [87] advocate that active engagement in rehabilitation can tap into the neural plasticity of human speech perception and adaptation to a range of listening environments. They believe this is best served through a blend of self-directed and clinician-supported approaches. There is, however, little evidence available on how frequent auditory training is required to facilitate the neuroplasticity required to establish a skill. Ericcson [88] indicated that a new task needed to be completed over 10,000 h before mastering a skill, and that performance level positively correlated with the time spent practicing! Regardless of the time spent, the nature of the task, the relevance and the goals will impact greatly on what is required for adult cochlear implant recipients to embrace and optimise their outcomes with their cochlear implants.

**Group Approaches**

In recent times during the COVID-19 pandemic, the use of digital connectivity became the primary means for communication across all age groups and for work, recreation, education and family life. Newly implanted cochlear implant recipients who were unable to attend in situ clinical sessions were still requiring rehabilitation with some clinics using a combination of Apps and in some clinics online training. Hearing Implants Australia [89] used telepractice to facilitate socialisation as well as auditory training opportunities between recipients in a group setting. Training needs of group participants were evaluated using the COSI before-hand and this helped establish streams of groups to enable recipients with similar goals to work together.

The groups factored in recommended principles advocated by Boothroyd [78]. As seen in Fig. 22.3 they captured the basic principles for providing a holistic approach to rehabilitation. Fourteen recipients across four states of Australia would attend these sessions at any one time (see Table 22.4).

**Table 22.4** Group therapy using telepractice [89]

| Principle | Example |
|---|---|
| Sensory management | Device usage and accessing digital technology and maximising the signal quality |
| Instructions | Presentation and discussion group on topic of interest, e.g. managing your device in background noise; importance of the "Men's shed programme" |
| Perceptual training | Auditory training exercises—Closed (bingo) and open set (trivia) |
| Counselling | Turn taking activities and sharing of experiences |

Whilst this procedure was not validated nor part of formal research, such initiatives can provide recipients with better connectivity to their devices and the confidence to use them in a range of listening situations, as reflected in the testimony of group members, some of whom also participated in remote programming of their devices during the COVID-19 pandemic (Video 22.4).

The goal of group intervention is to facilitate a successful transition to identifying oneself as hearing impaired without stigma. It achieves this goal by creating a group setting where people work together to generate localised normative practices that emotionally and practically support clients' social functioning and well-being. Furthermore, a shared identity emerges among clients in the programme. This identity is a basis for providing, receiving, and benefiting from social support. It provides individuals with the emotional, intellectual, and material resources to resist (i.e. question, challenge, and oppose) the stigmatisation they may experience and/or fear. It also provides a broader network of people who are ready to engage in processes of rejection and modification of negative stereotypes, a process that may become increasingly important in countries with aging populations.

## 22.17 Conclusion

Over more than 40 years there has been significant change as the cochlear implant has evolved from a research device to support lip-reading for profoundly deaf adults to a versatile hearing implant with thousands of recipients worldwide developing and maintaining typical listening, speech, language, and cognitive skills. In the earliest days, cochlear implant mapping was a lengthy and difficult task, driven by the clinician and isolated to specialised cochlear implant clinics. Recipients needed rehabilitation for their communication, however, very limited improvements in communication could be demonstrated, even with ongoing and sustained practice. Fast-forward to 2021, and we can see a reversal of the time and expectations around these tasks; programming cochlear implants have become faster, simpler and more accurate, and rehabilitation goals broader and greater as recipients and clinicians explore innovative ways to embark on a lifelong endeavour to improve and maintain communication and social skills. The ultimate shifts have been propelled along by the worldwide COVID-19 pandemic, where limitations on accessing services saw clinicians and recipients embrace programming and rehabilitation approaches that were online and self-directed. The range of recent advances has all served to prioritise the individual needs of the individual using a cochlear implant and place them at the very centre of their own care.

## Appendix

Websites for information regarding paediatric habiliation

- https://www.agbell.org/
- https://www.firstvoice.org.au/
- https://www.soundsteps.uk/
- https://avtdirect.com
- https://apps.apple.com/in/app/avtar-app/id1462413057
- https://play.google.com/store/apps/developer?id=avtar+,+Ritu+Nakra,avtar+app
- www.hearingfirst.org

Websites for auditory training for older children, teens and adults

- https://www.healthyhearing.com/report/51752-Exercise-your-ears-apps-and-games-to-keep-hearing-sharp
- https://www.hearinglink.org/your-hearing/implants/self-guided-rehabilitation/

## References


1. Psarros C, McMahon C. Tele-practice in audiology, Chapter 3. In: Houston KT, Rushbrooke E, editors. Evaluating the benefits of a tele-practice model. San Diego, CA: Plural; 2015.
2. Leigh JR, Moran M, Hollow R, Dowell RC. Evidence-based guidelines for recommending cochlear implantation for postlingually deafened adults. Int J Audiol. 2016;55(Suppl 2):S3–8. https://doi.org/10.3109/14992027.2016.1146415.
3. Newbold C, Richardson R, Seligman P, et al. Electrode stimulation causes rapid changes in electrode impedance of cell-covered electrodes. J Neural Eng. 2011;8(3)
4. Rance G, Dowell RC. Cochlear implantation for infants and children: advances. In: Clark GM, Cowan RSC, Dowell RC, editors. Speech processor programming. San Diego, CA: Singular Publishing Group; 1997. p. 147–70.
5. Museik F, Shinn J, Shermak G. Perspectives of the pure tone audiogram. J Am Acad Audiol. 2017;28:655–71.
6. Ling D. The six-sound test. In: Estabrooks W, editor. Auditory-verbal therapy and practice. Washington, DC: Alexander Graham Bell Association for the Deaf and Hard of Hearing; 2006. p. 207–310.
7. Gatehouse S, Noble W. The speech, spatial and qualities of hearing scale (SSQ). Int J Audiol. 2004;43(2):85–99. https://doi.org/10.1080/14992020400050014.
8. Botros A, Abrahams Y, Psarros C. Outcome focused fitting methodology using patient centred design. Suwanee: White Paper Cochlear; 2020.
9. Vaerenberg B, Smits C, De Ceulaer G, et al. Cochlear implant programming: a global survey on the state of the art. Sci World J. 2014;2014:501738. https://doi.org/10.1155/2014/501738.

10. Botros A, Banna R, Maruthurkkara S. The next generation of nucleus ® fitting: a multiplatform approach towards universal cochlear implant management. Int J Audiol. 2013;52:485–94.
11. NICE. All rights reserved. Subject to notice of rights. https://www.nice.org.uk/terms-andconditions# notice-of-rights page 30 of 30; 2020.
12. Incerti PV, Teresa YC, Ching SH, et al. Programming characteristics of cochlear implants in children: effects of aetiology and age at implantation. Int J Audiol. 2018;57:S27–40. https://doi.org/10.1080/14992027.2017.1370139.
13. Upson G, Rodriguez S. Clinical guidelines for adult Cochlear implantation. Perth: Health Networks Branch, Department of Health, Western Australia; 2013.
14. Diao M, Sun J, Tian F, et al. Cochlear implant device activation after 7 days in cochlear implant recipients. Eur Arch Otorhinolaryngol. 2018;276:1–7. https://doi.org/10.1007/s00405-018-5129-7.
15. Batuk MO, Yarali M, Cinar BC, et al. Is early Cochlear implant device activation safe for all on-the-ear and off-the-ear sound processors? Audiol Neurotol. 2019;24:279–84. https://doi.org/10.1159/000503378.
16. Hagr AR, Garadat S, Almomani M, Alsabellha R, Al-Muhawas F. Feasibility of one-day activation in cochlear implant recipients. Int J Audiol. 2015;54:1–6. https://doi.org/10.3109/14992027.2014.996824.
17. Mueller J, Reine CR. Quality standards for adults cochlear implantation. Cochlear Implants Int. 2013;14:S2.
18. Gordon KA, Cushing SL, Easwar V, Polonenko MJ, Papsin BC. Binaural integration: a challenge to overcome for children with hearing loss. Curr Opin Otolaryngol Head Neck Surg. 2017 Dec;25(6):514–9. https://doi.org/10.1097/MOO.0000000000000413.
19. Sharma A, Glick H. Cortical neuroplasticity in hearing loss: why it matters in clinical decision-making for children and adults Hear Rev. https://www.hearingreview.com/hearing-loss/hearing-disorders/apd/cortical-neuroplasticity-hearing-loss-matters-clinical-decision-making-children-adults, 2018.
20. Polonenko MJ, Papsin BC, Gordon KA. Limiting asymmetric hearing improves benefits of bilateral hearing in children using cochlear implants. Scientific Report in Nature; 2018.
21. Au A, Dowell RC. Evidence based criteria for bilateral cochlear implantation in adults. Am J Audiol. 2019;28(3S):775–82.
22. Buchman C, Gifford R, Haynes D, et al. Developing international consensus on the use of unilateral cochlear implants for bilateral severe, profound, or moderate sloping to profound sensorineural hearing loss in adults. Delphi Consensus Group on Cochlear implantation in adults. Poste presented at CI2019: 16th symposium on Cochlear implants in children, July 11–13, 2019, Hollywood, FL, USA, 2019. https://adulthearing.com/. Accessed 18 Mar 2021.
23. World Health Organisation. International classification of functioning, disability, and health. Geneva, Switzerland: World Health Organisation; 2001.
24. Punte AK, van der Heyning P. Quality standards for minimal outcome measurements in adults and children. Cochlear Implants Int. 2013;2:S39–42.
25. Adunka OF, Gantz BJ, Dunn C, et al. Minimum reporting standards for adult Cochlear implantation. Otolaryngol Head Neck Surg. 2018;159(2):215–9. https://doi.org/10.1177/0194599818764329.
26. Danemark B, Kramer S, Hickson L, et al. Development of ICF core sets for hearing loss. Oldenberg, Germany: International Collegium of Rehabilitative Audiology; 2009.
27. Psarros C. Improving efficiencies and effectiveness of CI Service delivery: the role of value stream mapping, presentation at CI2018 emerging issues, Washington, DC, 2018.
28. Eikelboom RH, Jayakody DMP, Swanepoel DW, et al. Validation of remote mapping of cochlear implants. J Telemed Telecare. 2014;20(4):171–7. https://doi.org/10.1177/1357633X14529234.
29. Frank K, Pengelly M, Zerfoss S. Telemedicine offers remote cochlear implant programming. Voices. 2006;13(1):16–9.
30. Psarros C, Van Wanrooy E. Tele-practice in audiology, Chapter 4. In: Houston KT, Rushbrooke E, editors. Remote programming in cochlear implants. San Diego, CA: Plural; 2015.

31. Sato AF, Clifford LM, Silverman AH, et al. Cognitive-behavioral interventions via telehealth: applications to pediatric functional abdominal pain. Child Health Care. 2009;38(1):1–22. https://doi.org/10.1080/02739610802615724.
32. Houston KT, Stredler-Brown A, Alverson DC. More than 150 years in the making: the evolution of telepractice for hearing speech and language services. Volta Rev. 2012;112(3):195–205.
33. McCarthy M, North J. RIDBC teleschool: guiding principles for tele-practice. Sydney: North Rocks Press; 2012.
34. Cullington H, Kitterick P, deBold L, et al. Personalised long-term follow-up of cochlear implant patients using remote care, compared with those on the standard care pathway: study protocol for a feasibility randomised controlled trial BMJ. Open. 2016;6:e011342. https://doi.org/10.1136/bmjopen-2016-011342.
35. Cullington H, Kitterick P, Weal M, et al. Feasibility of personalised remote long-term follow-up of people with cochlear implants: a randomised controlled trial. BMJ Open. 2018;8:e019640. https://doi.org/10.1136/bmjopen-2017-019640.
36. Shallop JK, Beiter AL, Goin DW, et al. Electrically Evoked Auditory Brain Stem Responses (EABR) and Middle Latency Responses (EMLR) obtained from patients with the nucleus multichannel Cochlear implant. Ear Hear. 1990;11(1):5–15.
37. Abbas PJ, Brown CJ, Shallop JK, et al. Summary of results using the nucleus CI24M implant to record the electrically evoked compound action potential. Ear Hear. 1999;20(1):45–59.
38. Game CJA, Gibson WPR, Pauka CK. Electrically evoked auditory brainstem potentials. Ann Otol Rhinol Layrngol. 1987;14(3):370–4.
39. Boisvert I, Reis M, Dowell RC. Cochlear implant outcomes: a scoping review. PLoS One. 2020;15(5):e0232421. https://doi.org/10.1371/journal.pone.0232421.
40. McKay C, Chandoun K, Akhourn H. Can ECAP measures be used for totally objective programming of Cochlear implants? J Assoc Res Otolaryngol. 2013;14(6):879–90.
41. de Vos, JJ.; Biesheuvel, JD; Briaire, JJ1; et al. Use of electrically evoked compound action potentials for Cochlear implant fitting: a systematic review. Ear Hear. 2018, 39(3), p 401-411. https://doi.org/10.1097/AUD.0000000000000495.
42. Botros A, Psarros C. Neural response telemetry reconsidered: I. The relevance of ECAP threshold profiles and scaled profiles to cochlear implant fitting. Ear Hear. 2010;31(3):367–79. https://doi.org/10.1097/AUD.0b013e3181c9fd86.
43. Finke M, Billinger M, Büchner A. Toward automated Cochlear implant fitting procedures based on event-related potentials. Ear Hear. 2017;38(2):e118–27. https://doi.org/10.1097/AUD.0000000000000377.
44. Somers B, Long CJ, Francart T. EEG-based diagnostics of the auditory system using cochlear implant electrodes as sensors. Sci Rep. 2021;11:5383. https://doi.org/10.1038/s41598-021-84829-y.
45. Gee AH, Zhao Y, Treece GM, et al. Practicable assessment of cochlear size and shape from clinical CT images. Sci Rep. 2021;11:3448. https://doi.org/10.1038/s41598-021-83059-6.
46. Eyles JA, Boyle PJ, Burton MJ, et al. Characteristic frequency mapping in subjects using the Nucleus 22 channel cochlear implant system with partial and full insertion. Ann Otol Rhinol Laryngol. 1995;166:356–8.
47. Greenwood DD. A cochlear frequency-position function for several species – 29 years later. J Acoust Soc Am. 1990;87(6):2592–605.
48. Grasmeder ML, Verschuur CA. Optimizing frequency to electrode allocation for individual cochlear implant users. J Acoust Soc Am. 2014;136:3313.
49. Ali H, Noble JH, Gifford RH, et al. Image-guided customization of frequency-place mapping in cochlear implants. In: 2015 IEEE international conference on acoustics, speech and signal processing (ICASSP), vol. 2015. QLD, Australia: South Brisbane; 2015. p. 5843–7. https://doi.org/10.1109/ICASSP.2015.7179092.
50. Lambriks LJG, van Hoof M, deBruyne J, et al. Evaluating hearing performance withcochlear implants within the same patient using daily randomization and imaging base fitting - the ELEPHANT study. Trials. 2020;21:564. https://doi.org/10.1186/s13063-020-04469-x.

51. Alnafjan FF, Allan SM, McMahon CM, et al. Assessing cochlear length using cone beam computed tomography in adults with cochlear implants. Otol Neurotol. 2018;39(9):e757–64. https://doi.org/10.1097/MAO.0000000000001934.
52. Zhao Y. Automatic techniques for cochlear implant CT image analysis submitted as part of doctoral thesis. Nashville Tennessee: Vanderbilt University; 2018.
53. Magrabi F, Habli I, Sujan M, et al. Why is it so difficult to govern mobile apps in healthcare? BMJ Health Care Inform. 2019;26:e100006. https://doi.org/10.1136/bmjhci-2019-100006.
54. https://www.tga.gov.au/medical-device-cyber-security-consumer-information. Accessed 11 Mar 2021
55. Meeuws M, Pascoal D, Bermejo I, et al. Computer-assisted C1 fitting: is the learning capacity of the intelligent agent FOX beneficial for speech understanding? Cochlear Implants Int. 2017;18(4):198–206.
56. Bennett RJ, Jayakody DMP, Eikelboom RH, et al. A prospective study evaluating cochlear implant management skills: development and validation of the Cochlear implant management skills survey. Clin Otolaryngol. 2016;41(1):51–8. https://doi.org/10.1111/coa.12472.
57. Galvin K, Gajadeera E. A proposed long-term programming schedule for adults using cochlear implants paper presented at APSCI 2019. Tokyo: Japan; 2019.
58. Hayton J, Dimitriou D. What's in a word? Distinguishing between habilitation and re-habilitation vision. Rehab Int. 2019;10(1):1–4. https://doi.org/10.21307/ijom-2019-007.
59. Hickson L, Meyer C, Lovelock K, et al. Factors associated with success with hearing aids in older adults. Int J Audiol. 2014;53(Suppl 1):S18–27.
60. Sharma SD, Cushing SL, Papsin BC, et al. Hearing and speech benefits of cochlear implantation in children: a review of the literature. Int J Pediatr Otorhinolaryngol. 2020;133:109984. https://doi.org/10.1016/j.ijporl.2020.109984.
61. Ching TC, Zhang VW, Flynn C, et al. Factors influencing speech perception in noise for 5-year-old children using hearing aids or cochlear implants. Int J Audiol. 2018;57:S70–80. https://doi.org/10.1080/14992027.2017.1346307.
62. Kishida Y, Kemp C. Improving parents' interactions with children with hearing loss using data-based feedback. Int J Disabil Dev Educ. 2020; https://doi.org/10.1080/1034912X.2020.1767761.
63. Lone Percy-Smith L, Lindbjerg Tønning T, Lignel Josvassen J, et al. Auditory verbal habilitation is associated with improved outcome for children with cochlear implant. Cochlear Implants Int. 2018;19:1.
64. Holden L, Finley C, Firszt J, et al. Factors affecting open-set word recognition in adults with Cochlear implants. Ear Hear. 2013;34(3):342–60. https://doi.org/10.1097/AUD.0b013e3182741aa7.
65. Tang L, Thompson C, Clark JH, et al. Rehabilitation and psychosocial determinants of cochlear implant outcomes in older adults. Ear Hear. 2017;38(6):663–71. https://doi.org/10.1097/AUD.0000000000000445.
66. Stropahl M, Besser J, Launer. Auditory training supports auditory rehabilitation: a state-of-the-art review. Ear Hear. 2020;41(4):697–704. https://doi.org/10.1097/AUD.0000000000000806.
67. Witkins BR. Listening theory and research: the state of the art. Int List Assoc J. 1990;4(1):7–32. https://doi.org/10.1207/s1932586xijl0401_3.
68. Janusik LA. Building listening theory: the validation of the conversational listening span. Commun Stud. 2007;58(2):139–56. https://doi.org/10.1080/10510970701341089.
69. Pisoni DB, Broadstock A, Wucinich T, et al. Verbal learning and memory after Cochlear implantation in post-lingually deaf adults: some new findings with the CVLT-II. Ear Hear. 2018;39(4):720–45. https://doi.org/10.1097/AUD.0000000000000530.
70. Dillon H, James A, Ginis J. Client oriented scale of improvement (COSI) and its relationship to several other measures of benefit and satisfaction provided by hearing aids. J Am Acad Audiol. 1997;8(1):27–43.
71. Lenarz T, Muller L, Czerniejewska-Wolska H, et al. Patient-related benefits for adults with Cochlear implantation: a multicultural longitudinal observational study. Audiol Neurotol. 2017;22:61–73. https://doi.org/10.1159/000477533.

72. Martin J. Quality standards for (re)habilitation. Cochlear Implants Int. 2013;14(Suppl 2):S34–8.
73. Pichora-Fuller MK, Kramer SE, Eckert MA, et al. Hearing impairment and cognitive energy: the framework for understanding effortful listening (FUEL). Ear Hear. 2016;37(Suppl 1):5S–27S. https://doi.org/10.1097/AUD.0000000000000312.
74. Erber N. Communication therapy for adults with sensory loss. Melbourne: Clavis; 1996.
75. Henry B, Pedley K, Fu QJ. Adult Cochlear implant home-based auditory training guide for clinicians. Sydney: Cochlear Limited; 2015. https://doi.org/10.13140/RG.2.1.2707.1208.
76. De Filippo CL, Scott BL. (1978) a method for training and evaluating the reception of ongoing speech. J Acoust Soc Am. 1978;63(4):1186–92. https://doi.org/10.1121/1.381827.
77. Plant G, Levitt H. Optimizing performance in adult Cochlear implant users through clinician directed auditory training. Semin Hear. 2015;36(4):296–310.
78. Boothroyd A. Adult aural rehabilitation: what is it and does it work? Trends Amplif. 2007;11(2):63–71. https://doi.org/10.1177/1084713807301073.
79. Grenness C, Hickson L, Laplante-Levesque A, et al. Patient-centred audiological rehabilitation: perspectives of older adults who own hearing aids. Int J Audiol. 2014;53(Suppl 1):S60–75.
80. Ferguson M, Maidment D, Henshaw H, et al. Evidence-based interventions for adult aural rehabilitation: that was then, this is now. Semin Hear. 2019;40(1):68–84. https://doi.org/10.1055/s-0038-1676784.
81. Reis M, Boisvert I, Beedell E, et al. Auditory training for adult Cochlear implant users: a survey and cost analysis study. Ear Hear. 2019;40(6):1445–56. https://doi.org/10.1097/AUD.0000000000000724.
82. Dunn C, Karsten S. Best practice for cochlear implantation: the evaluation process presentation at CI2018 ACI. Washington, DC: Alliance; 2018.
83. McDermott HJ. Music perception with Cochlear implants: a review. Trends Amplif. 2004;8(2):49–82. https://doi.org/10.1177/108471380400800203.
84. Gfeller K, Driscoll V, Schwalje A. Adult Cochlear implant recipients' perspectives on experiences with music in everyday life: a multifaceted and dynamic phenomenon. Front Neurosci. 2019;13:1229.
85. Giorgos Dritsakis G, van Besouw RM, O'Meara A. Impact of music on the quality of life of cochlear implant users: a focus group study. Cochlear Implants Int. 2017;18(4):207–15. https://doi.org/10.1080/14670100.2017.1303892.
86. Olson A, Williams R, Livingston E, et al. Review of auditory training Mobile apps for adults with hearing loss. September: Perspectives of the ASHA Special Interest Group Report; 2018.
87. Drouin JR, Theodore RM. Leveraging interdisciplinary perspectives to optimize auditory training for cochlear implant users. Lang Linguist Compass. 2020;14:e12394. https://doi.org/10.1111/lnc3.12394.
88. Ericsson K, Krampe R, Tesch-Romer C. The role of deliberate practice in the acquisition of expert performance. Psychol Rev. 1993;100:393–406.
89. Hearing Implants Australia. Catalyzing the dormant innovation in cochlear implants Paper presented at the CI Global Futures Forum August 2020. https://adulthearing.com/no-touch-pathways-webinar/, 2020.

# Cochlear Implant Reliability

# 23

Manfred Pieber and Sandra DeSaSouza

## 23.1 Introduction

Reliability of a certain system or component describes the ability of a system or component to perform its required functions under stated conditions, within specified performance limits, for a specified period of time. This ability is often quantified in terms of probability. Other concepts that are linked to the topic of reliability and that are often discussed together are availability, maintainability, and safety.

High reliability performance is an important basic feature of medical devices as a failure may result in serious patient harm. Therefore, patients, clinicians, payors, and above all regulators are demanding from medical device manufacturers that their medical devices are safe and effective, and reliable throughout the product life cycle. For manufacturers, high quality standards and good reliability performance are not only a matter of ethics and regulatory obligations, but are also helping to reduce the overall costs for the company by speeding up all necessary steps before market approval, and by stabilizing operations in the long run after market approval.

The topic of reliability and reliability engineering emerged in the early twentieth century, with the development of sophisticated statistical methods and probabilistic models. The focus was first on process control in production, but soon also moved

---

**Supplementary Information** The online version contains supplementary material available at [https://doi.org/10.1007/978-981-19-0452-3_23].

---

M. Pieber (✉)
MED-EL GmbH, Innsbruck, Austria
e-mail: manfred.pieber@medel.com

S. DeSaSouza

ENT Department, Jaslok Hospital & Research Centre, Mumbai, Maharashtra, India

Breach Candy Hospital and Desa Hospital, Mumbai, Maharashtra, India


S. DeSaSouza (ed.), *Cochlear Implants*,
https://doi.org/10.1007/978-981-19-0452-3_23

to product design and development. A major driver behind the new technical field was the military during the Second World War, as failures were extremely costly and dangerous. Shortly after the Second World War, the first professional societies for reliability engineering were founded (e.g., the IEEE Reliability Society, in 1948). These societies offered a platform for all researchers and practitioners in this field to publish and to discuss their discoveries and fostered the development of standardization. From the late 1960s onward, reliability engineering principles were also applied to medical devices [1]. A first standard on assessing and reporting the reliability performance of cardiac pacemakers was published already in 1986 and updated since then several times.

As medical devices became more complex and were used more widely in more critical therapies, many governments around the world regulated their design, manufacture, use, and sale, including requirements for quality and reliability. In 1976, the Medical Device Amendments to the Federal Food, Drug and Cosmetic Act empowered the US Food and Drug Administration (US FDA) to regulate medical devices during their design and development phases to ensure their safety and effectiveness. It created a risk-based classification system for all medical devices, established the regulatory pathways for new medical devices to get to market (premarket approval and premarket notification), and defined several key postmarket requirements (registration and listing of devices with the US FDA, Good Manufacturing Practices, and adverse event reporting). In 1990, the US Congress passed the Safe Medical Devices Act, which helped to strengthen the role of the US FDA and further improved postmarket surveillance of devices. In order to guide manufacturers in their design and development process, the US FDA regularly updates a comprehensive list of recognized consensus standards, which can be used by the manufacturers to demonstrate conformity in their product approval process.

Similar regulations concerning medical devices have also been established in other countries. For example, in the countries of the European Union, the Council Directive 90/385/EEC on active implantable medical devices came into effect in 1990, followed by the Medical Device Directive 93/42/EEC; both were replaced by the Medical Device Regulation 2017/745 in 2017. Similar to the USA, the European regulations are harmonized with a comprehensive list of normative standards. Manufacturers seeking device approval in the European market must show compliance to these standards.

## 23.2 Technical Standards for Cochlear Implants

Today, a comprehensive list of technical standards exists for medical devices, for example the IEC 60601 standard family for the safety and essential performance of medical electrical devices or the IEC 60068 standards for environmental testing of electrotechnical products, both published by the International Electrotechnical Commission (www.iec.ch). IEC 60601 was first published in 1977, was regularly updated, and consists of nearly 100 distinct documents. These standards typically contain technical specifications relevant for the design and development of devices, and test methods to be used for verification and validation testing of the devices.

Another series of standards is the ISO 14708 standard family for implants for surgery—active implantable medical devices, which consists of seven separate parts. It is published by the International Organization for Standardization (www.iso.org). ISO 14708-1, the first part of the series, describes general requirements for safety, marking, and information to be provided by the manufacturer, and was first published in 2000 and updated in 2014. ISO 14708-7, the seventh part of the series, describes requirements for cochlear and auditory brainstem implant systems. This standard was first published in 2013 and was updated in 2019. ISO 14708-7 builds on the European standard EN 45502-2-3 and on the US standard ANSI/AAMI CI68. EN 45502-2-3 was the first standard that was dedicated to the specific requirements of cochlear implants. It was published in 2006 by CENELEC, the European Committee for Electrotechnical Standardization (www.cenelec.eu), and subsequently revised in 2010. ANSI/AAMI CI86 was first published in 2017, by the American National Standards Institute (www.ansi.org) and the Association for the Advancement of Medical Instrumentation (www.aami.org). It is also a dedicated standard for cochlear implants which was developed by a committee assembled with technical experts from the manufacturers, universities, the US FDA, and representatives from medical societies. The standard was written with a focus on the total product life cycle, with requirements for long-term safety and effectiveness as well as device reliability.

## 23.3 Requirements Relevant for Cochlear Implant Reliability

Cochlear implants are complex pieces of engineering. A great variety of knowledge is needed for the design and development, as well as the manufacturing of the devices: from mechanical engineering and material science to biomedical and electrical engineering and software engineering. Furthermore, in order to create devices that are effective in the treatment of hearing loss, a good understanding of the application of the devices and the environment in the human body is also very important. Cochlear implant manufacturers are reliant on a good and close collaboration with clinical professionals like surgeons and audiologists, and on the input from experts in basic science in the area of biology, biochemistry, physics, and psychoacoustics, to name just a few disciplines.

This complexity is also an important factor in the assessment of the reliability of implants. After approximately 50 years of electrical stimulation of the inner ear, the knowledge about failure modes and failure mechanisms has significantly increased and has led to numerous improvements in device design. However, the reliability assessment also showed that treatment failures are depending not only on the device, but also on how the devices are used by surgeons and audiologists. And of course, the patients with their different etiologies, potential comorbidities, and behavior among many other characteristics are important to consider. In many cases, a complex mixture of all these factors contributes to complications with cochlear implants [2].

The following pages will provide an insight into the technical specifications and requirements, as described in the standards EN 45502-2-3, ANSI/AAMI CI86 and ISO 14708-7, which are relevant for cochlear implant design, with an emphasis on implant reliability. The clinical relevance of these requirements will be explained and for some requirements supported by examples from the literature. The focus will be on requirements from ANSI/AAMI CI86, because this standard covers the area of implant reliability in the most comprehensive way.

### 23.3.1 Protection of the Implant from Mechanical Forces

The standards require that the cochlear implant housing and the antenna coil are immune to mechanical impact stresses during normal use, including trauma during a patient's accident. This requirement is verified with a special impact test: the impact energy of the striking hammer is defined to be 2.5 J and to be applied at various places on the surface of the cochlear implant (Fig. 23.1). This test and the so-called pillow test are demonstrated in the video (in the supplement) (courtesy of Oticon Medical). The test is passed if the device under test still complies with the manufacturer's design specifications and fulfills the hermeticity requirements; also,

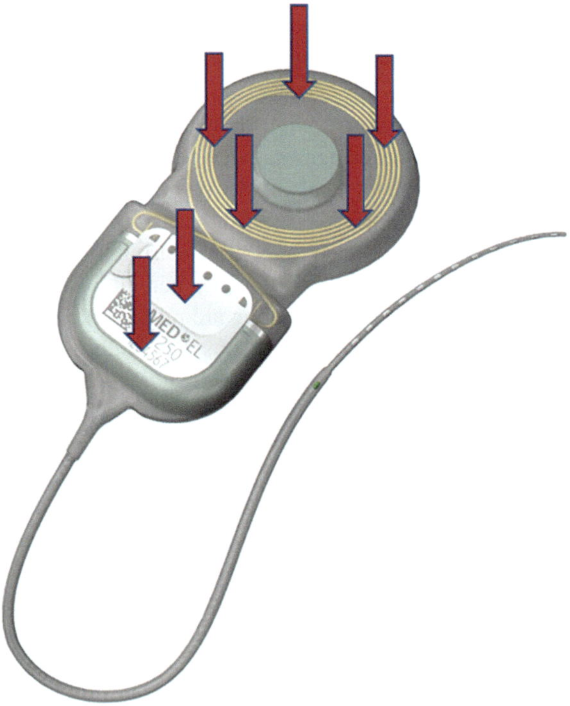

**Fig. 23.1** Approximate locations for mechanical impact testing

the antenna coil magnet may not be partially or fully dislodged from its magnet pocket. These tests are considered to simulate situations in which the device receives direct mechanical impact through the skin because of falls or collisions by the user or incidental direct external strikes delivered to the device (e.g., by bats or balls).

In the early days of commercial cochlear implantation, housing breakages following head trauma were common failures. The number of such cases was significantly higher with children than with adults [3–6]. The reason for the higher incidence of these failures in children is considered a consequence of them receiving the cochlear implant often before they learn to walk or at a very young age when they are physically most active. After the requirement for mechanical impact stress testing on the implant housing came into effect in a stepwise approach from 2010 onward, all cochlear implant manufacturers modified their designs accordingly. MED-EL introduced a new implant with titanium housing, the Concerto, into the European market in 2010, the second generation of titanium implants after the Sonata, and subsequently discontinued the marketing and sales of the older ceramic implant series Combi 40+ and Pulsar. One research study that analyzed the type and incidence of cochlear implant failures for MED-EL implants between 2003 and 2013 found a statistically significant reduction in this specific failure mechanism from the older generation ceramic Combi 40+ implants to the newer generation Sonata implants, made of titanium, in the population of children [6]. The impact stress requirement for the antenna coil was introduced with the ANSI/AAMI CI86 standard in 2017. Magnet displacement due to impact was reported in two case reports [7, 8], and for a few patients in one clinical review study [9]. Antenna coil breakages seem to be similarly rare.

Another important mechanical requirement concerns the robustness of electrode leads and arrays. Electrode leads should be able to withstand the tensile forces and the flexural stresses that might occur during or after implantation, without fracture of any wire or deterioration in any functional electrical insulation. This test is demonstrated in the video (in the supplement) (courtesy of Oticon Medical). The integrity of the electrode wires is determined by measuring the impedances of each wire. Upon passing the tests on tensile forces, it should be ascertained that the electrode will not be damaged with normal handling during the surgery as well as that the electrode lead may withstand the elongation that might be experienced in children during the skull growth period [10–12]. The tests on flexural stresses are designed to simulate any adverse handling prior to implantation, and micromovements of the electrode lead after implantation, especially in the region of the temporalis muscle. The defined minimum requirement to withstand at least 100,000 flex cycles is considered appropriate, if the surgeons are following the recommended clinical practice of properly immobilizing the implant within a bony bed.

Modern cochlear implant electrodes are very delicate structures, with wires thinner than human hair. This is necessary to design electrode arrays with a diameter of less than 1 mm at the basal end of the electrode, and a tip diameter of less than 0.5 mm, which is one precondition to achieve atraumatic insertion of the array into the human cochlea. It is no surprise that these parts of the cochlear implant are extremely vulnerable to mechanical forces. Several studies concluded that electrode failure is among the most frequent causes of device failure in cochlear implants [13, 14]. The described failures range from a single wire breakage which occurs in approximately 10% of patients and which is generally not associated with device explantation [15–17], to multiple wire breakages, which usually requires replacement of the cochlear implant [15, 18]. One Australian study looking into long-term performance with Nucleus electrode arrays demonstrated that newer array types had less failures compared to older electrode array models [19].

More recently, a new type of electrode failure has been described in the clinical literature, which manifests itself in an abnormal electrode impedance pattern, in some cases leading to relatively low impedances in several adjacent electrode channels and in other cases resulting in a "zig-zag" pattern of impedance values [15, 17, 20, 21]. Cullington [20] speculated that in these cases, the insulation between adjacent electrode wires was defect resulting in a "short circuit"-type behavior and low impedance values at the respective electrode channels. It is recommended to closely monitor these patients for a degradation in performance as this abnormal impedance pattern is difficult to detect using standardized test methods and degradation in performance may be an indicator for explantation [22].

In order to protect the electrode lead from mechanical forces and to prevent migration of the implant and the electrode lead, all manufacturers request some form of implant immobilization and electrode protection in their labeling. Many different methods for immobilizing the implant exist [23]: preparing a bony bed for the implant housing and a groove for the electrode lead; using sutures; placing the implant into a tight periosteal pocket; some MED-EL implants may also be fixated with small pins on the bottom of the housing; Oticon Medical implants feature screws for fixation. The electrode can be kept in place for example with bone paté and fibrin glue, by physically placing it into a split bony bridge [24], or by using a titanium clip [25]. Although some retrospective studies demonstrate less device failures and complications with preparing a bony bed and applying sutures for the implant as opposed to using the tight periosteal pocket technique [26], [27], previous and recent systematic reviews have not shown any evidence for a difference of both techniques regarding migration [23, 28]. Large prospective, longitudinal studies are needed to identify the safest and most reliable method for implant immobilization and electrode protection.

### 23.3.2 Protection of the Implant Electronics

The latest edition of ISO 14708-7 specifies requirements for the protection of the implant electronics from damage caused by electrostatic discharge and electromagnetic non-ionizing radiation. The test configuration for assessing the immunity of the implants was designed to be representative of real-life use. Non-implantable components of cochlear implant systems should also be included and the cochlear implant itself should be located inside a "head simulator." The aim of the tests is to prove that the implants do not cause unacceptable risk of harm to the patient, nor a long-term discomfort, because of susceptibility to interference to external electromagnetic fields under circumstances likely to be encountered in public access areas (such as power grid and transportation systems, mobile phones, induction stoves or induction heating systems, AM radio transmitters).

### 23.3.3 Protection of the Implant from Changes Caused by Medical Treatments

Magnetic resonance imaging (MRI) is a versatile imaging technique that is widely used for medical diagnosis and for staging and follow-up of a disease without exposing the body to ionizing radiation. However, the strong static and dynamic magnetic fields that are applied with an MRI machine may impact the integrity of the implant and potentially harm the patient. The risks to a patient with a cochlear implant undergoing an MRI examination range from magnetically induced torque and displacement force to the implant magnet, potentially resulting in magnet dislocation and painful experiences of the patient; gradient-induced vibration and heating; unintentional device output; implant magnet weakening; loss of implant functionality; and imaging artifact, which could result in the misinterpretation of test results or in a treatment delay. The standards describe requirements and test methods for each of these scenarios. Depending on the test results, manufacturers are mandated to include a declaration of safety to the labeling of the implants, which must contain a description of the conditions (clinical guideline) under which the MRI procedure can be conducted safely.

Prior to 2015, complications with MRI were frequently observed and reported, even with protective head bandages applied to the patient according to manufacturer information prior to the examination [9, 29–32]. The complication rates ranged between 10% and 20% with patients mostly reporting discomfort and pain, which was in some cases strong enough to stop the examination. Pain was mostly related to torque and displacement force to the implant magnet which was left *in situ* prior to the MRI; this occurred only with older implant models of Advanced Bionics and Cochlear, which featured a removable magnet placed in a soft silicone rubber pocket. Magnet displacement must be resolved with repositioning surgery, which carries a risk of infection and potentially long hearing downtime [33]. Today, all cochlear implant manufacturers offer solutions with modified magnet designs, which are approved for MRI examinations under certain conditions; however, these are different for each device, and consultation of manufacturer guidelines is recommended. Srinivasan, So [34] provide a good overview on the current products and the respective manufacturer guidelines [34]. Several experimental studies have demonstrated the safety of one of these modern designs [35–37], and first clinical studies have proven its usefulness and safety in clinical care [38, 39].

Other medical treatments that are covered in the standard are the usage of ultrasonic diagnostic equipment, therapeutic ionizing radiation, external defibrillators, and high-power electrical fields applied directly to the patient (as used for example in surgical diathermy). For most of these treatments, the manufacturer is obliged to provide guidance to the medical professional in the labeling documentation of the device.

### 23.3.4 Interaction Between the Implant and the Human Body

Cochlear implants interact in many ways with the surrounding tissue of the human body. The mechanical properties of the implant and its shape and size but also the material of the implant may cause a reaction from the surrounding bone and tissue, which in turn might lead to the device becoming unstable or dysfunctional. It goes without saying that the materials which are in permanent contact to tissue and bone must be biocompatible and that the implant must be delivered to the operating room in a sterilized container. Despite these preconditions for a successful qualification of any medical implant, when assessing clinical publications on cochlear implant complications, infections, skin and wound problems, and even device extrusion are frequent causes for interruption of the therapy [40–45]. Most of these cases are classified as minor complications, without the need for surgical intervention. Explantation of the device for this reason was only necessary in approximately 1% of the total implant population. Weder, Shaul [45] could demonstrate in their study of Nucleus implants that the rate of severe infections decreased after the year 2000. The authors hypothesize that besides improvements of surgical practice also modifications to the implant surface and shape (wider recesses and less steep sides of the implant housing) led to this positive trend. This finding is supported by the study of Jiang, Gu [41] for a wide range of devices.

Bacterial infections may also become life-threatening, if they enter the inner ear via the electrode and lead to bacterial meningitis. Several studies [46, 47] were initiated by the US Center for Disease Control and Prevention (US CDC), the US FDA, and several health departments in 2002, after a relatively large number of cases with post-implantation bacterial meningitis were reported to the US FDA by one manufacturer, which led to a voluntary device recall by the manufacturer later that year. The study by Reefhuis, Honein [46] indeed showed that the incidence of meningitis caused by *Streptococcus pneumoniae* was more than 30 times the incidence in a cohort of the same age in the general US population and that post-implantation bacterial meningitis was strongly associated with the use of the recalled device. In an update to this study, Biernath, Reefhuis [47] concluded that continued monitoring and prompt treatment of bacterial infections remain important in the longer follow-up of patients, and vaccination recommendations for all potential recipients of implants continue to apply. Bacterial meningitis should remain a concern for the clinician, although by following good clinical practice pre-, intra-, and post-operatively, and using modern cochlear implant designs, the risk for severe harm to the patient from bacterial meningitis has become very low [44, 48, 49].

The electrode array in the inner ear is not only a potential source for infection, but may also cause trauma to the tissue within the cochlea during the insertion. It is obvious that the potential for trauma depends not only on the skills of the surgeon, but also to a large degree on the mechanical characteristics of the electrode array. Trauma to the tissue within the cochlea is known to cause loss of residual low-frequency hearing, which may limit the patient's benefit for speech recognition [50]. This results in several design conflicts: the electrode should be as soft as possible, but at the same time it should be rigid enough for safe and reliable surgical handling; the electrode should be long enough to stimulate neural cells across a large frequency spectrum, but its diameter should not exceed the diameter of the *scala tympani* (ST), especially when getting closer to the apex [51]. A literature review recently investigated two specific problems that may occur during electrode insertion as reported by clinical studies with different commercially available electrode types: scalar deviation and electrode array tip fold-over [52]. Scalar deviation occurs if the electrode array dislocates from the ST, its preferred location for the surgical placement, to the *scala vestibuli* (SV). Scalar deviation is considered highly traumatic to the cochlea structures (Grade 3 on Eshraghi's scale of electrode insertion intra-cochlear trauma [53]). Electrode array tip fold-over is a different form of intra-cochlear complication, where the tip of the electrode gets stuck with any of the intra-cochlear structures and further pushing the electrode deeper makes it folded over. This may be corrected intra-operatively if detected, but damage to the intra-cochlear structures may prevail. Both problems are visualized in Fig. 23.2.

In their study, Dhanasingh and Jolly [52] compared two groups of commercially available electrode arrays: pre-curved type electrode arrays (including Advanced Bionics' Mid-Scala and Helix arrays, and Cochlear's Slim-Modiolar, Contour Advance, and Contour arrays) and straight lateral wall arrays (including Advanced Bionics' 1J array, Cochlear's Slim-Straight array, and MED-EL's Standard, Medium, Compressed, and FLEX electrode arrays). The analysis of 38 peer-reviewed publications revealed an approximately five times higher rate of both scalar deviation and tip fold-over with the pre-curved electrode arrays in comparison to the lateral wall electrode arrays. These findings were confirmed in a recently conducted meta-analysis; the differences of both array types are statistically significant [54]. Jwair, Prins [54] conclude that lateral wall electrode arrays should be the preferred option for cochlear implantation if the surgeon wants to minimize clinically relevant intra-cochlear trauma. In several recent prospective and retrospective studies of the Slim-Modiolar electrode array, translocations were still discovered [55–57]. While Australian researchers found no scalar translocations with this new product in their cohort of 120 adult patients, they experienced tip fold-over in 8 patients. Three of them had to be explanted and reimplanted with a different device [58].

Another potential problem of the electrode array is migration, which refers to an electrode array that post-operatively over time slipped partly or completely out of

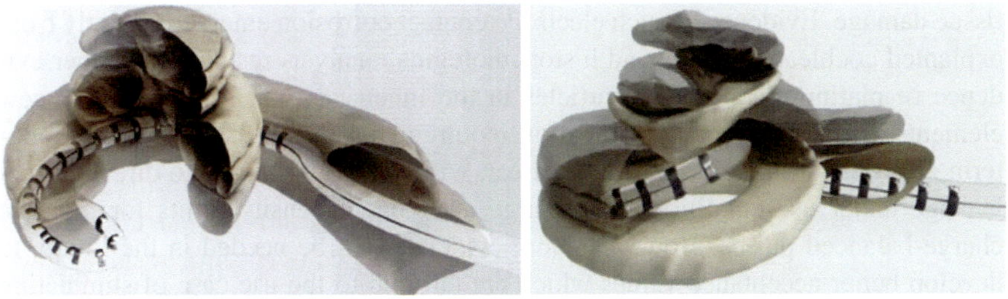

**Fig. 23.2** Visualization of electrode tip fold-over (left) and scalar deviation (right) (Dhanasingh and Jolly [52])

the cochlea. The movement of the electrode array usually does not damage the inner structures of the cochlea, but it may induce pain and facial nerve stimulation [59], and it is often only discovered indirectly by a degraded hearing performance which may make revision surgery necessary. During this procedure, the electrode array may be re-inserted deeper into the cochlea in many cases; rarely, though, an explantation and subsequent reimplantation with a new implant will be necessary. This complication is occurring more frequently with lateral wall electrodes, as several studies showed [60–62]. The underlying mechanisms for electrode migration are not yet fully understood. One retrospective review study found a potential association with cochlear ossification [63]. Proper fixation of the electrode lead outside the cochlea, e.g., in a bone groove, seems to be the best preventive strategy, and should be used routinely in all patients [33, 60].

While the human body in general is a quite stable environment for a device like a cochlear implant, the natural moisture inside the body poses a threat to any active implantable medical device. The body fluids are conducting electricity, which is the fundamental principle of why cochlear implants function at all, but electrical current flow may cause corrosion and other undesired effects to the electronic circuits, and the current may also spread and unintendedly stimulate other nearby neural structures. In order to prevent moisture from entering the implants and from destroying the electronics, the implant housings must be hermetically sealed from the body fluids. The most critical component to achieve this goal is the connector between electrode wires and implant electronics. The design of such a connector is a challenging task for the engineers, as the mechanical dimensions of the current implant housings are so small. A set of tests and strict acceptance criteria with an upper limit of moisture content inside the implant housing over the useful life of the device are defined in the ANSI/AAMI CI 86 standard. If the design or a process in manufacturing does not meet these specifications, the implant will fail over time. This has happened several times in the history of cochlear implants and has unfortunately led to at least three Field Corrective Actions with voluntary device recalls over the past 20 years. A paper by Hildrew and Molony [64] describes the clinical experience with one of these products [64].

Electrode contact corrosion may occur at the interface to the neural structures inside the cochlea, if direct current (DC), even at small levels but for a sustained period, is presented to the electrodes. The contacts will start to dissolve, and platinum ions and atoms will disintegrate into the inner ear and may potentially cause tissue damage. Evidence of such electrode contact corrosion emerged recently from explanted cochlear implants and histopathological analysis resulted in further evidence of platinum-containing particles in the inner ear [65, 66]. Therefore, new elements in the design and verification requirements were defined on safe, long-term electrical stimulation of the inner ear, with specifying limits to direct current leakage under use conditions and charge and charge density limits for biphasic charge-balanced pulses. However, more evidence will be needed in the future, to develop better acceptance values which are tailored to the use case of stimulating the inner ear and to modern cochlear implants.

As mentioned above, as an undesired side effect of the therapy with cochlear implants, other neural structures nearby the human cochlea may be stimulated as well. The result of such "misguided" electric current can be, for example, pain, vertigo, and facial nerve stimulation. Pain from stimulation is a rare complication and therefore not often reported in the literature. Anand, Devi [67] published a report on two patients, who could not tolerate their cochlear implant due to pain when switched on; the pain could be resolved by tympanic neurectomy [67]. Changes to the vestibular system which are caused by the cochlear implantation surgery are reported frequently in the literature. A recent literature review on this topic in pediatric patients confirmed previous findings on adults that cochlear implantation surgery is associated with a statistically significant decrease in vestibular evoked myogenic potential (VEMP) responses post-operatively [68]. Vertigo induced by the electrical stimulation of the cochlear implant is less frequently described and the few studies that exist are mostly case reports which do not have conclusive results [69–71].

Facial nerve stimulation is also a well-known complication of cochlear implantation and restricts the optimal use of the implant as it requires in most cases reprogramming of the stimulating strategy [72]. In very few cases, the side effects are so severe that only explantation (and potentially reimplantation) may help. The reported incidence varies widely, which may be related to insensitive detection methods that only capture the more severe cases. Some etiologies such as cochlear malformation and otosclerosis have been associated with a higher rate of facial nerve stimulation, and lateral wall electrodes seem to cause this complication more frequently due to their position inside the cochlea [73]. In a recent retrospective study comparing patients who suffer from facial nerve stimulation to a control group without facial nerve stimulation, a statistically significant difference was observed in the thickness but not in the density of the bone between the upper basal turn of the cochlea and the labyrinthine segment of the facial nerve [74]. This finding may be important for the counseling of future patients.

Finally, in order to ensure a lifelong therapy, the cochlear implant has to be designed to be removed and replaced by a similar device in the future, in case of failure, without any degradation in performance to the patient and without any additional harm. This was important to be demonstrated already early in the history of cochlear implantation [75], in order to convince regulators, clinicians, and of course patients to accept the risk of cochlear implantation at a time when implant failure was much more common than today. Since then, clinicians have been regularly conducting studies to assess the outcome of their patients after reimplantation and the results have been generally encouraging also with the latest generations of devices [76–80]. A recent study of Advanced Bionics patients who were implanted as children and decided to undergo explantation and reimplantation surgery as young adults in order to benefit from the latest technology showed also stable results [81].

### 23.3.5 Patient Selection and Surgery Related Problems

Cochlear implant candidates with certain etiologies or with comorbidities like obesity or diabetes may benefit less from the treatment or experience a higher risk for complications. Comprehensive and honest counseling by a multidisciplinary clinical team is the key to set realistic expectations for the candidates and to guide them in their decision-making process. The manufacturer must provide information on the devices and the indications and contraindications in the labeling and may support the clinician in the counseling process. Complications that are related to the etiology or to comorbidities of the patient and that may occur during surgery and at later stages of the treatment are cerebrospinal fluid gusher, delayed wound healing, recurring cholesteatoma, recurring otitis media, allergic reactions, or simply poor patient performance.

Surgical complications may be related to difficult medical conditions of the patient but may also be caused by human error. Manufacturers must provide information on specific details of their device design and how these details correspond to the common surgical technique for cochlear implantation, but the surgeon will always be the authority with final responsibility for the surgical procedure; if warranted, the surgeon may also decide to implant the device off-label (deliberately not following the instructions for use from the manufacturer). Common surgical complications that are observed in the clinics are facial nerve palsy and injury of the chorda tympani, peripheral vestibular function loss, vascular complications, and damage to the dura and intracranial complications. Some of these complications may resolve over time; others may disable the patient permanently. Candidates need to be made aware of these risks prior to surgery.

One possibility to further improve the surgical procedures and the surgical skills is to introduce and adhere to quality management guidelines for cochlear implantation, to attend educative courses, and to participate in regular practical trainings. Surgical societies usually offer such guidelines and training opportunities in most of the high-income countries. In order to assure high quality standards also in low- and medium-income countries, international ENT societies like the International Federation of ORL Societies (www.ifosworld.org), international collaborative networks like the HEARRING group (www.hearring.com), and also individual ENT departments at leading universities started initiatives for knowledge sharing and training. And of course, implant manufacturers not only offer guidance in the form of product labeling but also provide clinical professionals with a large range of training courses on best practice with their devices.

## 23.4 Clinical Follow-Up

Clinical follow-up of patients with cochlear implants is very important, especially in the first year after the operation. In the follow-up consultations, the cochlear implant surgeon and the audiologist should check the wound healing process and the skin flap, measure electrode impedances, select the best operating parameters for the implant to optimize the device mapping, and assess the hearing outcome of the patient. This should be done regularly and all the information obtained should be added to the patient records. If a patient experiences a problem with his cochlear implant, it is important to perform a functional evaluation of the implant *in vivo* in addition to other subjective and objective tests of implant functionality. As per ANSI/AAMI CI86, implant manufacturers are required to provide device-specific procedures and tools to enable the clinician to manage these suspicious cases. Tools currently available from each manufacturer range from impedance telemetry to monitor the function of the electrode channels; measurement of evoked compound action potentials (ECAP) to measure the health of the electrode-neural interface; electrocochleography (ECochG); and more sophisticated integrity tests which are often performed in collaboration with experts of the manufacturer. It must be noted though that these tools are designed to work within a specified range under normal conditions, which may not deliver correct results in all patients [82].

During clinical follow-up, also the external components of a cochlear implant system should be checked regularly, and the patient should be trained by the clinician on how to correctly use and maintain the external components. This will ensure that the cochlear implant system is working as intended for a long time.

## 23.5 Testing of Explanted Devices and Reliability Reporting

ANSI/AAMI CI86 is also setting out a clear guideline for manufacturers on how to test explanted and returned implants and what kind of information shall be shared by clinic and manufacturer for the investigation of an explanted device. This is important to determine the root cause of the failure which may then be used by the manufacturer to improve the device design or by the clinician to adapt the clinical procedures. The tests contain non-destructive analysis steps, like visual inspection and basic electrical tests (e.g., link integrity testing, basic functionality tests, simulated clinical testing). If it is suspected that the device may have failed or may have significantly contributed to the treatment failure, then destructive analysis is conducted subsequently, including hermeticity tests, residual gas analysis, and a detailed inspection of the electronic assembly with electric measurements at certain test points which are defined by the manufacturer. These tests are subsequently the basis for classifying the explanted device depending on the established failure mode and failure mechanism. ANSI/AAMI CI86 defines several categories for failure classification, which are shown in Fig. 23.3.

In addition to the test protocol and failure classification scheme, the reliability calculation method and the reporting method are clearly specified in ANSI/AAMI CI86. For each implant type, an actuarial analysis shall be conducted based on the theory of Kaplan and Meier [83]; the calculation method is described in detail also in the Annex of ISO 5841-2. Global field data shall be used to calculate cumulative removal percentages for each implant type, for the failure categories explanted for medical reason (MRE), device failure explants (DFE), and inconclusive failure analysis (INC) (Fig. 23.3). The patient population shall be stratified into children

Categories not included in reliability reporting

- Unrelated Medical Explants[a]
- Elective Upgrade Explant[a]

Categories included in reliability reporting

- Explanted for Medical Reason (MRE) – device in specification
    - o MRE Type A: infection, CSF leakage, meningitis, skin flap complication, misplaced electrode array electrode migration implant migration / extrusion, other
    - o MRE Type B: pain / burning, dizziness, anomalous percepts, performance issues, extracochlear stimulation, other
    - o MRE Type C: surgical error, device damage
- Device Failure Explants (DFE) – device out of specification
    - o Electronic component / assembly
    - o Electrode / electrode lead
    - o Receiver coil
    - o Magnet issue
    - o Excess moisture in the device
    - o Case damage
    - o Feed-through damage
    - o Obsolescence (unsupported device)
    - o Manufacturing process error
    - o Unknown mechanism
    - o Other
- Inconclusive (INC) – device must pass all tests

[a]device must pass functional tests

**Fig. 23.3** Classification of explanted devices for manufacturer reliability reporting (reproduced from ANSI/AAMI CI86)

who were implanted before the age of 10 years and all other patients, who are labeled "adults." A report, containing the results of these calculations, shall be published semi-annually, at the end of the first and third quarter of the calendar year.

The intention behind all these specifications was to establish uniform guidelines for cochlear implant manufacturers on how to classify failures and how to calculate and report reliability numbers in order to increase transparency. Before, manufacturers had established their own methodology based on ISO 5841-2, a standard developed for cardiac pacemakers. This standard has some important limitations, for example, permitting subjectivity in the inclusion of data and not differentiating the patient population by age. Therefore, a direct quantitative comparison of reliability data across manufacturers was impossible. This was also demonstrated in a recent analysis, which showed that the reliability data reported from clinical studies do not fit the data presented by cochlear implant manufacturers [84, 85].

Before the standardization committee started working on ANSI/AAMI CI86 in 2011, the limitations of the then established reliability reporting methods had been recognized not only by regulatory authorities but also by clinicians, who were proposing a failure classification scheme to be applied in addition to the rules as laid out in ISO 5841-2 [86]. However, the proposal of Battmer, Backous [86] was lacking transparency as well, because medical-related explantations were still excluded from being reported and failure classification did not follow a root-cause analysis but rather a clinical assessment, depending on the patient performance after successful reimplantation. Nevertheless, most of the manufacturers followed the suggested reporting principles of Battmer, Backous [86] and clinicians used it frequently to classify device failures in their studies. Another methodology for classifying suspected device failures was discussed in 2005 during a consensus workshop [87]. According to the statement by Balkany, Hodges [87], suspected device failures are classified as "soft" failures, whereas confirmed device failures are classified as "hard" failures. This was never adopted by manufacturers but is still widely used in clinical reliability reports [88].

## 23.6 Implant Reliability Performance

Some cochlear implant manufacturers recently began to report their reliability numbers following the requirements of ANSI/AAMI CI86. However, as not all manufacturers are yet compliant and because the data and the applied methodology have not yet been scrutinized by the FDA in an audit, it is still considered too early to use the currently available data from the manufacturers to be presented here. In order to obtain an insight into the reliability performance of current cochlear implants, it is therefore still recommended to rely on clinical studies based on the following quality factors:

- The completeness of data, especially with regard to the inclusion of all explantations or revisions irrespective of the root cause for failure or whether the patients were reimplanted after the explantation or not.
- The mean duration of follow-up, which should be at least several years. Cochlear implant patients experience a significantly higher failure rate during the first half year post-implantation, which is mainly attributable to medical-related complications [89]; however, to also cover device-related failures, a longer observation period is warranted.
- The analysis should be stratified into subgroups of different device models and patient populations by age. The total number of subjects in each subgroup should at least be 500, as complications and failures in general are rare.
- The results should ideally be presented as cumulative survival rates (CSR) or cumulative failure percentages (CFP), in order to fully capture the temporal characteristics of implantations and explantations. If this is not possible, then at least the mean or median follow-up time for each subgroup should be provided.
- Collaboration with the manufacturer of the devices included in the study is recommended, in order to obtain a deeper understanding of the failure modes and to improve the overall quality of the study.

The best way to meet these requirements are analyses of large registries. The US FDA has established a large database for postmarket surveillance in the 1990s, the

Manufacturer and User Facility Device Experience (MAUDE) database, which is publicly accessible (https://www.fda.gov/medical-devices/device-advice-comprehensive-regulatory-assistance/medical-device-databases). Manufacturers are mandated to report events to this database if their medical device or the malfunction of their medical device may have caused or contributed to a death or serious injury of a patient. However, the US FDA recognizes that there are several limitations to this passive surveillance system and that neither the incidence nor prevalence of such reported events may be determined from the database alone. The structural limitations of the MAUDE database were also described by Tambyraja, Gutman [90]. In Europe, together with the introduction of the new Medical Device Regulation, a new registry for medical devices will become available by 2022, the European Database for Medical Devices (EUDAMED), which will have a similar functionality as the MAUDE database.

There are efforts underway in the USA, mainly driven by the clinical community, to establish a registry which is dedicated to cochlear implants and allows for better data analysis [91]. But so far, this registry has not been used for an analysis of reliability performance. In France, a National Registry for Cochlear Implants (EPIIC) was already established in 2011 in a collaborative effort between the French Higher Health Authority (HAS), the French CI clinics, and the cochlear implant manufacturers. Recently, for the first time, a series of publications documented the current status of cochlear implantation in France based on findings from the EPIIC, including one publication on explantations and reimplantations [92] and one publication on complications [93].

The study of Hermann, Coudert [92] aimed to determine the frequency and the causes of cochlear explantations with subsequent reimplantations, after a 5-year follow-up of the patients included in the EPIIC. The study was conducted prospectively on 5051 patients (3178 adults and 1873 children) enrolled in the registry at 30 French CI clinics between January 2012 and December 2016. Assuming a constant number of annual implantations, the mean duration of follow-up of these patients would be 2.5 years. The explantation and reimplantation rate in this study was 1.96% for the total population, with 1.16% for adults and 3.31% for children ($p < 0.00001$). According to the study authors, 46.4% of the explantations were linked to a malfunction of the device, which was more common in children (53%) than in adults (18%, $p < 0.01$). In 39.3% of cases, the explantation was caused by medical or surgical reasons and in 14.1% the root cause for explantation could not be determined. Although theoretically possible, the authors decided not to extract data related to different implant brands or models, or the different implant clinics. Therefore, a more detailed analysis is not available.

The second study based on EPIIC was aimed at evaluating peri- and post-operative complications related to cochlear implantation. The study was conducted retrospectively, for all patients who underwent cochlear implantation at 31 French CI clinics between January 2012 and December 2016; 3483 adults and 2245 children were included in the study. Parent, Codet [93] found out that the total complication rate was 6.84%. Intraoperative complications were reported in 58 patients (1.01%), with no significant difference between adults and children. Post-operative complications were grouped into four different categories (local, device-related, cochleo-vestibular, lesions of adjacent structures), and were reported in 334 cases for 265 patients. Local complications (infections, scarring, pain, and hematoma) accounted for 43% of the detected post-operative complications. Their risk of occurrence was similar in the pediatric and adult population (2.67% and 2.38%, $p = 0.49$). Device-related complications were significantly higher for children (2.00%) than adults (0.80%, $p < 0.0001$), which was due to a significantly higher risk of trauma-related breakdown of the device (1.16% for children vs. 0.03% for adults, $p < 0.0001$). In contrast, cochleo-vestibular complications (dizziness, vertigo, and tinnitus) were observed significantly more often in adults (1.72%) than in children (0.40%, $p < 0.0001$). Also, complications related to lesions of adjacent structures occurred significantly more often in adults (0.83%) than children 0.36%, $p = 0.028$), which was mostly due to facial paralysis. Regarding their analysis of different etiologies, the only patient group associated with more complications than the largest group of patients with unknown etiology was the group with cochlear malformation ($p = 0.02$). 11.6% of the operations were done in an outpatient setting with no difference in the complication rate compared to the group of patients who were hospitalized, neither for adults nor for children. Parent, Codet [93] conclude that cochlear implantation is a safe technique with a low incidence of complications and can be offered safely to patients of all age groups.

These registry studies are extremely valuable as they deliver highly credible information because of the large cohort of patients. It will be interesting to see follow-up studies in some years from now in order to learn more about long-term reliability performance and about the advancement of technology and clinical procedures. The only possibility to match the patient numbers of such a large registry study is to form a multicenter study group. The HEARRING group (www.hearring.com) is an independent network of world-leading CI clinics and experts who decided in 2014 to conduct a large multicenter study on the type and incidence of cochlear implant failures, involving 2 HEARRING clinics in collaboration with MED-EL [6]. The retrospective database study included 11,662 cochlear implantations which were performed between January 2003 and April 2013. Over these 10 years, 6200 devices were implanted in adults and 5462 devices were implanted in children, with a mean duration of follow-up of 46.16 months. The methods of ANSI/AAMI CI86 were used for the failure analysis. The total failure rate for all devices and subjects was 2.41% and was significantly worse for children than adults (3.90% vs. 1.10%). This was mostly related to a significantly higher proportion of device failure explantations in children than in adults, irrespective of device type, and significantly higher medical-related explantations in children than in adults for ceramic implants. The higher number of device failures in children was caused by trauma-related breakages of the housing (in ceramic implants) or the electrodes (for all implant types). The higher number of medical-related explantations in children with ceramic implants was linked to a higher proportion of electrode damage from fatigue wire breakage after insufficient implant immobilization. The mean annual failure rate for all subjects and devices was 0.63% (1.03% for children, 0.28% for adults), with better values for newer generations of implants (Combi 40+ 0.90%; Pulsar 0.57%; Sonata 0.46%; Concerto 0.39%). Table 23.1 summarizes the results.

**Table 23.1** Reliability performance of 24 HEARRING clinics with MED-EL cochlear implants (reproduced from Van de Heyning, Atlas, et al. [6])

| Population | Number of implants | Mean follow-up years | Reimplantation | | Mean annual failure rate | Cumulative survival rate | |
|---|---|---|---|---|---|---|---|
| | | | Number | % | % | 5-year, % | 10-year, % |
| Total | 11,662 | 3.85 | 281 | 2.41 | 0.63 | na | na |
| Adults | 6200 | 3.89 | 68 | 1.10 | 0.28 | na | na |
| Children | 5462 | 3.80 | 213 | 3.90 | 1.03 | na | na |
| *Combi 40+* | | | | | | | |
| Total | 1695 | 6.66 | 102 | 6.02 | 0.90 | na | na |
| Adults | 695 | 7.62 | 20 | 2.88 | 0.38 | 97.8[a] | 96.5[a] |
| Children | 1000 | 5.92 | 82 | 8.20 | 1.39 | 92.7[a] | 88.3[a] |
| *Pulsar* | | | | | | | |
| Total | 4822 | 4.69 | 129 | 2.68 | 0.57 | na | na |
| Adults | 2491 | 4.90 | 30 | 1.20 | 0.25 | 98.6[a] | na |
| Children | 2331 | 4.40 | 99 | 4.25 | 0.97 | 95.1[a] | na |
| *Sonata* | | | | | | | |
| Total | 3196 | 2.87 | 42 | 1.31 | 0.46 | na | na |
| Adults | 1918 | 2.89 | 15 | 0.78 | 0.27 | 99.0[a] | na |
| Children | 1278 | 2.82 | 27 | 2.11 | 0.75 | 96.8[a] | na |
| *Concerto* | | | | | | | |
| Total | 1949 | 1.04 | 8 | 0.41 | 0.39 | na | na |
| Adults | 1096 | 1.00 | 3 | 0.27 | 0.27 | na | na |
| Children | 853 | 1.12 | 5 | 0.59 | 0.53 | na | na |

*na* not available
[a]Values estimated from the graphs in the paper

A similar, although single-center study was conducted on Nucleus implants by a group of researchers at the Sydney Cochlear Implant Center, with the support of Cochlear Corporation [14]. In a retrospective review over a period of 30 years, between January 1982 and June 2011, Wang, Wang [14] aimed to characterize revision cochlear implant surgery and to quantify rates of revision and device failure at their center. During the study period, 2827 cochlear implantations were performed in 2311 patients, with a median follow-up time of 4.8 years. 191 patients had to undergo 235 revision surgeries; the overall revision rate was 8.3%. The most common indication for revision surgery was device failure (57.8%), followed by migration/extrusion (23.4%), infection/wound complication (17.0%), and poor outcome/secondary pathology (6.4%). The two most common reasons for device failure were electrode array damage (48.1%) and loss of hermetic seal (45.5%). The cumulative revision rate for all devices at all ages increased linearly by approximately 1% per year, and it was significantly higher in children. After 10 years, the difference of cumulative revision rates between adults and children was 5% ($p = 0.008$). The risk for device explantation decreased significantly with more recently performed implantations and with newer generations of implants ($p = 0.0001$). Table 23.2 shows the cumulative revision rates for various types of Nucleus implants that were implanted during the study period.

**Table 23.2** Reliability performance of the Sydney Cochlear Implant Center with Nucleus cochlear implants (reproduced from Wang, Wang et al. [14])

| | | Reimplantation | | Cumulative survival rate | |
|---|---|---|---|---|---|
| Population | Number of implants | Number | % | 5-year, % | 10-year, % |
| Total | 2827 | 235 | 8.31 | 95.0[a] | 90.0[a] |
| Adults | na | 108 | 6.5 | 96.4[a] | 91.6[a] |
| Children | na | 127 | 10.8 | 93.7[a] | 87.1[a] |
| CI 22 | 352 | na | na | 91.8[a] | 83.2[a] |
| CI 24 | 794 | na | na | 92.3[a] | 89.4[a] |
| CI 24RE | 1091 | na | na | 96.1[a] | na |
| CI 512 | 519 | na | na | na | na |
| CI 422 | 6 | na | na | na | na |

*na* not available
[a]Values estimated from the graphs in the paper

Another, recently published study by a group of Canadian researchers from London Health Sciences Center stands out because the authors used also the ANSI/AAMI CI86 methodology for analyzing and reporting their data [94]. The objective of their study was to perform an institutional assessment of device failures and cochlear reimplantation rates over a 30-year period and to conduct a detailed literature review in order to compare their data. Between January 1988 and March 2017, 804 cochlear implantations were performed in adult (488 implants) and pediatric (316 implants) patients with implants from Advanced Bionics, Cochlear, and MED-EL. The institutional reimplantation rate was 2.9%, with rates of 8.2%, 6.1%, and 1.1% obtained for Advanced Bionics, Cochlear, and MED-EL, respectively. This difference in reliability performance across manufacturers is statistically significant ($p < 0.0001$). However, these results show rather a comparison of different implant generations, as all implants from Advanced Bionics and Cochlear were implanted before 2005, and MED-EL implants were used in the center from 2002 onward. Two other factors contributing to the relatively poor values for the Advanced Bionics implants in this study are the relatively low number of Advanced Bionics devices operated in this clinic and that the device failures of Advanced Bionics implants were related to faults in the hermetic seal of the implants, which resulted in a device recall by the manufacturer in 2004. Looking at device failure rates separately, there was a significant difference between the failure rates in the pediatric (2.8%) and adult (1.0%) populations ($p = 0.02$). This was mainly caused by the trauma-related failures in the pediatric group. Lane, Zimmerman [94] also conducted a literature review which revealed favorable results for their center, for both medical-related failures and device failures. They speculate that these results may be secondary to their surgical technique of drilling the bony bed for the implant housing and the electrode lead channel, their fixation method of the implant, and the low infection rate. Table 23.3 provides more details to this study.

Finally, another interesting and methodologically suitable long-term study was published recently by a group of researchers from the Samsung Medical Center in Korea, with the objectives of analyzing the revision surgery rate, the reasons for

**Table 23.3** Reliability performance at the London Health Sciences Center (reproduced from Lane, Zimmerman et al. [94])

| | | Reimplantation | | Cumulative survival rate | |
|---|---|---|---|---|---|
| Population | Number of implants | Number | % | 5-year, % | 10-year, % |
| Total | 804 | 23 | 2.86 | 98.5[a] | 97.0[a] |
| Adults | 488 | 9 | 1.84 | na | na |
| Children | 316 | 14 | 4.43 | na | na |
| *Advanced Bionics* | | | | | |
| Total | 49 | 4 | 8.16 | 98.2[a] | 94.4[a] |
| Adults | 40 | 4 | 10.00 | 98.0[a] | 94.0[a] |
| Children | 9 | 0 | 0 | 100.0 | 100.0 |
| Clarion 1.2 | 14 | na | na | 100.0 | 88.2 |
| Clarion CII | 1 | na | na | 100.0 | 100.0 |
| HiRes 90k | 34 | na | na | 97.3 | 97.3 |
| *Cochlear* | | | | | |
| Total | 214 | 13 | 6.07 | 97.4[a] | 95.0[a] |
| Adults | 115 | 3 | 2.61 | 99.1[a] | 98.4[a] |
| Children | 99 | 10 | 10.10 | 94.4[a] | 94.4[a] |
| CI 22M | 76 | na | na | 95.2 | 94.0 |
| CI 24M | 41 | na | na | 97.7 | 97.7 |
| CI 24R/RE | 96 | na | na | 99.0 | 95.9 |
| CI 522 | 1 | na | na | 100.0 | na |
| *MED-EL* | | | | | |
| Total | 541 | 6 | 1.11 | 99.0[a] | 99.0[a] |
| Adults | 333 | 2 | 0.60 | 99.3[a] | 99.3[a] |
| Children | 208 | 4 | 1.92 | 98.0[a] | 98.0[a] |
| Combi 40+ | 22 | na | na | 100.0 | 100.0 |
| Pulsar | 118 | na | na | 98.3 | 98.3 |
| Sonata | 167 | na | na | 99.4 | 99.4 |
| Concerto | 179 | na | na | 97.5 | na |
| Synchrony | 55 | na | na | na | na |

*na* not available

[a]Values estimated from the graphs in the paper

revision surgery, and device failure and survival rates of different device models [95]. The retrospective cohort study looked at implantations in 925 patients, which were performed between October 2001 and March 2019. 202 of these are adults (20 years of age and older according to the authors), and 723 are children. 43 of these patients underwent revision surgery (4.6%). Device failure was the most common reason (65%), followed by flap-associated problems (9.3%) and migration of the implant (9.3%). Overall, the 10-year cumulative survival rate of cochlear implantation was 94.4%. Several recalls were issued by manufacturers during the study period, which influenced the results. According to the authors, no meaningful differences in device failures were found among CI manufacturers or devices if the recalled devices were excluded from the analysis. Table 23.4 provides more detailed information on each of the implanted devices.

**Table 23.4** Reliability performance at the Samsung Medical Center (reproduced from Kim, Kim et al. [95])

| Population | Number of implants | Mean follow-up years | Reimplantation Number | Reimplantation % | Mean annual failure rate % | Cumulative survival rate 5-year, % | Cumulative survival rate 10-year, % |
|---|---|---|---|---|---|---|---|
| Total | 925 | 7.1 | 43 | 4.65 | 0.65 | na | na |
| *Advanced Bionics* | | | | | | | |
| Total | 146 | 11.5 | 9 | 6.16 | 0.53 | 94.48 | 93.8[a] |
| Clarion CII | 4 | 15.5 | 0 | 0 | na | 100.0 | 100.0 |
| HiRes 90k | 142 | 11.4 | 9 | 6.34 | 0.55 | 94.32 | 93.60 |
| *Cochlear* | | | | | | | |
| Total | 506 | 7.5 | 27 | 5.34 | 0.71 | 94.95 | 93.8[a] |
| CI 24R | 49 | 15.1 | 0 | 0 | na | 100.0 | 100.0 |
| CI 24RE | 159 | 10.2 | 9 | 5.66 | 0.55 | 94.34 | 94.34 |
| CI 422 | 185 | 4.6 | 4 | 2.16 | 0.47 | na | na |
| CI 512 | 66 | 7.9 | 13 | 19.70 | 2.49 | 83.33 | na |
| CI 522 | 30 | 1.0 | 1 | 3.33 | 3.33 | na | na |
| CI 532 | 17 | 0.5 | 0 | 0 | na | na | na |
| *MED-EL* | | | | | | | |
| Total | 270 | 4.1 | 7 | 2.59 | 0.63 | 96.93 | na |
| Pulsar | 1 | 6.5 | 0 | 0 | na | 100 | na |
| Sonata | 60 | 6.8 | 2 | 3.33 | 0.49 | 96.67 | na |
| Concerto | 178 | 3.8 | 4 | 2.25 | 0.59 | 97.55 | na |
| Synchrony | 31 | 0.6 | 1 | 3.23 | 5.38 | na | na |
| *Oticon* | | | | | | | |
| Neuro Zti | 3 | 0.5 | 0 | 0 | na | na | na |

*na* not available
[a]Values estimated from the graphs in the paper

A direct comparison of the results of these studies proves to be difficult. The studies were conducted over different study periods, with different device generations from different device manufacturers, and with different follow-up times of the included patients. Also, not all studies separately investigated children and adults, and if they did so, the authors used different criteria for stratification. Considering all these differences, the most reasonable method seems to be the analysis and comparison of CSR values of implant models of the same generation.

The CSR for the Nucleus CI 24RE can be derived from the publications of Wang, Wang [14] and Kim, Kim [95]; the 5-year values provided in the publications are at 96.1% and 94.34%, respectively, for the adults and children combined. The variation may be explained by the relatively higher proportion of pediatric patients in the Kim, Kim [95] study. The study of Lane, Zimmerman [94] documents a 5-year CSR value of 99.0% for the CI 24RE combined with the CI 24R implant which may be related to the relatively higher proportion of adult patients in their clinical cohort.

Values for MED-EL's Sonata and the Pulsar implants are available from the papers of Van de Heyning, Atlas [6], Lane, Zimmerman [94] and Kim, Kim [95]. The 5-year CSR values for the Sonata for all age groups combined range from 96.67% (Kim, Kim [95]) to 99.4% (Lane, Zimmerman [94]), which reflects the spread of values in the Van de Heyning, Atlas [6] publication between children and adults. The 5-year values for the Pulsar are in the range of 95.17% (children, Van de Heyning, Atlas [6]) and 98.65% (adults, Van de Heyning, Atlas [6]), with the values in the Lane, Zimmerman [94] paper for the total population being at 98.3%. Also the MED-EL data suggest that the difference in CSR values between the clinics is mainly related to the different populations in both studies (the Korean clinic is mainly implanting children, while the Canadian clinic is mainly implanting adults). When comparing the implant models with each other, both MED-EL implants show very similar values to the Nucleus CI24RE, by an estimated 1–2% difference after 5 years of implant use.

For the comparison of the Nucleus CI 422 and the MED-EL Concerto implant, the papers by Kim, Kim [95] and Lane, Zimmerman [94] can be used. Both show approximately the same 5-year CSR value for the Concerto at 97.5%, which corresponds to a reimplantation rate of 2.25% for a mean follow-up time of 3.8 years according to Kim, Kim [95]. The reimplantation rate for the Nucleus CI 422 is at 2.16% with a slightly longer mean follow-up time of 4.6 years (Kim, Kim [95]). Also in this comparison, the Nucleus CI 422 is very similar in its reliability performance to the MED-EL Concerto.

## 23.7 Conclusions

Cochlear implantation is in general a well-established and highly reliable clinical procedure, with annual failure rates between 0.5% for adults and 1.0% for children. Long-term studies demonstrate that the devices of the same generation but made by different manufacturers show approximately comparable reliability performance and that the devices and the surgical procedure are getting safer and more reliable over the years. This is not surprising, as manufacturers constantly improve their devices in order to meet the regulations and to be compliant with the latest technical standards. After all, manufacturers have an ethical responsibility toward the patients and the clinicians to further improve their products and to inform the public honestly about potential risks of the treatment.

## References


1. Dhillon BS. Medical device reliability and associated areas. CRC Press LLC; 2000. 240 p.
2. Causon A, Verschuur C, Newman TA. Trends in cochlear implant complications: implications for improving long-term outcomes. Otol Neurotol. 2013;34(2):259–65.
3. Weise JB, Muller-Deile J, Brademann G, Meyer JE, Ambrosch P, Maune S. Impact to the head increases cochlear implant reimplantation rate in children. Auris Nasus Larynx. 2005;32(4):339–43.

4. Cote M, Ferron P, Bergeron F, Bussieres R. Cochlear reimplantation: causes of failure, outcomes, and audiologic performance. Laryngoscope. 2007;117(7):1225–35.
5. Masterson L, Kumar S, Kong JH, Briggs J, Donnelly N, Axon PR, et al. Cochlear implant failures: lessons learned from a UK centre. J Laryngol Otol. 2012;126(1):15–21.
6. Van de Heyning P, Atlas M, Baumgartner W-D, Caversaccio M, Gavilan J, Godey B, et al. The reliability of hearing implants: report on the type and incidence of cochlear implant failures. Cochlear Implants Int. 2020;21(4):228–37.
7. Migirov L, Kronenberg J. Magnet displacement following cochlear implantation. Otol Neurotol. 2005;26(4):646–8.
8. Stokroos RJ, van Dijk P. Migration of cochlear implant magnets after head trauma in an adult and a child. Ear Nose Throat J. 2007;86(10):612–3.
9. Hassepass F, Stabenau V, Maier W, Arndt S, Laszig R, Beck R, et al. Revision surgery due to magnet dislocation in cochlear implant patients: an emerging complication. Otol Neurotol. 2014;35(1):29–34.
10. Eby TL, Nadol JB Jr. Postnatal growth of the human temporal bone. Implications for cochlear implants in children. Ann Otol Rhinol Laryngol. 1986;95(4 Pt 1):356–64.
11. Simms DL, Neely JG. Growth of the lateral surface of the temporal bone in children. Laryngoscope. 1989;99(8):795–9.
12. Dahm MC, Shepherd RK, Clark GM. The postnatal growth of the temporal bone and its implications for cochlear implantation in children. Acta Oto-Laryngologica. 1993;113(Suppl 505):4–39.
13. Gosepath J, Lippert K, Keilmann A, Mann WJ. Analysis of fifty-six cochlear implant device failures. ORL J Otorhinolaryngol Relat Spec. 2009;71(3):142–7.
14. Wang JT, Wang AY, Psarros C, Da Cruz M. Rates of revision and device failure in cochlear implant surgery: a 30-year experience. Laryngoscope. 2014;124(10):2393–9.
15. Carlson ML, Archibald DJ, Dabade TS, Gifford RH, Neff BA, Beatty CW, et al. Prevalence and timing of individual cochlear implant electrode failures. Otol Neurotol. 2010;31(6):893–8.
16. Goehring JL, Hughes ML, Baudhuin JL, Lusk RP. How well do cochlear implant intraoperative impedance measures predict postoperative electrode function? Otol Neurotol. 2013;34(2):239–44.
17. Harris JM, Neault MW, O'Neill EE, Griffin AM, Kawai K, Kenna MA, et al. Incidence, time course, and implications of electrode abnormalities in pediatric cochlear implant recipients. Ear Hear. 2021;42(2)
18. Zeitler DM, Budenz CL, Roland JT Jr. Revision cochlear implantation. Curr Opin Otolaryngol Head Neck Surg. 2009;17(5):334–8.
19. Newbold C, Risi F, Hollow R, Yusof Y, Dowell R. Long-term electrode impedance changes and failure prevalence in cochlear implants. Int J Audiol. 2015;54(7):453–60.
20. Cullington HE. Managing cochlear implant patients with suspected insulation damage. Ear Hear. 2013;34(4):515–21.
21. Gärtner L, Büchner A, Illg A, Lenarz T. Hidden electrode failure in a cochlear implant user. Laryngoscope. 2021;131(4):E1275–E8.
22. Lewkowitz A, Harris J, Licameli G. CIs with known potential for failure: monitoring and management in children. Hear J. 2020;73(9):9–10.
23. de Varebeke SP, Govaerts P, Cox T, Deben K, Ketelslagers K, Waelkens B. Fixation of cochlear implants: an evidence-based review of literature. B-Ent. 2012;8(2):85–94.
24. Lenarz T, Stöver T, Buechner A, Lesinski-Schiedat A, Patrick J, Pesch J. Hearing conservation surgery using the Hybrid-L electrode. Results from the first clinical trial at the Medical University of Hannover. Audiol Neurootol. 2009;14(Suppl 1):22–31.
25. Cohen NL, Kuzma J. Titanium clip for cochlear implant electrode fixation. Ann Otol Rhinol Laryngol Suppl. 1995;166:402–3.
26. Pamuk AE, Pamuk G, Jafarov S, Bajin MD, Sarac S, Sennaroglu L. The effect of cochlear implant bed preparation and fixation technique on the revision cochlear implantation rate. J Laryngol Otol. 2018;132(6):534–9.

27. Stern Shavit S, Weinstein EP, Drusin MA, Elkin EB, Lustig LR, Alexiades G. Comparison of cochlear implant device fixation-well drilling versus subperiosteal pocket. A cost effectiveness, case-control study. Otol Neurotol. 2021;42(4):517–23.
28. Markodimitraki LM, Strijbos RM, Stegeman I, Thomeer H. Cochlear implant fixation techniques: a systematic review of the literature. Otol Neurotol. 2021;
29. Kim BG, Kim JW, Park JJ, Kim SH, Kim HN, Choi JY. Adverse events and discomfort during magnetic resonance imaging in cochlear implant recipients. JAMA Otolaryngol Head Neck Surg. 2015;141(1):45–52.
30. Carlson ML, Neff BA, Link MJ, Lane JI, Watson RE, McGee KP, et al. Magnetic resonance imaging with cochlear implant magnet in place: safety and imaging quality. Otol Neurotol. 2015;36(6):965–71.
31. Young NM, Rojas C, Deng J, Burrowes D, Ryan M. Magnetic resonance imaging of cochlear implant recipients. Otol Neurotol. 2016;37(6):665–71.
32. Pross SE, Ward BK, Sharon JD, Weinreich HM, Aygun N, Francis HW. A prospective study of pain from magnetic resonance imaging with cochlear implant magnets in situ. Otol Neurotol. 2018;39(2):e80–e6.
33. Leinung M, Loth A, Gröger M, Burck I, Vogl T, Stöver T, et al. Cochlear implant magnet dislocation after MRI: surgical management and outcome. Eur Arch Otorhinolaryngol. 2020;277(5):1297–304.
34. Srinivasan R, So CW, Amin N, Jaikaransingh D, D'Arco F, Nash R. A review of the safety of MRI in cochlear implant patients with retained magnets. Clin Radiol. 2019;74(12):972.e9–e16.
35. Wolf-Magele A, Schnabl J, Hirtler L, Heinz G, Sprinzl GM. MRI safety with cochlear implants up to three Tesla – experiences by performing an in vitro test. J Otol Rhinol. 2016;5(4)
36. Canzi P, Aprile F, Simoncelli A, Manfrin M, Magnetto M, Lafe E, et al. MRI-induced artifact by a cochlear implant with a novel magnet system: an experimental cadaver study. Eur Arch Otorhinolaryngol. 2020;
37. Eerkens HJ, Smits C, Hofman MBM. Cochlear implant magnet dislocation: simulations and measurements of force and torque at 1.5T magnetic resonance imaging. Ear Hear. 2021;
38. Todt I, Tittel A, Ernst A, Mittmann P, Mutze S. Pain free 3 T MRI scans in cochlear implantees. Otol Neurotol. 2017;38(10):e401–e4.
39. Young NM, Hoff SR, Ryan M. Impact of cochlear implant with diametric magnet on imaging access, safety, and clinical care. Laryngoscope. 2021;131(3):E952–e6.
40. Hansen S, Anthonsen K, Stangerup SE, Jensen JH, Thomsen J, Caye-Thomasen P. Unexpected findings and surgical complications in 505 consecutive cochlear implantations: a proposal for reporting consensus. Acta Otolaryngol. 2010;130(5):540–9.
41. Jiang Y, Gu P, Li B, Gao X, Sun B, Song Y, et al. Analysis and management of complications in a cohort of 1,065 minimally invasive cochlear implantations. Otol Neurotol. 2017;38(3):347–51.
42. Olsen LB, Larsen S, Wanscher JH, Faber CE, Jeppesen J. Postoperative infections following cochlear implant surgery. Acta Otolaryngol. 2018;138(10):956–60.
43. Petersen H, Walshe P, Glynn F, McMahon R, Fitzgerald C, Thapa J, et al. Occurrence of major complications after cochlear implant surgery in Ireland. Cochlear Implants Int. 2018;19(6):297–306.
44. Nisenbaum EJ, Roland JT, Waltzman S, Friedmann DR. Risk factors and management of postoperative infection following cochlear implantation. Otol Neurotol. 2020;41(7):e823–e8.
45. Weder S, Shaul C, Wong A, O'Leary S, Briggs RJ. Management of severe cochlear implant infections-35 years clinical experience. Otol Neurotol. 2020;41(10):1341–9.
46. Reefhuis J, Honein MA, Whitney CG, Chamany S, Mann EA, Biernath KR, et al. Risk of bacterial meningitis in children with cochlear implants. N Engl J Med. 2003;349(5):435–45.
47. Biernath KR, Reefhuis J, Whitney CG, Mann EA, Costa P, Eichwald J, et al. Bacterial meningitis among children with cochlear implants beyond 24 months after implantation. Pediatrics. 2006;117(2):284–9.
48. Reefhuis J, Whitney CG, Mann EA. A public health perspective on cochlear implants and meningitis in children. Otol Neurotol. 2010;31(8):1329–30.

49. Lalwani AK, Cohen NL. Does meningitis after cochlear implantation remain a concern in 2011? Otol Neurotol. 2012;33(1):93–5.
50. Bas E, Dinh CT, Garnham C, Polak M, Van de Water TR. Conservation of hearing and protection of hair cells in cochlear implant patients' with residual hearing. Anat Rec (Hoboken). 2012;295(11):1909–27.
51. Dhanasingh A, Jolly C. An overview of cochlear implant electrode array designs. Hear Res. 2017;356:93–103.
52. Dhanasingh A, Jolly C. Review on cochlear implant electrode array tip fold-over and scalar deviation. J Otol. 2019;14(3):94–100.
53. Eshraghi AA, Yang NW, Balkany TJ. Comparative study of cochlear damage with three perimodiolar electrode designs. Laryngoscope. 2003;113(3):415–9.
54. Jwair S, Prins A, Wegner I, Stokroos RJ, Versnel H, Thomeer H. Scalar translocation comparison between lateral wall and perimodiolar cochlear implant arrays – a meta-analysis. Laryngoscope. 2020;
55. Durakovic N, Kallogjeri D, Wick CC, McJunkin JL, Buchman CA, Herzog J. Immediate and 1-year outcomes with a slim modiolar cochlear implant electrode array. Otolaryngol Head Neck Surg. 2020;162(5):731–6.
56. Heutink F, Verbist BM, Mens LHM, Huinck WJ, Mylanus EAM. The evaluation of a slim perimodiolar electrode: surgical technique in relation to intracochlear position and cochlear implant outcomes. Eur Arch Otorhinolaryngol. 2020;277(2):343–50.
57. Liebscher T, Mewes A, Hoppe U, Hornung J, Brademann G, Hey M. Electrode translocations in perimodiolar cochlear implant electrodes: audiological and electrophysiological outcome. Z Med Phys. 2020;
58. Shaul C, Weder S, Tari S, Gerard JM, O'Leary SJ, Briggs RJ. Slim, modiolar cochlear implant electrode: Melbourne experience and comparison with the contour perimodiolar electrode. Otol Neurotol. 2020;41(5):639–43.
59. Rivas A, Marlowe AL, Chinnici JE, Niparko JK, Francis HW. Revision cochlear implantation surgery in adults: indications and results. Otol Neurotol. 2008;29(5):639–48.
60. Dietz A, Wennstrom M, Lehtimaki A, Lopponen H, Valtonen H. Electrode migration after cochlear implant surgery: more common than expected? Eur Arch Otorhinolaryngol. 2016;273(6):1411–8.
61. Mittmann P, Rademacher G, Mutze S, Ernst A, Todt I. Electrode migration in patients with perimodiolar cochlear implant electrodes. Audiol Neurootol. 2015;20(6):349–53.
62. Rader T, Baumann U, Stover T, Weissgerber T, Adel Y, Leinung M, et al. Management of cochlear implant electrode migration. Otol Neurotol. 2016;37(9):e341–8.
63. Connell SS, Balkany TJ, Hodges AV, Telischi FF, Angeli SI, Eshraghi AA. Electrode migration after cochlear implantation. Otol Neurotol. 2008;29(2):156–9.
64. Hildrew DM, Molony TB. Nucleus N5 CI500 series implant recall: hard failure rate at a major Cochlear implantation center. Laryngoscope. 2013;123(11):2829–33.
65. Clark GM, Clark J, Cardamone T, Clarke M, Nielsen P, Jones R, et al. Biomedical studies on temporal bones of the first multi-channel cochlear implant patient at the University of Melbourne. Cochlear Implants Int. 2014;15(Suppl 2):S1–15.
66. Nadol JB Jr, O'Malley JT, Burgess BJ, Galler D. Cellular immunologic responses to cochlear implantation in the human. Hear Res. 2014;318:11–7.
67. Anand V, Devi MK, Kannan T, Chenniappan S. Laser tympanic neurectomy for post-cochlear implant pain: a new technique. Cochlear Implants Int. 2016;17(2):105–8.
68. Yong M, Young E, Lea J, Foggin H, Zaia E, Kozak FK, et al. Subjective and objective vestibular changes that occur following paediatric cochlear implantation: systematic review and meta-analysis. J Otolaryngol Head Neck Surg. 2019;48(1):22.
69. Jin Y, Shinjo Y, Akamatsu Y, Yamasoba T, Kaga K. Vestibular evoked myogenic potentials of children with inner ear malformations before and after cochlear implantation. Acta Otolaryngol. 2009;129(11):1198–205.
70. Coordes A, Basta D, Gotze R, Scholz S, Seidl RO, Ernst A, et al. Sound-induced vertigo after cochlear implantation. Otol Neurotol. 2012;33(3):335–42.

71. le Nobel GJ, Hwang E, Wu A, Cushing S, Lin VY. Vestibular function following unilateral cochlear implantation for profound sensorineural hearing loss. J Otolaryngol Head Neck Surg. 2016;45(1):38.
72. Alzhrani F, Halawani R, Basodan S, Hudeib R. Investigating facial nerve stimulation after cochlear implantation in adult and pediatric recipients. Laryngoscope. 2021;131(2):374–9.
73. Seyyedi M, Herrmann BS, Eddington DK, Nadol JB Jr. The pathologic basis of facial nerve stimulation in otosclerosis and multi-channel cochlear implantation. Otol Neurotol. 2013;34(9):1603–9.
74. Kasetty VM, Zimmerman Z, King S, Seyyedi M. Comparison of temporal bone parameters before cochlear implantation in patients with and without facial nerve stimulation. J Audiol Otol. 2019;23(4):193–6.
75. Hochmair-Desoyer I, Burian K. Reimplantation of a molded scala tympani electrode: impact on psychophysical and speech discrimination abilities. Ann Otol Rhinol Laryngol. 1985;94(1 Pt 1):65–70.
76. Dillon MT, Adunka OF, Anderson ML, Adunka MC, King ER, Buchman CA, et al. Influence of age at revision cochlear implantation on speech perception outcomes. JAMA Otolaryngol Head Neck Surg. 2015;141(3):219–24.
77. Sterkers F, Merklen F, Piron JP, Vieu A, Venail F, Uziel A, et al. Outcomes after cochlear reimplantation in children. Int J Pediatr Otorhinolaryngol. 2015;79(6):840–3.
78. Manrique-Huarte R, Huarte A, Manrique MJ. Surgical findings and auditory performance after cochlear implant revision surgery. Eur Arch Otorhinolaryngol. 2016;273(3):621–9.
79. Patnaik U, Sikka K, Agarwal S, Kumar R, Thakar A, Sharma SC. Cochlear re-implantation: lessons learnt and the way ahead. Acta Otolaryngol. 2016;136(6):564–7.
80. Reis M, Boisvert I, Looi V, da Cruz M. Speech recognition outcomes after cochlear reimplantation surgery. Trends Hear. 2017;21:2331216517706398.
81. Holcomb MA, Burton JA, Dornhoffer JR, Camposeo EL, Meyer TA, McRackan TR. When to replace legacy cochlear implants for technological upgrades: Indications and outcomes. Laryngoscope. 2019;129(3):748–53.
82. Walshe P, Thapa J, Ramli RR, Glynn F, Simoes-Franklin C, Reilly RB, et al. The usefulness integrity testing in children: a single institution experience of 86 tests over a period of 20 years. Clin Otolaryngol. 2018;
83. Kaplan EL, Meier P. Nonparametric estimation from incomplete observations. JASA. 1958;53(282):24.
84. O'Neill G, Tolley NS. Cochlear implant reliability: on the reporting of rates of revision surgery. Indian J Otolaryngol Head Neck Surg. 2020;72(2):257–66.
85. O'Neill G, Tolley NS. Cochlear implant reliability: reporting of device failures. Indian J Otolaryngol Head Neck Surg. 2020;72(3):326–8.
86. Battmer RD, Backous DD, Balkany TJ, Briggs RJ, Gantz BJ, van Hasselt A, et al. International classification of reliability for implanted cochlear implant receiver stimulators. Otol Neurotol. 2010;31(8):1190–3.
87. Balkany TJ, Hodges AV, Buchman CA, Luxford WM, Pillsbury CH, Roland PS, et al. Cochlear implant soft failures consensus development conference statement. Otol Neurotol. 2005;26(4):815–8.
88. Ulanovski D, Attias J, Sokolov M, Greenstein T, Raveh E. Pediatric Cochlear implant soft failure. Am J Otolaryngol. 2018;39(2):107–10.
89. Lander DP, Durakovic N, Kallogjeri D, Jiramongkolchai P, Olsen MA, Piccirillo JF, et al. Incidence of infectious complications following cochlear implantation in children and adults. JAMA. 2020;323(2):182–3.
90. Tambyraja RR, Gutman MA, Megerian CA. Cochlear implant complications: utility of federal database in systematic analysis. Arch Otolaryngol Head Neck Surg. 2005;131(3):245–50.
91. Schafer EC, Grisel JJ, de Jong A, Ravelo K, Lam A, Burke M, et al. Creating a framework for data sharing in cochlear implant research. Cochlear Implants Int. 2016;17(6):283–92.

92. Hermann R, Coudert A, Aubry K, Bordure P, Bozorg-Grayeli A, Deguine O, et al. The French National Cochlear Implant Registry (EPIIC): cochlear explantation and reimplantation. Eur Ann Otorhinolaryngol Head Neck Dis. 2020;137(Suppl 1):S45–9.
93. Parent V, Codet M, Aubry K, Bordure P, Bozorg-Grayeli A, Deguine O, et al. The French Cochlear Implant Registry (EPIIC): cochlear implantation complications. Eur Ann Otorhinolaryngol Head Neck Dis. 2020;137(Suppl 1):S37–43.
94. Lane C, Zimmerman K, Agrawal S, Parnes L. Cochlear implant failures and reimplantation: a 30-year analysis and literature review. Laryngoscope. 2020;130(3):782–9.
95. Kim SY, Kim MB, Chung WH, Cho YS, Hong SH, Moon IJ. Evaluating reasons for revision surgery and device failure rates in patients who underwent cochlear implantation surgery. JAMA Otolaryngol Head Neck Surg. 2020;146(5):414–20.

# Cochlear Implants: Recent Advances and New Horizons

# 24

Anandhan Dhanasingh and Claude Jolly

## 24.1 Introduction

Cochlear implants (CI) and the surgical procedure to implant have reached its maturity (in 2021) after 35 years of continuous research and development efforts. As young clinicians are emerging in the CI field, continuous education and training is necessary to keep them well-trained. This is where a scientific collaboration between the experienced clinicians and the CI manufacturers comes in where the CI manufacturer sponsors the training workshop on several occasions and experienced clinicians share their experience with the young clinicians. By and large, CI manufacturers take responsibility for directing the CI field to the next level and that is what CI field has evidenced in the last 30 years in fine-tuning the electrode array design to be highly atraumatic, implant stimulator case getting better with hermiticity, implant magnet becoming MRI compatible, and audio processors becoming aesthetically appealing and advanced with connectivity features. This chapter canvases through the recent advances (2021) and new horizons that could be expected in the CI field and from the CI manufacturers' point of view.

## 24.2 Recent Advances

In the year 2021 as it stands, the CI field has seen several new developments that have been recently made to the clinical application, and this section covers the key new developments and concepts in CI that are well accepted by the clinicians and patients.

**Supplementary Information** The online version contains supplementary material available at [https://doi.org/10.1007/978-981-19-0452-3_24].

A. Dhanasingh (✉) · C. Jolly
MED-EL Medical Electronics, Innsbruck, Austria
e-mail: Anandhan.dhanasingh@medel.com; claude.jolly@medel.com


S. DeSaSouza (ed.), *Cochlear Implants*,
https://doi.org/10.1007/978-981-19-0452-3_24

### 24.2.1 Thin Electrodes

It is clearer than ever before that preserving the intra-cochlear structures is one of the several steps that aims to reverse the CI in the future, when pharmaceutical agents take over the CI in restoring hearing in hearing loss subjects. The electrode array that goes inside the cochlea must be optimal in cross-sectional size and overall volume to safely fit inside the scala tympani (ST) compartment. MED-EL GmbH from Austria came up with the concept of FLEX electrode design. FLEX electrodes incorporate wave-shaped platinum-iridium wires that run through the central core of the electrode and platinum contacts slightly recessed from the surface of the electrode array making the electrode array highly flexible and are reported atraumatic as it is evidenced from the recent literature [1]. Cochlear Corporation from Australia has introduced the slimmer version of its pre-curved and straight electrodes under the commercial name Slim-Modiolar and Slim-Straight electrode. They claim that the slimmer version of their electrode has resulted in better hearing preservation rates [2]. Advanced Bionics LLC from the USA has recently introduced the SLIM-J lateral wall-type electrode which is a slimmer version of the 1J electrode. Mid-Scala is also a slimmer version of the HELIX electrodes. Oticon Medicals (previously called as Neurelec) based in France has come up with the EVO electrode which is again a slimmer version of its previous generation electrode. The aim of all these flexible and slimmer electrodes is to avoid electrode scalar deviation and tip fold-over which could cause damage to the intra-cochlear structures. The electrode insertion procedure as prescribed by the CI manufacturers and how good it is followed by the CI surgeons play a role in the proper placement of the electrode inside the ST. Figure 24.1 captures the electrode types and variants that are currently in clinical use.

### 24.2.2 Single-Unit Processor

The comfort of wearing the audio processor depends mainly on its aesthetic design and how practical it is to use. The duration of the usage of audio processor among

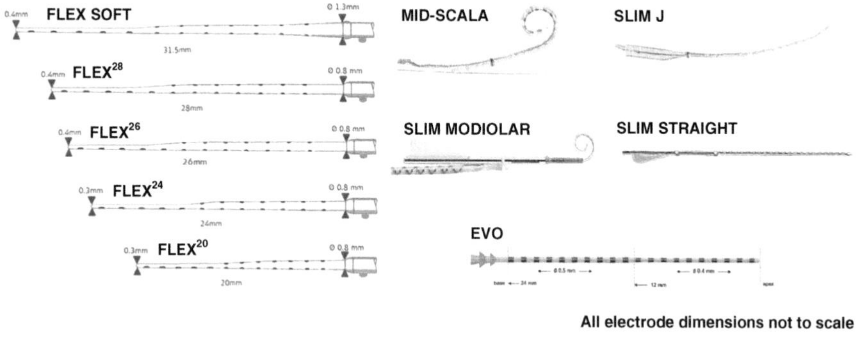


**Fig. 24.1** Latest electrode arrays that are currently (2021) available in the market

several other factors influences the hearing performance of the CI users [3]. The latest development in the audio processor is the single-unit processor that combines the battery pack, processing unit, and the external transmission coil in one unit. This solves several practical issues with *behind-the-ear* (BTE) processor in individuals wearing eyeglasses. Also, the single-unit processor goes invisible if it gets covered by hair. Other advantage is that it eliminates issues related to the cable that connects the processing unit with the external transmission coil. MED-EL GmbH started commercializing its single-unit processor under the name RONDO from 2013, and in the year 2021, they released the latest version RONDO 3. Cochlear Corporation came up with the single-unit processor under the commercial name KANSO in the year 2016. KANSO 2 is their latest version that was introduced in the year 2020. No other CI manufacturers have the single-unit processor at least till the year 2020, but it might come soon. Figure 24.2 shows the single-unit processor from two different CI brands.

Wireless charging of the audio processor battery (MED-EL), water-resistant protective case, and connectivity with external devices are some of the key accessories that come with the single-unit audio processor. Research studies have shown that the single-unit processors provide similar if not superior hearing performance compared to the BTE processor [4].

### 24.2.3 Otologic Preplanning Tool

Standard DICOM viewer to analyze the computer tomography (CT) and magnetic resonance imaging (MRI) images for any anatomical abnormalities was the standard of care until 2018. In 2018, CAScination AG, a Swiss company in collaboration with MED-EL, introduced OTOPLAN, a preplanning otological software tool

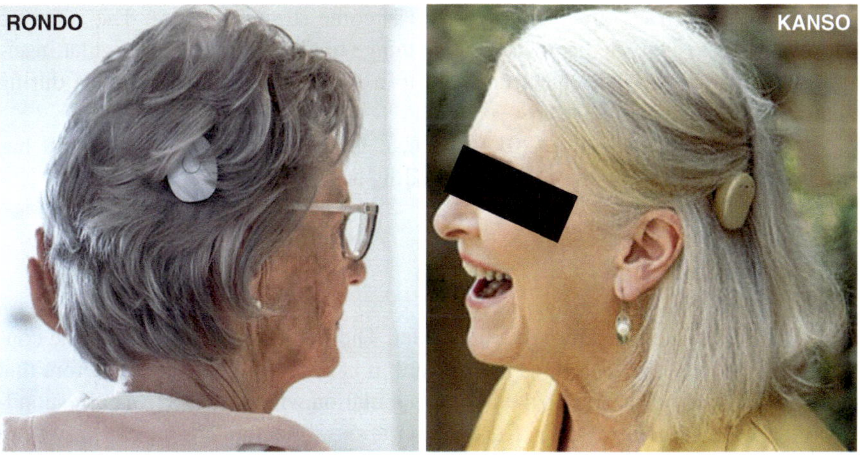




**Fig. 24.2** Single-unit processor from two different CI brands

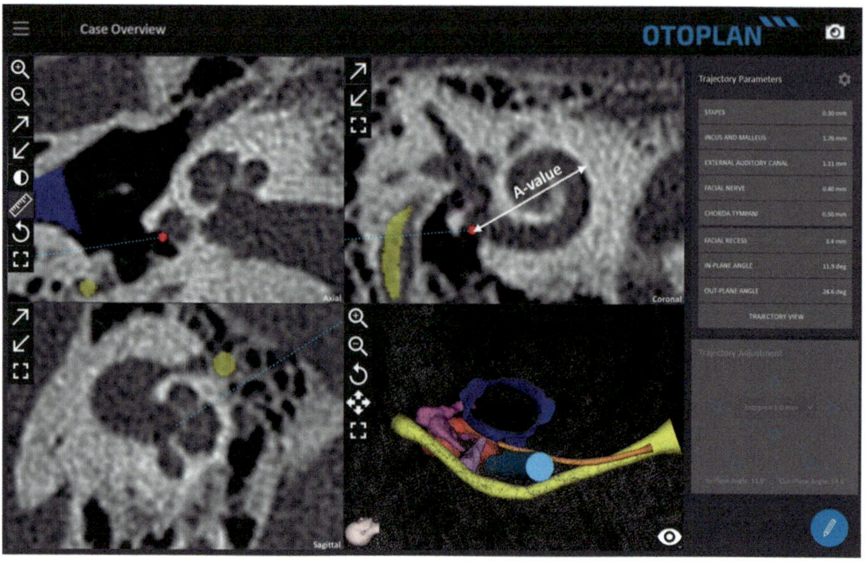


**Fig. 24.3** Preplanning software tool—OTOPLAN

that simplified the process of analyzing pre- and postoperative clinical images with few clicks on a touch screen as shown in Fig. 24.3. The software tool has several features including the estimation of the space between the facial nerve and the chorda tympani to reach the middle-ear space and to access the cochlea for the electrode insertion. The software also provides the possibility to estimate the cochlear size based on the A-value of the cochlea, which is widely used in the CI field. This software presents the cochlear size and corresponding frequency map with which choosing the electrode array length would become straightforward. The software also allows us to analyze the postoperative image to find out the exact angular insertion depth covered by the electrode and to assign the center frequencies during audio processor fitting.

From the recent literature (2019–2020), it is obvious that the OTOPLAN has been widely accepted by the CI field spreading across the world [5–9].

### 24.2.4 Personalized CI

Personalized CI is a concept rather a product. The world is moving toward the concept of personalization and so as the CI field. It is clearer now than ever before that the cochlear size varies among the human population which will have a corresponding effect on the frequency map. Recent reports show that the A-value can vary from a minimum of 7.4 mm to a maximum of 10.4 mm, and the corresponding cochlear duct length varies from 26.8 mm to 39.3 mm [10]. Figure 24.4 displays the classification of cochlear size based on the A-value. The hearing level of the cochlea is

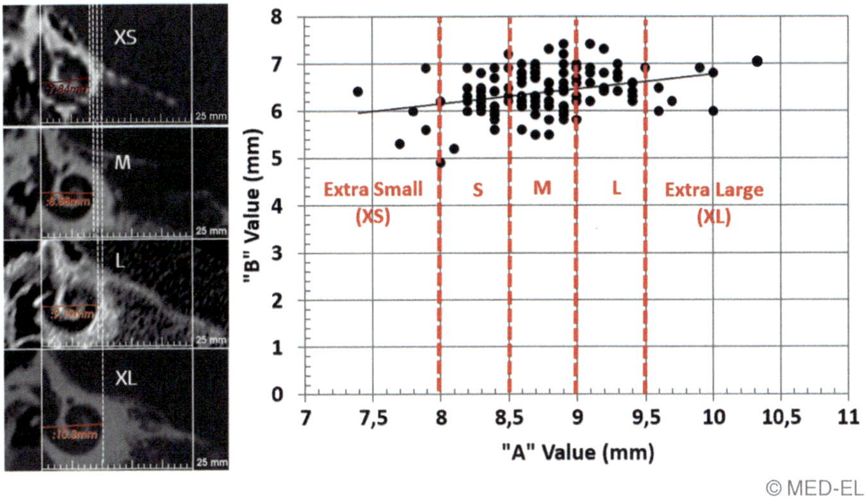


**Fig. 24.4** Classification of the cochlear size based on the A-value of the cochlea

identified from the audiogram, and the stability of the low-frequency (LF) residual hearing is seen from the patients' audiological history. With the cochlear size and the level of hearing loss information, the electrode array length can be optimally chosen matching the exact cochlear needs. For patients with highly stable LF residual hearing, a shorter electrode could be a safe choice from the surgeon's point of view, whereas in patients with progressive hearing loss, an electrode array length to cover the entire frequency range would be a better choice as per the recent reports from Japan [11]. It is a common belief in the CI field that a pre-curved electrode is a better electrode choice in patients with expected facial nerve stimulation (FNS). However, the recent report shows that the electrode type does not have an influence on suppressing the facial nerve stimulation [12].

The personalization is also possible with the signal processing strategy, as the concepts like triphasic pulse stimulation, bimodal delay compensation, and anatomy-based fitting (ABF) are currently available for the audiologist to choose the best suitable ones for their patients' need.

Triphasic pulse stimulation (TPS) is mainly suggested for patients with expected facial nerve stimulation. Figure 24.5 illustrates the difference between the biphasic and triphasic pulse. TPS reduces the intensity of the current spread, thereby avoiding the current spread from reaching the facial nerves [13, 14].

Bimodal delay compensation is mainly for patients who use conventional hearing aids (HA) on one ear and CI on the other ear. It is a known fact that the HA takes much more time to process the acoustic signal and to amplify them than natural hearing, whereas the CI audio processor processes the acoustic signal much faster than natural hearing. This could create a mismatch in the hearing perception by the patients. To minimize such a mismatch, the bimodal delay compensation can be applied to delay the CI processing artificially, thereby matching the CI with HA [15, 16].

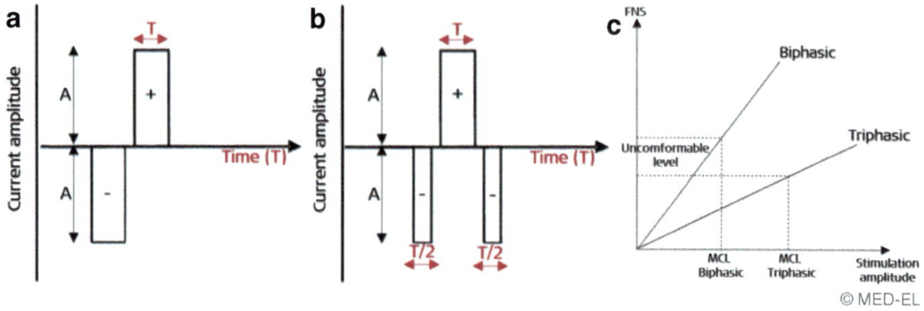


**Fig. 24.5** Balanced biphasic pulse stimulation (**a**) and triphasic pulse stimulation (**b**) showing two negative phases of duration (*T*/2) and one positive phase duration (*T*) (image courtesy of MED-EL). Model of expected benefit with triphasic pulse stimulation on FNS (**c**)

ABF is another new concept that allows us to assign the center frequencies to each of the stimulating channels, based on its anatomical position visualized from postoperative imaging and considering the patient's individual frequency map.

The strength of the magnet that comes in the external transmission coil can also be personalized as per the need that depends on the thickness of the skin flap. Aesthetically appealing audio processor covers, water wear, clips for body worn processor for pediatrics, and additional receiver like ROGER for classroom-type special environments can all be brought under the personalization concept.

### 24.2.5 Endoscope in CI

Endoscopic ear surgery (EES) has gained significant attraction during the last decade, and in CI, the endoscopic visualization is helpful in difficult cases when the full exposure of the middle-ear structures and the round window (RW) region is not available through standard mastoidectomy-posterior tympanotomy approach. The first advantage of EES is the endoscopic magnification, which is the growth of the visual field as the endoscope approaches near the object of interest. The second is the unique ability to visualize over the corners with the angled endoscopes. Both features contribute to the benefit of obtaining a panoramic view of the anatomical structures, which may not be possible with the direct line of vision of the microscope [17]. EES can be applied not only in the conventional CI, but also in other alternative CI approaches like Veria technique and robot-assisted CI. The endoscopic step also permitted the transmastoid/suprameatal microscopic step to be performed more safely even in subjects with unfavorable conditions such as a sclerotic mastoid, by knowing the exact location of the anatomical structures going into the tympanic cavity such as the course of the facial nerve [18]. Figure 24.6 shows a sample endoscopic view of the RW region obtained with a 0°, 4 mm rigid endoscope inserted through the facial recess (right ear).

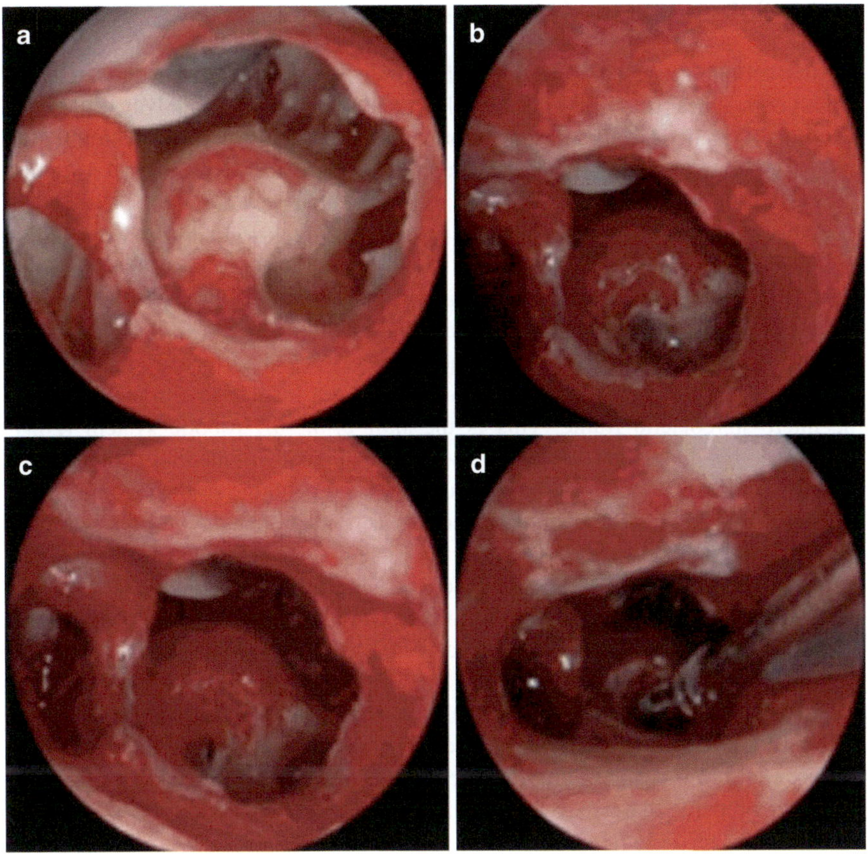


**Fig. 24.6** Endoscopic view of the round window (RW) region obtained with a 0°, 4 mm rigid endoscope inserted through the facial recess (right ear). RW region (**a**), RW membrane after removing the niche (**b**), membranous cochleostomy (**c**), electrode insertion (**d**)

## 24.3 New Horizons

The future of CI is going to be exciting as the CI field is learning a lot from other fields. The indications of CI are getting more liberal, and patients with better LF hearing but who do not benefit from the conventional HAs are now considered for CI. Both CI manufacturers and CI surgeons share the responsibility of preserving the LF residual hearing for the overall success of CI. The precision of the CI surgery both in drilling the mastoid to reach the cochlea and in inserting the electrode, adding pharmaceuticals, and predicting the progressiveness of hearing loss through genetic testing are some of the possibilities of preserving the LF residual hearing and certainly the CI field is marching toward it. Totally implantable cochlear implant (TICI) is another concept that could be successful in the future. This section captures the highlights of these topics.

### 24.3.1 Robot-Assisted CI Surgery

The first robotic-assisted CI surgery in patient was reported in 2014 by Prof. Labadie and his colleagues from the Vanderbilt University, USA [19]. This involves the identification of a safe linear trajectory through the facial recess targeting the ST from the pre-operative image. A customized micro-stereotactic frame needs to be designed, constructed, and sterilized to constrain a surgical drill along the desired trajectory. All these procedures need to be done during the CI surgery which could be seen as challenging.

In 2017, Prof. Caversaccio and his colleagues from the Bern University, Switzerland, reported with optimized techniques including nerve monitoring during robotic drilling to safely pass through the facial recess and perform a robotic access to the middle-ear cavity [20]. This technique did not involve in situ fabrication of the micro-stereotactic frame. This is the *state-of-the-art* robotic system (2021) developed by CAScination AG, Switzerland, and commercially named as HEARO. Figure 24.7a shows the computer-assisted planning of the drilling trajectory, and Fig. 24.7b shows the robot arm in action drilling the straight tunnel to reach the middle-ear space.

In 2018, Prof. Topsakal and colleagues from UZA Antwerp University Hospital, Belgium, performed the first HEARO robotic CI procedure in a patient, and to date (2020) more than 20 patients have received a CI using this minimally invasive HEARO system.

This system was CE marked in the year 2020 to be clinically applied in the European Union and in countries that accept the CE mark. The robotic-assisted CI surgery could well be the future for which the CI surgeons and the CI manufacturers should be prepared to develop the surgical skills and CI device, respectively.

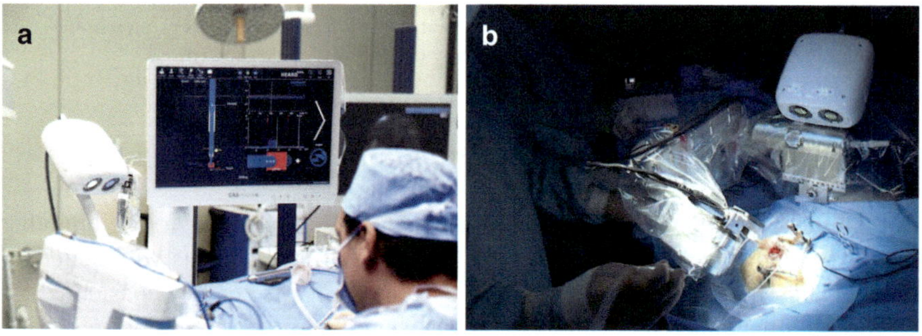




**Fig. 24.7** HEARO robotic system showing the computer control (**a**) and the robotic arm in action (**b**)

### 24.3.2 Robot-Assisted Electrode Insertion

With the robot-assisted CI surgery (drilling through facial recess) picking up its pace, the robot-assisted electrode array insertion is slowly coming to the forefront. The encouraging reason for the robot-assisted electrode insertion is that scientific reports favor the chances of preserving residual hearing with slow insertion of electrode array [21]. Collin SAS from France recently introduced a robotic system capable of inserting the electrode array at a constant speed uniformly throughout the full insertion of the electrode array. Commercially, this robotic system is named as RobOtol® as shown in Fig. 24.8. The system gives surgeons the control to stop the insertion process at any time and to adjust the insertion speed as per the surgical situation. At present (2020), this system is at the early stage of becoming the standard of use. Certainly, automated electrode insertion procedure could eliminate several non-uniformities in the handling of electrodes by surgeons which could be claimed as one reason for the variability in the hearing preservation results so far reported in the literature [22].

### 24.3.3 Augmented CI

Augmented CI is a term coined by Dr. Ingeborg Hochmair, the CEO of MED-EL, in making the CI treatment enriched with pharmaceuticals that can be released from the CI into the cochlea before, during, or for a short time after the implant surgery, or is chronically eluted from the electrode over a defined period of time [23]. To the best of authors' knowledge, almost all major CI manufacturers are making every

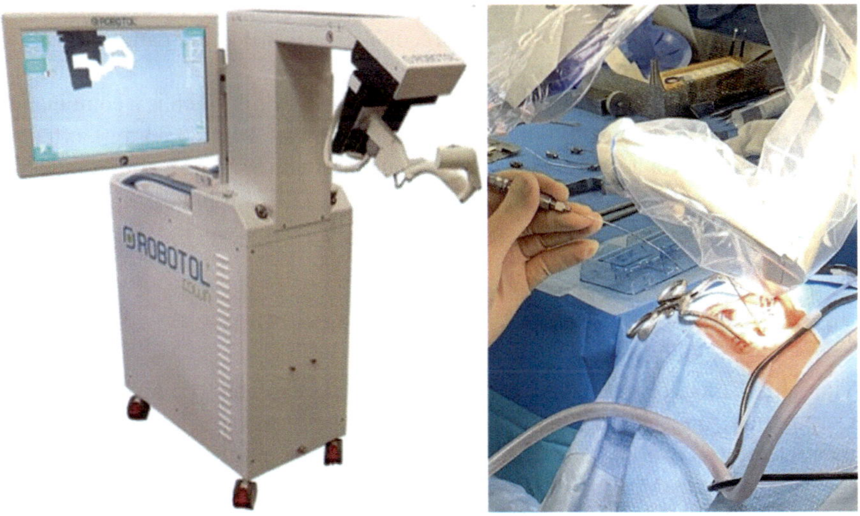


**Fig. 24.8** RobOtol system and Prof. Remi Marianowski from CHRU Brest, France, controlling RobOtol system in electrode insertion

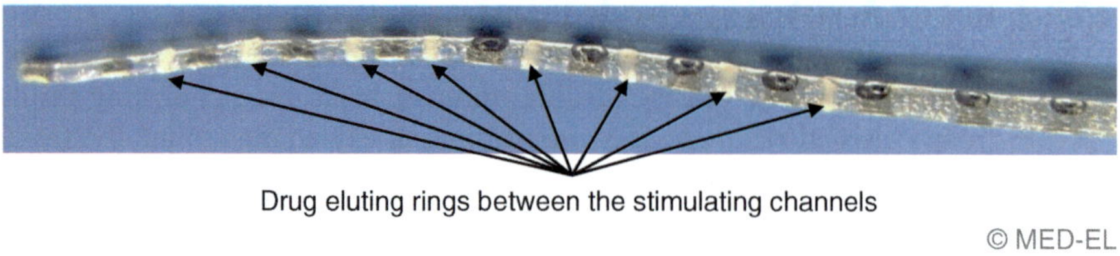


**Fig. 24.9** Electrode array with drug-eluting rings between the stimulating channels

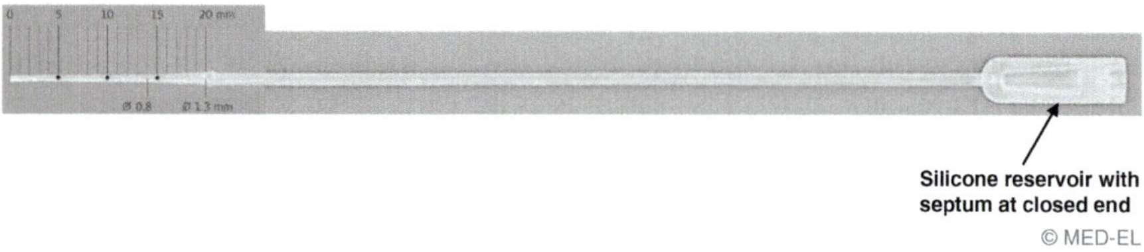


**Fig. 24.10** Inner-ear catheter designed by MED-EL to deliver pharmaceutical agents of surgeon's choice right before the electrode array insertion

effort and collaborating with the clinicians to understand and to bring the drug-eluting CI electrode into clinical use. In June 2020, the first-in-human intra-cochlear implantation of corticosteroid-eluting electrode designed by MED-EL as shown in Fig. 24.9 was implanted by Prof. Lenarz and his colleagues from Hannover, Germany.

Considering the individualized CI concept under the augmented CI topic, depending on the needs of the patients, the pharmaceutical agents should be selected. Inner-ear catheter as shown in Fig. 24.10 is a device that offers the possibility to deliver the pharmaceutical agents of surgeon's choice inside the patient's cochlea right before the CI electrode array insertion.

Recently, supplementary intake of antioxidant (ACEMg), which is a combination of (vitamin A) β-Carotene (3.0 mg), (vitamin C) ascorbic acid (83.33 mg), (vitamin E) DL-α-tocopherol acetate (44.5 mg), and magnesium (52.5 mg), all in one tablet was found to protect residual hearing in CI patients [24]. All in all, augmented CI, without a doubt, will certainly be a future topic of importance in the CI field.

### 24.3.4 Totally Implantable Cochlear Implant (TICI)

Though TICI was reported earlier in the year 2008 as a research device by Cochlear Corporation [25], still (2021) it is not commercially made available by any CI manufacturers. Two key challenges why TICI has not gained importance yet are the battery life and the efficacy of the subcutaneous microphone. Recently in the year 2020, MED-EL as the second CI manufacturer came up with an advanced version of TICI that was implanted in a patient by Prof. Lefebvre in Belgium.

Other than CI manufacturers, university research groups like Massachusetts Institute of Technology/Harvard Medical School have reported on the development of fully implantable CI (FICI) using piezoelectric middle-ear sensor [26]. TICI, if made reliable, could minimize several wearing discomforts involved with the *behind-the-ear* (BTE) audio processor including swimming under water, hearing while taking bath, and sweat-related issues in tropical places. TICI would enable continuous usage of CI, and this could improve the overall hearing performance and resulting language development especially in pediatrics. TICI is designed with the possibility of using the *behind-the-ear* (BTE) processor if the internal battery runs out of energy.

### 24.3.5 Genetics in CI

Half of the congenital hearing loss (HL) is genetic with more than 400 known syndromes with HL as a feature and more than 100 known genes that have HL as the only clinical manifestation. Most cases of congenital HL are identified soon after birth via newborn hearing screening (NBHS). However, many HL cases only become apparent later in life due to the expression of late-onset HL mutations or following an environmental insult, like antibiotic use or head trauma, in the genetically predisposed patient. A genetic screening panel that incorporates a population's common HL genes could hence represent an effective adjunct test to newborn screening, improving the time of diagnosis and treatment [27].

In 2020, Dr. Yoshimura, Prof. Usami, and their colleagues from Japan carried out genetic testing that has the potential to impact hearing preservation, following CI [28]. They identified the cause of HL in 21 families, and 19 patients out of those received a genetic diagnosis, with the CDH23 gene most frequently implicated, followed by ACTG1, mit1555A>G, MYO7A, MYO15A, SLC26A4, and TMPRSSS3. Additionally, two patients were diagnosed with otosclerosis and congenital diaphragmatic hernia (Fig. 24.11).

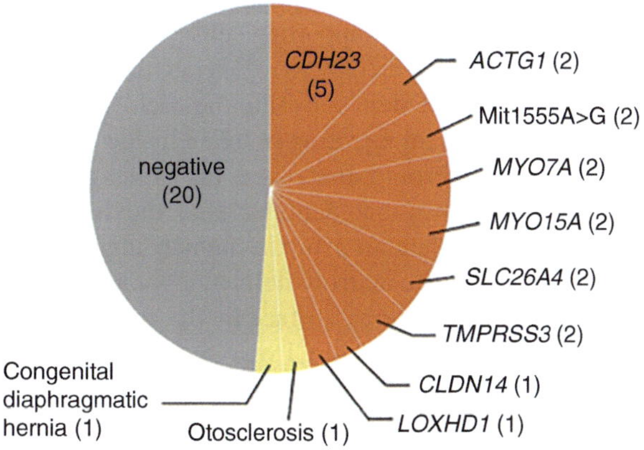


**Fig. 24.11** From a patient population of $n = 41$, orange indicates genetic causes of HL, yellow indicates other causes, and gray indicates unknown

Out of all the above mentioned genes, they found that patients who had pathogenic variants in the CDH23, MYO7A, or MYO15A gene showed statistically better hearing preservation scores compared with patients with HL due to other causes.

In the same year, a report on concurrent hearing and genetic screening of neonates by Prof. Dai, Prof. Han, and their colleagues from the two biggest hospitals in Beijing, China, was published, showing the importance of genetic screening in the early identification of late development of hearing loss in children [29].

The study included 180,469 infants born in Beijing between April 2013 and March 2014 with the last follow-up on February 24, 2018. Hearing screening was performed using transiently evoked otoacoustic emission (TEOAE), and dried blood spots were collected for genetic screening using DNA microarray platform to identify nine variants in four genes, GJB2, SLC26A4, mtDNA 12SrRNA, and GJB3. The important finding from this mega-study is that infants with pathogenic combinations of GJB2 variants and SLC26A4 variants may pass newborn hearing screening, and most of them will develop hearing loss at an early age (<5 years old).

These two recent studies show that newborn genetic screening clearly shortens the time to diagnosis and intervention, reveals the etiology of genetic deafness, and ensures timely habilitation of infants and young children. Genetic testing for the identification of future HL will take a key position in the future of the CI.

### 24.3.6 Stem-Cell Research in CI

Hearing is affected by the loss or dysfunction of the sensory cells. The loss of sensory cells would lead to the degeneration of neuronal cell bodies that are present within central modiolus trunk. The stem cell therapy aims to regenerate the lost sensory and the neuronal cell bodies. In 1993, the hair cell regeneration in response to aminoglycoside ototoxicity was reported to occur in the vestibular sensory epithelia of adult mammals. In mammalian vestibule, hair cell regeneration seems to originate from supporting cells that reenter the cell cycle when neighboring hair cells are dying and mitotic supporting cells seem to divide asymmetrically, generating new hair cells and supporting cells [30–34]. These findings encouraged several studies on stem cell therapy to regenerate the cochlear sensory cells.

The delivery of stem cells into the cochlea might require opening the cochlea followed by careful injection or taken inside by some means. In 2016, there was a report from Prof. Lenarz and his colleagues from the Hannover Medical School, Germany, that demonstrated the first application of the autologous stem-cell transplantation to the human inner ear in combination with the CI electrode. The bone marrow-derived mononuclear cells (BM-MNC) were coated on to the electrode array surface by the application of fibrin glue creating a biohybrid CI. This biohybrid CI was implanted in three patients providing the initial safety data and taking one step closer to the routine clinical application of the stem cells [35].

## 24.4 Conclusion

The CI field had evidenced continuous innovation in the last 35 years with fruitful scientific collaboration between the clinicians and the CI manufacturers making the CI reach its maturity. The experienced clinicians and researchers have created the platform for the next generation to take the learnings from the past and move the CI field to the next level. Personalized CI treatment would certainly be the future which would include genetic testing, robotic-assisted CI surgery, and electrode insertion along with the addition of pharmaceutical agents enabling the CI recipients to get the best benefit from the overall CI treatment. Stem cell-based CI treatment is slowly emerging with the aim of reversing the CI by regenerating the lost sensory cells.

## References

1. Dhanasingh A, Jolly C. Review on cochlear implant electrode array tip fold-over and scalar deviation. J Otolaryngol. 2019;14(3):94–100.
2. https://pronews.cochlearamericas.com/is-hearing-preservation-possible-with-the-slim-modiolar-electrode/
3. Fu QJ, Galvin JJ III. Maximizing cochlear implant patients' performance with advanced speech training procedures. Hear Res. 2008;242(1–2):198–208.
4. Dazert S, Thomas JP, Büchner A, Müller J, Hempel JM, Löwenheim H, Mlynski R. Off the ear with no loss in speech understanding: comparing the RONDO and the OPUS 2 cochlear implant audio processors. Eur Arch Otorhinolaryngol. 2017;274(3):1391–5.
5. Andersen SAW, Bergman M, Keith JP, Powell KA, Hittle B, Malhotra P, Wiet GJ. Segmentation of temporal bone anatomy for patient-specific virtual reality simulation. Ann Otol Rhinol Laryngol. 2020;3:3489420970217.
6. Lovato A, Marioni G, Gamberini L, Bonora C, Genovese E, de Filippis C. OTOPLAN in cochlear implantation for far-advanced otosclerosis. Otol Neurotol. 2020;41(8):e1024–8.
7. Lee SY, Jung Bae Y, Carandang M, Kim Y, Hee Han J, Huh G, Song JJ, Koo JW, Ho Lee J, Ha Oh S, Choi BY. Modiolar proximity of slim modiolar electrodes and cochlear duct length: correlation for potential basis of customized cochlear implantation with perimodiolar electrodes. Ear Hear. 2020;
8. Almuhawas FA, Dhanasingh AE, Mitrovic D, Abdelsamad Y, Alzhrani F, Hagr A, Al SA. Age as a factor of growth in mastoid thickness and skull width. Otol Neurotol. 2020;41(5):709–14.
9. Lovato A, de Filippis C. Utility of OTOPLAN reconstructed images for surgical planning of cochlear implantation in a case of post-meningitis ossification. Otol Neurotol. 2019;40(1):e60–1.
10. Khurayzi T, Dhanasingh A, Almuhawas F, Alsanosi A. Shape of the cochlear basal turn: an indicator for an optimal *electrode-to-modiolus* proximity with precurved electrode type. Ear Nose Throat J. 2021;100(1):38–43.
11. Yoshimura H, Moteki H, Nishio SY, Usami SI. Electric-acoustic stimulation with longer electrodes for potential deterioration in low-frequency hearing. Acta Otolaryngol. 2020;140(8):632–8.
12. Ahn JH, Oh SH, Chung JW, Lee KS. Facial nerve stimulation after cochlear implantation according to types of nucleus 24-channel electrode arrays. Acta Otolaryngol. 2009;129(6):588–91.
13. Alhabib SF, Abdelsamad Y, Yousef M, Alzhrani F. Performance of cochlear implant recipients fitted with triphasic pulse patterns. Eur Arch Otorhinolaryngol. 2020;

14. Braun K, Walker K, Sürth W, Löwenheim H, Tropitzsch A. Triphasic pulses in cochlear implant patients with facial nerve stimulation. Otol Neurotol. 2019;40(10):1268–77.
15. Zirn S, Arndt S, Aschendorff A, Wesarg T. Interaural stimulation timing in single sided deaf cochlear implant users. Hear Res. 2015;328:148–56.
16. Seebacher J, Franke-Trieger A, Weichbold V, Zorowka P, Stephan K. Improved interaural timing of acoustic nerve stimulation affects sound localization in single-sided deaf cochlear implant users. Hear Res. 2019;371:19–27.
17. Güneri EA, Olgun Y. Endoscope-assisted cochlear implantation. Clin Exp Otorhinolaryngol. 2018;11(2):89–95.
18. Marchioni D, Soloperto D, Guarnaccia MC, Genovese E, Alicandri-Ciufelli M, Presutti L. Endoscopic assisted cochlear implants in ear malformations. Eur Arch Otorhinolaryngol. 2015;272(10):2643–52.
19. Labadie RF, Balachandran R, Noble JH, Blachon GS, Mitchell JE, Reda FA, Dawant BM, Fitzpatrick JM. Minimally invasive image-guided cochlear implantation surgery: first report of clinical implementation. Laryngoscope. 2014;124(8):1915–22.
20. Caversaccio M, Gavaghan K, Wimmer W, Williamson T, Ansò J, Mantokoudis G, Gerber N, Rathgeb C, Feldmann A, Wagner F, Scheidegger O, Kompis M, Weisstanner C, Zoka-Assadi M, Roesler K, Anschuetz L, Huth M, Weber S. Robotic cochlear implantation: surgical procedure and first clinical experience. Acta Otolaryngol. 2017;137(4):447–54.
21. Rajan GP, Kontorinis G, Kuthubutheen J. The effects of insertion speed on inner ear function during cochlear implantation: a comparison study. Audiol Neurootol. 2013;18(1):17–22.
22. Fabie JE, Keller RG, Hatch JL, Holcomb MA, Camposeo EL, Lambert PR, Meyer TA, McRackan TR. Evaluation of outcome variability associated with lateral wall, mid-scalar, and perimodiolar electrode arrays when controlling for preoperative patient characteristics. Otol Neurotol. 2018;39(9):1122–8.
23. Dhanasingh A, Hochmair I. Thirty years of translational research behind MED-EL. Acta Otolaryngol. 2021; In-press.
24. Scheper V, Schmidtheisler M, Lasch F, von der Leyen H, Koch A, Schwieger J, Büchner A, Lesinski-Schiedat A, Lenarz T. Randomized placebo-controlled clinical trial investigating the effect of antioxidants and a vasodilator on overall safety and residual hearing preservation in cochlear implant patients. Trials. 2020;21(1):643.
25. Briggs RJ, Eder HC, Seligman PM, Cowan RS, Plant KL, Dalton J, Money DK, Patrick JF. Initial clinical experience with a totally implantable cochlear implant research device. Otol Neurotol. 2008;29(2):114–9.
26. https://www.e4ent.com/news/fully-implantable-cochlear-implant-fici-piezoelectric-middle-ear-sensor/
27. Rudman J, Liu XZ. Genetics of hearing loss. Hear J. 2019;72(4):6–9.
28. Yoshimura H, Moteki H, Nishio SY, Miyajima H, Miyagawa M, Usami SI. Genetic testing has the potential to impact hearing preservation following cochlear implantation. Acta Otolaryngol. 2020;140(6):438–44.
29. Dai P, Han DM, et al. Concurrent hearing and genetic screening of 180,469 neonates with follow-up in Beijing, China. Am J Hum Genet. 2019;105(4):803–12.
30. Warchol ME, Lambert PR, Goldstein BJ, Forge A, Corwin JT. Regenerative proliferation in inner ear sensory epithelia from adult guinea pigs and humans. Science. 1993;259:1619–22.
31. Forge A, Li L, Corwin JT, Nevill G. Ultrastructural evidence for hair cell regeneration in the mammalian inner ear. Science. 1993;259:1616–9.
32. Hawkins JE Jr, Johnsson LG, Stebbins WC, Moody DB, Coombs SL. Hearing loss and cochlear pathology in monkeys after noise exposure. Acta Otolaryngol. 1976;81:337–43.
33. Raphael Y, Altschuler RA. Reorganization of cytoskeletal and junctional proteins during cochlear hair cell degeneration. Cell Motil Cytoskeleton. 1991;18:215–27.
34. Lee DH. The past, present and future of cochlear stem cell research: we have no conclusion but now we have hope. Korean J Audiol. 2010;14(3):163–72.
35. Roemer A, Köhl U, Majdani O, Klöß S, Falk C, Haumann S, Lenarz T, Kral A, Warnecke A. Biohybrid cochlear implants in human neurosensory restoration. Stem Cell Res Ther. 2016;7(1):148.

GPSR Compliance

*The European Union's (EU) General Product Safety Regulation (GPSR) is a set of rules that requires consumer products to be safe and our obligations to ensure this.*

*If you have any concerns about our products, you can contact us on ProductSafety@springernature.com*

In case Publisher is established outside the EU, the EU authorized representative is:

Springer Nature Customer Service Center GmbH
Europaplatz 3
69115 Heidelberg, Germany

**Batch number: 10726058**

Printed by Printforce, the Netherlands